Intestinal Failure

A DOCTOR OR HEALTH WORKER'S OATH

I promise to treat all patients equally, with humanity, respect and to the best of my ability.
I shall listen to their story, keep their confidences and be honest at all times.
I shall strive to bring hope, however small.
I shall endeavour to improve my knowledge, and to be aware of new treatments.
I shall admit that which I do not know and shall not be afraid to seek help from those who do.
I shall willingly teach my skills to others.

In memory of my father, Jon Nightingale, who died in August 1997 of motor neurone disease.

Intestinal Failure

Edited by

Jeremy M D Nightingale MD MRCP

Consultant Gastroenterologist
Gastroenterology Centre
Leicester Royal Infirmary
Leicester

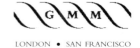

LONDON • SAN FRANCISCO

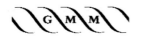

Greenwich Medical Media Limited
137 Euston Road
London
NW1 2AA

870 Market Street, Ste 720
San Francisco
CA 94109

ISBN 1 900 151 936

First published 2001

Visit our website at:
www.greenwich-medical.co.uk

Distributed worldwide by Plymbridge Distributors Ltd and in the USA by Jamco Distribution
Typeset by Phoenix Photosetting, Chatham, Kent
Printed by MPG Books Ltd, Bodmin, Cornwall

Contents

Section 5: TREATMENT OF INTESTINAL FAILURE

Section 6: OUTCOME OF INTESTINAL FAILURE

Section 7: PROBLEMS OF TREATMENT

Section 8: SURGICAL TREATMENT OF INTESTINAL FAILURE

APPENDICES

Contributors

Simon P Allison MD, FRCP
Consultant Physician and Professor in Clinical Nutrition
Department of Diabetes Endocrinology and Nutrition
Clinical Nutrition & Investigation Unit
Queen's Medical Centre
Nottingham, UK

Michael C Allwood BPharm, PhD, FRPharm SGB
Pharmacy Academic Practice Unit
University of Derby
Kingsway
Derby, UK

Christine Blanshard, MA, MD, MRCP
Consultant Gastroenterologist
Department of Gastroenterology
Homerton Hospital
London, UK

Michael F Byrne MA, MRCP
Registrar and Lecturer in Gastroenterology
Beaumont Hospital
Dublin, Ireland

Gordon L Carlson MD, FRCS
Consultant Surgeon and Honorary Senior Lecturer
University of Manchester
Intestinal Failure Unit
Hope Hospital
Salford, UK

Paola Domizio FRCPath
Senior Lecturer and Honorary Consultant Histopathologist
Department Histopathology
St Bartholomew's Hospital
West Smithfield
London, UK

Hamish D Duncan MD, MRCP
Consultant Physician and Gastroenterologist
Department of Medicine
Queen Alexandra Hospital
Cosham, Portsmouth, UK

Jacqueline Edington BSc, DPhil SRD RPHNutr
Senior Clinical Nutrition Manager
Medical Division
Abbott Laboratories
Maidenhead, UK

Marinos Elia MD, FRCP
Head of Adult Clinical Nutrition and Honorary
Consultant Physician
Dunn Clinical Nutrition Centre
Addenbrooke's Hospital
Cambridge, UK

Alastair Forbes MD, FRCP
Consultant Gastroenterologist
Northwick and St Mark's Hospital NHS Trust
Harrow, UK

Robert A Goodland PhD
Histopathology Unit
Imperial Cancer Research Fund
London, UK

Gill Hardy PhD, FRSC
Professor of Pharmaceutical Nutrition
School of Biological Sciences
Oxford Brookes University
Oxford, UK

Xavier Hébuterne MD, PhD
Gastroenterology and Nutrition
Professor of Nutrition
Nutrition Support Unit
Archet Hospital, France

Susan M Hill DM, MRCP, MRCPCH, DCh
Consultant Paediatric Gastroenterologist and Honorary
Senior Lecturer
Gastroenterology Unit
Institute of Child Health and Great Ormond Street
Hospital for Children NHS Trust
Guilford Street, London, UK

Stephanie Hughes RGN, DipN, BSc (Hons)
Colorectal Specialist Nurse
Intestinal Failure Unit and Department of Surgery
Hope Hospital
Greater Manchester, UK

Ann J Hunter FRCP, MRCPath
Consultant Haematologist
Leicester Royal Infirmary NHS Trust
Leicester, UK

Miles H Irving D.Sc(Hon) MD ChM FRCS
FACS(Hon)
Ex-Professor of Surgery
Department of Surgery
Clinical Sciences Building
Hope Hospital
Salford, UK

Khursheed N Jeejeebhoy MDE, PhD
St Michael's Hospital
Gi Div
Toronto
Ontario
Canada

Palle Bekker Jeppesen MD, PhD
Department of Medical Gastroenterology
Section of Gastroenterology
Rigshopitalet
Blegdansvej
Copenhagen, Denmark

Martin J Lee BSc MRPharms MBA
Pharmacy Department
Derbyshire Royal Infirmary NHS Trust
Derby, UK

John E Lennard-Jones MD, FRCP, FRCS
Emeritus Professor of Gastroenterology
The Royal London Hospital Medical College
Emeritus Consultant Physician
St Mark's Hospital London
Northwick and St Mark's Hospital NHS Trust
Watford, UK

Sarah G Long RGN, RSCN
Senior Nutrition Nurse Specialist
Gastroenterology Unit
Institute of Child Health and Great Ormond Street
Hospital for Children NHS Trust
Guilford Street, London, UK

Sally Magnay RGN
Clinical Nurse Specialist
John Radcliffe Hospital
Headington, Oxford, UK

Joanne E Martin PhD, FRCPath
Professor of Histopathology
Departments of Morbid Anatomy and Histopathology
Institute of Pathology
The Royal London Hospital
London, UK

Alistair S McIntyre MD, FRCP
Consultant Gastroenterologist
Wycombe Hospital
High Wycombe
Buckinghamshire, UK

Ann Mensfoth SRD
Senior Dietitian(Home Enteral Nutrition Service)
Fosse Health Trust
Leicester Royal Infirmary
Leicester, UK

Bernard Messing MD
Service d'Hépato-Gastro-Entérologie et d'Assistance
Nutritive
Hôpital Lariboisiére-Saint-Lazare
Ambroise Paré
Paris Cedex, France

Peter J Milla MSc, FRCP, FRCPCH
Professor of Paediatric Gastroenterology and Nutrition
Hon. Consultant Paediatric Gastroenterologist
Gastroenterology Unit
Institute of Child Health
London, UK

Per B Mortensen MD PhD
Head of the Department of Medical Gastroenterology
Rigshospitalet
Blegdamsvej
Copenhagen, Denmark

Frank Murray MD, FRCP
Consultant Physician and Gastroenterologist
Beaumont Hospital
Dublin, Ireland

Anne Myers RGN, BA (Hons)
Lead Nurse for Intestinal Failure
Intestinal Failure Unit and Department of Surgery
Hope Hospital
Greater Manchester, UK

Jeremy M D Nightingale MD, MRCP
Consultant Gastroenterologist
Gastroenterology Centre
Leicester Royal Infirmary
Leicester, UK

Kenneth O'Byrne BAO, MD, DCHM, MRCPI
Senior Lecturer in Oncology
University Department of Oncology
Leicester Royal Infirmary NHS Trust
Leicester, UK

Chris R Pennington MD, FRCP
Professor of Gastroenterology
Directorate of General Medicine
Ninewells Hospital and Medical School
Dundee, UK

Ray J Playford PhD, MRCP
Professor of Gastroenterology
Department of Gastroenterology
Royal Postgraduate Medical School
Hammersmith Hospital
London, UK

A Graham Pockley PhD
Reader, Section of Surgery
Division of Clinical Sciences (NGH)
Clinical Sciences Centre
Northern General Hospital
Sheffield, UK

Jeremy Powell-Tuck MD, FRCP
Senior Lecturer in Human Nutrition and Honorary
Consultant Physician
Rank Department of Human Nutrition
St Bartholomew's and the Royal London School of
Medicine and Dentistry
Royal London Hospital, London, UK

Edgar Pullicino FRCP, PhD
Department of Gastroenterology and Clinical Nutrition
St Luke's (Teaching) Hospital
G'Mangia, Malta

Eamonn MM Quigley MD, FRCP, FACP, FACG
Professor of Medicine and Human Physiology
Head of the Medical School
Nutrition of Ireland
Cork, Ireland
Professor (Adjunct) of Medicine and Physiology
University of Nebraska Medical Center, Omaha, USA

David M Richards MD, FRCS
Consultant General and Colorectal Surgeon
The Royal Oldham Hospital
Oldham
Greater Manchester, UK

David BA Silk MD FRCP
Consultant Physician and Gastroenterologist
Department of Gastroenterologist and Nutrition
Central Middlesex Hospital NHS Trust
London, UK

John Snowden MD, MRCP, MRCPath
Consultant Haematologist
Leicester Royal Infirmary
Leicester, UK

Robin C Spiller MD, FRCP
Reader in Gastroenterology
Division of Gastroenterology
School of Medical and Surgical Sciences
University Hospital
Nottingham, UK

Williams P Steward PhD, FRCP, FRCP (C)
Head of Department and Professor of Oncology
University Department of Oncology
Leicester Royal Infirmary
Leicester, UK

Charles RV Tomson DM, FRCP
Consultant Renal Physician
The Richard Bright Renal Unit
Southmead Hospital
Westbury-on-Trym
Bristol, UK

Jon S Thompson MD, FACP
Professor of Surgery and chief,
Department of Surgery
General and Gastrointestinal Surgery
University of Nebraska Medical Center
Omaha, USA

Carolyn Wheatley
Chairperson to PINNT and member of LITRE committee
Christchurch
Dorset, UK

David L Wingate DM, FRCP
Professor of Gastrointestinal Science and Director of Science
Research Unit
St Bartholomew's and the Royal London Hospitals
Science Research Unit
London, UK

Susanne Wood RGN Dip N
Lecturer Practitioner in Nutrition Support Nursing
Kingston Hospital
Kingston
Surrey, UK

Richard F M Wood MD, FRCS
Professor of Surgery
Section of Surgery
Division of Clinical Sciences (NGH)
Clinical Sciences Centre
Northern General Hospital
Sheffield, UK

Preface

This international multiauthor textbook brings the subject of intestinal failure in adults and children to a wide readership. Doctors, nurses, dietitians, pharmacists, research workers and patients have written the chapters to give practical advice and knowledge from different viewpoints. All issues relating to the provision of nutritional support in hospitals and in the community are included.

Appendices 1–3 facilitate quick measurements of a patient's nutritional state without needing to perform calculations.

This book should provide an essential source of reference to all members of a nutrition support team (clinicians, dietitians, nurses and pharmacists) and to specialist workers/researchers in the field.

Any comments, corrections, additional information or suggestions for inclusion in a future edition should be sent to the editor.

Jeremy Nightingale
May, 2001

Acknowledgements

I thank all the contributors, many of whom have helped review other chapters and whose contributions have, on occasions, been incorporated into other chapters. I also thank the following for invaluable assistance.

Tom Alun-Jones FRCS
Moira Currie SRD
Simone Daly
Judith Dunn RGN
Helen Ghandi RGN
Mohammed Ghatei PhD
Carol Glencourse SRD
Michael Green MRCP FRCPCH
John Kennedy RGN DPSN
Patricia Kilby
Kim Krarup MRCP FRCR
Leona Laderman
Tracey Lovejoy SRD

Nora Naughton, Project Manager
Peter Rodgers MRCP FRCR
Gavin Robertson FRCS
Pauline Robinson SRD
Christine Russell SRD
Atul Sinha MRCP
Jonathan Shaffer FRCP
Gavin Smith, Book Publisher
Iain Stephenson MRCP
Ruth Swan, Copy-editor
Moira Taylor PhD SRD DADP

The Oley Foundation
214 Hun Memorial, A-28
Albany Medical Center
Albany, NY 12208-3478
USA
Tel: (518) 262-5079
Fax: (518) 262-5528

Foreword

To have been party to the recognition of a new specialty, encourage its development, see it acknowledged as a specialty in its own right and then bring it to a maturity and set it on its future path, all within the space of 30 years, must be regarded as both an awe inspiring experience and a privilege.

Such has been the experience of the team of authors that have contributed to this unique volume. It is remarkable that it is only 30 years since Dudrick, Wilmore, Vars and Rhoads showed that children could grow and mature normally when sustained by parenteral nutrition alone. From this classic study has developed the whole field of intestinal failure and its treatment.

This book brings together those who were the pioneers, those who refined the techniques that enabled patients to receive safe enteral and parenteral nutrition outside the hospital and those who now have the task of taking the management of intestinal failure to the next stages. The assembled chapters reveal a remarkable record of international interdisciplinary collaboration between scientists and clinicians, doctors and nurses, health economists and those with expertise in the relatively new discipline of the measurement of

quality of life. What is most gratifying, however, is the inclusion of an authoritative and scientifically rigorous expression of the patient perspective. The management of intestinal failure was arguably the trailblazer in demonstrating that successful outcomes could only be obtained if the patient was incorporated as an integral part of the therapeutic team.

Jeremy Nightingale has performed an outstanding service to gastroenterology by bringing together a group of authors who provide not only an authoritative, current statement on the total management of patients with intestinal failure but also a record of the development of this specialty which will act as a reliable reference for many years to come.

This book sets the seal on Intestinal Failure as a distinct specialty and will act as a standard text for those who need to know how to deal with patients afflicted with this difficult but fascinating condition

Professor Sir Miles Irving
D.Sc(Hon) MD ChM FRCS FACS(Hon)
Newcastle Upon Tyne
May, 2001

Introduction
Definition and classification of intestinal failure

DEFINITION

Intestinal failure (IF) occurs when there is reduced intestinal absorption so that macronutrient and/or water and electrolyte supplements are needed to maintain health and/or growth. Undernutrition and/or dehydration result if no treatment is given or if compensatory mechanisms do not occur.

CLASSIFICATION

Severity
The severity of intestinal failure can be graded according to the method by which macronutrients/fluid are given.

Severe IF: parenteral nutrition and/or parenteral saline are required because health cannot be sustained by exposing the small bowel mucosa to more, continuous or altered nutrients and/or electrolytes.

Moderate IF: an enteral tube is used for the administration of macronutrients and/or a glucose/saline solution.

Mild IF: dietary adjustments, oral nutrients and/or a glucose/saline solution (or sodium chloride supplements) are needed.

A patient may change, due to compensatory mechanisms, from having severe to mild IF with time. For example a patient who has had a massive small intestinal resection, and in whom intestinal adaptation has occurred, may with careful dietary advice and appropriate drug therapy be able to stop parenteral nutrition.

Underlying diagnoses
IF can be acute or chronic (Fig. 1).

Acute IF may be reversible (within 6 months) and has surgical causes (e.g. enterocutaneous fistula, obstruction or ileus) and medical ones (enteritis due to chemotherapy or acute irradiation damage, or infrections including HIV).

Chronic IF can be due to gastrointestinal resection(s) short bowel or gastrectomy) gut bypass (as in the surgery for obesity) or small bowel dysfunction

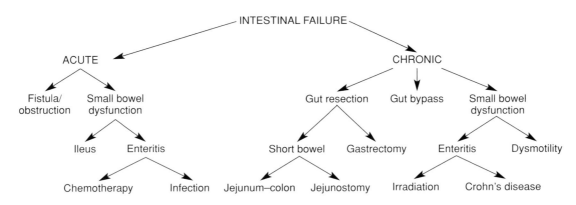

Figure 1

(pseudo-obstruction or a chronic enteritis such as Crohn's disease, irradiation, microvillus atrophy or autoimmune enteropathy). The remaining gut function of patients who have had a total or partial gastrectomy is often so disordered that nutrient supplements are needed; hence their inclusion.

This definition and classification of IF encompasses a broader spectrum of patients than that of Fleming and Remington who defined IF as a 'reduction in functioning gut mass below the minimum amount necessary for adequate digestion and absorption of nutrients'.[1] This was commonly interpreted as patients needing parenteral nutrition to sustain their life often for prolonged periods and in a specialized unit. It made no mention of patients whose main problem was of salt and water loss from either a jejunostomy or a high output enterocutaneous fistula. The new definition and classification proposed for this book includes patients with many underlying diagnoses, many of whom will be managed in non-specialist hospitals and without the need for parenteral nutrition.

This book does not discuss gastrointestinal diseases, which cause a reversible IF, but for which there are specific non-surgical treatments. Examples include gluten, cow's milk or soya free diets for coeliac disease, milk or soya food sensitive enteropathies respectively, or antibiotic treatment for bacterial overgrowth, giardia, Whipples' disease or tropical sprue.

REFERENCE

1. Fleming CR, Remington M. Intestinal failure. In: Hill G. L. (ed), Nutrition and the Surgical Patient. New York: Churchill Livingstone, 1981: 219–235.

Jeremy Nightingale

Section 1

Background

1

Historical overview

J. E. Lennard-Jones

*T*he term 'intestinal failure' was used by Irving and colleagues in the title of a paper published in 1980.[1] In the following year, a book chapter by Fleming and Remington gave the first definition as a 'reduction in functioning gut mass below the minimal amount necessary for adequate digestion and absorption of nutrients'.[2] Irving and his colleagues popularized the term when they described their work in a specially designated 'Intestinal Failure Unit' for the treatment of complex intestinal disorders.[3] A key feature of this unit was the ability to provide safe, effective, long-term parenteral nutrition. The phrase 'intestinal failure' began in surgical practice as a unifying concept for apparently different conditions all of which have the common feature that the normal absorptive function of the small intestine is impaired, usually to such an extent that parenteral feeding is needed.[3] It is now recognized that some patients can also be treated by giving extra or special nutrients via the intestine. The definition of intestinal failure in this book as 'reduced gastrointestinal absorption to the extent that macronutrient and/or fluid supplements are required' widens the concept to include the need for enteral or parenteral supplements to maintain a normal nutritional state. Malabsorption of a single nutrient, such as Vitamin B[12], or the need for a special diet to exclude a damaging component such as gluten, is not included within this definition.

Loss of intestinal absorptive function can be complete or partial. Intestinal failure may be described as *acute* when it is reversible and due to such surgical conditions as intra-abdominal sepsis and ileus, a high volume entero-cutaneous fistula, intestinal obstruction or temporary severe malabsorption after extensive small bowel resection or it can be due to chemotherapy. If long-term treatment over weeks, months, or longer is required intestinal failure can be described as *chronic*, especially if continued treatment is needed at home.

PARALLEL DEVELOPMENTS

Developments in different disciplines since the middle years of this century have led to our current understanding and treatment of intestinal failure. First, the application to both normal subjects and those with intestinal resection of new laboratory techniques, has advanced understanding of small intestinal function. Second, the scope of surgical treatment has extended to include more complex operations on the intestine so that intestinal failure occurs more frequently, and is often more severe, than hitherto. During the same

time period medical causes of intestinal failure have been recognized. Third, clinical necessity has stimulated the application of innovative techniques to treat the condition in the short- or long-term. These parallel developments in time will be described sequentially in the following review.

ADVANCES IN KNOWLEDGE

Sites of nutrient absorption

Many of the laboratory measurements, now regarded as routine, were developed at the beginning of the second half of the twentieth century. For example, a widely used method for measurement of fat in faeces was first reported in 1949 and microbiological techniques for the measurement of folic acid or vitamin B[12] in blood were devised in 1956 and 1961 respectively. Radio-isotope methods for measuring vitamin B[12] absorption were developed in the late 1950s. By the early 1960s it became apparent, mainly as a result of studying patients with either proximal or distal malabsorption due to disease or resection, that carbohydrate, protein and most water-soluble vitamins are absorbed proximally by the jejunum, whereas fat is absorbed over a longer length of intestine.[4,5] The length of intestine over which fat is absorbed increases as more fat is taken by mouth. As a result, fat malabsorption occurs when distal small intestine is resected and a critical fat intake is exceeded.[6]

It was through studies of patients with ileal resection that the distal site of vitamin B12 absorption was detected.[4] The need of patients with distal ileal resection for parenteral supplements of vitamin B12 is now well recognised.

Dilution of nutrients by digestive secretions

Intubation experiments in normal subjects published in 1957 showed that when a liquid test meal containing a non-absorbed marker is drunk, most carbohydrate and protein is absorbed within 100 cm of the duodeno-jejunal junction.[7] These experiments and others performed during the next decade also drew attention to the three to five-fold dilution of food by digestive secretions during its passage through the stomach and duodenum.[8] This dilution is detectable in most normal subjects at a distance of at least 200 cm from the duodeno-jejunal flexure. Thus dilution of a meal is likely in the effluent of a jejunostomy sited

200 cm or less from the flexure with the result that the patient may lose more fluid from the stoma than is taken by mouth.

Fluid and electrolyte fluxes

Sophistication of intubation experiments to enable study of a segment of small intestine demonstrated large fluid and electrolyte shifts in both directions across the normal jejunal mucosa. In this way it was shown between the 1960s and early 1980s that the jejunal mucosa can maintain only a small electrochemical or osmotic gradient between the lumen and blood as compared with the ileum or, even more so, the colon.[9,10] Furthermore, in 1963 the coupling of sodium and glucose transport across the jejunal mucosa was revealed.[11–13]

Effect of malabsorption on the colon

The localization of bile salt re-absorption to the distal ileum was recognized in the mid-1960s; depletion of the bile salt pool as a result of distal ileal resection and the adverse effect of bile salts on the colonic mucosa were recognized soon after. Likewise, the stimulation of colonic peristaltic motor activity and inhibition of water and electrolyte absorption by long-chain fatty acids entering the colon was shown in the 1970s and 1980s to be a potential factor in causing diarrhoea in patients with a short small intestine anastomosed to colon.[14,15] The mechanism of increased oxalate absorption by the colon in patients with a short gut, leading to hyperoxaluria and oxalate renal stones, was unravelled in the 1970s as due to a combination of colonic calcium binding by long-chain fatty acids and the effect of a higher than normal concentration of bile salts on the colonic mucosa.[16]

Adaptation of the residual small intestine after a partial resection

Experiments in animals, dating from the early years of the century, but particularly from the late 1960s onwards, have shown that when a length of small intestine is resected, with anastomosis of the proximal jejunal and distal ileal segments, marked hypertrophy with increased absorptive function of the distal ileum occurs.[17] It seems that the distal ileum which plays little part in normal nutrient absorption has a capacity for increasing its absorptive role when nutrients reach

it due to proximal resection of intestine. Functional investigation in man has shown increased absorption of water, sodium, glucose and calcium in the jejunum,[18–20] but villous hyperplasia has not been demonstrated in man when distal intestine is resected with formation of a terminal jejunostomy.[21]

DEVELOPMENT OF SURGICAL PRACTICE

Extensive resection

The first resection in man of more than 200 cm of small intestine has been attributed to Koberle in 1880, and 55 of such operations were reported up to 1912.[22] Most such operations until the middle years of the century were performed as an emergency for removal of non-viable intestine infarcted due to strangulation or volvulus. Thus, in a 1935 review of 257 cases the commonest reasons for resection were volvulus in 76 and strangulated hernia in 45 (Table 1.1).[23] Mesenteric artery or vein occlusion constituted only 13% of the cases at that time, whereas by 1969 the proportion had risen to 48%.[24] This change may reflect a decreased incidence of hernial strangulation, increasing age of

Table 1.1 – Reasons for 'extensive' and 'massive' intestinal resections in adults in 1912 and 1935

Flint 1912: 'Extensive' intestinal resection [22]	
Strangulated hernia	19
Tumour	10
Gangrene	4
Adhesions/bands	4
Tuberculosis	3
Uterine perforation	3
Other	6
Unknown	6
Total	55
Haymond 1935: 'Massive' intestinal resection [23]	
Volvulus	76
Strangulated hernia	45
Mesenteric thrombosis	34
Tuberculosis	16
Mesenteric tumours	14
Uterine perforation	11
Adhesions/bands	7
Other	54
Total	257

the population and the fact that surgeons became willing to resect a long length of infarcted intestine in the knowledge that treatment was now available to compensate for the resulting malabsorption.

Extensive small bowel resection for vascular insufficiency of the central portion of the small bowel usually spares the proximal and distal ends. Such operations lead to removal of mid-small bowel with jejuno-ileal anastomosis and retention of the colon. The distal ileum has considerable potential for adaptation and the colon, with its capacity for avid absorption of sodium and water, prevents severe fluid and sodium depletion. These cases, with a reasonable good prognosis, still occur but the knowledge that parenteral therapy is available (see below) now allows surgeons to resect even the whole small bowel for a condition such as desmoid tumour of the mesentery. There are now also many people in whom the residual intestine is limited to a relatively short length of residual jejunum ending in a stoma.

Construction of a stoma

The surgery of ulcerative colitis was greatly facilitated by the development and introduction of an everted mucosal ileostomy in 1952 and the development of satisfactory appliances adherent to the skin during the same period.[25] From time to time colectomy for ulcerative colitis is complicated by a vascular accident which leads to loss not only of the colon but also a large part of the small bowel with creation of a terminal jejunostomy.

This operation may be needed electively for the treatment of Crohn's disease when there is extensive involvement of both small and large bowel. Thus in a series reported in 1992 of 86 patients each with less than 200 cm of small bowel remaining, 38 had a jejunostomy as the result of surgical treatment for Crohn's disease or ulcerative colitis.[26]

Entero-cutaneous fistula

A high volume entero-cutaneous fistula is similar in its effluent to a high jejunostomy, but is often complicated by sepsis. While maintaining nutrition parenterally, surgeons can now delay definitive operation for a high-volume entero-cutaneous fistula until sepsis is dealt with, the anatomical situation is defined and the patient's general condition is optimal. Treatment in this way has greatly reduced the mortality of this dangerous condition.

Characterization of resection

The term 'extensive' small bowel resection was reserved in the earlier literature to describe removal of at least 200 cm. This length was chosen because it was believed to represent about one-third of the small intestinal length and experimental work suggested that up to this proportion can be removed without detriment to weight and strength. These observations failed to take account of the variable length of the human small intestine. In 1935, Haymond[23] drew attention to this variability and observed correctly that 'a resection of a large amount in one individual would constitute a different percentage of the total length in another'. Before closing the abdomen after a resection, surgeons should thus measure the length of residual intestine along the anti-mesenteric border, and define the proportions of proximal and distal intestine.

Follow-up observations have shown the prognostic importance of these records. Patients with less than 200 cm of small bowel remaining fall into three groups: those with an anastomosis between residual jejunum and ileum proximal to an intact colon; those with anastomosis of small bowel to colon; and those with a terminal small intestinal stoma.[26] The prognosis as regards the need for long-term parenteral therapy depends in each group on the length of residual small bowel but those with a colon can tolerate shorter lengths of small bowel than those with a jejunostomy.

Surgical treatment of intestinal failure

Although procedures[27,28] have been performed with some success to lengthen a short residual intestine or delay passage of its contents to allow absorption to occur, the main hope of surgical advance centres on intestinal transplantation.[29] Rejection of the graft remains a problem but the successful result when an identical twin was the donor points to the success of surgical technique; the problem to be overcome is immunological.[30]

RECOGNITION OF MEDICAL CAUSES OF INTESTINAL FAILURE

A number of congenital disorders associated with intestinal failure were described during the 1970s and 1980s. For example, a rare congenital defect of intestinal villus formation in babies[31] and a number of different familial types of pseudo-obstruction have been identified.[32] The latter may present as a myopathy in which the intestine becomes wide, atonic and subject to bacterial overgrowth or as a disorder of the myenteric nerve plexus which leads to obstructive episodes without mechanical cause. Chronic pseudo-obstruction has also been recognized later in life secondary to a systemic disorder such as scleroderma or as a sporadic condition of unknown cause.

DEVELOPMENT OF TREATMENT

Enteral nutrition (Table 1.2)

The earliest enteral feeds were given rectally by enema. The ancient Egyptians gave wine, whey, milk and/or barley broth nutrient enemas.[33] John Hunter gave one of the earliest orogastric feeds documented in 1790 to a patient who had had a stroke. He used a pig bladder as a reservoir for an egg, water, sugar, milk or wine feed and this was squeezed into the stomach through a feeding tube, made by a watchmaker, consisting of a whale bone and eel skin.[33] Feeding tubes were at first large and made of rubber, gradually these have been refined to radio-opaque fine-bore tubes either made of polyvinyl chloride or polyurethane.[34] While the first gastrostomies and jejunostomies were fashioned at laparotomy, they are now placed using endoscopic and radiological techniques.[35–39]

In 1943 milk protein was used to make casein hydrolysates as the protein component of a feed, subsequently some feeds have been based on soya bean or

Table 1.2 – Key developments in enteral nutrition

BC	Nutrient enemas used by Ancient Egyptians[33]
1790	Oro-gastric feeding tube[33]
1867	Soft rubber tubing for gastric lavage[34]
1876	Surgical gastrostomy[35]
1885	Surgical feeding jejunostomy[36]
1910	Oro-duodenal feeding[33]
1943	Casein hydrolysates[33]
1952	Surgically placed needle jejunostomy[37]
1963	Chemically defined (elemental) diet for space travel[33]
1980	Endoscopic gastrostomy[38]
1981	Radiological gastrostomy[39]
1990s	Immunomodulation (glutamine, arginine and MCTs)

egg white. Carbohydrate was first given as glucose or sucrose, but in order to keep the osmolality low, glucose-polymer mixtures derived from the hydrolysis of corn starch were used.[33,40] Lipid as long-chain triglyceride was derived from soya, corn or safflower oils, and lipid as medium-chain triglyceride from coconut oil.

Parenteral nutrition (Table 1.3)

Fluid and electrolyte balance has been maintained in patients with intestinal failure since the earliest days of intravenous fluid administration. One of the earliest reports of giving intravenous nutrition was when three patients who had cholera and were considered about to die, were given intravenous fresh (still warm) cow's milk, two of these patients survived.[41] Isotonic, or slightly hypertonic, solutions of glucose were given by peripheral infusion but not enough to provide an adequate energy source because higher concentrations caused thrombosis of the vein. The problems to be solved before intravenous feeding could become a reality, were to devise solutions which provide in a non-irritant form amino-nitrogen for synthesis of protein and an adequate energy source.

Intact protein, other than human plasma or albumin, tends to be allergenic. These whole proteins were used in the first half of the twentieth century for temporary nutritional support but expansion of the circulating plasma volume and slow turnover of the protein were limiting factors. Early workers suggested that amino acid solutions might be effective but it was not until 1937 that an amino acid solution produced by hydrolysis of casein was first shown to be a practicable method of treatment.[43] By 1943, a review recorded treatment of at least 500 patients with this product and included a reference to combined treatment with a fat emulsion.[50] A casein enzymatic

Table 1.3 – Key developments in parenteral nutrition

1873	Milk infusions to treat cholera[41]
1898	Intravenous glucose[42]
1937	Protein hydrolysates (amino acids) infusions[43]
1952	Subclavian vein catheterization using infraclavicular approach[44]
1961	Lipid emulsion[45]
1968	Hypertonic glucose infused into a large vein[46]
1970	Long-term parenteral nutrition ('the artificial gut') using arterio-venous shunt[47]
1973	Teflon-cuffed tunnelled silicone rubber catheter[48]
1973	Peripheral feeding[49]

hydrolysate, in which amino acids and small peptides were separated from residual large peptides by dialysis, was widely used in Europe during the 1950s and 1960s, and a fibrin hydrolysate was used in America. Intensive work defined the optimal amino acid composition, including the ratio of essential to non-essential amino acids and the need to provide the amino acids in an L-form. It was recognized that a mixture of crystalline amino acids would have the advantage of providing flexible solutions of known composition and such a solution was first used clinically in 1940 for intravenous nutrition in children.[51] However, the initial technical difficulty, and thus high commercial cost, of such solutions delayed their introduction for routine use until the 1960s and early 1970s, since when they have superseded the use of protein hydrolysates.

A fat emulsion offered the possibility of a rich caloric source which would not be osmotically active. However, there were many initial difficulties. Low molecular weight triglycerides were found to be acutely toxic. Cotton seed oil and soya bean oil emulsions had low acute toxicity but the former gave rise to toxic effects when given to animals over a period up to 4 weeks. Soya bean oil stabilized with egg yolk phosphatides, which mimicked the structure of chylomicrons, proved non-toxic in animals and was used successfully in man for the first time during the early 1960s.[45] During a 1963 conference in London, Wretlind and Schuberth described their research on the experimental and clinical development of a clinically useful fat emulsion, a preparation still in use today. This was a major advance and, by combining a fat emulsion with a protein hydrolysate, enabled them to maintain satisfactory parenteral nutrition via a peripheral vein. There was an immediate surge of interest in this new technique.

Fructose, sorbitol and ethanol were all tested as possible alternative energy sources to glucose in early work, but all have disadvantages. Glucose is metabolically the most suitable compound but the quantity given was limited by the need to keep the volume of infusate physiological and avoid thrombosis of peripheral veins. Dudrick and colleagues overcame this problem in 1968 by infusing hypertonic glucose into a large central vein where the blood flow is adequate to dilute the solution and thus avoid local phlebitis and thrombosis.[46] This technique was widely adopted in America where fat emulsions were at that time unavailable, and administration of solutions through a central vein has been used by clinicians elsewhere, particularly for long-term parenteral feeding.

Since central venous catheters require skilled placement and are potentially dangerous, there has been a reversion for short term use to the original Swedish technique of peripheral parenteral feeding using a fat emulsion and relatively dilute glucose and amino acid solutions.

Some patients with chronic intestinal failure require prolonged, even life-long, parenteral feeding. There was excitement when the concept of an 'artificial gut' based on the experience of prolonged renal dialysis was introduced by Scribner and colleagues in 1970.[47] The original technique based on intermittent infusion via a peripheral arterio-venous fistula was unsuccessful. A technique of superior vena caval catheterization, adapted for home use by the design of a silicone rubber catheter with a Dacron cuff to seal and fix it within a skin tunnel, proved satisfactory and nine patients treated at home in America were reported in 1973.[48] In the same year, Jeejeebhoy and colleagues published details of 13 patients treated at home in Canada for up to 23 months.[52] In Britain, use of the technique was first mentioned in 1978 and 25 patients treated at different centres were described in 1980 at a conference held for the purpose.[53,54] Parenteral nutrition at home is now a standard technique in many countries for patients with long-standing intestinal failure who cannot be treated successfully using an enteral regime.

During the 1970s and 1980s much has been done to ensure that nutrient solutions are optimal in their ratio of energy to protein, mix of different amino acids, and content of vitamins and trace elements. The technique of fluid administration both in hospital and at home has been simplified and improved in safety. For example, the original need for multiple bottle changes and additions has been simplified by mixing most or all the ingredients in a single pouch or a bag containing 3 litres.[54] Sophisticated pumps have been developed to control the rate of flow and warn of air bubbles or line blockage. Air bubbles in the solution have been minimized by modifying the material used for manufacture of the bag. Most important of all, protocols have been developed to minimize infection and venous thrombosis so that the risk of these complications is now low when care is provided by an experienced team.

Resection and anastomosis

Metabolic studies of patients after resection date back at least to 1938. An example of an investigation aimed at improving management is a report in 1949 of giving a patient with short gut a liquid feed made up of protein hydrolysate, milk, cream and glucose compared with a normal diet.[55] The patient retained only 15 cm of jejunum anastomosed to transverse colon. She had lost weight from 64 kg to 42 kg, complained of weakness and dizziness (blood pressure 80/60), abdominal pain and bloating, and passed 3–6 stools daily. This is a vivid description of the chronic poor health of a patient at that time with a major resection of small intestine. The synthetic diet did not help her but it is interesting to note that she was taking only 1345 kcal daily in her normal diet which contained 48 g of fat.

It gradually became apparent that patients with a short small intestine in continuity with colon benefit from a low fat, high carbohydrate diet. Such patients need to eat more energy-giving foods than normal to compensate for malabsorption. A child reported in 1961 who had lost the whole of his jejunum and retained only 39 cm of ileum showed immediate improvement on a low fat, high protein, high carbohydrate diet. Weight loss was reversed, a growth spurt commenced and diarrhoea diminished.[56] Similarly, an adolescent who retained only 13 cm of jejunum and 5 cm of terminal ileum did well when dietary carbohydrate and protein were increased and part of the fat intake was replaced by medium-chain triglycerides.[57]

The work of Booth et al.[5] and Andersson et al.[58] during the 1960s and 1970s showed that a low fat diet decreases diarrhoea, loss of divalent cations (calcium and magnesium) and urinary oxalate. It is only in recent years that a further benefit of increased dietary carbohydrate has been demonstrated; unabsorbed carbohydrate entering the colon is fermented by colonic bacteria yielding short-chain fatty acids which are absorbed as a source of energy.[59]

Terminal jejunostomy

A patient who underwent an extensive small bowel resection in 1958 which left 120 cm of small bowel ending in a jejunostomy was troubled mainly by profuse drainage from the stoma.[60] When investigated in 1973, the jejunostomy effluent at times exceeded the volume of nutrients taken by mouth. Such profuse losses, with incipient sodium and magnesium deficiency, are a common problem in patients with a short gut and a jejunostomy.

Developments in treatment to minimize sodium losses from the jejunostomy have been threefold. First, it was shown that when such a patient drinks water, or

a dilute sodium solution, there is a net sodium loss from the jejunostomy.[61,62] When a normal person drinks water, sodium enters the upper intestine from the blood but this sodium is re-absorbed by the ileum or colon; in these patients it is lost from the body via the stoma. Second, the same research showed that the coupling of sodium and glucose absorption can be utilized to promote sodium absorption.[61,62] Thus such patients should restrict their water intake and substitute a glucose-electrolyte solution. Animal and human experiments showed that the concentration of sodium in this solution should be at least 90 mmol/L to promote sodium absorption in the upper gut.[63] Third, opiate drugs, such as codeine phosphate or loperamide can make a small contribution to reducing losses.[64,65] Lastly, drugs which reduce gastric,[66,67] or all digestive secretions[68,69] can benefit patients in whom the diluting effect of these digestive juices leads to a greater fluid output than taken by mouth.

Comparisons of oral intake and jejunostomy loss have shown that many patients absorb 60% or less of energy in their diet.[70] Thus, they need to eat more than normal or, if absorption is only about 30%, receive a parenteral supplement. In certain patients total jejunostomy loss exceeds the volume of food and fluid taken by mouth. Such patients cannot survive without parenteral supplements.[71] Unlike patients with an intact colon, fat is not deleterious to patients with a jejunostomy and is a valuable source of energy.[72-74]

CONCLUSION

The concept of intestinal failure, the reasons for it, physiological understanding of impaired intestinal absorption and the development of treatments have largely occurred during the last 30 years of this century. It is perhaps because this concept is relatively new that the term is not yet part of core medical teaching, as is the case with cardiac, respiratory, hepatic or renal failure. The following chapters do much to establish intestinal malabsorption, severe enough to require replacement therapy, as another universally recognized type of system failure.

REFERENCES
1. Milewski PJ, Gross E, Holbrook I, Clarke C, Turnberg LA, Irving MH. Parenteral nutrition at home in management of intestinal failure. *Br Med J* 1980; **1**: 1356–1357.

2. Fleming CR, Remington M. Intestinal failure. In: Hill GL (ed) *Nutrition and the Surgical Patient*. Churchill Livingstone: Edinburgh, 1981, Ch. 14, pp. 219–235.

3. Irving M, White R, Tresadern J. Three years' experience with an intestinal failure unit. *Ann R Coll Surg Engl* 1985; **67**: 1–5.

4. Booth CC. The metabolic effects of intestinal resection in man. *Postgrad Med J* 1961; **37**: 725–739.

5. Booth CC, Macintyre L, Mollin DL. Nutritional problems associated with extensive lesions of the distal small intestine in man. *Quart J Med* 1964; **33**: 401–420.

6. Booth CC, Alldis D, Read AE. Studies on the site of fat absorption: 2. Fat balances after resection of varying amounts of the small intestine in man. *Gut* 1961; **2**: 168–174.

7. Borgstrom B, Daalq A, Lundh G, Sjovall J. Studies of intestinal digestion and absorption in the human. *J Clin Invest* 1957; **36**: 1521–1536.

8. Fordtran JS, Locklear TW. Ionic constituents and osmolality of gastric and small intestinal fluids after eating. *Am J Dig Dis* 1966; **11**: 503–521.

9. Fordtran JS, Rector FC Jr, Ewton MF, Soter N, Kinney J. Permeability characteristics of the human small intestine. *J Clin Invest* 1965; **44**: 1935–1944.

10. Davis GR, Santa Ana CA, Morawski SG, Fordtran JS. Permeability characteristics of human jejunum, ileum, proximal colon and distal colon: results of potential difference measurements and unidirectional fluxes. *Gastroenterology* 1982; **83**: 844–850.

11. Schedl HP, Clifton JA. Solute and water absorption by the human small intestine. *Nature* 1963; **199**: 1264–267.

12. Fordtran JS, Rector FC Jr, Carter NW. The mechanisms of sodium absorption in the human small intestine. *J Clin Invest* 1968; **47**: 884–900.

13. Fordtran JS. Stimulation of active and passive sodium absorption by sugars in the human jejunum. *J Clin Invest* 1975; **55**: 728–737.

14. Ammon HV, Phillips SF. Inhibition of colonic water and electrolyte absorption by fatty acids in man. *Gastroenterology* 1973; **65**: 744–749.

15. Spiller RC, Brown ML, Phillips SF. Decreased fluid tolerance, accelerated transit, and abnormal motility of the human colon induced by oleic acid. *Gastroenterology* 1986; **91**: 100–107.

16. Dobbins JW, Binder HJ. Importance of the colon in enteric hyperoxaluria. *N Engl J Med* 1977; **296**: 298–301.

17. Bristol JB, Williamson RCN. Nutrition, operations, and intestinal adaptation. *J Parenter Enteral Nutr* 1988; **12**: 299–309.

18. Weinstein DL, Shoemaker CP, Hersh T, Wright HK. Enhanced intestinal absorption after small bowel resection in man. *Arch Surg* 1969; **99**: 560–562.

19. Dowling RH, Booth CC. Functional compensation after small-bowel resection in man. *Lancet* 1966; **1**: 146–147.

20. Gouttebel MC, Saint Aubert B, Colette C, Astre C, Monnier LH, Joyeux H. Intestinal adaptation in patients with short bowel syndrome. *Dig Dis Sci* 1989; **34**: 709–715.

21. O'Keefe SJD, Shorter RG, Bennet WM, Haymond MW. Villous hyperplasia is uncommon in patients with massive intestinal resection. *Gastroenterology* 1992; **102**: A231.

22. Flint JM. The effect of extensive resections of the small intestine. *Bull Johns Hopkins Hosp* 1912; **23**: 127–144.

23. Haymond HE. Massive resection of the small intestine. An analysis of 257 collected cases. *Surg Gynec Obstet* 1935; **693**: 705.

24. Simons BE, Jordan GL. Massive bowel resection. *Am J Surg* 1969; **118**: 953–959.

25. Brooke BN. The management of an ileostomy including its complications. *Lancet* 1952; **2**: 102–104.

26. Nightingale JMD, Lennard-Jones JE, Gertner DJ, Wood SR, Bartram CI. Colonic preservation reduces need for parenteral therapy, increases incidence of renal stones but does not change high prevalence of gallstones in patients with short bowel. *Gut* 1992; **33**: 1493–1497.

27. Mitchell A, Watkins RM, Collin J. Surgical treatment of the short bowel syndrome. *Br J Surg* 1984; **71**: 329–333.

28. Bianchi A. Longitudinal intestinal lengthening and tailoring: results in 20 children. *J R Soc Med* 1997; **90**: 429–432.

29. Grant D. Current results of intestinal transplantation. *Lancet* 1996; **347**: 1801–1803.

30. Calne RY, Friend PJ, Middleton S, Jamieson NV, Watson CJE, Soin A, Chavez-Cartaya R. Intestinal transplant between two of identical triplets. *Lancet* 1997; **350**: 1077–1078.

31. Philips AD, Jenkins P, Raafat F, Walker-Smith JA. Congenital microvillous atrophy. *Arch Dis Child* 1985; **60**: 135–140.

32. Anuras S, Christensen J. Recurrent or chronic intestinal pseudo-obstruction. *Clin Gastroenterol* 1981; **10**: 177–190.

33. Randall HT. Enteral nutrition: tube feeding in acute and chronic illness. *J Parenter Enteral Nutr* 1984; **8**: 113–136.

34. Rombeau JL, Barot LR. Enteral nutritional therapy. *Surg Clin North Am* 1981; **613**: 605–620.

35. Cunha F. Gastrostomy. Its inception and evolution. *Am J Surg* 1946; **72**: 610–634.

36. Torosian MH, Rombeau JL. Feeding by tube enterostomy. *Surg Gynecol Obstet* 1980; **150**: 918–927.

37. McDonald HA. Intrajejunal drip in gastric surgery. *Lancet* 1954; **I**: 1007.

38. Gauderer MWL, Ponsky JL, Izant RJ. Gastrostomy without laparotomy: a percutaneous endoscopic technique. *J Pediatr Surg* 1980; **15**: 872–875.

39. Preshaw RM. A percutaneous method for inserting a feeding gastrostomy tube. *Surg Gynecol Obstet* 1981; **152**: 658–660.

40. Silk DBA. Towards the optimization of enteral nutrition. *Clin Nutr* 1987; **6**: 61–74.

41. Hodder EM. Transfusion of milk in cholera. *Practitioner* 1873; **10**: 14–16.

42. Lilienfeld C. Versuche über intravenöse Ernahrung. *Zeitschriff fur Diatetische und Physikalische Therapie* 1899; **2**: 209–217.

43. Elman R. Amino-acid content of the blood following intravenous injection of hydrolysed casein. *Proc Soc Exp Biol Med* 1937; **37**: 437–440.

44. Aubaniac R. L'injection intraveineuse sous-claviculaire; avantages et technique. *Presse Méd* 1952; **60**: 1456.

45. Wretlind A. Fat emulsions. In: Lee HA (ed) *Parenteral Nutrition in Acute Metabolic Illness*. Academic Press: London, 1974, pp. 77–92.

46. Dudrick SJ, Wilmore DW, Vars HM, Rhoads JE. Long-term total parenteral nutrition with growth, development and positive nitrogen balance. *Surgery* 1968; **64**: 134–142.

47. Scribner BH, Cole JJ, Christopher TG. Long-term parenteral nutrition; the concept of an artificial gut. *JAMA* 1970; **212**: 457–463.

48. Broviac JW, Cole JJ, Scribner BH. A silicone rubber atrial catheter for prolonged parenteral alimentation. *Surg Gynec Obstet* 1973; **136**: 602–606.

49. Fox HA, Krasna IH. Total intravenous nutrition by peripheral vein in neonatal surgical patients. *Pediatrics* 1973; **52**: 14–20.

50. Editorial. Intravenous alimentation. *Br Med J* 1943; **1**: 416–417.

51. Shohi AT, Blackfan KD. The intravenous administration of crystalline amino acids to infants. *J Nutr* 1940; **20**: 305–316.

52. Jeejeebhoy KN, Zohrab WJ, Langer B, Phillips MJ, Kuksis A, Anderson GH. Total parenteral nutrition at home for 23 months, without complication, and with good rehabilitation. *Gastroenterology* 1973; **65**: 811–820.

53. Report. Home parenteral nutrition in England and Wales. *Br Med J* 1980; **281**: 1407–1409.

54. Powell-Tuck J, Farwell JA, Nielsen T, Lennard-Jones JE. Team approach to long-term intravenous feeding in patients with gastrointestinal disorders. *Lancet* 1978; **2**: 825–828.

55. Althausen TL, Uyeyama K, Simpson RG. Digestion and absorption after massive resection of the small intestine. 1. Utilization of food from a 'natural' versus a 'synthetic' diet and a comparison of intestinal absorption tests with nutritional balance studies in a patient with only 45 cm of small intestine. *Gastroenterology* 1949; **12**: 795–808.

56. Clayton BE, Cotton DA. A study of malabsorption after resection of the entire jejunum and the proximal half of the ileum. *Gut* 1961; **2**: 18–22.

57. Winawer SJ, Broitman SA, Wolochow DA, Osborne MP, Zamcheck N. Successful management of massive small-bowel resection based on assessment of absorption defects and nutritional needs. *N Engl J Med* 1966; **274**: 72–78.

58. Andersson H, Jagenburg R. Fat-reduced diet in the treatment of hyperoxaluria in patients with ileopathy. *Gut* 1974; **15**: 360–366.

59. Nordgaard I, Hansen BS, Mortensen PB. Colon as a digestive organ in patients with short bowel. *Lancet* 1994; **343**: 373–376.

60. Simko V, Linscheer WG. Absorption of different elemental diets in a short-bowel syndrome lasting 15 years. *Dig Dis* 1976; **21**: 419–425.

61. Griffin GE, Fagan EF, Hodgson HJ, Chadwick VS. Enteral therapy in the management of massive gut resection complicated by chronic fluid and electrolyte depletion. *Dig Dis Sci* 1982; **27**: 902–908.

62. Newton CR, Gonvers JJ, McIntyre PB, Preston DM, Lennard-Jones JE. Effect of different drinks on fluid and electrolyte losses from a jejunostomy. *J R Soc Med* 1985; **78**: 27–34.

63. Rodrigues CA, Lennard-Jones JE, Thompson DG, Farthing MJG. What is the ideal sodium concentration of oral rehydration solutions for short bowel patients? *Clin Sci* 1988; **74 (Suppl 18)**: 69.

64. Newton CR. Effect of codeine phosphate, Lomotil and isogel on ileostomy function. *Gut* 1978; **19**: 377–383.

65. Rodrigues CA, Lennard-Jones JE, Walker ER, Thompson DG, Farthing MJG. The effects of octreotide, soy polysaccharide, codeine and loperamide on nutrient, fluid and electrolyte absorption in the short bowel syndrome. *Aliment Pharmacol Ther* 1989; **3**: 159–169.

66. Jacobsen O, Ladefoged K, Stage JG, Jarnum S. Effects of cimetidine on jejunostomy effluents in patients with severe short-bowel syndrome. *Scand J Gastroenterol* 1986; **21**: 824–828.

67. Nightingale JMD, Walker ER, Farthing MJG, Lennard-Jones JE. Effect of omeprazole on intestinal output in the short bowel syndrome. *Aliment Pharmacol Ther* 1991; **5**: 405–412.

68. Ladefoged K, Christensen KC, Hegnhoj J, Jarnum S. Effect of a long acting somatostatin analogue SMS 201-995 on jejunostomy effluents in patients with severe short bowel syndrome. *Gut* 1989; **30**: 943–949.

69. Nightingale JMD, Walker ER, Burnham WR, Farthing MJG, Lennard-Jones JE. Octreotide (a somatostatin analogue) improves the quality of life in some patients with a short intestine. *Aliment Pharmacol Ther* 1989; **3**: 367–373.

70. Rodrigues CA, Lennard-Jones JE, Thompson DG, Farthing MJG. Energy absorption as a measure of intestinal failure in the short bowel syndrome. *Gut* 1989; **30**: 176–183.

71. Nightingale JMD, Lennard-Jones JE, Walker ER, Farthing MJG. Jejunal efflux in short bowel syndrome. *Lancet* 1990; **336**: 765–768.

72. Woolf GM, Miller C, Kurian R, Jeejeebhoy KN. Diet for patients with a short bowel: high fat or high carbohydrate? *Gastroenterology* 1983; **84**: 823–828.

73. Simko V, McCarroll AM, Goodman S, Weesner RE, Kelley RE. High-fat diet in a short bowel syndrome. Intestinal absorption and gastroenteropancreatic hormone responses. *Dig Dis Sci* 1980; **25**: 333–339.

74. McIntyre PB, Fitchew M, Lennard-Jones JE. Patients with a jejunostomy do not need a special diet. *Gastroenterology* 1986; **91**: 25–33.

2

Normal intestinal anatomy and physiology

J. Nightingale and R. Spiller

*T*he gastrointestinal tract is a complex system with diverse functions related to the interactions between food and the body. Although its prime functions are digestion and absorption, it is also a sophisticated immunological defence organ and the body's largest endocrine organ. It extends as a hollow muscular tube of variable calibre from the mouth to anus (Fig. 2.1). Its main function is to break large molecules into small soluble ones and then selectively to absorb water, macronutrients, minerals and vitamins. This all happens in a highly co-ordinated manner with information about the luminal content of any one area of the gut being transmitted both proximally and distally. Thus the distal bowel can prepare for a meal that is about to arrive and can regulate the rate at which chyme is delivered to it from the proximal gut. Mucosal nerves and endocrine cells sensitive to luminal contents relay information and instructions via the enteric nervous system and blood stream. The small intestine is also exposed to a wide range of food antigens and bacteria and thus contains a large amount of immunological tissue whose function is to protect the body against pathogenic bacteria while maintaining immune tolerance to food antigens.

OESOPHAGUS

The oesophagus is a muscular tube about 25 cm long; its function is to propel the food bolus from the pharynx to the gastric cardia. It is lined with a tough squamous epithelium. The upper two-thirds has striated voluntary skeletal muscle and the lower one-third involuntary smooth muscle.[1] About 2 kg of food and drink pass down it each day, diluted and lubricated by 500 ml of saliva from lingual, sublingual, sub-mandibular and parotid salivary glands. Food viscosity is reduced by the acts of chewing, dilution and swallowing.

STOMACH

The adult stomach is an acidic storage area that can hold up to 1.5 l;[1] it starts digestion and delivers partly processed food at a controlled rate into the duodenum. It consists of two functionally different parts: the fundus and the antrum.

The fundus is mainly a storage area in which gastric juice is secreted and mixed with food to begin digestion. In addition to the many mucus-secreting cells found throughout the stomach, the fundal parietal cells secrete 0.1 M hydrochloric acid and intrinsic factor. During fasting the gastric pH ranges from 1.8 to 2.0; addition of food buffers this, raising the gastric pH to 4–5. Acid kills most micro-organisms, denatures protein making it more susceptible to hydrolysis, and converts inactive pepsinogen to pepsin, which is the active form of the enzyme. Intrinsic factor, a muco-protein with a molecular weight of 55 000, binds B_{12} and this complex is absorbed in the distal 60 cm of ileum.[2] Fundal chief cells secrete pepsinogen and rennin. Pepsin is important in the breakdown of collagen, as it cleaves protein at the site of aromatic amino acids; rennin coagulates milk.

Partly digested food from the fundus enters the antrum. The antrum has less of a secretory role and is responsible for mixing food and grinding it into small particles. Repetitive antral contractions occurring at 3 per minute propel chyme towards the pylorus, whose closure causes frequent retrograde flow. This to-and-fro flow produces marked shearing that reduces food particles to less than 2 mm in diameter, a size at which they can pass through the pylorus into the duodenum. Thus the pylorus acts as a sieve.[3] Endocrine G cells in the antrum release gastrin, which stimulates the fundal parietal cells to secrete acid. The mixture of food, drink and secretion leaving the stomach is called chyme. Although the surface area of the stomach is small and the epithelium relatively impermeable, some molecules (e.g. alcohol and aspirin) can be absorbed from the stomach.

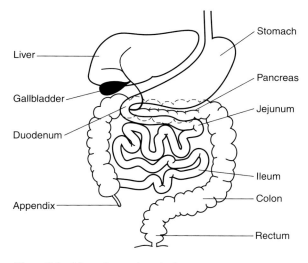

Liver

Gallbladder

Duodenum

Appendix

Stomach

Pancreas

Jejunum

Ileum

Colon

Rectum

Figure 2.1 – Normal gastrointestinal anatomy.

DUODENUM

The duodenum is the widest part of the small bowel. It is 20–25 cm long and extends from the pylorus to the duodeno-jejunal flexure. In its structure it is essentially the same as the jejunum in that a villus structure starts absorption, but it contains submucosal bicarbonate-secreting glands of Brunner. The alkaline secretion from these glands helps to neutralize the gastric acid. In the second part of the duodenum, alkaline pancreatico-biliary secretions are added to the chyme. The pancreatic enzymes are responsible for breaking macronutrients (protein, carbohydrate, lipid and nucleic acids) into smaller molecules (peptides, oligo/disaccharides, fatty acids/glycerol and nucleotides). Bile contains bile salts that aid lipid digestion and absorption; it also contains some end products of metabolism such as haemoglobin, cholesterol and some drugs. Bile is concentrated by the 7–10 cm long gallbladder which can hold 30–50 ml of fluid.[1] When lipid-containing chyme is within the duodenum, the gallbladder contracts and the sphincter of Oddi relaxes so that concentrated gallbladder bile is secreted into the duodenum.

VOLUME OF GASTROINTESTINAL SECRETIONS

The work of Borgström *et al.*[4] and Fordtran and Locklear[5] provides an estimate for the daily volume of intestinal secretions when a normal diet is consumed. They have shown, using non-absorbed markers in healthy subjects, that about 4.0 L of endogenous secretions pass the duodeno-jejunal flexure daily. This quantity is made up of about 0.5 L saliva, 1–2 L gastric juice[6] and 1.5 L of pancreatico-biliary secretions (0.6 L is pancreatic juice[7]). Thus, each day about 6 L of chyme pass the duodeno-jejunal flexure. The process of digestion usually adds further secretions in the upper jejunum, increasing the flow still further until the mid jejunum when absorption comes to predominate and flow decreases progressively until only 1–2 L enter the colon (Table 2.1).

JEJUNUM AND ILEUM

The proximal two-fifths of the small bowel is called the jejunum, and the distal three-fifths the ileum. The jejunum diameter is 4 cm, and that of the ileum 3.5 cm. The small intestinal absorptive area is vastly increased by the villi, there being 20–40 per mm of small bowel;[1] villi are longer and more numerous in the jejunum than in the ileum (Fig. 2.2). The endothelial cells that line the villus are made in the crypts and migrate to the villus tip from where they are shed; these cells have a life span of only 2–5 days. The jejunum has many circular folds and is thicker, more vascular and muscular than the ileum but it has few lymphatics. The ileum has few circular folds and it contains many lymphoid follicles.[1]

LENGTH OF THE SMALL INTESTINE

The normal human small intestinal length from the duodeno-jejunal flexure to the ileocaecal valve as measured at autopsy, by a small bowel enema or at surgery varies from about 275 to 850 cm (Table 2.2)[9–15] and is shorter in women. The full intestinal length is achieved by 10 years of age.[9] Congenital cases of

Table 2.1 – Approximate daily volume and composition of intestinal secretions produced in response to food

	Volume (litres)	pH	Na	K	Cl (mmol/L)	HCO$_3$	Mg	Ca
Saliva	0.5	7	45	20	44	60	0.7	1.3
Gastric juice	2.0	2	10	10	130	0	0.5	2.0
Pancreatic juice	0.6	8	140	10	30	110	0.2	0.3
Hepatic bile	0.9	7	145	5	100	28	0.6	2.5
Small bowel secretion	1.8★	7	138	6	141	<5	<0.1	2.5
Serum		7.4	140	4	100	24	1.0	2.4

★ This fluid is released and absorbed on the mucosa and rarely needs to be taken into account in calculating fluid losses. Estimates of its electrolyte composition are unreliable.[8]

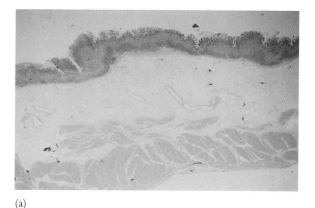

(a)

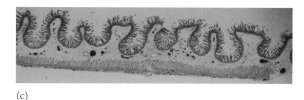

(b)

(c)

(d)

Figure 2.2 – Histological full-thickness sections of (a) stomach, (b) jejunum, (c) ileum and (d) colon. Kindly provided by P Domizio.

patients having problems due to a short length of intestine have been reported.[16] Radiological measurements of small bowel length give shorter results than those obtained at autopsy or surgery, partly because radiographs are only in two dimensions. A small bowel enema[14,15] causes bowel distension leading to overall shortening. The bowel may also be apparently shortened when measurements are made after passing a small flexible polyvinyl plastic tube through the nose to the caecum[12] as this causes the bowel to telescope around the tube.

An appreciation of the wide range of normal small intestinal length is important and emphasizes the need, after a bowel resection, to refer to the remaining length of small intestine rather than to the amount resected.

DIGESTION AND ABSORPTION IN THE SMALL INTESTINE

Water, sodium and chloride

Although some water and sodium may be absorbed before chyme reaches the jejunum in most normal subjects, a meal continues to be diluted by secretions at a distance of 100 cm distal to the duodeno-jejunal flexure.[4,5] This distance is clinically important: if a patient has a stoma situated in the upper 100 cm of jejunum, the volume that emerges from the stoma is likely to be greater than the volume taken by mouth. Such a patient will be in negative fluid and sodium balance after any food or drink.[17] Most meals have a low sodium content (10–40 mmol/L), generating a steep concentration gradient between the lumen and plasma. Sodium-rich salivary and pancreatico-biliary secretions raise the luminal level, as do intestinal secretions, so that the sodium concentration at the duodeno-jejunal flexure reaches about 90 mmol/L and increases further towards 140 mmol/L in the terminal ileum.[5]

Jejunal mucosa is more permeable to water, sodium and chloride than ileal mucosa. It allows back diffusion through leaky intracellular junctions so the jejunal contents become iso-osmolar. Thus water movements in response to an osmotic gradient in the jejunum are nine times as great[18] and sodium fluxes twice as great[19] as in the ileum. Sodium absorption in the jejunum can occur only against a small concentration gradient, depends upon water movement, and is coupled to the absorption of glucose and some amino acids.[20] When

Table 2.2 – Measured lengths of small intestine from the duodeno-jejunal flexure

Author	Date	Number	Sex	Small intestinal length mean	range (cm)
Autopsy★					
Bryant[9]	1924	160	Both	620	300–850
		27	M	650	460–810
		17	F	590	410–760
Underhill[10]	1955	100	Both	620	340–790
		65	M	640	490–790
		35	F	590	340–720
Surgery					
Backman and Hallberg[11]	1974	42	Both	660	400–850
		12	M	700	500–850
		20	F	620	400–780
Slater and Aufses†[12]	1991	38	Both	500	300–780
		14	M	540	330–780
		24	F	480	300–640
Radiological					
Intubation					
Hirsch *et al.*[13]	1956	10	Both	260	210–320
		6	M	260	220–320
		4	F	260	210–320
Small bowel enema					
Fanucci *et al.*[14]	1988	158	Both	290	160–430
Fanucci *et al.*[15]	1984	5	M	310	260–370
		5	F	260	230–280

★ Autopsy measurements from pylorus, all others from the duodeno-jejunal flexure (duodenum = 25 cm).
† 21 of these patients had small bowel and 4 others colonic Crohn's disease but their small intestinal lengths were not different from 13 patients without Crohn's disease.

the small bowel is intubated and perfused with solutions containing different amounts of sodium, absorption of sodium from the perfusate occurs if its sodium concentration is 90 mmol/L or more, while secretion of sodium into the lumen occurs if the concentration is less. Several studies have shown that maximal jejunal absorption of sodium from a perfused solution occurs at a concentration around 120 mmol/L.[21–23] In contrast, the ileum can absorb sodium against a concentration gradient, and movement of sodium is not coupled with glucose or other nutrients. The ileum is important in conserving sodium and water when the body becomes depleted since, unlike the jejunum, the ileal mucosa can increase its sodium absorption in response to aldosterone.[24] Some chloride is actively absorbed in the ileum in exchange for bicarbonate.

Macronutrients

The salivary, gastric and pancreatico-biliary secretions break large molecules (e.g. polypeptides, polysaccharides, nucleotides) into medium-sized ones (e.g. oligopeptides, oligosaccharides and nucleosides) within the gut lumen. They are not designed to create small molecules (e.g. amino acids, glucose or nucleic acids) as these would be hyperosmolar and thus cause water secretion and an osmotic diarrhoea. The final breakdown to small molecules occurs at the mucosal brush border immediately before absorption (Table 2.3). Intubation studies in healthy subjects have shown that most polysaccharides, proteins and fats are digested and absorbed within the upper 200 cm of the small intestine.[4] The site of absorption of a meal depends upon its nature: meat and salad are absorbed high in the

Table 2.3 – Content and function of most upper gastrointestinal secretions

Secretion	Content	Functions/released/activated by
Saliva	α-Amylase	Converts starch to oligosaccharides, maltose, maltotriose and α limit dextrins. Needs pH 7, inactive in gastric acid
	Lipase	From lingual glands, cleaves MCTG to MCFA/glycerol, acid stable
Gastric juice	HCl	Denatures protein, kills micro-organisms, activates pepsinogen released by gastrin, food, cholinergic agents and hypoglycaemia
	Pepsin(ogen)	Hydrolyses bonds by aromatic amino acids (tyrosine and phenylalanine) and leucine (collagen) at pH 2–3. Activated by acid
	Lipase	Cleaves MCTG to MCFA/glycerol, acid stable
	Intrinsic factor	Binds B_{12} and the complex is absorbed in the terminal ileum
	Gelatinase	Liquefies gelatine
Pancreatic juice	Bicarbonate	To neutralize acid and provide optimum pH for pancreatic enzymes, released by secretin
	α-Amylase	Starch to oligosaccharides, maltose, maltotriose and α limit dextrins
	Lipase	1 and 3 glycerol/fatty acid bonds hydrolysed, inhibited by acid
Endopeptidases	Trypsin(ogen)	Cleaves bonds next to arginine and lysine. It is activated by enterokinase an enzyme produced by duodenal mucosa and by itself. It activates all other pancreatic proteolytic enzymes
	Chymotrypsin(ogen)	Cleaves bonds by tyrosine, tryptophan, phenylalanine, methionine and leucine. Activated by trypsin
	(pro)Elastase	Cleaves bonds by alanine, glycine and serine, activated by trypsin
Exopeptidases	(pro)Carboxypolypeptidase A	Cleaves bonds by valine, leucine, isoleucine and alanine (contains zinc), activated by trypsin
	(pro)Carboxypolypeptidase B	Cleaves bonds by arginine and lysine
	DNA/RNAases	Nucleotides to nucleosides
	Esterase	Cleaves cholesterol esters
	(pro)Phospholipase A	Cleaves lecithin to lysolecithin
Bile	Bile salts (primary/secondary)	Bind fat to form globules; then, after lipase has acted, form small micelles which transport the lipid to the brush border
Mucosa★	Bicarbonate	Neutralizes acid generated in process of digestion
	Enterokinase	Activates trypsin
Disaccharidases		Disaccharides to monosaccharides
	Maltase	Maltose to glucose
	Isomaltase	Isomaltose to glucose
	Sucrase	Sucrose to glucose and fructose
	Lactase	Lactose to glucose and galactose
	Trehalase	Trehalose to glucose
	α-Dextrinase	α Limit dextrins to glucose
Exopeptidases		
	Aminopeptidase	Peptides to amino acids hydrolysis starting at amino end
	Dipeptidases	Dipeptides to amino acids
Nucleosidases		Cleave nucleoside to nucleic acid and hexose/pentose

( ): the name of the enzyme in its inactive secreted form.
★ Mucosal brush border (secretion of glycoprotein enzymes).

jejunum, while milk and doughnuts are absorbed more distally, after a large amount of water has been secreted.

Carbohydrate and protein

Saliva and gastric and pancreatico-biliary secretions break down carbohydrate and protein to oligo-saccharides and oligopeptides. The final stage of carbohydrate and protein digestion therefore occurs on the mucosal brush border where oligosaccharides are broken down to monosaccharides and oligopeptides are broken down to amino acids immediately before absorption. In the jejunum, glucose and galactose absorption is partly coupled with that of sodium;

fructose absorption occurs by an independent mechanism.

Protein is digested by enzymes that cleave protein either at specific points in the middle of proteins, endopeptidases (pepsin, trypsin, chymotrypsin and elastase), or work systematically from the ends, exopeptidases. Carboxypeptidases from pancreatic juice start at the carboxyl end while aminopeptidases on the brush border start at the amino end.

Lipid

Triglycerides and fatty acids separate into a lipid phase and do not contribute to the osmotic forces that dominate fluid flux across the small intestinal mucosa. Salivary and gastric lipase are active in the gastric juice and start digestion by splitting monoglycerides from triacylglycerol. Monoglycerides combine with bile salts to generate micelles. Shearing forces around the pylorus are believed to contribute to emulsification, the process that generates fatty droplets in the duodenum. This requires agents such as bile salts and lecithin to lower surface tension, thereby acting like soap and keeping the droplets in solution. The increased surface area of lipid is acted upon by co-lipase and lipase which cleave fatty acids from triglyceride mainly at the 1 and 3 positions. This enzymatic reaction continues as the products (free fatty acids and 2 monoglycerides) are immediately bound by bile salts to form micelles, allowing them to diffuse to the mucosal brush border for active absorption. There, fatty acid binding proteins allow removal of fatty acids from the micelles, which then diffuse back into the lumen to solubilize more lipid. The micelles protect the brush border from the damaging effects of free fatty acids.

The liver makes two bile acids, cholic and chenodeoxycholic acid. These are conjugated with glycine or taurine in the ratio 3:1. The taurine conjugates are more soluble and are present in a greater amount in people who eat meat than in vegetarians. Each day, one-third to one-quarter of the primary bile acids undergo anaerobic bacterial dehydroxygenation within the terminal ileum and colon. This dehydrogenation takes place at position 7 and results in the formation of the secondary bile acids, deoxycholic acid and a little relatively insoluble lithocholic acid respectively. Most lithocholic acid is sulphated and amidated and lost in the stool. Normal human bile therefore consists of 50% cholic acid, 39% chenodeoxycholic acid, 15% deoxycholic acid and 5% lithocholic acid. Each individual contains 3–5 g of bile salts that circulate through the entero-hepatic circulation 5–14 times daily. This circulation is important for the action of some drugs, such as loperamide, that enter it; if the entero-hepatic circulation is disrupted (e.g. by an ileal resection) higher than normal doses of loperamide are needed for the same effect. Cholesterol also undergoes secretion in the bile and reabsorption in the small intestine, the balance of which has an important effect on serum levels. Reabsorption can be reduced by poorly absorbed plant phytosterols such as sitosterol, which competitively inhibit cholesterol uptake into micelles.[25] Fibre supplementation reduces reabsorption of bile salts. Ispaghula and pectin are particularly effective, while bran is ineffective. This is important because bile salt excretion stimulates bile acid synthesis from cholesterol and hence lowers serum cholesterol.[26]

Long-chain fatty acids (C14–20) are absorbed and formed into chylomicrons which pass via the thoracic duct to the systemic circulation. Medium-chain fatty acids (C6–12) are absorbed in the small and large bowel and pass directly into the portal venous system; they are readily oxidized in the liver via a carnitine independent pathway.

Nucleotides

Deoxyribonucleic acid (DNA) and ribonucleic acid (RNA) are broken down to nucleosides by pancreatic DNA/RNA endonucleases and exonucleases, which cleave from either the middle or the end of the molecules respectively. Phosphodiesterase hydrolyses nucleotides from the 3′ end. The resulting nucleosides are split into nucleic acids and pentoses by nucleosidases at the brush border immediately before absorption.

Micronutrients

Vitamins

Water-soluble vitamins are actively absorbed from the upper intestine, with the exception of vitamin B_{12} which is selectively absorbed from the distal 60 cm of ileum.[2] The fat-soluble vitamins A, D, E and K, essential fatty acids and cholesterol do not have specific active uptake mechanisms but dissolve in the lipophilic centre of the micelles; this allows these hydrophobic molecules to diffuse through the aqueous chyme to reach the lipid outer membrane of the brush border into which these lipophilic substances readily diffuse.

Minerals

Magnesium. Magnesium is an important intracellular cation that is a cofactor for many enzymatic reactions; 50% is in bone. Each day, about 10–20 mmol of magnesium are consumed, of which about one-third is absorbed, principally by a gradient-driven saturable process occurring mainly in the distal small intestine and colon.[27] The proportion absorbed varies according to the amount of magnesium in the diet. When the total dietary magnesium is increased to 24 mmol in a healthy person only 24% is absorbed, while if the dietary intake is reduced to 1 mmol 76% is absorbed.[28] The jejunal absorption of magnesium, like that of calcium, is increased by 1,25-dihydroxychole-calciferol.[29] Magnesium in the circulation is 30% bound to albumin. The serum levels, however, are an unreliable index of magnesium status, and severe deficiency can occur when the serum levels are normal.[30] Under conditions of magnesium deprivation the kidney can reduce magnesium excretion to less than 0.5 mmol/d.[31] Aldosterone increases[32] and parathormone reduces renal magnesium excretion.[33] Very little magnesium is found in the intestinal secretions (Table 2.1).

Calcium. Of the calcium ingested, 30–80% is normally absorbed, mainly by active transport in the upper small intestine. The transport is facilitated by 1,25-dihydroxycholecalciferol, lactose and protein. Phosphates, phytates and oxalate form insoluble complexes with calcium and thus inhibit calcium absorption.

Iron. Normally, only 3–6% of the iron ingested is absorbed; this is sufficient to replace losses of 0.6 mg/d in men and 1.2 mg/d in women. Gastric acid dissolves insoluble iron salts and facilitates the reduction of ferric iron (Fe^{3+}) present in most food to ferrous iron (Fe^{2+}) which can be actively absorbed in the upper small bowel. This reduction depends on ascorbic acid, which is actively secreted in gastric juice, and other reducing agents in the diet. The amount of iron entering the circulation is carefully controlled. Only a small amount is allowed to enter the circulation, while the rest is bound to apoferritin to form ferritin within a mucosal cell. This poorly absorbable complex enters the gut lumen when the mucosal cell is shed and is thus lost from the body.

Zinc. Like iron and calcium, zinc is mainly absorbed in the upper small intestine; blood levels peak 2–3 hours after ingestion. Endogenous, particularly pancreatic, secretions contain substantial amounts of zinc. Intestinal luminal levels of zinc fall distally as it is actively absorbed, a process facilitated by the absorption of dipeptides. Once absorbed, it is bound to albumin and circulating macroglobulin. Excretion is via sweat and in urine and faeces. Zinc absorption is, like that of calcium, impaired by dietary phytate and oxalate.[34] Geophagia (ingestion of clay) is associated with severe zinc deficiency characterized by hypopituitarism and dwarfism.[35] Zinc deficiency is frequent in patients with Crohn's disease as there are excessive faecal losses together with a poor intake.[36]

Copper. This potentially toxic metal is rapidly absorbed and loosely bound to albumin. It is rapidly taken up by the liver and avidly secreted into the circulation bound to caeruloplasmin. Deficiency is extremely rare; it can cause a microcytic anaemia and twisted abdominal hair. The main clinical problem in copper metabolism is failure to excrete it adequately. Urine excretion is normally low and the main route of excretion is via bile where copper forms a complex with a fragment of caeruloplasmin which prevents its reabsorption. Defective excretion is seen in Wilson's disease, an autosomal recessive trait characterized by caeruloplasmin deficiency and hence an accumulation of copper in the liver with resulting fibrosis.

ILEOCAECAL VALVE

The ileocaecal valve consists of two semilunar flaps projecting into the lumen of the large bowel at the junction of the caecum and colon. Two main functions are classically attributed to the ileocaecal valve: (1) to control the passage of ileal contents into the caecum, so allowing adequate time for digestion and absorption; and (2), more importantly, to prevent the regurgitation of caecal contents into the small bowel.[37] These functions are questionable: in patients who had had a right hemicolectomy for localized colon cancer, transit of a scrambled egg meal from the small to large bowel was qualitatively and quantitatively the same as in healthy subjects.[38] The mean anaerobic bacterial count in the distal ileum is 10^4/ml compared with 10^8/ml in the caecum; the mean coliform content is 10^3/ml in the ileum and 10^6/ml in the caecum.[39] No major episodes of colo–ileal reflux occur when the ileocaecal valve has been removed,[38] thus the bacterial population in the ileum is unlikely to be changed. Ileal peristalsis is probably the main factor that keeps the number of bacteria in the small bowel so much lower than in the colon. The ileum can differentiate between liquid and solid but the ileocaecal junction cannot.[40]

COLON

The average length of the colon at autopsy is about 1.6 metres (range 1.0–3.3),[8,9] being longer in men than in women. The unstretched colon at colonoscopy is much shorter at about 0.9 metres. The colon has many haustra and its longitudinal muscle is reduced to three longitudinal bands (taeniae coli).[1] It has the functions of absorbing water (up to 6 litres/day),[41] sodium, minerals (e.g. magnesium and calcium), some vitamins and fermenting unabsorbed non-starch carbohydrate to short-chain fatty acids (acetate, propionate and butyrate). The appendix and terminal ileum may secrete antimicrobial substances to regulate the colonic bacterial flora. The functions of the right and left sides of the colon are different. The right side is mainly involved with water and sodium absorption and with fermentation; the left colon is largely a storage and propulsive organ. The colon avidly absorbs sodium and chloride against a high concentration gradient and so normal stool contains very little sodium and chloride.

Evidence that the colon can absorb nutrients and minerals comes from reports dating as far back as ancient Egypt of various mixed enema solutions containing such ingredients as milk, egg, beef broth, wine or brandy being used to give nutrition support,[42] and from the fact that magnesium poisoning can occur from magnesium sulphate enemas.[43]

GASTROINTESTINAL MOTILITY

The gut is innervated by the vagus nerve (parasympathetic) which contains 90% sensory (afferent) and 10% efferent neurones. Information travels from the gut lumen to the brain via mucosal free nerve endings and entero-endocrine cells. These cells, whose microvilli extend into the gut lumen, respond to a range of stimuli including bacteria toxins, pH, osmolality and lipid, as well as direct contact. Stretch of the gut wall may also activate tension receptors in the muscle layers. The gut is additionally innervated from the spinal (sympathetic) nerves. There is a complex interchange of information between the submucosal and myenteric plexus and the brain. The pattern of gastro-

intestinal motility depends upon whether an individual is in a fasted or fed state. The electrical activity recorded from the gut does not always correspond to the pressure activity.

Stomach and small intestine

Fasting

During fasting, three phases of pressure activity can be identified: during phase I there is no activity; irregular activity occurs during phase II; phase III is characterized by strong rhythmic contractions starting in the stomach and spreading distally. Phase III, also called the interdigestive migrating complex or migrating motor complex (MMC), occurs every 90 minutes (range 50–140) and lasts for 5–10 minutes in any one area; it takes about 90 minutes to reach the terminal ileum. Although the MMC shows great regularity in a trained laboratory dog, in man its frequency and form varies both between and within an individual.[44] Some MMCs start in the stomach while the majority commence in the mid-jejunum, many petering out before reaching the terminal ileum. The MMC is strongly propulsive and is thought to be responsible for clearing the last part of a meal from the stomach and small intestine, thus having a 'housekeeper' function.[45] Loss of the MMC is associated with small bowel bacterial overgrowth.[46]

Just before the MMC, there is an increase in the concentration of gastric acid and pepsinogen secreted, followed by an increase in the concentration of secreted pancreatic enzymes and bicarbonate.[47] These secretions may be the reason why, even in the fasting state, there is some output from a high jejunostomy.

Fed

In the fed stomach, a wave of depolarization (gastric slow wave or basic electrical rhythm) is associated with a peristaltic wave that starts in the mid-stomach and spreads to the pylorus every 20 seconds (3/min). Liquid from a mixed liquid and solid meal starts to empty as soon as it reaches the stomach, and 50% of 200 ml orange juice consumed with a pancake has left the stomach at 98 minutes. If the liquid is taken alone, the rate of gastric emptying is much faster. The solid emptying usually occurs in a linear fashion after a variable lag phase (usually 20–30 minutes) during which the meal remains in the fundus undergoing digestion and dilution by gastric secretions. Thus the time taken for 50% of a solid pancake to leave the stomach is 150 minutes.[48]

The frequency of the slow wave, which is now thought to originate in the interstitial cell of Cahal, varies from 12/min in the jejunum to 8/min in the ileum. Small bowel contractions can be segmental or peristaltic (rate 2–25 cm/s), peristalsis predominating in the duodenum while segmenting contractions predominate further distally. Peristalsis can cause very rapid transit if there is no inhibitory feedback from nutrients; thus water can reach the caecum in 15 minutes. Even with nutrients, the first part of a liquid meal can travel very rapidly, reaching the caecum in just 14 minutes for liquid and 24 minutes for solid.[48] This first sample then excites inhibitory feedback responses which slow gastric emptying to allow time for digestion and absorption. After the bulk of a meal has been emptied from the stomach, 'fasting' activity resumes.

Colon

Most of the time there is segmental contracting non-propulsive activity within the colon which allows mixing of the colonic contents and time for absorption. Several times a day, high-pressure propulsive peristaltic waves propel some of the colonic contents to the rectum ('mass movement'). Isotope studies have shown that the first part of a meal remains in the colon for a median of 31 hours (range 24–48). In normal subjects most of a meal will have left the bowel within 3 days of being eaten. Colonic transit is slower in women.[49] On a Western diet, stool weight is about 200 g/d.

Controlling mechanisms

The rate of gastric emptying is normally controlled by both neural and hormonal mechanisms so that chyme is delivered into the intestine at a rate optimal for digestion and absorption. There are at least four gastrointestinal sites which, depending on their luminal contents, may affect gastric emptying: the stomach itself, the proximal small bowel, the distal small bowel, and the colon and rectum. Large volume,[50] high nutrient density (e.g. lipid-based),[51] hyper- or hypo-osmolar solutions[52] or acid[53] meals all slow gastric emptying. A painful stimulus applied outside the gut will also delay gastric emptying,[54] as do various inflammatory cytokines released during infections. The upper small intestine regulates the rate of gastric emptying: studies in dogs have shown that the longer the length of duodenum and jejunum exposed to glucose,[55] acid[56] or lipid (sodium oleate),[57] the greater the delay in gastric emptying. An infusion into the human ileum of lipid,[58–60] protein hydrolysate[61] or carbohydrate[62,63] delays proximal small bowel transit, and lipid[59,64,65] and carbohydrate[66] also delay gastric emptying. The effect of nutrients in the ileum in delaying gastric emptying and small bowel transit is referred to as the 'ileal brake'.

Evidence for two mechanisms, one delaying gastric emptying and the other delaying small bowel transit, comes from experiments which show that intravenous naloxone prevents intralipid infused into the ileum from slowing small bowel transit but does not prevent it from slowing gastric emptying.[67,68]

Events within the colon affect the rate of gastric emptying. Balloon distension in the colon or rectum of animals[69–72] and man[73] causes a rapid inhibition of gastric and intestinal contractions and tone, so delaying gastric emptying and intestinal transit. This is probably the result of a neural mechanism as the effect in animals can be abolished by splanchnic nerve excision.[70,71] However, there is also a hormonal component as balloon inflation of the rectum causes delayed inhibition of motility in denervated jejunal loops.[72] When unabsorbed nutrients reach the colon in patients with jejunum anastomosed to colon, there is rapid slowing of gastric emptying;[48] this is probably caused by raised peptide YY levels[74] and is referred to as the 'colonic brake'.

GASTROINTESTINAL HORMONES

A hormone is a blood-borne chemical messenger that has an identifiable structure, is released in one part of the body and, after passing in the blood stream, has a physiological action in another part, even when all neural connections between the two parts have been severed. It should also be possible to inject the hormone and induce its physiological effects.

The various gastrointestinal hormones are described here in some detail not only because they are important in controlling the activity of the gut but because they are used and may be increasingly used in the future to treat some patients with intestinal failure. Most of the hormones fall into one of two families according to their molecular structure: the gastrin family (gastrin and cholecystokinin) or the secretin family (gastric inhibitory peptide, glucagons, secretin and vasoactive intestinal peptide). The hormones (Table 2.4), which all are produced in response to luminal stimuli, have four main areas of action: (1) to

Table 2.4 – Gastrointestinal hormones (table kindly completed with the help of Mohammed Ghatei, Hammersmith Hospital, London)

Hormone	Amino acids	$t_{1/2}$	Main site	Released by	Main functions
Gastrin	17/34	5/42	Antral G cells	Protein High serum calcium Pepsinogen secretion	Gastric acid secretion
Somatostatin	14/28	3	Antral/pancreatic D cells	Food (especially lipid) or acid in duodenum	Reduces salivary, gastric and pancreatico-biliary secretions Slows gastric emptying Slows small bowel transit Reduces portal blood flow 'Endocrine cyanide'
Cholecystokinin (CCK)	8/33	2/5	Duodenum/jejunum I cells	Lipid and protein	Pancreatic secretion (B) Gallbladder contraction (A) Inhibits gastric emptying Pancreatic growth Satiety and memory
Secretin	27	3	Duodenum/jejunum S cells	Acid Starvation	Pancreatic bicarbonate secretion Pancreatic growth Pepsinogen secretion
Gastric inhibitory peptide (GIP)	42	20	Duodenum/jejunum K cells	Lipid and carbohydrate	Inhibits gastric secretion Inhibits gastric motility 'Incretin'*
Motilin	22	4.5	Duodenum/jejunum M cells	High-fat meal Alkali	Increases gastric and small intestinal motility Causes MMC
Pancreatic polypeptide	36	7	Pancreas	Hypoglycaemia	Gallbladder relaxation Reduces pancreatico-biliary secretions (not HCO_3)
Vasoactive intestinal peptide (VIP)	28	<1	Upper small intestine, colon	Intraduodenal acid	Relaxes smooth muscle Increases blood flow, pancreatic HCO_3 secretion, intestinal secretions Inhibits gastric secretion
Neurotensin	13	1.5	Ileum N cells	Fatty meal in upper gut	Inhibits gastric secretion, pancreatic bicarbonate secretion Relaxes gallbladder Villus/crypt growth Glycogenolysis
Peptide YY (PYY)	36	9	Ileum/colon L cells	Lipid or bile salts in ileum/colon	Slows gastric emptying, small bowel transit 'Ileal and colonic brakes' Reduces gastric secretion, small bowel water/electrolyte absorption
Pancreatic glucagon	29	10	Pancreas A cells	Amino acids in duodenum Hypoglycaemia	Inhibits pancreatic secretion Relaxes smooth muscle Increases blood glucose
Glucagon-like peptide-1 (GLP-1)	31	4.5	Ileum/pancreas	Rapid gastric emptying Lipid and carbohydrate	Inhibits gastric secretion Inhibits gastric emptying 'Incretin'*
Glucagon-like peptide-2 (GLP-2)	33	2.5	Ileum/colon L cells	Nutrients in ileum/colon	Small and large bowel villus/crypt growth Reduces gastric antral motility
Enteroglucagon (glicentin)	69	NK	Ileum/colon L cells	Nutrients	Villus growth Slows gut transit

* An 'incretin' augments the rise in plasma insulin level after an oral glucose load.
NK = not known.

control gastric emptying or secretion (gastrin and somatostatin); (2) to regulate the rate of digestion (cholecystokinin, secretin, gastric inhibitory peptide and motilin); (3) to slow the rate of gastrointestinal transit (GLP-1, neurotensin and peptide YY); or (4) to promote intestinal growth (GLP-2, enteroglucagon and neurotensin). Only five − gastrin, secretin, CCK, GIP and motilin − are true hormones, the others being better regarded as neuromodulators with a principally local or paracrine action. The link with the nervous system is important and many hormones are released after vagal stimulation (e.g. gastrin, somatostatin, pancreatic polypeptide and VIP).

Gastrin

Gastrin exists as two forms produced by the G cells situated in the gastric antrum, duodenum and jejunum. Big gastrin, G34, is found mainly in the duodenum; it has plasma half-life $(t_\frac{1}{2})$ of 42 minutes and is the most abundant form in the circulation in the fasting state. Little gastrin, G17, which is mainly found in the gastric antrum, has a $t_\frac{1}{2}$ of 5 minutes and is a more powerful stimulus in causing gastric acid secretion. Gastrin release is caused by amino acids and peptides in the stomach and by vagal nerve stimulation as occurs with hypoglycaemia or hypercalcaemia. Both forms of gastrin are inactivated in the small bowel and kidney, which may in part explain the hypergastrinaemia seen after an extensive small bowel resection or in patients with renal failure. Gastrin stimulates gastric acid and pepsin secretion in the stomach partly by causing histamine release; it increases antral smooth muscle activity and may have a trophic effect. Excess gastrin gives rise to the Zollinger–Ellison syndrome which is characterized by duodenal and jejunal ulcers[75] and diarrhoea; the diarrhoea is the result of malabsorption caused by the excess gastric acid inhibiting pancreatic enzyme function and micelle formation.

Somatostatin

Somatostatin has been referred to as 'endocrine cyanide' as it reduces the circulating levels of all known gastrointestinal peptide hormones, most anterior pituitary hormones, and many others (e.g. calcitonin and renin). By endocrine, paracrine and neurotransmitter actions, it inhibits most gastrointestinal functions. It reduces gastric, pancreatic and biliary secretions[76] and reduces pentagastrin-stimulated salivary flow.[77] It slows small bowel transit, may delay gastric emptying, reduces gastrointestinal blood flow and reduces the absorption of carbohydrate, lipid and amino acids. Tumours that produce excess somatostatin (somatostatinomas) may give rise to a triad of diabetes, gallstones and malabsorption.[78]

Cholecystokinin

Cholecystokinin (CCK), which was shown to be the same as pancreozymin in 1966, is rapidly metabolized by the liver. It acts as a primary regulator of upper gastrointestinal function as it balances lipid and protein digestion with the rate at which they are delivered to the small intestine. It reduces the amount of chyme reaching the upper small intestine by causing satiety[79–81] and reducing gastric emptying, while at the same time promoting digestion by causing gallbladder contraction and pancreatic secretion.[82] There are two types of CCK receptors: CCK-A in the gallbladder, pancreas and intestine, while CCK-B predominates in the stomach and brain. Only the first eight amino acids are needed for potency at these receptors.

Secretin

Secretin was the first of all hormones to be discovered in 1902 by Baylis and Starling who observed bicarbonate and pancreatic secretions to occur from a denervated pancreas after acid was instilled into the duodenum, and after injections of small bowel extracts.[83] It is released by duodenal and jejunal mucosa in response to acid (pH <4.5),[84] starvation and alcohol. It is metabolized in the vascular system and kidneys.

Gastric inhibitory polypeptide

Gastric inhibitory polypeptide (GIP) was originally thought to be an 'enterogastrone' (a substance from the bowel that inhibits gastric activity) as it is released by fat, especially long-chain fatty acids derived from triglyceride hydrolysis,[85] glucose in the duodenum and to a lesser extent by amino acids. While it inhibits gastric acid secretion (also pepsin and gastrin secretion)[86] and gastric motility, these effects may not be of physiological importance in man.[87] Its main action is probably as an 'incretin' for, if GIP is infused together with glucose, a greater rise in plasma insulin occurs than if glucose alone is infused.[88] It is inactivated and cleared by the kidney.

Pancreatic polypeptide

Pancreatic polypeptide has actions directly opposite to those of CCK. It is released rapidly after a meal but its levels remain raised long after the other hormone levels have returned to normal and its role may be to promote the storage of bile and pancreatic enzymes before the next meal.[89] It is metabolized by the liver and excreted by the kidneys. Fasting levels of pancreatic polypeptide increase with age[90] and this could contribute to the increased incidence of gall-stones with age.

Motilin

Motilin release from the duodenum and proximal jejunum is stimulated by a high-fat meal and suppressed by a carbohydrate or protein meal.[91] Mixed meals thus have little overall effect on circulating motilin levels.[91] In man, unlike dogs, acid in the duodenum (not alkali) causes its release.[92] Motilin may inhibit gastric emptying at a high but physiological plasma level and promote it at a low level.[93] Motilin probably plays only a minor role in the control of normal gastric emptying; for acid infused into the duodenum or fat ingestion both delay gastric empty-ing yet cause motilin release.[91,92] Motilin, however, is the only gastrointestinal hormone that has been shown to increase the rate of gastric emptying.

Motilin may be responsible for inducing the MMC, as there is a cyclical rise in plasma levels before the complex occurs and an infusion of motilin causes them to occur with increased frequency.[94] Motilin analogues such as macrolide antibiotics (e.g. erythro-mycin) cause premature phase III-like intense con-tractions of the gastric antrum and small bowel. These contractions accelerate gastric emptying and may be used to treat gastroparesis; however, the intense cramps from the small bowel contractions and diarrhoea may cause the course of antibiotics to be aborted.

Vasoactive intestinal peptide

Vasoactive intestinal peptide (VIP) acts mainly as a neurotransmitter but has some hormonal actions. It is metabolized locally. It is a powerful smooth muscle relaxant, and thus systemically causes hypotension, flushing and tachycardia. Its main role may be to increase the blood flow to the gut following a meal. At high levels it inhibits gastric acid secretion while stimulating pancreatic bicarbonate and intestinal fluid secretion. Tumours producing VIP (vipomas) were first reported in 1958 and are an extremely rare cause of profuse watery diarrhoea with stool volumes of 2–11 l/24 h associated with hypokalaemia and achlor-hydria.[95] Symptoms may respond to injections of a long-acting synthetic somatostatin analogue, which will inhibit VIP secretion.

Neurotensin

Neurotensin is so named because it caused vaso-dilatation and hypotension in the rat; it also increased vascular permeability.[96] It is rapidly broken down into two fragments, each having a long half-life and being biologically active.[97] Neurotensin is found in N cells which are located mainly in the ileal mucosa; few are found in the jejunum and almost none in the colon.[98] The mechanism of neurotensin release is complex: lipid in any form taken orally or administered into the proximal jejunum causes a high and rapid rise in neurotensin levels, more so than if administered distally into the ileum.[99] It is probable that fat in the upper small intestine primes the ileal N cells by a neural or hormonal mechanism so that they can release neuro-tensin when exposed to this fat.[99] Neurotensin promotes small bowel growth.[100]

Peptide YY

Peptide YY has structural similarities to pancreatic polypeptide. It consists of 36 amino acids with a tyrosine at each end and hence was called peptide YY.[101] It is distributed throughout the small and large intestine from duodenum to rectum (there is none in the stomach) and increases in amount from the ileum to the rectum (concentrations: jejunum 5 pmol/g, terminal ileum 84 pmol/g, ascending colon 82 pmol/g, sigmoid 196 pmol/g and rectum 480 pmol/g[102]). It coexists in the L cells with GLP-2/enteroglucagon[103,104] and has a 70% sequence homology with the neuro-transmitter neuropeptide Y. High levels of peptide YY are observed in situations in which unabsorbed nutrients reach the colon, such as tropical sprue or chronic pancreatitis,[105] dumping syndrome[106] and after an ileal resection which leaves the colon in situ.[74,107] Low levels occur in jejunostomy and ileostomy patients as their colons have been removed.[74,107]

Peptide YY may be the major hormone responsible for the ileal and colonic brakes[60,74,108] which slow gastric emptying and small bowel transit when unabsorbed nutrients reach the ileum or colon. Although peptide YY is stored in the same cells as GLP-2/ enteroglucagon, it is unlikely to exert a major trophic effect on the gastrointestinal tract.[109]

An infusion of peptide YY at a level that reproduces post-prandial concentrations causes a sustained natriuresis, probably by reducing plasma renin and aldosterone.[110] Peptide YY abolished the flushing associated with a vipoma.[111]

Glucagon-like peptides

The existence of a bowel source of a glucagon was first realized in 1961 when the non-specific antisera for glucagon detected immunoreactive material in the gut as well as the pancreas.[112,113] The plasma levels of this 'enteroglucagon' were determined by measuring total glucagon-like immunoreactivity using antisera to the middle and N-terminal portion of the glucagon sequence. Pancreatic glucagon was measured with specific C-terminal directed antisera. The entero-glucagon levels were derived by subtracting the pancreatic glucagon level from the total glucagon-like immunoreactivity;[114] this value is higher than the pancreatic glucagon level.

The structure of human proglucagon (160 amino acids), the common precursor from which all glucagon-like molecules are post-synthetically modified, was determined in 1983.[115] The processing of the molecule is different in the pancreas and intestine. In the pancreas it is cleaved to produce glicentin-related pancreatic polypeptide (GRPP), pancreatic glucagon and a large fragment called the major proglucagon-derived fragment (MPGF). MPGF contains GLP-1 and GLP-2. In the intestine it is cleaved to produce glicentin (69 amino acids) or oxyntomodulin, both of which have glucagon activity and may be 'enteroglucagon', and the glucagon-like peptides (GLP-1 and GLP-2).[116,117]

Pancreatic glucagon. Pancreatic glucagon con-sists of 14 amino acids which are in the same position as in secretin, thus it can inhibit the pancreatic secretory response to secretin. It increases blood glucose by stimulating hepatic glycogenolysis. It is metabolized in the liver. Pancreatic glucagon is used therapeutically to relax the stomach for a barium study, and is used as a positive inotrope to treat β-blocker overdoses. Glucagonomas produce a mixture of products and are characterized by necrolytic migratory erythema, weight loss and diabetes.

Glucagon-like peptide-1 (GLP-1). GLP-1 immunoactivity is co-localized with glucagon in the pancreas and enteroglucagon in the ileum.[117] GLP-1 is secreted at the same time as pancreatic glucagon and enteroglucagon.[118] GLP-1 plasma levels rise most when gastric emptying is fast.[119] GLP-1 levels peaked 15 minutes after a solid meal and 15 minutes before insulin.[119] GLP-1 has been shown to stimulate insulin

release[120,121] and it is a more powerful 'incretin' than GIP.[120]

Glucagon-like peptide-2 (GLP-2). GLP-2 has been synthesized and its receptor characterized.[121] Its structure is highly conserved throughout all mammalian species (only 1 amino acid different in the rat). It is an enterocyte-specific growth hormone that in mice causes small and large bowel villus/crypt growth and increases small and large bowel length and weight. In mice, it also reduces body weight loss and restores mucosal integrity after colitis has been induced with dextran. In pigs, it reduces gastric antral motility.[122]

As GLP-2 stimulates mucosal growth, there is the opportunity to give it therapeutically to patients with a short bowel to promote adaptation, or to adults and children with intestinal damage (e.g. from ischaemia, irradiation, chemotherapy, severe coeliac disease, necrotizing enterocolitis or congenital microvillus atrophy).

Enteroglucagon. Enteroglucagon (glicentin or oxyntomodulin) is found in the L cells with PYY.[103,104] The greatest concentration is found in the ileum and colon (duodenum 15 pmol/g, jejunum 58 pmol/g, ileum 275 pmol/g, colon 179 pmol/g and rectum 96 pmol/g);[114] there is none in the fundus and antrum. High levels occur if there is a loss of small bowel absorptive surface area, such as in patients who have undergone small intestinal resection or jejuno-ileal bypass surgery for obesity.[123]

Much information about its role in man come from the study of a single patient with a tumour that secreted enteroglucagon; it caused villus hypertrophy and increased intestinal transit time.[124,125]

KINETIC ARCHITECTURE OF THE GUT

The proliferative zone is restricted to the basal two-thirds of the crypt in the small bowel and most of the colon, and to the neck region in the stomach (Fig. 2.3). A small number of cells at the base of this proliferative zone give rise to all the other epithelial cells[126] and can be regarded as the 'stem' cells.[127] These stem cells are of great significance as they may be the prime sites for growth control (and the main target for carcinogenesis) since they do not migrate, whereas their daughter cells are transitory and disposable. Stem cells may divide slowly and be extremely radio-

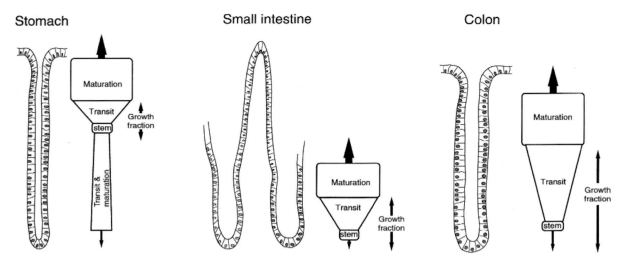

Figure 2.3 – Kinetic architecture of the main regions of the gastrointestinal tract. Kindly provided by RA Goodlad and RJ Playford.

sensitive; they may also be pre-programmed to self-destruct if their DNA template is badly damaged.[128] The daughter cells produced in the stem cell zone migrate up the crypt and undergo three or four 'transit' divisions before they leave the cell division cycle and differentiate to take on their functional role for their last few days before being lost. Cell death can either be a passive process, as in cell necrosis, or it can be the energy-requiring, active, gene-directed, endonuclease-activating process known as apoptosis.[129] Cell loss from the villus tip was once thought to be a passive sloughing of cells, but now is considered an active apoptotic process.

Crypt proliferation

Cell division can be divided into four phases, which make up the cell cycle. Chromosomes can readily be seen separating at mitosis, which is called the M phase. The daughter cells then enter the first portion of interphase, the post-mitotic, pre-synthetic gap called G_1. Cells can either remain in G_1 or go on to the next phase of the cell cycle, the S phase, in which DNA synthesis occurs. There is then a short, second gap phase, known as G_2, in which the cell prepares for mitosis and assembles the spindle proteins. The output of cells from the crypt depends on three main factors: (i) the duration of the cell cycle; (ii) the proportion of the crypt involved in proliferation, known as the growth fraction; and (iii) the size of the crypt. Proliferative activity is not constant: there are marked circadian rhythms in proliferative activity in the gut.

Some of these may be inherent but others appear to be coupled to the food intake pattern several hours previously and may be more pronounced in the colon.[130]

In addition to control of cell production in the crypts, the gut can also increase its cellularity by a process of crypt division or fission, in which a crypt can be seen to develop a septum at its end; the septum then enlarges until two new crypts are created. This process is known as the crypt cycle.[131] Increased crypt fission is seen in the adult after intestinal damage[132] and after intestinal resection.[133]

IMMUNOLOGICAL FUNCTIONS

The huge surface area necessary for absorption renders the gut vulnerable to invasion and necessitates a complex series of defences to exclude pathogens while allowing absorption and oral tolerance of dietary antigens. The importance of this function is underlined by the fact that diarrhoeal diseases in infancy remain the commonest cause of premature death world-wide. Further evidence of the importance of adequate mucosal immunity is seen in AIDS patients who frequently suffer debilitating wasting and diarrhoea from viral, bacterial and protozoal infections. Non-immune defences are also important; these include salivary lysozyme which attacks bacterial cell walls, lactoferrin which chelates iron, thereby preventing the growth of organisms that need it, destruction of ingested organisms by gastric acid and digestive proteases, together with exclusion of pathogens by the mucus barrier and effective clearing of gut contents by propulsive motility patterns. Bile salts and antibacterial peptides known as 'defensins' are also important, as are antibiotics secreted by the normal colonic flora.

Organization of the mucosal immune system

The mucosal immune system is provided by the gut-associated lymphoid tissue (GALT), which contains 10^{10} cells/metre and accounts for 80% of the total body immunocytes. This tissue can be divided into organized and diffuse compartments. The organized GALT comprises isolated lymphoid follicles and Peyer's patches, which are collections of follicles containing precursors of T- and B-cells, commonest in the terminal ileum and proximal colon. These respond to antigenic stimulation, increasing rapidly on exposure to bacteria following birth, peaking in adolescence, and declining gradually thereafter. The diffuse GALT includes immunologically committed T- and B-cells (plasma cells producing predominantly IgA immunoglobulin) found diffusely throughout the lamina propria and acting as the effector limb of the immune response.

Antigen sampling

Ingested bacteria, viruses and other dietary antigens are absorbed by specialized M cells that overlie the aggregates of ileal lymphoid tissue (Peyer's patches). These cells, which account for about 10% of epithelial cells overlying the follicles, are flattened and specially adapted to rapidly pinocytose bacteria and other dietary antigens and pass them to macrophages and lymphoid cells that lie within intraepithelial 'pockets' in the M cell. Some bacteria, such as Shigella, have taken advantage of this process and use the M cell to breach the gut barrier and subsequently spread from enterocyte to enterocyte.[134] Macrophages are the main but not the sole[135] antigen-presenting cells; they take up antigens and, after processing them, present them to T-cells bound to class II major histocompatibility complex (MHC) antigens on the macrophage surface. The T-cells have receptors, structurally similar to immunoglobulins, which recognize specific antigens. They are composed of two subunits, most commonly of α and β type or less commonly of γ and δ type. These bind to the antigen–MHC complex and are thereby activated, a process facilitated by CD8 or CD4

adhesion molecules which bind to a constant region of either the class I or II MHC molecules respectively. Class II MHC molecules are expressed on antigen-presenting cells (mainly macrophages but also some epithelial cells), but class I MHC may be expressed by almost any cell in the body. These bind 'foreign' or 'neo' antigens derived from the cytosol of infected or altered cells such as viral antigens or tumour products. This process of antigen presentation takes place mainly in the dome of the lymphoid follicle, after which antigen-specific T- and B-cell precursors migrate along the lymphatics to the mesenteric lymph nodes where they mature and clonally expand. Further migration via the thoracic duct allows distribution to the entire gut lymphoid tissue. This homing back to the gut depends on the expression of adhesion molecules, such as lymphocyte function antigen (LFA-1) on the lymphocyte and up-regulation of adhesion molecules known as 'addressins' such as VCAM-1 (vascular cell adhesion molecules) and ICAM-1 or 2 (intercellular adhesion molecules), on the endothelial cells in the lymphoid follicle.[136] There B-cells differentiate into plasma cells producing immunoglobulin, mostly IgA, while activated T-cells act as cytotoxic lymphocytes as well as T-helper cells facilitating immune response to further antigenic exposure.

Intraepithelial T-cells are predominantly CD8+ (cytotoxic phenotype) with only 10% being CD4+ (helper T-cells). Their role is unclear but they are markedly raised in coeliac disease, a condition in which the T-cell receptors are predominantly of the $\gamma\delta$ type rather than the more usual $\alpha\beta$ type. The significance of this finding is as yet unclear but it appears to be a marker of disease susceptibility, being found in asymptomatic relatives.[137]

COMPARATIVE ANATOMY

Plant-eating animals digest complex carbohydrate (e.g. cellulose) either in the upper gut or in the caecal/colonic area. Ruminants have an expanded lower end of the oesophagus that forms most of the four-chamber stomach (e.g. sheep and cattle); in plant-eating birds the mid-oesophagus expands to form the crop.[138] Non-ruminants (e.g. horses, rabbits and plant-eating birds) have a long blind-ending caecum. Protozoa, both in the rumen and caecum, assist bacteria in the fermentation of plant material. Animals that digest roots, nuts and wood (e.g. pigs and elephants) have long small and large intestines. Largely carnivorous animals such as dogs and cats have a relatively short small intestine, a very small caecum and a short muscular colon.[139] Man, as an omnivore, is similar to the pig, having a colon intermediate in size between that of herbivores and carnivores.

REFERENCES

1. Williams PL (ed) *Grays Anatomy*. Churchill Livingstone, New York, 1995.

2. Thompson WG, Wrathell E. The relation between ileal resection and vitamin B12 absorption. *Can J Surg* 1977; **20:** 461–464.

3. Meyer JH, Thomson JB, Cole MB. Sieving solid food by the canine stomach and sieving after gastric surgery. *Gastroenterology* 1979; **76:** 804–813.

4. Borgström B, Dahlqvist A, Lundh G, Sjövall J. Studies of intestinal digestion and absorption in the human. *J Clin Invest* 1957; **36:** 1521–1536.

5. Fordtran JS, Locklear TW. Ionic constituents and osmolality of gastric and small intestinal fluids after eating. *Am J Dig Dis* 1966; **11:** 503–521.

6. Carlson AJ. *The control of hunger in health and disease.* University of Chicago Press, Chicago, Illinois, 1916, pp 232–247.

7. McCaughan JM, Sinner BL, Sullivan CJ. The external secretory function of the human pancreas. Physiologic observations. *Arch Intern Med* 1938; **61:** 739–754.

8. Emonts P, Vidon N, Bernier JJ, Rambaud JC. Twenty-four hour intestinal water and electrolyte flow rates in normal man: assessment by the slow marker perfusion technique (author's translation). *Gastroenterol Clin Biol* 1979; **3:** 139–146.

9. Bryant J. Observations upon the growth and length of the human intestine. *Am J Med Sci* 1924; **167:** 499–520.

10. Underhill BML. Intestinal length in man. *Br Med J* 1955; **2:** 1243–1246.

11. Backman L, Hallberg D. Small intestinal length. An intraoperative study in obesity. *Acta Chir Scand* 1974; **140:** 57–63.

12. Slater G, Aufses AH Jr. Small bowel length in Crohn's disease. *Am J Gastroenterol* 1991; **8:** 1037–1040.

13. Hirsch J, Ahrens EH, Blankenhorn DH. Measurement of the human intestinal length in vivo and some causes of variation. *Gastroenterology* 1956; **31:** 274–284.

14. Fannucci A, Cerro P, Fannucci E. Normal small-bowel measurements by enteroclysis. *Scand J Gastroenterol* 1988; **23:** 574–576.

15. Fanucci A, Cerro P, Fraracci L, Ietto F. Small bowel length measured by radiology. *Gastrointest Radiol* 1984; **9:** 349–351.

16. Schalamon J, Schober PH, Gallippi P, Matthyssens L, Hollwarth ME. Congenital short bowel; a case study and review of the literature. *Eur J Pediatr Surg* 1999; **9:** 248–250.

17. Nightingale JMD, Lennard-Jones JE, Walker ER, Farthing MJG. Jejunal efflux in short bowel syndrome. *Lancet* 1990; **336:** 765–768.

18. Fordtran JS, Rector FC Jr., Ewton MF, Soter N, Kinney J. Permeability characteristics of the human small intestine. *J Clin Invest* 1965; **44:** 1935–1944.

19. Davis GR, Santa Aria CA, Morawski SG, Fordtran JS. Permeability characteristics of human jejunum, ileum, proximal colon and distal colon: results of potential difference measurements and unidirectional fluxes. *Gastroenterology* 1982; **83:** 844–850.

20. Fordtran JS, Rector FC Jr., Carter NW. The mechanisms of sodium absorption in the human small intestine. *J Clin Invest* 1968; **47:** 884–900.

21. Spiller RC, Jones BJM, Silk DB. A jejunal water and electrolyte absorption from two proprietary enteral feeds in man: importance of sodium content. *Gut* 1987; **28:** 681–687.

22. Sladen GE, Dawson AM. Inter-relationships between the absorptions of glucose, sodium and water by the normal human jejunum. *Clin Sci* 1969; **36:** 119–132.

23. Rodrigues CA, Lennard-Jones JE, Thompson DG, Farthing MJG. What is the ideal sodium concentration of oral rehydration solutions for short bowel patients? *Clin Sci* 1988; **74(suppl 18):** 69.

24. Levitan R, Goulston K. Water and electrolyte content of human fluid after d-aldosterone administration. *Gastroenterology* 1967; **52:** 510–512.

25. Heinemann T, KullakUblick GA, Pietruck B, Von Bergmann K. Mechanisms of action of plant sterols on inhibition of cholesterol absorption. Comparison of sitosterol and sitostanol. *Eur J Clin Pharmacol* 1991; **40:** S59–S63.

26. Spiller RC. Cholesterol, fibre, and bile acids. *Lancet* 1996; **347:** 415–416.

27. Kayne LH, Lee DBN. Intestinal magnesium absorption. *Miner Electrolyte Metab* 1993; **19:** 210–217.

28. Graham LA, Caesar JJ, Burgen ASV. Gastrointestinal absorption and excretion of magnesium in man. *Metabolism* 1960; **9:** 646–659.

29. Krejs GJ, Nicar MJ, Zerwekh JE, Norman DA, Kane MG, Pak CYC. Effect of 1,25-dihydroxyvitamin D3 on calcium and magnesium absorption in the healthy human jejunum and ileum. *Am J Med* 1983; **75:** 973–976.

30. Lim P, Jacob E. Magnesium status of alcoholic patients. *Metabolism* 1972; **21:** 1045–1051.

31. Shils ME. Experimental human magnesium depletion. I. Clinical observations and blood chemistry alterations. *Am J Clin Nutr* 1964; **15**: 133–143.

32. Horton R, Biglieri EG. Effect of aldosterone on the metabolism of magnesium. *J Clin Endocrinol Metab* 1962; **22**: 1187–1192.

33. Zofkova I, Kancheva RL. The relationship between magnesium and calciotropic hormones. *Magnes Res* 1995; **8**: 77–84.

34. Reinhold JG, Parsa A, Karimian N, Hammick JW, Ismail-Beigi F. Availability of zinc in leavened and unleavened wholemeal wheaten breads as measured by solubility and uptake by rat intestine in vitro. *J Nutr* 1974; **104**: 976–982.

35. Prasad AS, Halsted JA, Nadimi M. Syndrome of iron deficiency anemia, hepatosplenomegaly, hypogonadism, dwarfism and geophagia. *Am J Med* 1961; **31**: 532–546.

36. Nakamura T, Higashi A, Takano S, Akagi M, Matsuda I. Zinc clearance correlates with clinical severity of Crohn's disease. A kinetic study. *Dig Dis Sci* 1988; **33**: 1520–1524.

37. Phillips SF, Quigley EMM, Kumar D, Kamath PS. Motility of the ileocolonic junction. *Gut* 1988; **29**: 390–406.

38. Fich A, Steadman CJ, Phillips SF, Camilleri M, Brown ML, Haddad AC, Thomforde GM. Ileocolonic transit does not change after right hemicolectomy. *Gastroenterology* 1992; **103**: 794–799.

39. Bentley DW, Nichols RL, Condon RE, Gorbach SL. The microflora of the human ileum and intraabdominal colon: Results of direct needle aspiration at surgery and evaluation of the technique. *J Lab Clin Med* 1972; **79**: 421–429.

40. Hammer J, Camilleri M, Phillips SF, Aggarwal A, Haddad AM. Does the ileocolonic junction differentiate between solids and liquids? *Gut* 1993; **34**: 222–226.

41. Debongnie JC, Phillips SF. Capacity of the colon to absorb fluid. *Gastroenterology* 1978; **74**: 698–703.

42. Randall HT. Enteral nutrition: Tube feeding in acute and chronic illness. *J Parenter Enteral Nutr* 1984; **8**: 113–136.

43. Fawcett SL, Cousins RJ. Magnesium poisoning following enema of epsom salt solution. *JAMA* 1943; **123**: 1028–1029.

44. Kellow JE, Borody TJ, Phillips SF, Tucker RL, Haddad AM. Human interdigestive motility: Variations in patterns from esophagus to colon. *Gastroenterology* 1986; **91**: 386–395.

45. Itoh Z, Aizawa I, Sekiguchi T. The interdigestive migrating complex and its significance in man. *Clin Gastroenterol* 1982; **11**: 497–521.

46. Soudah HC, Hasler WL, Owyang C. Effect of octreotide on intestinal motility and bacterial overgrowth in scleroderma. *N Engl J Med* 1991; **325**: 1461–1467.

47. Vantrappen GR, Peeters TL, Janssens J. The secretory component of the interdigestive migrating motor complexes in man. *Scand J Gastroenterol* 1979; **14**: 663–667.

48. Nightingale JMD, Kamm MA, van der Sijp JRM *et al.* Disturbed gastric emptying in the short bowel syndrome. Evidence for a 'colonic brake'. *Gut* 1993; **34**: 1171–1176.

49. Kamm MA. The small intestine and colon: scintigraphic quantitation of motility in health and disease. *Eur J Nucl Med* 1992; **19**: 902–912.

50. Hunt JN, MacDonald I. The influence of volume on gastric emptying. *J Physiol* 1954; **126**: 459–474.

51. Hunt JN, Stubbs DF. The volume and energy content of meals as determinants of gastric emptying. *J Physiol* 1975; **245**: 209–225.

52. Hunt JN. Some properties of an alimentary osmoreceptor mechanism. *J Physiol* 1956; **132**: 267–288.

53. Hunt JN, Pathak JD. The osmotic effects of some simple molecules and ions on gastric emptying. *J Physiol* 1960; **154**: 254–269.

54. Thompson DG, Richelson E, Malagelada J-R. Perturbation of upper gastrointestinal function by cold stress. *Gut* 1983; **24**: 277–283.

55. Lin HC, Doty JE, Reedy TJ, Meyer JH. Inhibition of gastric emptying by glucose depends on length of intestine exposed to nutrient. *Am J Physiol* 1989; **256(Gastrointest Liver Physiol 19)**: G404–G411.

56. Lin HC, Doty JE, Reedy TJ, Meyer JH. Inhibition of gastric emptying by acids depends on pH, titratable acidity, and length of intestine exposed to acid. *Am J Physiol* 1990; **259(Gastrointest Liver Physiol 22)**: G1025–G1030.

57. Lin HC, Doty JE, Reedy TJ, Meyer JH. Inhibition of gastric emptying by sodium oleate depends on length of intestine exposed to nutrient. *Am J Physiol* 1990; **259(Gastrointest Liver Physiol 22)**: G1031–G1036.

58. Spiller RC, Trotman IF, Higgins BE *et al.* The ileal brake – inhibition of jejunal motility after ileal fat perfusion in man. *Gut* 1984; **25**: 365–374.

59. Holgate AM, Read NW. Effect of ileal infusion of intralipid on gastrointestinal transit, ileal flow rate, and carbohydrate absorption in humans after ingestion of a liquid meal. *Gastroenterology* 1985; **88**: 1005–1011.

60. Spiller RC, Trotman IF, Adrian TE, Bloom SR, Misiewicz JJ, Silk DBA. Further characterisation of the 'ileal brake' reflex in man – effect of ileal infusion of partial digests of fat, protein, and starch on jejunal motility and release of neurotensin, enteroglucagon, and peptide YY. *Gut* 1988; **29**: 1042–1051.

61. Read NW, McFarlane A, Kinsman RI et al. Effect of infusion of nutrient solutions into the ileum on gastro-intestinal transit and plasma levels of neurotensin and enteroglucagon. *Gastroenterology* 1984; **86**: 274–280.

62. Spiller RC, Trotman IF, Silk DBA, Lee YC, Ghatei MA, Bloom SR, Misiewicz JJ. Control of jejunal motility by ileal contents and hormones in man. *Gastroenterology* 1983; **84**: 1319.

63. Jain NK, Boivin M, Zinsmeister AR, Brown ML, Malagelada J-R, DiMagno EP. Effect of ileal perfusion of carbohydrates and amylase inhibitor on gastro-intestinal hormones and emptying. *Gastroenterology* 1989; **96**: 377–387.

64. Fone DR, Horowitz M, Read NW, Dent J, Maddox A. The effect of terminal ileal triglyceride infusion on gastroduodenal motility and the intragastric distri-bution of a solid meal. *Gastroenterology* 1990; **98**: 568–575.

65. Welch I McL, Cunningham KM, Read NW. Regulation of gastric emptying by ileal nutrients in humans. *Gastroenterology* 1988; **94**: 401–404.

66. Layer P, Zinsmeister AR, DiMagno EP. Effects of decreasing intraluminal amylase activity on starch digestion and postprandial gastrointestinal function in humans. *Gastroenterology* 1986; **91**: 41–48.

67. Read NW, Welch I McL. Naloxone prevents the effect of ileal lipid on small bowel transit but not on gastric emptying. *Gut* 1984; **25**: A1326.

68. Kinsman RI, Read NW. Effect of naloxone on feed-back regulation of small bowel transit by fat. *Gastroenterology* 1984; **87**: 335–337.

69. Pearcy JF, Van Liere EJ. Studies on the visceral nervous system. *Am J Physiol* 1926; **78**: 64–73.

70. Youmans WB, Meek WJ. Reflex and humeral inhibition in unanaesthetised dogs during rectal stimulation. *Am J Physiol* 1937; **120**: 750–757.

71. Morin G, Vial J. Champ de l'inhibition reflexe provoque de par la distension de l'intestin. *C R Soc Biol* 1934; **113**: 1540–1541.

72. Lalich J, Meek WJ, Herrin RC. Reflex pathways concerned in inhibition of hunger contractions by intestinal distension. *Am J Physiol* 1936; **115**: 410–414.

73. Youle MS, Read NW. Effect of painless rectal distention on gastrointestinal transit of solid meal. *Dig Dis Sci* 1984; **29**: 902–906.

74. Nightingale JMD, Kamm MA, van der Sijp JRM, Walker ER, Ghatei MA, Bloom SR, Lennard-Jones JE. Gastrointestinal hormones in the short bowel syndrome. PYY may be the 'colonic brake' to gastric emptying. *Gut* 1996; **39**: 267–272.

75. Zollinger RM, Ellison EH. Primary peptic ulcerations of the jejunum associated with islet cell tumours of the pancreas. *Ann Surg* 1955; **142**: 709–728.

76. Reichlin S. Somatostatin. *N Engl J Med* 1983; **309**: 1495–1501, 1556–1563.

77. Loguercio C, de Sio I, Romano M, del Vecchio Blanco C, Coltorti M. Effect of somatostatin on salivary secretion in man. *Digestion* 1987; **36**: 91–95.

78. Ganda OP, Weir GC, Soelderner JS et al. Somatostatinoma – a somatostatin containing tumour of the endocrine pancreas. *N Engl J Med* 1977; **297**: 1352–1357.

79. Sturdevant RAL, Goetz H. Cholecystokinin both stimulates and inhibits human food intake. *Nature* 1976; **261**: 713–715.

80. Muurahainen N, Kissileff HR, Derogatis AJ, Pi-Sunyer FX. Effects of cholecystokinin-octapeptide (CCK-8) on food intake and gastric emptying in man. *Physiol Behav* 1988; **44**: 645–649.

81. Lieverse RJ, Jansen JBMJ, Masclee AAM, Lamers CBHW. Satiety effects of cholecystokinin in humans. *Gastroenterology* 1994; **106**: 1451–1454.

82. Schmidt WE, Creutzfeldt W, Schleser A et al. Role of CCK in regulation of pancreaticobiliary functions and GI motility in humans: effects of loxiglumide. *Am J Physiol* 1991; **23**: G197–G206.

83. Baylis WM, Starling EH. The mechanism of pancreatic secretion. *J Physiol* 1902; **28**: 325–335.

84. Meyer JH, Grossman MI. Pancreatic bicarbonate response to various acids in the duodenum of dogs. *Am J Physiol* 1970; **219**: 964–970.

85. Ross SA, Shaffer EA. The importance of triglyceride hydrolysis for the release of gastric inhibitory poly-peptide. *Gastroenterology* 1981; **80**: 108–111.

86. Pederson RA, Brown JC. Inhibition of histamine, pentagastrin and insulin-stimulated canine gastrin secretion by pure 'gastric inhibitory polypeptide'. *Gastroenterology* 1972; **62**: 393–399.

87. Maxwell V, Shulkes A, Brown JC, Solomon TE, Walsh JH, Grossman MI. The effect of gastric inhibitory polypeptide on pentagastrin-stimulated acid secretion in man. *Dig Dis Sci* 1980; **25**: 113–116.

88. Dupre J, Ross SA, Watson D, Brown JC. Stimulation of insulin secretion by gastric inhibitory polypeptide in man. *J Clin Endocrinol Metab* 1973; **37**: 826–828.

89. Adrian TE, Greenberg GR, Bloom SR. Actions of pancreatic polypeptide in man. In: Bloom SR, Polak JM (eds) *Gut hormones*, 2nd edn. Churchill Livingstone, Edinburgh, 1981, pp 206–212.

90. Adrian TE, Bloom SR, Bryant MG, Polak JM, Heitz PH, Barnes AJ. Distribution and release of human pancreatic polypeptide. *Gut* 1976; **17:** 940–944.

91. Christofides ND, Bloom SR, Besterman HS, Adrian TE, Ghatei MA. Release of motilin by oral and intravenous nutrients in man. *Gut* 1978; **20:** 102–106.

92. Mitznegg P, Bloom SR, Domschke W, Domschke S, Wunsch E, Demling L. Release of motilin after duodenal acidification. *Lancet* 1976; **i:** 888–889.

93. Christofides ND, Long RG, Fitzpatrick ML, McGregor GP, Bloom SR. Effect of motilin on gastric emptying of glucose and fat in humans. *Gastroenterology* 1981; **80:** 456–460.

94. Vantrappen G, Janssens J, Peeters TL, Bloom SR, Christofides ND, Hellemans J. Motilin and the interdigestive migrating motor complex in man. *Dig Dis Sci* 1979; **24:** 497–500.

95. Verner JV, Morrison AB. Endocrine pancreatic islet disease with diarrhoea: report of a case due to diffuse hyperplasia of non-beta islet tissue with a review of 54 additional cases. *Arch Intern Med* 1974; **133:** 492–500.

96. Carraway R, Leeman SE. The isolation of a new hypotensive peptide, neurotensin, from bovine hypothalami. *J Biol Chem* 1973; **248:** 6854–6861.

97. Hammer RA, Carraway RE, Leeman SE. Elevation of plasma neurotensin immunoreactivity after a meal. Characterization of the elevated components. *J Clin Invest* 1982; **70:** 74–81.

98. Polak JM, Sullivan SN, Bloom SR, Buchan AMJ, Facer P, Brown MR, Pearse AGE. Neurotensin in human intestine: Radioimmunoassay and specific localisation in the N cell. *Nature* 1977; **270:** 183–185.

99. Wiklund B, Liljeqvist L, Rokaeus A. Studies in man on the mechanism by which fat increases the plasma concentration of neurotensin-like immunoreactivity. *Acta Chir Scand* 1986; **152(suppl 530):** 9–14.

100. Wood JG, Hoang HD, Bussjaeger LJ, Solomon TE. Neurotensin stimulates growth of small intestine in rats. *Am J Physiol* 1988; **255:** G813–G817.

101. Tatemoto K. Isolation and characterization of peptide YY (PYY), a candidate gut hormone that inhibits pancreatic exocrine secretion. *Proc Natl Acad Sci USA* 1982; **79:** 2514–2518.

102. Adrian TE, Ferri G-L, Bacarese-Hamilton, Fuessl HS, Polak JM, Bloom SR. Human distribution and release of a putative new gut hormone, Peptide YY. *Gastroenterology* 1985; **89:** 1070–1077.

103. Ali-Rachedi A, Varndell IM, Adrian TE, Gapp DA, Van Noorden S, Bloom SR, Polak JM. Peptide YY (PYY) immunoreactivity is co-stored with glucagon-related immunoreactants in endocrine cells of the gut and pancreas. *Histochemistry* 1984; **80:** 487–491.

104. Bottcher G, Sjolund K, Ekblad E, Hakanson R, Schwartz TW, Sundler F. Co-existence of peptide YY and glicentin immunoreactivity in endocrine cells of the gut. *Regul Pept* 1984; **8:** 261–266.

105. Adrian TE, Savage AP, Bacarese-Hamilton AJ, Wolfe K, Besterman HS, Bloom SR. Peptide YY abnormalities in gastrointestinal diseases. *Gastroenterology* 1986; **90:** 379–384.

106. Adrian TE, Long RG, Fuessl HS, Bloom SR. Plasma peptide YY (PYY) in dumping syndrome. *Dig Dis Sci* 1985; **30:** 1145–1148.

107. Adrian TE, Savage AP, Fuessl HS, Wolfe K, Besterman HS, Bloom SR. Release of peptide YY (PYY) after resection of small bowel, colon or pancreas in man. *Surgery* 1987; **101:** 715–719.

108. Pironi L, Stanghellini V, Miglioli M *et al.* Fat-induced ileal brake in humans: a dose-dependent phenomenon correlated to plasma levels of peptide YY. *Gastroenterology* 1993; **105:** 733–739.

109. Savage AP, Gornacz GE, Adrian TE, Ghatei MA, Goodlad RA, Wright NA, Bloom SR. Is raised plasma peptide YY after intestinal resection in the rat responsible for the trophic response? *Gut* 1985; **26:** 1353–1358.

110. Playford RJ, Mehta S, Upton P *et al.* Effect of peptide YY on human renal function. *Am J Physiol* 1995; **268:** F754–F759.

111. Mehta S, Upton P, Rentch R *et al.* Preliminary report: role of peptide YY in defence against diarrhoea. *Lancet* 1990; **335:** 1555–1557.

112. Unger RH, Eisentraut AM, Sims K, McCall MS, Madison LL. Sites of origin of glucagon in dogs and humans (abstract). *Clin Res* 1961; **9:** 53.

113. Ungar RH, Ketterer H, Eisentraut AM. Distribution of immunoassayable glucagon in gastrointestinal tissues. *Metabolism* 1966; **15:** 865–867.

114. Ghatei MA, Bloom SR. Enteroglucagon in man. In: Bloom SR, Polak JM (eds) *Gut hormones*, 2nd edn. Churchill Livingstone, Edinburgh, 1981, pp 332–338.

115. Bell GI, Sanchez-Pescador R, Laybourn PJ, Najarian RC. Exon duplication and divergence in the human preproglucagon gene. *Nature* 1983; **304:** 368–371.

116. Orscov C, Holst JJ, Poulsen SS, Kirkegaard P. Pancreatic and intestinal processing of proglucagon in man. *Diabetologia* 1987; **30:** 874–881.

117. Dunphy JL, Fuller PJ. Enteroglucagon, bowel growth and GLP-2. *Mol Cell Endocrinol* 1997; **132:** 7–11.

118. Orskov C, Holst JJ, Knuhtsen S, Baldissera FGA, Poulsen SS, Nielsen OV. Glucagon-like peptides GLP-1 and GLP-2, predicted products of the glucagon gene, are secreted separately from pig small intestine but not pancreas. *Endocrinology* 1986; **119:** 1467–1475.

119. Miholic J, Orskov C, Holst JJ, Kotzerke J, Meyer HJ. Emptying of the gastric substitute, glucagon-like peptide-1 (GLP-1), and reactive hypoglycaemia after total gastrectomy. *Dig Dis Sci* 1991; **36:** 1361–1370.

120. Kreymann B, Ghatei MA, Williams G, Bloom SR. Glucagon-like peptide-17-36: A physiological incretin in man. *Lancet* 1987; **2:** 1300–1304.

121. Druker DJ. Glucagon-like peptide 2. *Trends Endocrinol Metab* 1999; **10:** 153–156.

122. Wojdemann M, Wettergren A, Hartmann B, Holst JJ. Glucagon-like peptide-2 inhibits centrally induced antral motility in pigs. *Scand J Gastroenterol* 1998; **33:** 828–832.

123. Bloom SR, Polak JM. Plasma hormone concentrations in gastrointestinal disease. *Clin Gastroenterol* 1980; **93:** 785–798.

124. Gleeson MH, Bloom SR, Polak JM, Henry K, Dowling RH. Endocrine tumour in kidney affecting small bowel structure, motility, and absorptive function. *Gut* 1971; **12:** 773–782.

125. Bloom SR. An enteroglucagon tumour. *Gut* 1972; **13:** 520–523.

126. Cheng H, Leblond CP. Origin, differentiation and renewal of the four main epithelial cell types of the mouse small intestine. V. Unitarian theory of the origin of the four epithelial cell types. *Am J Anat* 1974; **144:** 537–562.

127. Potten CS, Loeffler M. A comprehensive model of the crypts of the small intestine of the mouse provides insight into the mechanisms of cell migration and the proliferative hierarchy. *J Theor Biol* 1987; **127:** 381–391.

128. Hall PA, Watt FM. Stem cells: the generation and maintenance of cellular diversity. *Development* 1989; **106:** 619–633.

129. Alison MR, Sarraf CE. Apoptosis: a gene-directed programme of cell death. *J R Coll Physicians Lond* 1992; **26:** 25–35.

130. Goodlad RA, Wright NA. The effects of starvation and refeeding on intestinal cell proliferation in the mouse. *Virch Arch Cell Pathol* 1984; **45:** 63–73.

131. Totafumo J, Bjerknes M, Cheng H. The crypt cycle: Crypt and villus production in adult intestinal epithelium. *Biophys J* 1987; **52:** 279–294.

132. Cairnie AB, Millen BH. Fission of crypts in the small intestine of the irradiated mouse. *Cell Tissue Kinet* 1975; **8:** 189–196.

133. Cheng H, McCulloch C, Bjerknes M. Effects of 30% intestinal resection on whole population cell kinetics of mouse intestinal epithelium. *Anat Record* 1986; **215:** 35–41.

134. Wassef JS, Keren DF, Mailloux JL. Role of M cells in initial antigen uptake and in ulcer formation in the rabbit intestinal loop model of shigellosis. *Infect Immun* 1989; **57:** 858–863.

135. Geppert TD, Lipsky PE. Antigen presentation by cells that are not of bone marrow origin. *Reg Immunol* 1989; **2:** 60–71.

136. Salmi M, Jalkanen S. Regulation of lymphocyte traffic to mucosa-associated lymphatic tissues. *Gastroenterol Clin North Am* 1991; **20:** 495–510.

137. Holm K, Maki M, Savilahti E, Lipsanen V, Laippala P, Koskimies S. Intraepithelial gamma delta T-cell-receptor lymphocytes and genetic susceptibility to coeliac disease. *Lancet* 1992; **339:** 1500–1503.

138. Duke GE. Gastrointestinal physiology and nutrition in wild birds. *Proc Nutr Soc* 1997; **56:** 1049–1056.

139. Wrong OM, Edmonds CJ, Chadwick VS. The large intestine: Its role in mammalian nutrition and homeostasis. MTP Press, 1981.

Section 2

Acute intestinal failure

3

Surgical causes and management

Gordon Carlson

*A*cute intestinal failure has been recognized as a specific clinical entity for many years[1], and occurs when there is a potentially reversible cause (see Preface). In surgical patients acute intestinal failure is usually associated with enterocutaneous fistulas, intestinal obstruction and ileus. In these circumstances, fluid and electrolyte absorption, as opposed to nutrient absorption, may be the principal clinical problem.

Most cases of acute intestinal failure are short lived, require artificial nutritional support for fewer than 14 days and are managed in non-specialized units. Although the incidence of acute intestinal failure in these circumstances is unknown, it is extremely common and, of course, the vast majority of such cases present to and are managed in non-specialized units. When one restricts an epidemiological assessment to those cases in which referral to a specialist intestinal failure unit is made, the annual incidence of intestinal failure requiring specialist treatment is slightly in excess of 5.5 new patients per million population.[2] This figure may be an underestimate of the true incidence of acute intestinal failure associated with intestinal fistula, complex metabolic derangement or postoperative abdominal sepsis, as many of these cases are managed with difficulty in non-specialist centres.

In the UK, future estimates of the incidence of acute intestinal failure are likely to be more accurate since the introduction of the centrally funded National Specialist Commissioning Advisory Group

Table 3.1 – Causes of acute intestinal failure. Adapted from Pettigrew and Hill 1984[16]

When the gastrointestinal tract is 'blocked'
   Mechanical obstruction
   Paralytic ileus
   Intestinal pseudo-obstruction

When the intestinal tract is too short
   Massive resection
   Internal or external fistulas

When the intestinal tract is inflamed
   Inflammatory bowel disease
   Severe infective enteritis
   Radiotherapy
   Chemotherapy

When the gastrointestinal tract fails to function adequately for other reasons
   Intra-abdominal sepsis
   Multiple organ failure
   Acute pancreatitis

(NSCAG). It funds those cases of acute intestinal failure requiring management by a limited number of specialized intestinal failure units (Table 3.2).

Table 3.2 – Criteria for referring patients with acute intestinal failure to a specialist unit

Persistent intestinal failure beyond 6 weeks complicated by venous access problems
Multiple fistulas within a totally dehisced abdominal wound
Total or near total (< 30 cm remaining) enterectomy
Recurrent venous access problems due to sepsis or thrombosis
Persistent severe abdominal sepsis
Persistent nutritional or metabolic problems associated with a high output stoma or fistula
Any patient with an intestinal fistula beyond the expertise of the referring hospital

AETIOLOGY AND PATHOGENESIS

Acute intestinal failure occurs as a consequence of conditions which primarily or secondarily affect the gastrointestinal tract (Table 3.1). Within a specialized intestinal failure unit, the most common underlying condition responsible for intestinal failure is Crohn's disease (Fig. 3.1), and the principal reason for acute intestinal failure is intestinal fistula(s) (Fig. 3.2). This population of patients is very different to that seen in

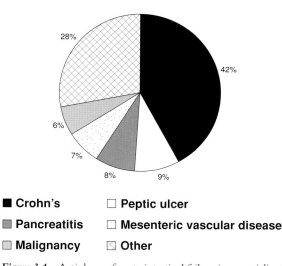

- ■ Crohn's
- □ Peptic ulcer
- ▨ Pancreatitis
- □ Mesenteric vascular disease
- ▨ Malignancy
- ⊠ Other

Figure 3.1 – Aetiology of acute intestinal failure in a specialized unit. Adapted from Scott *et al.*[2]

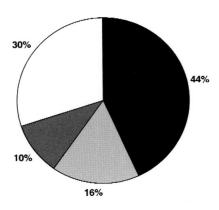

■ Fistula □ Short Bowel ■ Sepsis □ Other

Figure 3.2 – Clinical problems leading to acute intestinal failure. Adapted from Scott *et al.*[2]

Table 3.3 – Factors indicating an enterocutaneous fistula is unlikely to close spontaneously

- Distal bowel obstruction
- Diseased bowel at the fistula site (e.g. Crohn's, irradiation or malignancy)
- Discontinuity of the bowel ends
- Abscess at the site of the fistula or continuing sepsis
- Mucocutaneous continuity (i.e. bowel mucosa is visible on the surface of the abdomen
- Multiple (complicated) fistulas

most hospitals, because most of the cases (62%) referred to specialized units will need surgical treatment.[2]

Intestinal fistulas

A fistula is defined as an abnormal communication between two epithelialized surfaces. A fistula communicating with a hollow viscus is called an internal fistula and one communicating with the skin an external fistula. A fistula can be single or complicated. An intestinal fistula is said to have a high output if more than 500 ml is produced in 24 h.

Enterocutaneous fistulas most commonly result as a postoperative complication from either partial breakdown of an intestinal anastomosis or injury to the gut during abdominal closure (82%). Death from enterocutaneous fistulas is most commonly due to sepsis, though some are due to electrolyte imbalance, undernutrition, massive bleeding or the underlying disease. Spontaneous closure of a fistula may occur within 6 weeks of its first appearance in up to 60% of patients. Table 3.3 lists some of the factors that make spontaneous closure unlikely. Although there is little published evidence, the chance of spontaneous closure of a fistula may be reduced if a patient is undernourished, septic (as indicated by a low serum albumin or transferrin) or has another systemic problem (e.g. cardiac, respiratory, renal or hepatic failure).

In many cases the pathogenesis of acute intestinal failure is multifactorial and complex. For example, many patients with an intestinal fistula also have an intra-abdominal abscess. In some cases, an intestinal fistula may have developed as a consequence of impaired anastomotic healing because the anastomosis was constructed within a pre-existing abscess cavity (typically in Crohn's disease) or in a patient with established sepsis.[3]

There is evidence that intestinal function is impaired in sepsis, as a consequence of mucosal oedema,[4] defective enterocyte maturation[5] and down-regulation of nutrient transporters.[6] When combined with the increased metabolic demand and impaired fuel utilization associated with sepsis[7] the presence of impaired intestinal function may lead rapidly to a state of cachexia not unlike that observed in advanced malignant disease.[8] In addition nutritional support, however aggressive, is unlikely to be successful in the restoration of lean body mass in the presence of sepsis.[9] A major priority in managing the patient with acute intestinal failure is therefore to detect and eradicate sepsis. Other factors may also be of importance in the development or maintenance of acute intestinal failure, particularly in the setting of critical illness: Changes in intestinal motility undoubtedly occur and although their aetiology is unclear, may cause difficulty with enteral feeding. In general, reduced intestinal motility is observed,[10] possibly as a consequence of impaired absorption of fluid, altered nervous and regulatory peptide control of motility patterns,[11] decreased intestinal blood flow[12] and bacterial colonization of the small intestine (which may itself develop as a consequence of impaired motility[13]). In addition, handling of the gut at surgical operation may result in ileus because of the development of an inflammatory response within the intestinal muscle.[14] Finally, other factors that may contribute to impaired motility are pulmonary and liver disease and centrally acting sedative and narcotic drugs.[15] The net effect of these changes, which may disturb gastric and colonic motility to a greater extent than small intestinal motility is to cause abdominal distension, nausea and vomiting.

MANAGEMENT

The initial priorities in the management of the patient with acute intestinal failure are the detection and management of sepsis and the institution of nutrition and metabolic support (Table 3.4). It is important to note that the management of sepsis is of overwhelming importance because inadequately treated sepsis is the most common cause of death in patients with complicated acute intestinal failure. In the management of intestinal fistulas, control of sepsis has been shown to be the major determinant of successful outcome.[17]

Table 3.4 – Principles of managing a high output enterocutaneous fistula

- Treat sepsis
- Reduce fistula output (similar treatment to high output jejunostomy)
- Care of fistula site
- Nutritional support
- Psychological support
- Define anatomy
- Elective surgery

Diagnosis and management of abdominal sepsis

The diagnosis of sepsis should be entertained in any patient with a history of gastrointestinal surgery who is failing to make satisfactory progress. Renewed consideration should be given to the presence of sepsis in any patient who requires postoperative artificial nutritional support, unless this has been commenced as part of planned postoperative care. Although swinging pyrexia, leucocytosis and abdominal signs are classical features of sepsis, they are not invariably present. Hypoalbuminaemia, hyponatraemia or unexplained jaundice may be more subtle signs of abdominal sepsis and should lead to a careful search for a septic focus. In some cases this may prove to be within the chest or urinary tract or may relate to central venous lines but the abdomen should be suspected whenever abdominal surgery has been performed.

Initial imaging with ultrasound scan may be of value in the detection of subphrenic or pelvic collections and plain chest radiography may show elevation of the diaphragm and basal collapse with a 'sympathetic' pleural effusion indicative of a subphrenic abscess. Ultrasound may be difficult to perform and interpret, however, in the postoperative patient where the presence of drains or stomas make scanning technically difficult and gaseous distension of the abdomen creates an image of poor quality.[18] Computed tomography (CT) is, in general, the most effective imaging modality (Fig. 3.3) and, if combined with oral contrast, will distinguish intra-abdominal or pelvic abscesses from immotile, fluid-filled loops of bowel.[19,20] The diagnostic accuracy of CT scanning in abdominal sepsis is of the order of 97%. Radiolabelled leucocyte scanning usually takes too long to organize and perform to be entirely satisfactory and also has a lower specificity than CT. It may, however, be of particular value in cases where an abnormality is suspected and may allow more detailed, focused imaging with CT or magnetic resonance imaging at the site of a suspected 'hot spot'. Finally, it is important to emphasize that it may be necessary to undertake diagnostic laparotomy if the clinical features of sepsis are convincing despite negative imaging.

Once a focus of abdominal or pelvic sepsis has been diagnosed, prompt drainage is mandatory. Antibiotic therapy may be of value in the management of patients with sepsis but it will not lead to the resolution of sepsis unless combined with treatment of the abscess cavity itself. Fortunately, in many cases percutaneous drainage of abscesses is possible under radiological guidance because as abscess cavities enlarge they tend to assume a globular shape and push neighbouring structures aside.[20] Large drains (8–10 F) can be inserted into abscess cavities under local anaesthetic (Fig. 3.4). If several drains are inserted simultaneously, the cavity can be irrigated regularly with saline to ensure adequate and prolonged drainage. In general, the drains are kept in place and a contrast study performed through one of them to ensure that the abscess cavity has collapsed prior to drain removal.

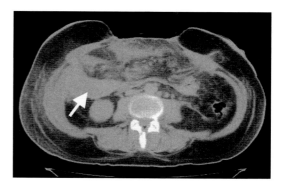

Figure 3.3 – CT scan showing intra-abdominal abscess (arrowed).

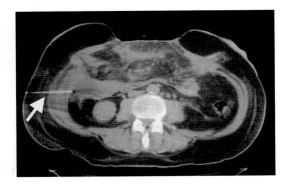

Figure 3.4 – CT scan showing percutaneous drainage (arrowed) of intra-abdominal abscess shown in Fig. 3.3.

In some cases, percutaneous drainage of abscesses is likely to be ineffective. This is particularly likely where a CT scan has shown multiple interloop abscesses, or where the pus is of particularly thick consistency (for example in infected pancreatic necrosis). In such cases and in sepsis associated with anastomotic dehiscence surgical exploration will be required. In the latter case, adequate control of sepsis is unlikely to be achieved simply by drainage without either exteriorizing the bowel ends or at the very least producing a defunctioning proximal stoma.

Where intra-abdominal contamination is severe and sepsis continues, with further collections of infected fluid, or where the underlying focus of sepsis cannot be removed (for example in necrotizing pancreatitis), further attempts to deal with sepsis are necessary. A variety of approaches have been advocated, including radical peritoneal debridement[21] and continuous post-operative peritoneal lavage,[22] neither of which has been shown to be effective. Other options include repeated laparotomies, either on demand or as planned procedures. Controlled trials of repeated planned laparotomy for severe abdominal sepsis have not shown that it improves survival[23] and the therapeutic value of each successive operation diminishes[24] with an associated risk of intestinal injury, leading to secondary intestinal fistula formation. An alternative approach in such cases is to leave the abdomen open (lapar-ostomy)[25] and simply pack the abdominal cavity with saline-soaked sterile gauze rolls (Fig. 3.5), changing the packs on a daily basis. Alternatively, the abdomen can be closed temporarily using a prosthetic mesh with a nylon zip allowing easy re-inspection of the abdominal cavity while minimizing the risk of secondary damage to the viscera associated with

packing.[26] Either technique allows regular inspection of the abdominal contents and prompt drainage of further septic foci. Leakage from open loops of bowel within the laparostomy can be controlled with the use of suction catheters placed within the wound. The abdomen is allowed to heal by secondary intention and, initially, fistulating loops of bowel become fixed within a dense mass of granulation tissue (Fig. 3.6). Intestinal continuity can generally be safely established by a further laparotomy undertaken 6 months later when the peritoneal cavity has become re-established[27] and the best indication of this is prolapse of the fistulating bowel segments (Fig. 3.7).

In the presence of an intestinal fistula, maintenance of skin integrity is of major importance and should be considered at an early stage. The output of intestinal fistulas, particularly from the proximal gastrointestinal tract may be massive and if inadequately controlled, may cause widespread skin destruction. It is important

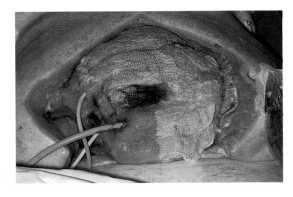

Figure 3.5 – Newly-created laparostomy wound.

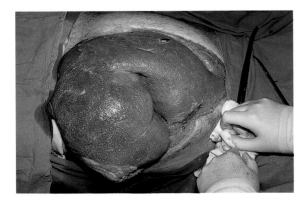

Figure 3.6 – Laparostomy wound after 6 weeks, showing viscera covered with dense granulation tissue.

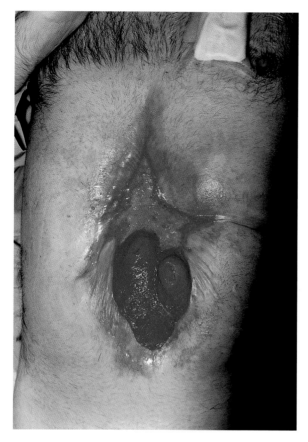

Figure 3.7 – Prolapse of a fistula within a completely healed laparostomy wound.

therefore to involve a stoma nurse specialist in the care of such patients. Fortunately, a wide variety of stoma and fistula appliances are presently available. Large Eakin bags can be cut to suit the shape of the abdominal wall and, when combined with suction catheters and Stomahesive® paste, will control the vast majority of fistulas. In certain cases it may be almost impossible to adequately control the output of a fistula. This is, for example, likely to be the case where a high output fistula has developed in the base of a deep or an irregularly shaped wound. In these circumstances, repeated failed attempts to keep a bag on a fistula may be extremely demoralizing and under these circumstances it may be preferable to fashion a proximal loop jejunostomy in the left upper quadrant. While this will produce a very high output proximal stoma, it will, at least be possible to control the output with a stoma bag, which is vastly preferable to an uncontrollable fistula with extensive skin excoriation.

Nutritional support

In general, the aim of nutritional support in the patient with acute intestinal failure is to provide at least basal requirements of energy and nitrogen until normal diet can be tolerated. Nutritional intervention should be considered whenever:[28]

- Starvation for longer than 5 days is expected or has occurred, whether as a result of impaired intake or gastrointestinal disease.

- The underlying disease has led to an increase in nutritional requirements beyond that which can be provided by a 'normal diet'.

- Nutritional depletion already existed prior to the onset of acute gastrointestinal failure.

The vast majority of patients with acute intestinal failure will require nutritional support. In most cases, this will only be necessary until intestinal function has returned to normal. In patients with proximal intestinal fistulas, however, nutritional support is likely to be required until the fistula has closed spontaneously or until optimal conditions for surgery to close the fistula have been achieved. In the case of the patient with a combination of a fistula and a laparostomy, this may take more than 6 months and under these circumstances it may be appropriate, in an otherwise fit individual with satisfactory home circumstances, to discharge the patient on home parenteral nutrition, pending definitive surgery.

Enteral nutrition

As a general principle, the enteral route should be used for nutritional support whenever possible. Enteral feeding is safer, more physiological, may preserve intestinal mucosal integrity and is certainly far less expensive than parenteral nutrition. There is no evidence to suggest that enteral nutrition is inferior to parenteral nutrition in the maintenance of nutritional status or in allowing the spontaneous closure of enterocutaneous fistulas, provided enteral feed can be delivered to healthy intestine.[29] In acute intestinal failure, however, enteral feeding may be impractical or inappropriate. Although postoperative 'ileus' generally affects predominantly the stomach and colon, rather than the small intestine, the resulting abdominal distension may cause intolerance of enteral feeding, with nausea and vomiting. One study of aggressive early postoperative enteral feeding after upper gastrointestinal surgery has suggested that the resulting abdominal distension may lead to respiratory impairment.[30] Nevertheless, successful enteral feeding has been achieved early in the postoperative period.[31] A combination of nasoenteric tube, prokinetic drugs and thoracic epidural analgesia (allowing the avoidance of opiates) may make enteral nutrition easier to tolerate[32,33] and studies have also indicated that enteral feeding may even be safe and effective in acute pancreatitis.[34] Enteral nutrition may prove satisfactory in patients with a low output distal ileal or colonic fistula but is inappropriate when there is obstruction or a fistula of the upper gastrointestinal tract, unless access can be gained to the gut below the diseased segment. It may be possible to place an enteral feeding tube directly into the small intestine through an entero-cutaneous fistula. The output of the fistula can be collected, mixed with enteral feed and infused into the distal, healthy gut, but the technique is demanding for nursing staff, aesthetically unpleasant and has consequently not proved popular in the UK.

Parenteral nutrition

For the majority of patients with acute intestinal failure, parenteral nutrition will be the preferred modality of nutritional support. This may either be because of the presence of disease of the intestine, which precludes satisfactory enteral nutrition, an inability to tolerate enteral nutrition or altered nutritional requirements such as those associated with severe sepsis or injury.

If the anticipated period of nutritional support is fewer than 14 days, parenteral nutrition can be provided safely via a peripheral vein. The chief attraction of peripheral total parenteral nutrition (TPN) is that it requires little in the way of special expertise and is not associated with the potential morbidity of central venous cannulation. The ability to provide TPN for prolonged periods via the peripheral route is limited by the development, in many cases, of thrombophlebitis.[35] This can be minimized by the use of lipid-containing regimens[36] (which have a lower osmolality than glucose-based regimens and are therefore less irritant to venous endothelium), by adding heparin and hydrocortisone to the feed and by the application of nitrate patches to promote venodilatation at the feeding site.[37] While standard intravenous cannulae can be used, purpose-designed peripheral feeding lines, which are of extremely small calibre and made of inert polyurethane are available and have been used with success.[36,38] Despite these manoeuvres it may not be possible to administer more than 3 litres of TPN without phlebitis because of the flow rates required in small veins. Central venous TPN is therefore recommended in patients with large fluid requirements or acutely ill adult patients, who may have energy requirements greater than 2000 kcal/day. Central venous TPN is also necessary where it is evident that a prolonged period of parenteral feeding is likely to be required. While central venous access for feeding can be obtained via a peripheral vein and peripherally inserted central venous catheters (PICCs) have been shown to provide a safe and effective means of venous access for parenteral nutrition,[39] they have not generally proved popular in the UK.

The ability to manage complex cases of acute intestinal failure associated with abdominal sepsis or fistulas is, to a very considerable extent, dependent upon the ability to provide complication-free parenteral nutrition. Irrespective of the route chosen for venous access, a strict aseptic technique is essential. The lines used for nutritional support should be set aside for this purpose alone and maintained by dedicated nursing teams according to a strict aseptic protocol. It has clearly been established that under these conditions, catheter-related sepsis rates are negligible.[2]

Definitive treatment

Once sepsis has been excluded or eradicated and nutritional and metabolic support initiated, the management of acute intestinal failure is directed at the underlying cause. Clearly, definitive treatment will depend upon the exact cause of intestinal failure. In many cases, the cause will be self-limiting (for example in paralytic ileus, severe infective diarrhoea or uncomplicated acute pancreatitis) and recovery can be expected. Aggressive medical therapy may be required to deal with the underlying cause in some cases (e.g. high-dose steroid therapy for Crohn's disease, or anticoagulation for patients who have sustained a mesenteric vascular occlusion because of thrombophilia). In patients with an intestinal fistula who have acute intestinal failure, a definitive treatment plan can only be produced once the anatomy of the fistula is determined. This will require careful planning and meticulous radiological assessment. The most useful investigations are fistulography (in which fistula openings are catheterized and contrast medium injected) and barium contrast studies. Intravenous urography or endoscopic retrograde cholangio-pancreatography may also be required, depending upon the anatomy of the fistula. Many fistulas (possibly up to 60%) will close spontaneously within 4–6 weeks of supportive treatment. Where spontaneous closure is thought likely, oral fluids and diet should be curtailed until closure has occurred. The role of other agents in promoting fistula closure is controversial. Octreotide, an analogue of somatostatin, has been used in patients with external biliary, pancreatic and intestinal fistulas and has been said, on the basis of uncontrolled trials, to reduce fistula output and enhance the rapidity of fistula closure.[40,41] It seems unlikely that octreotide will help fistula closure where local factors are in favour of continued fistula patency, however, and, in addition, the use of octreotide is not supported by the findings of more carefully designed randomized trials which have failed to show evidence of benefit.[42–44] Definitive surgical treatment for acute intestinal failure attributable to intestinal fistulas will be required if spontaneous fistula closure does not occur. Internal fistulas will not, in general, close spontaneously. External gastrointestinal fistulas are unlikely to close spontaneously if the factors outlined in Table 3.3 are present.

Patients who are referred to a specialized unit for management have usually selected themselves by virtue of the underlying pathology or failure of spontaneous fistula closure. The exact nature of surgery required will depend upon the anatomy and aetiology of the fistula but the general principles are as follows: attempts to deal definitively with the fistula should not be made until the patient is well, free from sepsis and adequately nourished. It is desirable to leave at least 3 months between the previous laparotomy and definitive surgical treatment to allow for softening of adhesions within the abdomen. This may necessitate discharging the patient on home parenteral nutrition. Re-operative surgery of this nature is extremely technically demanding and adequate amounts of time should be set aside. Sharp, rather than blunt dissection is required to avoid tearing the bowel at the site of adhesions and segments of bowel with fistulas should be resected rather than bypassed. Intestinal anastomosis should only be attempted if the patient is free from sepsis, undernutrition and local conditions are entirely favourable. It is particularly important to avoid leaving an anastomosis within an old abscess cavity as this will inevitably lead to re-fistulation. In patients with a jejunostomy and an intact colon, consideration should be given to intestinal re-anastomosis, even if it will not prevent the need for long-term parenteral nutrition. Once intestinal continuity is restored the additional absorptive area of the colon may reduce fluid and electrolyte requirements and thus the frequency and/or volume of TPN required. Diarrhoea is often surprisingly easy to control with loperamide, codeine phosphate and/or cholesytramine.

OUTCOME OF TREATMENT FOR ACUTE INTESTINAL FAILURE

Acute intestinal failure varies widely in nature, from transient postoperative ileus after major abdominal surgery, to life-threatening abdominal sepsis with multiple intestinal fistulas. Generalized statements about outcome are therefore unlikely to be helpful. Prior to the antibiotic era and the use of nutritional support, the mortality associated with the development of an entero-cutaneous fistula was in excess of 60%, with many patients succumbing to the combined effects of sepsis and undernutrition.[45] Prior to the advent of safe parenteral nutrition,[46] it proved impossible to maintain nutritional status in patients who had undergone massive enterectomy, and death inevitably resulted from progressive inanition.

The prognosis for patients with even the most complex manifestations of acute intestinal failure has improved considerably over the last three decades, as a result of improvements in surgical technique, intensive care medicine, antimicrobial chemotherapy, stoma/skin care and nutritional support. The principle factors which now adversely affect outcome are sepsis (which if severe is still associated with a mortality in excess of 30%), co-morbidity and underlying disease. A large prospective study of 300 admissions with intestinal failure to a specialized unit over a 7-year period recorded a mortality rate of 13%. The major adverse prognostic factors on admission were increasing age and hypoalbuminaemia, the latter indicative of severe sepsis.[47] The healthcare costs associated with the management of patients with complicated acute intestinal failure have not been published but may be considerably in excess of £60 000 per consultant episode in the UK[48] and it is appropriate that expertise be concentrated in a small number of specialized units. The multifaceted nature of the problems faced by patients with acute intestinal failure makes a team approach to management mandatory and it is important to note that nurses, dieticians, pharmacists and physiotherapists are all essential, in addition to medical practitioners, for a successful outcome.[49]

REFERENCES

1. Fleming CR, Remington M. Intestinal failure. In: Hill GL (ed) *Nutrition and the Surgical Patient*. Churchill Livingstone: Edinburgh, 1981, pp. 219–235.

2. Scott NA, Leinhardt DJ, O'Hanrahan T, Finnegan S, Shaffer JL, Irving MH. Spectrum of intestinal failure in a specialised unit. *Lancet* 1991; **337**: 471–473.

3. Irving MH, Carlson GL. Enterocutaneous fistulas. *Surgery* 1998; **16**: 217–220.

4. Hersch M, Gnidec AA, Bersten AD, Trosler M, Rutledge FS, Sibbald WJ. Histologic and ultra-structural changes in non-pulmonary organs during early hyperdynamic sepsis. *Surgery* 1990; **107**: 397–410.

5. Rafferty JF, Noguchi Y, Fischer JE, Hasselgren PO. Sepsis in rats stimulates cellular proliferation in the mucosa of the small intestine. *Gastroenterology* 1994; **107**: 121–127.

6. Gardiner K, Barbul A. Intestinal amino acid absorption during sepsis. *J Parenter Enteral Nutr* 1993; **17**: 277–283.

7. Little RA, Carlson GL. Insulin resistance and tissue fuels. In: Kinney JM, Tucker HN (eds) *Organ Metabolism and Nutrition. Ideas for Future Critical Care*. Raven Press: New York, 1994: pp. 49–68.

8. Carlson GL, Irving MH. Infection, recognition and management in critically ill surgical patients. In: Hanson G (ed) *Critical Care of the Surgical Patient*. Chapman & Hall: London, 1997, pp. 273–290.

9. Streat SJ, Beddoe AH, Hill GL. Aggressive nutritional support does not prevent protein loss despite fat gain in intensive care patients. *J Trauma* 1987; **27**: 262–266.

10. Dive A, Moulert M, Jonard P, Jamart J, Mahiev P. Gastroduodenal motility in mechanically ventilated critically ill patients: a manometric study. *Crit Care Med* 1994; **22**: 441–447.

11. Thompson J. The intestinal response to critical illness. *Am J Gastroenterol* 1995; **90**: 190–200.

12. Dahn MS, Lange P, Lobdell K, Hans B, Jacobs LA, Mitchell RA. Splanchnic and total body consumption differences in septic and injured patients. *Surgery* 1987; **101**: 69–80.

13. Marshall SC, Christou NV, Meakins JL. The gastro-intestinal tract: the undrained abscess of mutiple organ failure. *Ann Surg* 1993; **218**: 111–119.

14. Kalff JC, Schraut WH, Simmons RL, Bauer AJ. Surgical manipulation of the gut elicits an intestinal muscularis inflammatory response resulting in post-surgical ileus. *Ann Surg* 1998; **228**: 652–663.

15. Schiller L. Drug-induced changes in bowel function. *Contemp Gastroenterol* 1989; **2**: 29–35.

16. Pettigrew RA, Hill GL. Therapeutic nutrition. In: Bouchier IAD, Allan RN, Hodgson HJF, Keighley MRB (eds) *Textbook of Gastroenterology*. Baillière-Tindall: London, 1984, pp. 1227–1245.

17. Soeters PB, Ebeid AM, Fischer JE. Review of 404 patients with gastrointestinal fistulas: impact of parenteral nutrition. *Ann Surg* 1979; **190**: 189–202.

18. Knochel JQ, Kochler PR, Lee TG, Welch DM. Diagnosis of abdominal abscesses with computed tomography, ultrasound and indium-111 leucocyte scans. *Radiology* 1980; **137**: 425–432.

19. Gerzof SG, Johnson WC. Radiologic aspects of diagnosis and treatment of abdominal abscesses. *Surg Clin N Am* 1984; **64**: 53–65.

20. Gerzof SG, Oates ME. Imaging techniques for infections in the surgical patient. *Surg Clin North Am* 1988; **68**: 147–166.

21. Polk HC, Fry DE. Radical peritoneal debridement for established peritonitis. The results of a prospective randomised clinical trial. *Ann Surg* 1980; **192**: 350–355.

22. Jennings WC, Wood CD, Guernsey JM. Continuous postoperative peritoneal lavage in the treatment of peritoneal sepsis. *Dis Col Rectum* 1982; **25**: 641–643.

23. Hau T, Ohmann C, Womershauser A, Wacha H, Yang Q. Planned relaparotomy vs relaparotomy on demand in the treatment of intraabdominal infections. The peritonitis study group of the surgical infection society – Europe. *Arch Surg* 1995; **130**: 1193–1196.

24. Anderson ID, Fearon KCH, Grant IS. Laparotomy for abdominal sepsis in the critically ill. *Br J Surg* 1996; **83**: 535–539.

25. Mughal MM, Bancewicz J, Irving MH. 'Laparostomy': a technique for the management of intractable intra-abdominal sepsis. *Br J Surg* 1986; **73**: 253–259.

26. Walsh GL, Chiasson P, Hedderich G, Wexler MJ, Meakins JL. The open abdomen. The Marlex mesh and zipper technique: a method of managing intra-peritoneal infection. *Surg Clin North Am* 1988; **68**: 25–40.

27. Scripcariu V, Carlson G, Bancewicz J, Irving MH, Scott NA. Reconstructive abdominal operations after laparostomy and multiple repeat laparotomies for severe intra-abdominal infection. *Br J Surg* 1994; **81**: 1475–1478.

28. Chandran VP, Sim AJ. Nutritional support in acute intestinal failure. *Baillière's Clin Gastroenterol* 1991; **5**: 841–860.

29. Voitk AJ, Echave V, Brown RA, McArdle AH, Gurd FN. Elemental diet in the treatment of fistulas of the alimentary tract. *Surg Gynecol Obstet* 1973; **137**: 68–72.

30. Watters JM, Kirkpatrick SM, Norris SB, Shamji FM, Wells GA. Immediate postoperative enteral feeding results in impaired respiratory mechanics and decreased mobility. *Ann Surg* 1997; **226**: 369–377.

31. Beier-Holgersen R, Boesby S. Influence of post-operative enteral nutrition on postsurgical infections. *Gut* 1996; **39**: 833–835.

32. Kehlet H, Rung GW. Postoperative opioid analgesia: time for a reconsideration? *J Clin Anaesth* 1996; **8**: 441–445.

33. Kehlet H. Balanced analgesia: a prerequisite form optimal recovery. *Br J Surg* 1998; **85**: 3–4.

34. Windsor AC, Kanwar S, Li AG *et al.* Compared with parenteral nutrition, enteral feeding attenuates the acute phase response and improves disease severity in acute pancreatitis. *Gut* 1998; **42**: 431–435.

35. May J, Murchan P, MacFie J, Sedman P, Donat R, Palmer D, Mitchell CJ. Prospective study of the aetiology of infusion phlebitis and line failure during peripheral parenteral nutrition. *Br J Surg* 1996; **83**: 1091–1094.

36. Willams N, Wales S, Irving MH. Prolonged peripheral parenteral nutrition with an ultrafine cannula and low osmolality feed. *Br J Surg* 1996; **83**: 114–116.

37. Tighe MJ, Wong C, Martin IG, McMahon MJ. Do heparin, hydrocortisone and glyceryl trinitrate influence thrombophlebitis during full intravenous nutrition via a peripheral vein? *J Parenter Enteral Nutr* 1995; **19**: 507–509.

38. Plusa SM, Horsman R, Kendall Smith S, Webster N, Primrose JN. Fine bore cannulas for peripheral intra-venous nutrition: polyurethane or silicone? *Ann R Coll Surg Edin* 1998; **80**: 154–156.

39. Alhimyary A, Fernandez C, Picard M, Tierno K, Pignatone N, Chan HS, Malt R, Souba W. Safety and efficacy of total parenteral nutrition delivered via a peripherally inserted central venous catheter. *Nutr Clin Pract* 1996; **11**: 199–203.

40. Tassiopoulos AK, Baum G, Halverson JD. Small bowel fistulas. *Surg Clin N Am* 1996; **76**: 1175–1181.

41. Paran H, Neufeld D, Kaplan O, Klausner J, Freund U. Octreotide for treatment of postoperative alimentary tract fistulas. *World J Surg* 1995; **19**: 430–433.

42. Sancho JJ, di Costanzo J, Nubiola P, Larrad A, Beguiristain A, Roqueta F, Franch G, Oliva A, Gubern JM, Sitges-Serra A. Randomized double-blind placebo-controlled trial of early octreotide in patients with postoperative enterocutaneous fistulas. *Br J Surg* 1995; **82**: 638–641.

43. Carlson GL, Scott NA, Irving MH, Sancho JJ, Sitges Serra A. Somatostatin in gastroenterology. More studies needed. *Br Med J* 1994; **309**: 604–605.

44. Scott NA, Finnegan S, Irving MH. Octreotide and postoperative enterocutaneous fistulae: a controlled prospective study. *Acta Gastroenterologica Belgica* 1993; **56**: 266–270.

45. Edmunds LF, Williams GM, Welch CE. External fistulas arising from the gastrointestinal tract. *Ann Surg* 1960; **152**: 445–473.

46. Dudrick SJD, Wilmore DW, Vars HM, Rhoads JE. Can intravenous feeding as the sole means of nutrition support growth in the child and restore weight loss in an adult? An affirmative answer. *Ann Surg* 1969; **169**: 974–984.

47. Elebute EA, Stoner HB. The grading of sepsis. *Br J Surg* 1983; **70**: 29–31.

48. Shaffer JL, Bradley A. Personal communication, 1998.

49. Irving MH, White R, Tresadern J. Three years' experience with an intestinal failure unit. *Ann R Coll Surg Engl* 1985; **67**: 1–5.

4

Care of Intestinal Stoma and Enterocutaneous Fistula

Stephanie Hughes, Anne Myers and Gordon Carlson

*P*atients with acute intestinal failure complicated by the presence of an intestinal stoma or entero-cutaneous fistula should be managed by a multi-disciplinary team. Unsatisfactory care of stomas and fistulas may result in physical discomfort and mental trauma to the patient[1] and may prejudice nutritional support, surgical treatment or spontaneous fistula closure. This chapter outlines the fundamental principles of management of patients with intestinal stomas and enterocutaneous fistulas in the setting of the patient with intestinal failure.

DEFINITIONS AND PRINCIPLES OF TREATMENT

Intestinal stoma

An intestinal stoma is a surgically created opening of the gut on to the body surface. The nomenclature used to describe a stoma depends on the precise site of the gastrointestinal tract brought up to form the opening (e.g. jejunostomy, ileostomy or colostomy[2]). A stoma is defined as an end stoma (in which the bowel at the site selected is divided and brought up to the skin) or a split/loop/defunctioning stoma when the bowel is not divided but simply opened (Fig 4.1). A defunctioning stoma is intended for a few weeks often to defunction an anastomosis distal to it (e.g. an anterior resection or the rectum or ileoanal pouch). In each case, the bowel is ideally brought out through the rectus abdominis muscle to minimize the chance of a parastomal hernia developing,[3] and then sutured to the skin after an approximately 2.5 cm circular area of skin has been removed. Large bowel stomas (colostomies) are generally sutured flush with the skin, whereas small bowel stomas (ileostomy, jejunostomy, duodenostomy) have an everted 2.5–3.0 cm spout. This modification, devised by Brooke, enables the corrosive effluent to be kept away from the skin and appliances to be kept on with relative ease[4].

Enterocutaneous fistula

An enterocutaneous fistula is an abnormal communi-cation between the gastrointestinal tract and the skin. Enterocutaneous fistulas may develop as result of complications of surgery or as a result of intrinsic disease of the gastrointestinal tract (e.g. in Crohn's disease, malignancy or diverticular disease of the colon). Enterocutaneous fistulas (Fig. 4.1) are classified according to the site of origin and attachments, the number of openings, the orientation with respect to the long axis of the intestinal tract and the presence of an associated abscess cavity. When more than one organ system is involved, fistulas are described as com-plex. For example, a fistula arising from the side of the terminal ileum and passing directly to the skin of the abdomen would be described as a simple lateral ileal fistula (Fig. 4.2A). A similar track passing from the side of ileum into an abscess cavity, and the bladder then to the skin is described as a complex lateral ileovesico-cutaneous fistula (Fig. 4.2B). Fistulas that arise perpendicular to the long axis of the gut are referred to as end fistulas and most commonly arise from the duo-denal stump after a Polya gastrectomy. Intestinal fistu-las are most commonly caused by an anastomotic leak, trauma, inflammatory bowel disease, malignant disease, diverticular disease of the colon, or as a consequence of radiotherapy.[5]

The key principles in the management of a patient with an enterocutaneous fistula is the adequate treat-ment of abdominal sepsis, this is the most common cause of death.[6] Sepsis should be suspected and rigorously looked for in all patients with an intestinal fistula, by a combination of ultrasound, contrast-enhanced CT scanning and radioisotope imaging. Where possible, sepsis should be managed by per-cutaneous drainage, but in some cases, notably those in which sepsis has arisen due to anastomotic dehiscence, a laparotomy will be required for drainage of abscesses and creation of a proximal defunctioning stoma to divert the faecal stream. In cases of severe abdominal sepsis with multiple or recrudescent abscess cavities, a laparostomy may be required to allow adequate drainage[7] (see Chapter 3).

Once sepsis has been treated, attention is given to skin care, nutritional and metabolic support. Many fistulas will heal spontaneously provided there is no continuity between the gut mucosa and the skin, no disease at the site of the fistula (for example Crohn's disease), no distal obstruction and no intervening undrained abscess cavity.[5] In such cases enteral nutritional support with a low residue diet is appro-priate for low output (< 200 ml/day) fistulas in the distal ileum or colon, whereas patients with high out-put (> 500ml/day) fistulas, which are typically found in the proximal small bowel will usually require parenteral nutrition. It is the authors' preference to restrict such patients to sips of fluid only if contrast radiology suggests that a fistula is likely to close spontaneously. Where closure is unlikely, prevention of oral intake is unnecessary and such patients can be

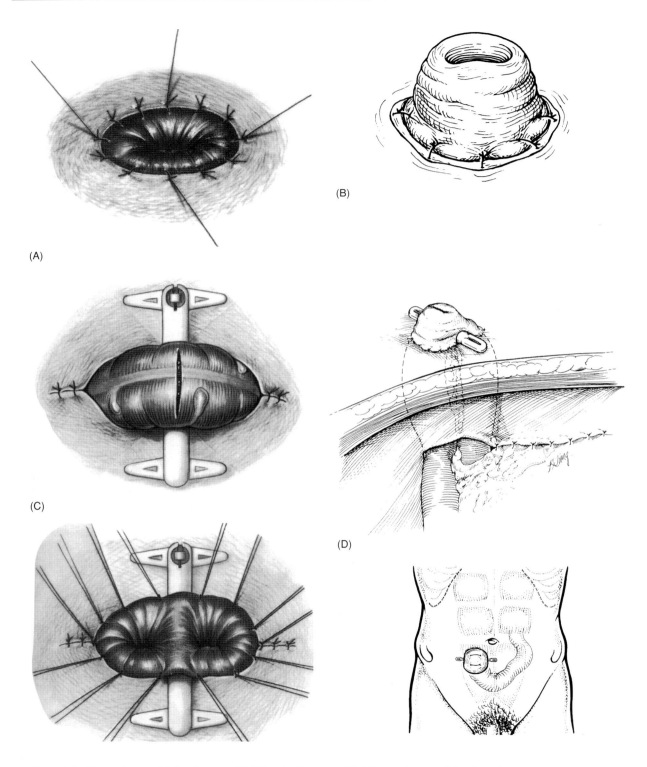

Figure 4.1 – Types of stoma (A) A colostomy, (B) A Brooke ileostomy, (C) A loop colostomy, (D) a loop ileostomy.

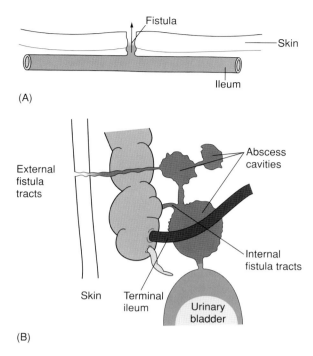

Figure 4.2 – Classification of intestinal fistulas, showing (A) a simple lateral ileocutaneous fistula track and (B) a complex track involving skin and bladder with intervening abscess cavities.

allowed relatively unrestricted access to fluids and diet, provided fluid intake is not excessive and does not make local management of the fistula impossible. The same principles apply to the management of the high output fistula as the high output stoma (restriction of oral fluid intake and the use of oral glucose–electrolyte solutions, drugs that reduce motility and intestinal or secretions). Although initial studies suggested that octreotide might aid the spontaneous closure of fistulas,[8] randomized controlled trials have failed to support this[9] and it seems likely that spontaneous fistula closure is related primarily to anatomical considerations. For this reason, octreotide is not routinely used in the management of patients with intestinal fistulas.[10]

MANAGEMENT OF THE PATIENT WITH A STOMA/FISTULA

Psychological support and training of the patient should, if possible, begin prior to surgery that results in a stoma. The Stoma Care Nurse, in conjunction with the multidisciplinary team, will make a significant contribution at this time of preparation.

Choosing the stoma site

The Stoma Care Nurse should discuss the planned surgery with the patient, using diagrams to explain what a stoma is, how it will affect their life, how it is managed and how to manage problems. The ideal site for the stoma is selected after careful evaluation of the patient. A flat area of normal skin contour, below the belt or waistline (except for a transverse colostomy) is chosen away from bony prominences (iliac crest or costal margin), surgical scars/skin folds/creases and unobscured by pendulous breasts. The optimal site avoids places where clothing grips the abdomen or where the bag would be conspicuous or easily damaged. The site chosen is marked with indelible ink and should be just medial to the linea semilunaris. The patient is asked to sit, bend, stand and walk to check the suitability of position (it may be useful to apply a pouch if difficulties are evident or if the patient requests). A reserve site may also be chosen.

Aims of long-term care

The experience of gastrointestinal illness and surgery associated with the formation of a stoma or the development of a fistula constitutes a major upheaval in a patient's life[11] The aim of caring for a patient with a stoma and/or a fistula is to allow a relatively good quality of life by preventing physical and psychological stress; this means ensuring a comfortable stoma that does not leak and is not malodorous or easily visible. The patient should be given advice about the practical aspects of caring for and living with a stoma so that they can return to a full independent home and work life[12] Controlling stoma and/or fistula output enables patients to gain confidence, increase self-esteem/ dignity and resume independence.

Skin care

Care of the skin around a stoma or fistula is perhaps the most important component of nursing care. The principal objective is to keep the effluent away from the skin. The more proximal in the gut a fistula, the more likely its output is to discharge corrosive fluid with activated pancreatic enzymes that can cause painful skin destruction (Fig. 4.3).

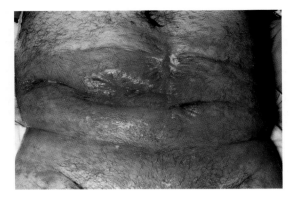

Figure 4.3 – Extensive skin damage resulting from a high output fistula with inadequate skin protection.

An initial assessment of the stoma/fistula and surrounding skin should first be made noting approximate measurements, skin condition/degree of excoriation, description of output and any associated nursing implications (e.g. pain). Skin contours are noted for creases where leakage could occur. It is often helpful to photograph the wounds at this time. This information, together with accurate measurements of stoma output, allows the stomatherapist to select the most appropriate appliance thus enabling collection of the effluent and controlling the problems of leakage and odour. The patient, in turn, gains comfort, confidence and independence. Key aspects of management of the patient with an intestinal stoma or fistula are the selection of appropriate equipment and the adoption of suitable management techniques.

Equipment

The carer/nurse must determine the size/type of appliance and initially the frequency of bag emptying and changing. The aim is to keep the equipment and procedures simple and allow for the patient to choose their preferences. Complex ritualistic procedures must be avoided. In the United Kingdom appliances for stoma care are exempt from prescription charges for patients with a permanent stoma but not a temporary stoma.

Stoma/fistula bags   A well-fitting adhesive appliance will protect the skin, remove unpleasant odours, reduce risk of cross-infection, allow assessment of fluid losses, preserve dignity and allow the patient mobility and rest.[1] There are many types of stoma and fistula appliances available and the manufacturers also produce accessories to treat damaged skin, produce an even body contour (thus allowing better fitting of a stoma appliance) and deodorize offensive exudates. Immediately postoperatively a clear, unvented, drainable standard bag on which the aperture is cut to fit the stoma is used so that the viability of the stoma can be monitored and stool/air output can be observed. As the stomal output becomes regular and predictable a one- or two-piece bag can be used. The former attaches directly to the skin and may be closed or drainable. A closed bag is often appropriate for a colostomy, which is typically changed twice a day. A drainable appliance is appropriate for ileostomies/jejunostomies or for colostomies with a fluid output. Flatus valves (vent/charcoal filter), to allow escape of gases, are now present in most drainable pouches whilst they have been present in closed pouches for a number of years. Two-piece appliances have a flange that can stay on the skin for 3–4 days and are fitted with either a drainable or closed bag. Drainable pouches should be changed every 24–72 hours. Bags for use over an established stoma have a pre-cut aperture, come as three sizes (mini, midi or maxi) and are opaque. Most bags hold about 200–300 ml of fluid.

Extensive wound areas require a large 'wound manager' pouch or an Eakin device (Fig. 4.4) These can be adapted to the size and shape of any wound and are drained continuously. Planned stomas that are of routine size are more easily catered for, but stomas that have become flush or have retracted, can be successfully managed with the use of convex flanges incorporated within the bags. Pouches should be kept in a cool place out of direct sunlight.

Adhesive flanges   An appliance usually sticks to the skin by a cohesive seal. Clean, warm, dry skin is needed. If the skin is itchy, Caladryl® can be used and helps both with itching and adhesion.

Filling pastes/wafers/dressings   There are many hydrocolloid pastes that can be used to fill defects in a wound (e.g. Stomahesive®, Orobase®, Granuflex®, Dansac®). Wafers are compressed thin (1.3-mm thick) squares made of gelatin, pectin, sodium carboxymethylcellulose and polisobutylene. They are available in varying sizes/makes, e.g. Comfeel/Stomahesive® and can be used to cover and fill defects. Wafers may be used to help adherence of the appliance and may act as barriers between the bag/skin. The flanges of a stoma bag can safely cover the top of wounds.

Absorbent dressings with associated barrier creams are inadequate for outputs of more than 20 ml per day.

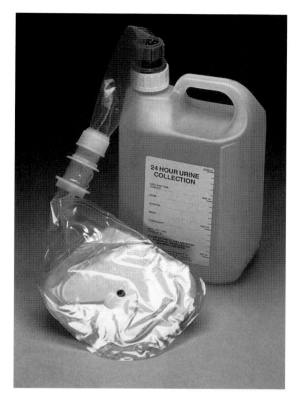

Figure 4.4 – The Eakin bag, attached via a 'megostomy' tube, to a collection bottle, known as the Greensmith device.

Appropriate well-fitting/constructed stoma appliances cut to fit the area and so cover exposed skin enable successful management.[13]

Techniques

Fitting an appliance over a stoma   The old appliance/flange is peeled from the skin gently by easing the skin away. The surrounding skin is then cleaned using soft gauze and warm water and the area dried well with gauze, a soft towel or white kitchen roll. Water alone is adequate for this purpose. However, if desired, an unperfumed, gentle soap could be used. It is not necessary to use lotions or skin preparations. Direct contact with the intestinal mucosa should be avoided. An appliance of the correct size is selected or the new flange is cut to size. The backing is peeled off and applied gently to the abdomen over the stoma area. The clip is applied if a drainable pouch is used.

An ileostomy bag is usually emptied 5–6 times/24 h (total volume is about 500–800 ml/24 h) and most patients do this once during the night. If the patient has a high stoma output the flange/bag/dressing change is undertaken when the output is likely to be lowest or when help is available (for list of equipment see Table 4.1). Following drainage of the pouch, the end of the appliance is cleaned with water/toilet tissue and the clip re-applied. Some patients flush inside the bag with water using a syringe or small spray bottle. Odour powders/deodorant sprays may be used at this time. The pouch is subsequently changed as required. In hot conditions this may need to be undertaken more frequently as the flange can 'melt' and thus leak.

Table 4.1 – Key equipment for dressing a complex high output enterocutaneous fistula

Gauze for cleaning
Warm water
Hair dryer
Suction equipment
Wound manager
Hydrocolloid filling paste/wafers
Suitable drainage appliance
A drainable collection device

Fitting an appliance over a complex fistula   The area should be cleaned with warm water and dried thoroughly with soft gauze or the use of a hair dryer. Shaving of body hair may be necessary to optimise adhesion and prevent discomfort. Excoriated skin should have Orahesive® powder applied sparingly. It is often helpful in caring for large fistula wounds to make a template of the area with a piece of clear plastic material. This assists with cutting the base/flange of the pouch and is useful in observing the healing process, as smaller templates will be required probably weekly. Crevices or creases of intact skin can be filled with Stomahesive® paste (it may be helpful to use a syringe to insert) or pieces of Cohesive® seals to even the site (Fig. 4.6). A warm hair dryer will harden the paste following moulding and if necessary more paste can then be applied to facilitate adhesion. It may be necessary to cover this area with a sheet of Stomahesive® or Comfeel® cut to fit, but the base of an Eakin pouch alone is usually quite adequate. The immediate edge around the stoma/fistula should be piped with soft paste to help adhere and prevent leakage of the effluent between the surfaces. The readily prepared pouch should now be applied, firmly moulding it to the surface and ensuring that no creases occur during the procedure (Fig. 4.7). The patient should be encouraged to rest for approximately 30 minutes to promote adhesion of the appliance.

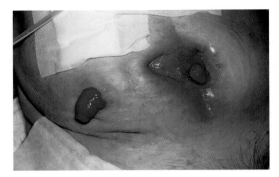

Fig 4.5

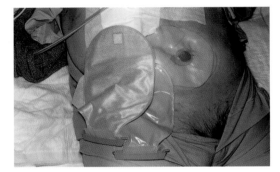

Fig 4.6

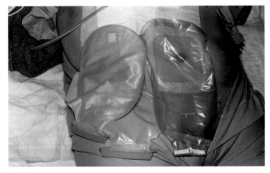

Fig 4.7

Figure 4.5–4.7 – Applying a bag to an intestinal fistula.

The technique used should be fully documented so that other team members can maintain the prescribed care. The area should be regularly inspected and any evidence of pain, burning of the skin, leakage, odour or detachment of the appliance should be investigated and treated appropriately. This usually requires pouch replacement. The plan of nursing care should be evaluated regularly and changes made as required. The patient with extensive fistula formation may not be able to participate in any practical aspects of the skin care until their general condition is improved or surgery to treat the underlying problem is undertaken. However, wherever possible the patient should be encouraged to begin to participate in caring for their stoma and so in turn gain independence, autonomy and sense of well-being. The plan to teach and involve the patient with their care should begin following discussion between the stomatherapist, nurses and, most importantly, the patient.

Some fistulas lie in large irregular cavities, which make them exceptionally difficult to manage. Such fistulas may require a short-term treatment of sump suction until the area shrinks to manageable dimensions. This is applied via a catheter incorporated within the pouch, through which low-grade continuous suction can be applied. This treatment should not be prolonged because the creation of a negative pressure at the cutaneous surface of a fistula may prevent spontaneous closure and the treatment also restricts mobilization.[14]

The ultimate goal of management is for the patient to be able to care for themselves. This may not always be possible, however. Depending upon the patient's individual circumstances, close relatives may need to undertake patient care or the patient may request they be at least made aware of the needs that may be required. Practical skills should be demonstrated to the patient with careful explanations that can be easily understood. Patients should be reassured that they will not be discharged from hospital until they or their carers can cope with the required stoma care. Following a period of observation, patient participation should be encouraged and this can be gradually increased. Continuous assessment is required and the nurse must continue to support the patient even when full independence in stoma care is achieved. The patient should be informed of all aspects of stoma care from the obtaining of supplies to the disposal of appliances and should be made aware of the availability of self-help associations who can assist in the rehabilitation or with welfare issues.

Emptying drainage bags Stoma bags and pouches should be regularly emptied to prevent excessive accumulation of effluent because the weight of the fluid can dislodge the bag. Appliances cannot be flushed down the toilet. Faecal matter is instead emptied and the pouch wrapped in a plastic bag or newspaper for disposal. High output fistulas/stomas (over 500 ml/24 h) may require frequent drainage and this can disturb sleep, thus adding to stress. To prevent this, a secondary drainage container allowing continuous gravity drainage of stoma bags into a plastic bottle (Fig. 4.9) can be used. This apparatus (known as a 'megostomy' or 'Greensmith device') was invented by the husband of a patient with a high output stoma and has improved considerably the quality of life of many patients with a short bowel. The device can be placed adjacent to the bed or carried in a simple carrier bag during mobilization.[9]

THE NORMAL STOMA

All stomas are oedematous after surgery and shrink over the first 1–2 postoperative weeks. This results in a requirement for a smaller template.

Colostomy

A colostomy generally begins to act 2–5 days after surgery. Flatus, followed by watery faeces, will first become apparent but with the introduction of oral fluids and diet the effluent will become solid. The volume of output will be influenced by the diet, the presence of coexisting intestinal disease and the precise location of the stoma with respect to the colon. In general, colostomy output varies between 200 and 600 ml/24 h.

Ileostomy

An ileostomy generally starts to work within 24 hours. During the first week, an output of about 1.2 litres of watery stool is expected and this falls for the second week to about 600 ml daily of porridge-like stool. The output initially rises as food is taken. A normal ileostomy may reduce its output over the following few months.

Jejunostomy

The output from a jejunostomy increases dramatically after food/fluid is taken orally and may reach more than 6 litres if less than a metre of jejunum remains. Patients with a jejunostomy are likely to require continued intravenous fluid and electrolyte therapy in order to prevent metabolic complications. It should be stressed that excessive thirst due to dehydration should be treated with oral fluid restriction (typically to < 1500 ml/day) and the loss replaced intravenously. Allowing such patients unrestricted access to oral fluids results in a vicious cycle in which excessive fluid intake results in increasing fluid output from the stoma and greater thirst. It is important to remember that 1 litre of jejunostomy fluid contains 100 mmol/L sodium and this amount must be replaced, together with 20–40 mmol of potassium. In patients with a newly-created jejunostomy, careful attention to monitoring of fluid and electrolyte balance should be given. Although daily plasma measurements are of value, homeostatic mechanisms result in failure of plasma measurements to detect dehydration or electrolyte depletion until late in their evolution. A more useful and more acceptable means of monitoring the patients fluid and electrolyte status is to perform at least twice-weekly measurement of urinary sodium concentration in such patients. The finding of a urinary sodium of less than 20 mmol/L in such patients implies sodium depletion and a need for further assessment. Further aspects of the medical treatment of the patient with a high output stoma is discussed in Chapter 24.

Diet with a stoma

Patients with stomas can be reassured that they will not have to make major modifications to their diet. Some foods, however, may cause discomfort or even intestinal obstruction, malodorous flatulence or diarrhoea and may be best avoided, although patients will ultimately determine their dietary preferences on an individual basis.

Nuts and fibrous foods such as dried fruits (e.g. raisins and sultanas) and 'pithy' fruit (e.g. orange) may cause discomfort or even obstruction in patients with an ileostomy. Other foods that may be partly digested include celery, coconut, coleslaw (raw cabbage), sweetcorn, orange, mushroom, nuts, peas, popcorn, pineapple, relishes (e.g. chutney), seeds and skins (e.g. apples/pears). Foods that may cause flatulence/malodour are generally avoided (asparagus, baked beans, cabbage, broccoli, brussel sprouts, fish, cauliflower, eggs, beer, carbonated beverages, onions and parsnips).

Reduction of odour

Deodorizing tablets or drops can be put into a stoma bag if there is perceived to be a major problem of malodour. Neutralizing sprays can also be used. If there is a malodorous wound it may be redressed with a charcoal- or metronidazole-based dressing. Some foods may cause flatulence (e.g. brassicas such as sprouts) and the diet can be restricted if desired.

Training of patient/carer

The patient and/or their carer must learn how to empty the stoma bag, use the pouch clip and change and dispose of a one- or two-piece appliance. They need to know how to look after the peristomal skin and cope with leakage, flatus or malodour. They also need to identify a reliable source of supply of stoma care products.

Irrigation

Some patients try to regulate their colostomy output by irrigation, enabling 'continence'. It is undertaken every 24–48 hours, cleansing the colon. One litre of warm water is inserted slowly (over 15 minutes) via a cone on the end of soft tubing sited 5–10 cm up the stoma. After a brief period a long drainable pouch is connected over the stoma allowing faeces and water to drain into the toilet. The procedure is time-consuming and not very popular in the United Kingdom.[17] It should **not be** used for an ileostomy.

Leakage from a stoma/fistula

There are many reasons for leakage (Table 4.2). While the stoma site and complications relating to it may be responsible, a poor technique is often the culprit. This may be due to poor vision or manual dexterity, an overfull appliance, one that has been left on for too long or alternatively changed too frequently. An uneven skin surface due to sitting in one position for a long time or changing weight (increase, decrease or pregnancy) may affect the way an appliance fits, thus making it liable to leak. Pancaking of solid stool at the top of a stoma can cause leakage. It can be helped by putting baby oil onto the inside top of the appliance, covering the filter or an adhesive bar can be placed on the outside of stoma to form a bridge. This prevents both pancaking and also the stoma bag sticking to the

Table 4.2 – Reasons for stomal leakage

1. Badly sited stoma on bony prominence, skin creases, dips or scars
2. Stoma shrinkage, retraction, prolapse, or peristomal herniation
3. Poor technique (can be due to poor vision or manual dexterity)
4. Weight change (gain or loss)
5. Pancaking
6. Peristomal skin allergy or granulation tissue

stoma. Peristomal skin irritation can be due to allergy to plaster or the appliance adhesive and a change of these may help. The hairs around an appliance may need to be shaved. Fungal infections frequently occur on moist, warm peristomal skin. Granulation at the stoma edge is harmless but can cause bleeding or prevent bag application. This responds to cautery with a silver nitrate pencil.

Activities

A patient may cover their stoma with a minibag for swimming or sexual intercourse. A bag is usually changed after swimming. Participation in most sports is possible though heavy contact sports (e.g. rugby) should be avoided and weight-lifting may make a stoma more likely to prolapse. When flying, it is helpful and reassuring for the patient to carry spare stoma bags in both the aeroplane hold and in the hand luggage. The insurance company should be told of the stoma. During the flight a good fluid and salt intake needs to be ensured as patients with a stoma may be at increased risk of dehydration.

Psychological care

Psychological care is an integral part of the management of patients with stomas and fistulas. This is especially important in the patient who presents with a fistula after repeated failed surgical procedures. In such cases there may be complete loss of confidence in the carers and a state of profound depression and withdrawal. Interestingly, few, if any, clinical psychologists have specific experience in the problems faced by such patients and are unable to relate to the unique problems associated with complex and repeated surgery, multiple fistulas and stomas and prolonged hospitalization. In general, trained members of nursing staff have proven to be the most effective source of psychological support. The patient should be given sufficient information at all times to be aware and actively engaged in their treatment plan. This may include explanations of investigative procedures, surgical options, intended outcomes and any possible complications. It is necessary to repeat these discussions several times so that uncertainty can be avoided. Family members should also be included whenever this is thought to be appropriate. The availability of the spouse or partner is of vital importance and their support is invaluable in offsetting the initial feelings of shame and mutilation felt by many patients.[15] Education should be given to the relatives so that the sharing relationship is allowed to continue, and the family need to behave normally and demonstrate continued acceptance of the patient, promoting positive attitudes and dispelling possible feelings of rejection or revulsion.[12] The new body image can be difficult to accept but if there is time for the consideration of change then mental adjustment will be easier. However, sudden developments, as in the occurrence of a fistulae or emergency surgery requiring a stoma can give rise to rejection, denial and the problems of withdrawal. Other factors influencing body image are the visibility of the change and its encroachment on lifestyle.[16] Encouragement and allowing ample opportunities to talk will be much needed for both parties and they should be encouraged to voice concerns and fears. Reassurance regarding the progress or possible outcomes will be constantly required and the nurse must answer honestly but never offer false or premature reassurance.[12] When the patient is discharged the stomatherapist and the district nurses will maintain continuity of care, and supportive counselling will still be required. Certain problems only become evident on discharge from hospital, especially relating to difficulties in personal or sexual relationships. These may require expert help from marriage guidance or psychosexual counsellors though the nurse can help assess the situation and make arrangements for referral if appropriate.

THE COMPLICATED STOMA

Specific medical and nursing care may be required to manage the stoma when complications occur. The principal general complication associated with creation of a stoma relates to fluid and electrolyte balance in patients with a high output proximal stoma. This is discussed above and in Chapter 16. Local complications associated with stoma formation may be apparent early or late in the postoperative period. Complications of stomas are common and 20–30% of patients will require further surgery within 5 years for a problem with the stoma.

Early

In the first days after surgery, local complications relating to the blood supply of the stoma and its attachment to the skin are common. These include obstruction from torsion or oedema of the stoma (especially in the presence of a loop ileostomy), bleeding, retraction, necrosis and peristomal infection. Infection is surprisingly uncommon without an element of necrosis at the mucocutaneous junction.

These complications may require further surgery. Necrosis of the stoma (Fig. 4.8) may be managed conservatively, provided that the patient is systemically well, has no signs of spreading peritonitis and viable mucosa is identifiable outside the patients' abdominal wall. This can usually be easily ascertained by gently inserting an endoscope into the stoma or even using a lubricated test-tube and shining a torch along it for illumination. When conservative management is successful, the stoma generally heals with stenosis (Fig. 4.9) and may require subsequent refashioning.

Late

Local complications that develop in the weeks or months after fashioning a stoma, generally relate to stoma care itself, the development of a parastomal hernia or intestinal disease.

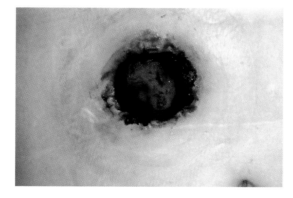

Figure 4.8 – Superficial necrosis of a colostomy. Viable mucosa can clearly be seen within the deeper tissues of the stoma.

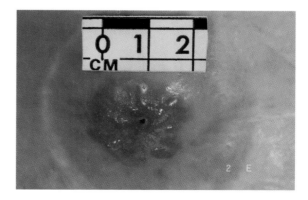

Figure 4.9 – Stenosis of the stoma following superficial necrosis.

Skin damage

Skin excoriation can happen within half an hour of exposure to jejunostomy/ileostomy fluid, Stoma-hesive® can be applied to the area to help healing and to protect the skin. Ulceration around a stoma may be due to a poorly fitting stoma appliance but in patients with inflammatory bowel disease, pyoderma gangrenosum (Fig. 4.10) or Crohn's disease of the skin should be suspected, the latter in the presence of typical 'punched out' ulcers.

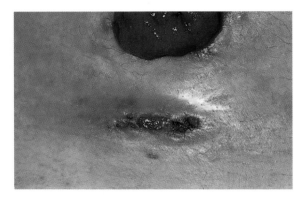

Figure 4.10 – Pyoderma gangrenosum around an ileostomy.

Bowel damage

Ulceration, excessive granulation tissue and bleeding from the mucosa, usually of an ileostomy, are common complaints and may be attributable to a poorly fitting stoma appliance (Fig. 4.11). In patients with Crohn's disease, recrudescence of disease within the stoma may

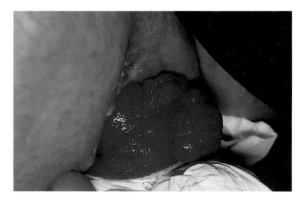

Figure 4.11 – Granulations and superficial ulceration of an ileostomy, due to a poorly fitting stoma appliance.

occur and present with pain, bleeding and visible ulceration. In severe cases, the associated stricturing may lead to intestinal obstruction. A biopsy may be required to establish a definitive diagnosis.

Herniation

Parastomal herniation is common around an end colostomy particularly if a stoma brought out is lateral to the rectal sheath and if the abdominal musculature is very weak as often occurs in the elderly. A parastomal hernia may predispose to intestinal obstruction and strangulation, is disfiguring for the patient and may make it difficult to fit an appliance. Parastomal hernias are, however, difficult to correct surgically. A variety of surgical approaches may be adopted ranging from local suture repair and mesh repair to laparotomy and transposition of the stoma, depending upon the size of the hernia and the age and condition of the patient. The long-term results of repair are poor, with up to 50% of patients reporting a recurrence of their hernia. In general, surgical repair of a parastomal hernia is avoided unless the hernia prevents the fitting of a stoma appliance or is narrow-necked and symptomatic.

Prolapse

Prolapse of a stoma is generally associated with the development of a parastomal hernia and is characterized by an 'elephant's trunk-like' everted protrusion of the stoma. This may prevent satisfactory fitting of an appliance and is especially common in patients with a transverse loop colostomy, which should therefore be avoided if at all possible. Surgery is usually required to refashion the stoma and usually dividing the bowel and converting the loop to an end stoma.

Stenosis and retraction

These complications both result from defective surgical technique. Stenosis results from circumferential fibrosis at the mucocutaneous junction, most commonly as a secondary consequence of ischaemia and necrosis. This may respond to repeated dilatation (usually under general anaesthesia) but frequently requires refashioning. It must be remembered that refashioning an ilesotomy may involves a considerable amount of bowel being resected (> 5 cm) and this can be very important if the patient has intestinal failure. Retraction occurs when insufficient bowel has been mobilized to allow the mucosa to be sutured to the skin edge without tension. In the absence of impaired vascularity (as opposed to stenosis) the bowel does not become necrotic but the opening of the stoma lies in a depression. This leads to leakage under the flange, which may then lift off. Persistent leakage, which cannot be compensated for by the use of an appropriate appliance, is an indication for surgical refashioning of the stoma.

REFERENCES

1. Forbes A, Myers C. Enterocutaneous fistulae and their management. In: Myers C (ed) *Stoma Care Nursing. A Patient-centred Approach*. Arnold, London, 1996, pp. 63–77.

2. Irving MH, Hulme O. Intestinal stomas. In: *ABC of Colo-Rectal Disease*. BMJ Publishing Group, London, 1993, pp. 68–70.

3. Nicholls RJ. Surgical procedures. In: Myers C (ed) *Stoma Care Nursing. A Patient-centred Approach*. Arnold, London, 1996, pp. 90–122.

4. Brooke BN. The management of an ileostomy including its complications. *Lancet* 1952; **2**: 102–104.

5. Irving MH, Carlson GL. Enterocutaneous fistulas. *Surgery* 1998; **vol**: 217–220.

6. Soeters PB, Ebeid AM, Fischer JE. Review of 404 patients with gastrointestinal fistulas. Impact of parenteral nutrition. *Ann Surg* 1979; **190**: 189–202.

7. Carlson GL Irving MH. Infection: recognition and management of infection in surgical patients. In:

Hanson G (ed) *Critical Care of the Surgical Patient – a Companion to Bailey and Loves' Surgery*. Chapman and Hall Medical, London, 1997, pp. 273–290.

8. Torres AJ, Landa JI, Morenzo-Azcoita M, *et al*. Somatostatin in the management of gastrointestinal fistulas. *Arch Surg* 1992; **127**: 97–100.

9. Scott NA, Irving MH. *Gastrointestinal Fistulae*. Sandoz, 1989.

10. Carlson GL, Scott NA, Irving MH, Sancho JJ, Sitges-Serra A. Somatostatin in gastroenterology. More studies needed. *Br Med J* 1994; **309**: 604.

11. Model G. A new image to accept. *Professional Nurse*. 1990; **March** 310–314.

12. Elcoat C. Stoma care, taking an holistic approach. *Nursing Times* 1998; **84**: 57–60.

13. Gross E, Irving M. Protection of the skin around intestinal fistulas. *Br J Surg* 1977; **64**: 258–263.

14. Blower AL, Irving MH. Enterocutaneous fistulas. *Surgery* 1992; **12**: 27–31.

15. Wade B. Nursing care of the stoma patient. *Surgical Nurse* 1989; **25**: ix–xii.

16. Morrall SE. The shock of the new; altered body image after creation of a stoma. *Professional Nurse*. 1990; **July**: 531–534.

17. McCahon S. Faecal stomas. In: Porrett T, Daniel N (eds) *Essential Coloproctology for Nurses*. 1999, pp. 165–187.

5

Chemotherapy and haemopoietic stem cell transplantation

W. Steward, A. Hunter, K. O'Byrne and J. Snowden

INTRODUCTION

*T*he use of cytotoxic drugs in the treatment of malignant and non-malignant conditions has increased exponentially in the last 20 years. There will be a further marked increase in their use in the future both because of a steady rise in the incidence of neoplasia and as a result of the availability of new, more effective anticancer agents. With the development of new protocols and drugs, survival rates have increased such that 52% of all patients with malignancy will be alive 5 years after diagnosis[1] (Table 5.1).

Unfortunately, all chemotherapy drugs produce side effects; these vary both in severity and according to the predominant types of target cell. Toxicity limits both the dose and the frequency of administration and may reduce the potential to cure some patients. Historically, effects on the bone marrow were of most concern but the recent availability of haemopoietic growth factors, stem cell support and improved protocols of care with newer antibiotics have reduced concerns about myelosuppression. Gastrointestinal toxicity has increasingly become a clinical problem and frequently limits the amount of chemotherapy that can be given. High-dose chemotherapy with bone marrow or stem cell support is now frequently used in the treatment of haematological and solid tumours, and in these

situations gastrointestinal toxicity is of great concern as it causes severe morbidity for the patients and occasional mortality. It may be further complicated by graft-versus-host-disease (GVHD), which can follow allogeneic bone marrow transplantation.

A review of all the individual cytotoxic drugs and their effects on the gut is beyond the scope of this book. This chapter describes the general issues associated with these agents and discusses the role of the gastroenterologist and nutrition team in the care of patients who receive them, with special reference to patients having a bone marrow or stem cell transplant.

MECHANISMS OF ACTION OF CYTOTOXIC DRUGS

Malignant cells exhibit four main characteristics that distinguish them from their normal counterparts. Their proliferation is uncontrolled and although its rate may not be greater than that of normal cells, it is continuous, resulting in ever-increasing cell numbers.[2] Malignant cells lack normal function and they are able to invade surrounding tissue and form distant metastases.

Table 5.1 – Use of chemotherapy in adult neoplasia

Tumour type	Aim of treatment	Outcome
Hodgkin's disease	Cure	>85% 5-year survival stage I/II
		>50% 5-year survival stage III/IV
		Median survival 7–10 years
Leukaemia	Cure	Depends on type
		30–50% 5-year survival
Lung		
• small cell limited	Cure	20% 2-year survival
• small cell extensive	Palliation	Median survival 10 months
• non-small cell	Palliation	Median survival 10 months
Colon/rectal		
• localized	Cure	50% 5-year survival
• metastatic	Palliation	Median survival 14 months
Breast		
• localized	Cure	>60% 5-year survival
• metastatic	Palliation	Median survival 14 months
Gastric cancer, metastatic	Palliation	Median survival 6–8 months
Pancreatic cancer, inoperable	Palliation	Median survival 6 months
Ovarian cancer		
• early stage	Cure/palliation	75% 5-year survival
• advanced stage	Prolongation of survival	Median survival 18 months

Anticancer drugs exert their effects in a limited number of ways and lead to damage to cells. Their benefit results from the fact that repair of damage is more rapid in normal than malignant cells, such that intermittent administration will lead to a steady reduction in the malignant population while, it is hoped, leaving the population of normal cells relatively unchanged.[3] Most cytotoxic drugs interfere with DNA or protein synthesis but other mechanisms of action are increasingly utilised as rational drug development attempts to target specific differences in malignant cells but leave normal cells relatively spared (Fig. 5.1). Cytotoxic drugs are often classified, according to their mechanisms of action, into several groups.

Alkylating agents. These drugs bind covalently with DNA, interfering with its replication. Examples include the nitrogen mustards, cyclophosphamide, melphalan and chlorambucil.

Antimetabolites. These block metabolic pathways involved with DNA synthesis. They include the folate antagonist, methotrexate, and pyrimidine analogues such as 5-fluorouracil and cytosine arabinoside.

Cytotoxic antibiotics. These agents are among the most commonly used in oncology and are derived from microbes. They have pleiotropic effects, including alkylating activity and inhibition of topoisomerases. Examples include the anthracyclines doxorubicin and daunorubicin.

Agents that target the mitotic spindle. Most drugs in this class are derived from plants. They exert their action through alteration of microtubule function and thereby interfere with mitosis. Vincristine and vinblastine disrupt the mitotic spindle; newer agents, which include the taxanes, prevent microtubule disassembly.

Topoisomerase inhibitors. These agents inhibit either topoisomerase 1 or 2 and thereby prevent DNA replication. Etoposide and irinotecan are important examples of this class of compound.

Hormones. Glucocorticoids such as prednisolone and dexamethasone are frequently incorporated into cancer chemotherapy regimens. They exert a direct antitumour effect in most lymphoid malignancies and reduce inflammatory responses to tumours. They are also widely utilised to reduce nausea and vomiting. Some steroid-based hormones are used to treat specific tumours, e.g. prostatic malignancy.

Hormone antagonists. Hormonal antagonists such as tamoxifen may be used to treat hormone-responsive tumours, which include breast and prostatic malignancies. These agents have a favourable therapeutic ratio causing minimal normal tissue toxicity.

Differentiation and immune modifiers. Some drugs, such as retinoic acid, exert their effect by altering the cellular response to certain stimuli and promote differentiation of malignant cells. Other agents, including α-interferon, may promote an immune response to some malignancies and lead to cell death and tumour regression.

Miscellaneous drugs. A number of cytotoxic agents exist which do not easily fit into a specific classification but promote cell death by a variety of mechanisms, many of which are still poorly understood. These agents include the platinum derivatives, cisplatin and carboplatin, procarbazine and hydroxyurea.

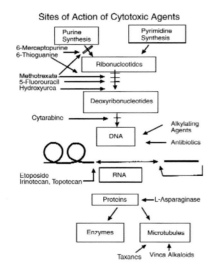

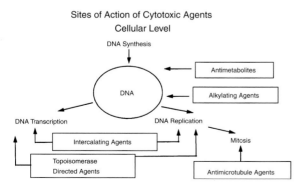

Figure 5.1 – Sites of action of cytotoxic agents.

Chemotherapy is rarely prescribed as a single agent, but usually takes the form of combination regimens, which are administered intermittently rather than on a continuous basis. When combinations are used, individual agents are chosen on the basis of having different mechanisms of action and, preferably, different patterns of toxicity.[4]

EFFECT OF CHEMOTHERAPY ON NORMAL TISSUES

Cytotoxic agents generally have greater toxicity for cells that have higher rates of proliferation. Cell turnover varies between normal tissue types and is particularly high in the haemopoietic system and gastrointestinal tract. The effect of most cytotoxic drugs is not limited to malignant cells but is also seen in those normal cells that are undergoing division. It is the toxicity profile of individual drugs that is dose-limiting and governs how the agent is used.

The kinetics of chemotherapeutic agents frequently follow a dose-response curve similar to that seen with many drugs (Fig. 5.2a). The effects on normal tissues may be represented in similar graphs (Fig. 5.2b). The respective position of organs changes for different drugs. For tumour cell types in which cell death can be significantly increased with doses not limited by gut or other organ toxicity, the use of haemopoietic sparing techniques may offer significant improvement in survival rates (Fig. 5.2c). In cancers where tumour sensitivity is less than gut sensitivity to cytotoxic drugs, little benefit will be seen (Fig. 5.2d). The haemopoietic sparing techniques currently in use include treatment with haemopoietic growth factors, such as granulocyte colony-stimulating factor (G-CSF) and granulocyte-macrophage colony-stimulating factor (GM-CSF), and haemopoietic stem cell transplantation, which is discussed later in this chapter.

The bone marrow is exquisitely sensitive to chemotherapy, and even low doses can result in marked neutropenia and thrombocytopenia. With recent improvements in the ability to support patients successfully through myelosuppressive episodes, escalation in the dose of drugs administered has been possible.[5] It is anticipated that this will be reflected in an improvement in antitumour effect and prolonged survival times. This change in practice has heightened the impact of such treatment on the gut and focused attention on the gastrointestinal system.

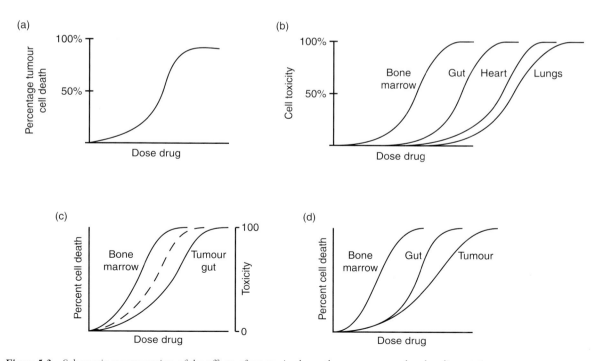

Figure 5.2 – Schematic representation of the effects of cytotoxic chemotherapy on normal and malignant tissue.

THE EFFECT OF CHEMOTHERAPY ON THE GASTROINTESTINAL TRACT

Anorexia, cachexia and malnutrition may be prominent presenting features of malignancy, causing morbidity and mortality in patients who have advanced disease.[6] Treatment of the malignancy with chemotherapy can worsen the cachexia and malnutrition, further compromising the nutritional status of the patient.[7] The undifferentiated cells of the small intestine have a high proliferative potential and it is these that are most damaged by cytotoxic drugs.[8] The antimetabolites, such as cytosine arabinoside and methotrexate, have been shown to block DNA synthesis in the gastrointestinal epithelium of animals and humans within a few hours of exposure.[9]

The effects of chemotherapy on the gastrointestinal system are wide-ranging and can be divided into several categories:

1. nausea and vomiting

2. direct cytotoxic effect on the mucosal cells of the intestine

3. motility effects due to damage to the innervation of the gut

4. damage to mucin production and reduced production of other intestinal secretions

5. effects on the liver with consequent alteration in the absorption of nutrients in the small intestine.

Nausea and vomiting

The nausea and vomiting induced by chemotherapy occurs when the vomiting centre in the medullary reticular formation is stimulated by the chemoreceptor trigger zone (CTZ) in the area postrema of the fourth ventricle.[10] Stimuli to the vomiting centre may also arise from afferent fibres located in the cerebral cortex, gastrointestinal tract (particularly the duodenum), heart, and vestibular apparatus. The CTZ is the predominant site of action initiating emesis caused by cytotoxic agents.

Nausea and vomiting are the most common early manifestations of the toxicity caused by chemotherapy, and repeated studies have shown them to be the most distressing side effects – more so than alopecia, for example.[11] If the patient is fit, there may be no serious consequences, but in those who are already debilitated or malnourished following surgery and/or radio-

therapy the addition of drug-related emesis may cause further marked deterioration in the clinical condition unless intensive nutrition support is provided.

Different chemotherapy drugs vary markedly in their emetogenic potential.[12] Nitrogen mustard, cisplatin, dacarbazine and streptozotocin induce vomiting in all patients, whereas oral chlorambucil, melphalan and busulfan usually produce little nausea and vomiting. Nausea and vomiting induced by antimetabolite drugs often depends on dose and schedule. Methotrexate given in conventional doses rarely produces vomiting whereas high-dose infusions given to patients with osteosarcoma or to prevent CNS disease in lymphoma and leukaemia cause vomiting in the majority of patients. 5-Fluorouracil causes minimal toxicity when given as a single weekly bolus, but when it is administered on 5 consecutive days, as is common in North America, it produces vomiting in up to 90% of patients.[13]

In most patients, emesis commences within 1–6 hours of administration and subsides after 24–36 hours. Occasionally, delayed emesis may occur 24 or more hours after administration and may persist for up to a week. Less frequently, chronic nausea and vomiting may follow chemotherapy and can be particularly difficult to treat. Once patients have experienced nausea and vomiting they may develop similar anticipatory symptoms before subsequent courses of treatment.

The management of emesis caused by chemotherapy has improved dramatically in the last 10 years. The availability of serotonin antagonists including ondansetron and granisetron combined with dexamethasone has resulted in excellent control in the majority of patients, even with the most emetogenic regimens.[14] Metoclopramide with or without steroids is used for less emetogenic agents. The aim of therapy should be to prevent emesis from the first course in order to avoid subsequent anticipatory symptoms.

Direct cytotoxic effects on the mucosal cells of the intestine

A direct effect on mucosal cells can affect any part of the bowel and may severely compromise dietary intake. The antimetabolites and anthracycline antibiotics are the agents that most commonly damage the gastrointestinal mucosa. Symptoms usually occur 5–7 days after exposure and may last for 1–2 weeks.

The degree of damage varies according to the dose and schedule of administration of many of these drugs.

The toxicity of methotrexate to the gastrointestinal epithelium, for example, depends on the duration of exposure rather than on peak concentrations.[15] Toxicity may be increased if there are effusions but can be reduced if folinic acid rescue is given within 42 hours of administration.[16] Prior irradiation injury may worsen the effect.

5-Fluorouracil is one of the most commonly used anticancer drugs and is given to patients with malignancies involving the gastrointestinal tract and breast. If given on a daily schedule for 5 consecutive days it can produce severe mucosal damage, resulting in profound mucositis and leading to bloody diarrhoea.[17] Patients who develop this are profoundly unwell and require intensive support. Mortality may result from septicaemia and renal failure. When this agent is given on a once-weekly basis, on the other hand, gastrointestinal toxicity is rare.[18]

Even when mucosal damage is relatively mild, serious morbidity may ensue. Local infection with organisms such as *Candida* and herpes virus, particularly in the mouth, may cause pain and reduce subsequent oral intake, further compromising the patient's nutritional status.[19] It is essential that the clinician is aware of this and that advice is given about topical mouth care with the provision, where appropriate, of antifungal and antiviral therapy. For some patients, intravenous nutrition support may be indicated if pain prevents swallowing.

Motility effects resulting from damage to the innervation of the gut

The vinca alkaloids (particularly vincristine) frequently cause autonomic nerve dysfunction leading to colicky abdominal pain and constipation.[20] Occasionally an ileus may occur, especially in elderly patients, and can be fatal.[21] The onset of symptoms usually occurs soon after drug administration, frequently within 3 days, and may be associated with peripheral neuropathy. Up to one-third of patients receiving vincristine may develop constipation, the incidence rising as the cumulative dose increases.[22] It is important to provide prophylactic laxatives. Patients who develop an ileus should be managed conservatively with careful monitoring of fluid balance.

Malabsorption

Preclinical data from animals exposed to chemotherapy have revealed frequent observations of structural changes in the small intestine with associated malabsorption and decreased disaccharidase activity.[23] In one study, patients receiving single-agent methotrexate underwent a small intestinal biopsy.[24] Ultrastructural changes were seen, including swollen mitochondria and abnormalities of the Golgi apparatus and endoplasmic reticulum. A reduction in serum vitamin B_{12} and xylose absorption has also been demonstrated in patients receiving L-asparaginase and methotrexate respectively.[25,26] The mitotic count within crypts appears to reduce markedly during chemotherapy and to recover to pretreatment levels during the same period that haematological recovery occurs. This effect has been shown to be associated with malabsorption in some studies,[27] although results are variable and may be a manifestation of the underlying cachexia syndrome associated with many malignancies rather than a direct effect of the chemotherapy.

EFFECTS OF CHEMOTHERAPY ON RADIATION TOXICITY

The use of radiotherapy in patients who are also receiving chemotherapeutic agents must be carefully considered as damage to normal tissue can be significantly increased.[28] Damage to all tissues may be increased but the skin and mucous membranes are most susceptible. Doxorubicin is most frequently implicated, but enhancement of irradiation injury to the oesophagus and gastrointestinal tract has also been reported with actinomycin D, bleomycin, 5-fluorouracil and vinblastine.[29] Although enhancement of toxicity is greater when both chemotherapy and radiotherapy are given concomitantly, actinomycin D and doxorubicin may produce a 'recall phenomenon'. This may occur at a site that has previously been irradiated when one of these drugs is given weeks or months later.[30] The dose of radiotherapy must be carefully monitored in this situation to avoid severe toxicity. The site most frequently affected is the oesophagus, particularly when radiotherapy is given for lung cancer with concurrent combination chemotherapy that includes doxorubicin. Severe oesophagitis may occur and result in a stricture.

The combination of chemotherapy with abdominal radiotherapy, for example for pelvic malignancy, may result in severe acute enteritis. Small bowel obstruction may follow. Doxorubicin, actinomycin D and 5-fluorouracil produce the most severe gastrointestinal toxicity.

NUTRITION SUPPORT

Under-nutrition (protein–energy malnutrition) is common in patients with malignancy and may produce a syndrome termed 'cancer cachexia'.[31] This appears to be mediated by a variety of cytokines: TNF-α is frequently implicated.[32] It most often affects proteins and calories, but deficiencies of vitamins and trace minerals are common.[33] Studies have demonstrated a relationship between weight loss and a lower chance of responding to treatment.[34] In order to improve the ability of patients to tolerate the toxicity of therapies and thereby improve survival, several groups have reported the results of trials examining the role of nutrition support in patients with malignant disease.[35–37] Five-year survival rates may be up to 50% lower for patients with weight loss at the time of diagnosis compared with those who have retained their previous weight.[38]

Metabolic abnormalities in patients with cancer cachexia have been reported to include marked alterations of lipid, carbohydrate and protein metabolism.[39] Energy stores are diminished and total body water is increased. Of particular interest is the marked reduction of glutamine levels in patients with cancer cachexia.[40] Malignant cells extract glutamine with higher efficiency than any other cell in the body and this may affect normal protein synthesis.[41]

The observation that cancer cachexia leads to significant morbidity and may worsen mortality has led several centres to evaluate the use of aggressive nutrition support during administration of chemotherapy.[42–47] Unfortunately, trials to date have revealed conflicting results and none has shown significant survival benefits for patients receiving either parenteral or enteral nutrition. Gastrointestinal toxicity has been improved in two randomised studies [42,43] but was worse in one.[44]

Although many trials have not demonstrated a clear benefit for enteral nutrition in cancer patients, most of these have, unfortunately, been poorly designed. Nutrition support should be considered for patients with cachexia and increasing weight loss if aggressive therapy is to be offered. Enteral nutrition is the preferred form of feeding if the gastrointestinal tract is functional and may be achieved by the use of nasogastric tubes or gastrostomy or jejunostomy feeding catheters. Parenteral nutrition (PN) should only be used in selected patients (Box 5.1). The indications for PN may include severely malnourished patients who are responding to chemotherapy and in whom gastro-

---

Box 5.1 – Reasons for giving parenteral nutrition to patients with malignancy (a predicted 'long' survival with a good quality of life is desirable before starting parenteral nutrition)

Gastrointestinal toxicity (mucositis/enterocolitis)
Bowel obstruction
Prolonged ileus
High-output enterocutaneous fistula
Malabsorption
Graft-versus-host-disease (GVHD)

---

intestinal or other toxicities preclude adequate enteral intake for more than one week. PN may also be considered for patients whose severe cachexia is the primary reason for failure of restoration of performance status and in whom treatment-associated toxicities prevent the use of enteral nutrition. There should be a reasonable expectation that antitumour therapy will produce a response and improve survival. Some patients may develop diffuse intra-abdominal malignancy and this may cause malabsorption or obstruction. The decision to provide PN for such patients depends primarily on the underlying tumour type and the likelihood of it responding to chemotherapy. Chemoresponsive diseases such as germ cell tumours, lymphomas and ovarian cancers may reduce rapidly in volume with chemotherapy, and recovery can be enhanced by a period of PN. Similarly, patients who have developed severe, prolonged mucositis and enterocolitis as a result of radiotherapy may benefit from support with PN. For patients who are markedly malnourished and, as a result, are felt to be poor risks for chemotherapy, the use of enteral nutrition should be considered as the improvement in nutritional status may allow its subsequent use. There is no evidence that PN is superior to enteral nutrition in the majority of such patients.

The use of PN in the peri-operative setting has been examined in several studies and, again, conflicting results have been obtained. Patients seem to benefit from PN after the development of a prolonged ileus following an abdominal procedure: if the patient has been unable to resume oral intake 7 days after surgery, PN may be considered. Lean body mass may be maintained as a result, improving quality of life and allowing a more rapid return to normal activities.[44]

Cancer patients who undergo multiple bowel resections may develop the problems of a short bowel. Prolonged home PN may be required for those patients who are potentially cured by their surgery (e.g. desmoid disease) (Ch. 26). Several different formulations of PN solutions are available and have been used in trials in cancer patients.

SPECIFIC NUTRITIONAL PROBLEM

Chylous ascites or chylothorax

Chylous ascites or a chylous pleural effusion most commonly results from malignancy, especially lymphoma.[48,49] A chylous leak can also result from surgery or radiotherapy,[50] and is also relatively common after an abdominal aortic aneurysm repair[51] or an anterior spinal operation.[52] The leak can be from the thoracic duct, cisterna chyli or its intestinal tributaries. Normally, about 1.5–2.0 litres of chyle pass through the thoracic duct each day (about 90 ml/h fasting and 230 ml/h after a meal); its movement is dependent upon the negative intrathoracic pressure, with backflow being prevented by valves. Chyle is a milky, odourless alkaline fluid containing at least 200 kcal/l. It contains protein of an amount greater than 30 g/l, which is about half that of the plasma, lipid which is mostly triglyceride 4–40 g/l, though there is some cholesterol and phospholipid, and cells which are predominantly lymphocytes. To confirm that a fluid is chylous the protein content should be more than half that of plasma, the lipid content should be greater than that of plasma, and fat globules and predominantly lymphocytes should be seen on microscopy.

The initial principles of treating a chylous leak are to slow the production of chyle, to prevent pulmonary or vascular complications caused by increased intra-abdominal pressure or lung compression, and to maintain the patient's nutritional status. If the leak does not close spontaneously, the site of the leak may be localised and surgical or radiological methods used to try and stop it. Chylous flow can be reduced by giving a high-protein diet that is low in fat but contains medium-chain triglycerides (MCT); an MCT with a short chain length (C8) is less likely to appear in the ascites or effusion than one of a longer length (C10).[53] MCT may be given in enteral feeding. Total parenteral nutrition with no oral intake is also effective but entails the risks associated with parenteral nutrition. Other medical treatments that have been tried include subcutaneous octreotide[54] and intravenous etilefrine (a sympathomimetic drug).[55] A high intra-abdominal pressure may help to reduce chylous flow and thus drainage is only necessary if major problems (usually respiratory) are occurring. If the leak continues for longer than a month, a lymphangiogram may be done to help localise it. Surgery can be performed to ligate the thoracic duct or lymphatic vessels. A leaking lymphatic duct can also be obliterated by cisterna chyli puncture and microcoil embolisation.[56] Peritoneovenous shunting has been performed but is complicated by shunt occlusion because of the viscosity of chyle; sepsis and disseminated intravascular coagulation are also common.

BONE MARROW AND HAEMOPOIETIC STEM CELL TRANSPLANTATION (HSCT)

The potential of cytotoxic drugs to kill cancer cells is dose-limited by toxicity to vital organs, in particular the bone marrow. The administration of much higher doses of chemotherapy and radiotherapy to achieve a higher cancer cell kill rate is made possible by the use of haemopoietic stem cell transplantation or 'rescue'. The use of HSCT is associated with profound effects on the gastrointestinal tract.

Gastroenterologists and the nutrition team are frequently involved in the management of such complications. The aim of this section is to provide the gastroenterology team with a practical understanding of HSCT (see Box 5.2), its gastrointestinal complications and their management (see Box 5.4). Further details of HSCT can be obtained from larger texts and reviews.[57–59]

Terminology

There are three types of HSCT:

1. Allogeneic HSCT, in which stem cells are transplanted from a donor to a recipient. The donor may be a relative, usually an HLA-matched sibling, or a matched unrelated donor (MUD) from a panel such as the Anthony Nolan Bone Marrow Trust. Graft-versus-host disease (GVHD), effectively 'rejection in reverse', is a common sequel to allogeneic HSCT. It may be defined as acute or chronic and has a spectrum of severity from subclinical to life-threatening. The combination of GVHD and slow immune reconstitution largely explain the relatively high treatment-related morbidity and mortality (10–50%) associated with allogeneic HSCT. Allogeneic HSCT may also be complicated by graft rejection mediated by residual host lymphocytes.

2. Autologous HSCT, in which the patient's own stem and progenitor cells are used for haemopoietic rescue after high-dose chemotherapy and/or radiotherapy. Although not strictly a form of transplantation, the procedure follows similar principles to allogeneic HSCT. Autologous HSCT is not associated with GVHD or significant risk of graft rejection, and immune reconstitution is relatively quick. Overall, the treatment-related mortality is 3–5%. The stages of an autologous HSCT are summarised in Box 5.2.

Box 5.2 – Stages of an autologous peripheral blood stem cell transplant (timings of different stages are examples and not necessarily accurate for all procedures)

2–4 months before transplant
A double-lumen long-term central venous (Hickman-type line) catheter is
inserted (platelets $>50 \times 10^9/l$) and intermediate-dose chemotherapy is often given for several cycles to debulk disease. Ideally the patient should be in remission before stem cell harvest and transplant.

1 month before transplant
Haemopoietic growth factors, e.g. granulocyte colony-stimulating factor (G-CSF), are given. Peripheral blood stem cells (CD34+) are harvested from peripheral blood using leucapheresis. They are then frozen in liquid nitrogen and may be stored for many years, if necessary.

−2 to −7 days
Conditioning with myeloablative dose of chemotherapy ± total body irradiation.

Day 0
Transplantation – infusion of haemopoietic stem cells via central catheter.

Day +5–15
Mucositis, diarrhoea and leucopenia.

Day +15 onwards
Recovery expected with resumption of a normal oral intake providing there are no other complications.

Day +30 onwards
Removal of central line.

1–18 months
Immunity gradually restored.

Syngeneic HSCT. This is occasionally performed when identical twin donors are available.

Sources of haemopoietic stem cells (HSC)

HSC may be obtained from:

1. Bone marrow obtained by direct aspiration from the iliac crests and sternum under general anaesthetic.

2. Peripheral blood stem cells (PBSC) obtained following the administration of recombinant haemopoietic cytokines (usually G-CSF) with or without chemotherapy and collected with a cell separator machine ('leucapheresis'). In addition to the avoidance of a general anaesthetic and pain related to harvesting, PBSC have important advantages over bone marrow including faster neutrophil and platelet recovery and improved immune reconstitution.

3. Umbilical cord blood, which is rich in haemopoietic progenitors. This use has been largely restricted to paediatric patients because of the relatively small numbers of HSC available.

Indications for HSCT

Malignancy is the indication for the majority of patients undergoing HSCT (Box 5.3). Both autologous

---

Box 5.3 – Indications for haemopoietic stem cell transplantation

Malignant disease
Acute myeloid leukaemia
Acute lymphoblastic leukaemia
Chronic myeloid leukaemia
Non-Hodgkin's lymphoma
Hodgkin's disease
Myeloma
Neuroblastoma

Bone marrow or immune failure
Severe aplastic anaemia
Severe combined immunodeficiency

Haemoglobinopathies
Thalassaemia major
Sickle cell disease

Other (developmental)
Autoimmune diseases
Solid tumours (teratoma, breast)

---

and allogeneic HSCT are routinely used in a number of conditions depending on the type of tumour, the age of the patient, and donor availability. Other indications include diseases that affect the haemopoietic stem cell population such as thalassaemia, aplastic anaemia and severe combined immune deficiency. In these conditions, allogeneic HSCT is the only therapeutic option. There is also increasing interest in the use of autologous HSCT in patients with severe autoimmune and inflammatory disorders such as multiple sclerosis, rheumatoid arthritis, scleroderma and systemic lupus erythematosus.

Conditioning

The conditioning therapy or preparative regimen, which is common to all types of transplant procedure, has several roles:

- to reduce or eradicate the abnormal cell population
- to 'make space' within the bone marrow for the new cells to grow
- to immunosuppress the patient to prevent graft rejection.

Following conditioning, the peripheral blood counts fall dramatically and a period of pancytopenia follows which lasts between 7 and 28 days depending on the type of transplant and source of stem cells. Supportive measures to prevent anaemia, bleeding and infection are important. Other potential complications arise from the toxicity of the conditioning regimens and may occur early or late following transplant.

Principles of the HSCT procedure

1. Consideration of the patient for HSCT.

2. Assessment of patient suitability:
   - understanding procedure and consent
   - fitness to undergo the procedure, e.g. respiratory and renal reserve
   - treatment of identified problems
   - attention to nutritional aspects.

3. Development of an individual patient transplant protocol.

4. Pre-transplant conditioning therapy: chemotherapy with or without radiotherapy, i.e. total body irradiation, total lymphoid irradiation, irradiation to sites of bulk disease.

5. Infusion of HSC.

6. Post-transplant care, immediate and long-term.

Gastrointestinal complications of HSCT

From a practical point of view, the gastrointestinal complications of HSCT (Box 5.4) can be divided into early (before 2–3 weeks) and late (after 2–3 weeks). The early complications relate largely to the effect of high-dose cytotoxic therapy on the gastrointestinal tract and therefore are similar for both autologous and allogeneic HSCT. The late complications are more common in allogeneic transplantation, with the occurrence of graft-versus-host disease and slow immune reconstitution.

Box 5.4 – Gastrointestinal effects of HSCT

Before transplant
Poor nutritional status
Infections (herpes simplex, hepatitis C, bacterial overgrowth)

Conditioning
Emesis (Mallory–Weiss tears)
Oesophagitis

After transplant
1–3 weeks
Delayed emesis
Infections: viral (e.g. hepatitis), bacterial or fungal
Mucositis
Ileus
Bleeding
Cholestasis secondary to drugs (e.g. cyclosporin A)

>2–3 weeks
Nausea, vomiting, anorexia
Long-term diarrhoea (malabsorption or disaccharidase deficiency)
GVHD
Opportunistic infections (fungal, herpes and cytomegalovirus)
Gallstones
Iron overload
Poor saliva production
Reduced/altered taste sensation

Early complications

Nausea and vomiting. As discussed earlier in relation to standard-dose cytotoxic therapy, nausea and vomiting may accompany HSCT. Particular attention must be paid to antiemetic therapy as high doses of cytotoxic therapy are given prior to HSCT. Serotonin antagonists are routinely used and are usually supplemented with metoclopramide and dexamethasone. The latter is useful in controlling the delayed emesis associated with drugs such as cyclophosphamide and may be continued for several days after the therapy is stopped.

Other medications commonly used following HSCT may also be associated with nausea. These include antibiotics such as nystatin, co-trimoxazole and imipenem and GVHD prophylaxis with cyclosporine and methotrexate.

Opportunistic infections of the oesophagus and stomach may lead to nausea and vomiting. Although such infections are often prevented in many patients with the routine use of prophylactic antifungal and antiviral drugs, upper gastrointestinal endoscopy may confirm herpetic or candidal infections in the early post-transplant period. Nausea is a common accompaniment of systemic sepsis, especially if the patient is hypotensive.

Problems lower in the gastrointestinal tract may result in nausea and vomiting. Obstruction is rare, but ileus may follow electrolyte imbalance, sepsis or use of drugs such as opiates.

Mucositis. Mucositis is an inevitable complication of the intense cytotoxic regimens and may be better referred to as mucosal barrier injury.[60] The entire gastrointestinal tract may be affected, although symptoms arise principally in the mouth, pharynx and upper oesophagus as pain and dysphagia, and in the lower gastrointestinal tract as diarrhoea, bloating, pain and perianal (and vaginal) soreness.

There are four phases: inflammatory, epithelial, ulcerative and healing. The oral mucosa is white and areas of slough may be seen. Distinct ulcers are common but should be swabbed to exclude super-added infections, especially of viral origin. Bleeding may occur into these areas and so platelet support is a vital part of the supportive care. Pain is less commonly associated with the stomach and intestinal damage but diarrhoea, nausea, bloating and ileus are common manifestations. Bleeding is an unusual but potentially very serious side effect. During this period most patients will often be unable to swallow fluids or solids.

Management of mucositis is predominantly aimed at symptom control and prevention of infections. Use of analgesic mouthwashes is often followed by topical measures such as lignocaine lozenges, but ultimately many patients depend on opiate analgesia given orally or as an infusion. Patient-controlled analgesia is often usefully employed. Diarrhoea is controlled with the careful use of antidiarrhoeals such as loperamide and codeine phosphate, although it is important to exclude infection before these are prescribed. The risks of infection occurring with breakdown of mucosal barriers are reduced with antiseptic mouthwashes and, in many units, antibiotics such as colistin and ciprofloxacin, antifungals such as nystatin and fluconazole, and antivirals such as acyclovir are used for gut decontamination and systemic prophylaxis. A number of approaches have been employed to modify locally the effect of cytotoxic therapy on the mouth including ice, saliva reduction (e.g. hyoscine) and prostaglandins, although their role remains unclear. Novel agents, such as keratinocyte growth factor, interleukin 11 and the chemoprotectant amifostine, are under investigation.[61,62]

As a consequence of the mucositis and neutropenia, infections are common. Bacteria cross the damaged mucosal barrier, quiescent viral infections (e.g. herpes simplex or cytomegalovirus) may reactivate, and fungal overgrowth (e.g. Candida) may occur. The time to heal will vary depending on conditioning protocol, the general fitness and nutritional status of the patient, and the nature of any infections that occur, but is usually within 2–3 weeks. Once healed, most patients complain that the mucosa of their mouth feels 'thin' and they are unable to tolerate alcohol or spicy food for about 6–12 months. There is also a loss of taste, which takes 6–12 weeks to recover. Those patients who have undergone total body irradiation have the added complication of reduced salivary secretion. The saliva produced is thick and does not function. Disaccharidase deficiency in the small bowel may persist.

Infective and neutropenic colitis. The differential diagnosis of diarrhoea in the early post-transplant period is complex, and several pathologies may exist concomitantly. Infective colitis may occur in the early post-transplant period but, given that patients are usually nursed in isolation with a 'clean food' or 'neutropenic' diet, the incidence of organisms traditionally associated with 'food poisoning' is low. The precise nature of clean food diets differs between institutions, but generally consists of freshly cooked food and avoidance of salads, unfresh and reheated food. An example is given in Table 5.2. In the past, food for neutropenic patients was often irradiated, although many centres no longer regard this as necessary.

The use of broad-spectrum antibiotics means that *Clostridium difficile* infection is relatively common. This presents as watery diarrhoea, often with a high pyrexia, in the neutropenic patient. Treatment is with metronidazole as a first-line agent, oral vancomycin being reserved for the more resistant cases (to reduce the generation of vancomycin-resistant enterococci).

Neutropenic colitis (also known as ileocaecal syndrome or 'typhlitis') is a rare complication thought to be caused by direct bacterial invasion of the colonic or caecal mucosa, resulting in a toxic mucosal necrosis.[63] The patient complains of symptoms of pain and tenderness in the right iliac fossa. Treatment is principally supportive with broad-spectrum antibiotics, limited oral intake and growth factors to tide the patient over until neutrophil recovery occurs. In severe cases, megacolon and perforation can occur. Surgical intervention with subtotal colectomy and defunctioning colostomy may be necessary although the risks will naturally be high in such patients. In some cases, clostridial super-infection may produce a necrotising fasciitis requiring surgical intervention, high-dose penicillin and hyperbaric oxygen therapy.

Gastrointestinal bleeding. Patients may be profoundly thrombocytopenic for at least 14 days and for up to several weeks post transplant. During this period they are dependent on platelet transfusions to maintain platelet counts above $10–20 \times 10^9/l$. These levels usually prevent spontaneous bleeding if the patient is stable; however, they are often insufficient if the patient is unstable or has an injury. Following HSCT, the potential for such injuries to the gastro-intestinal tract is high. Complications such as mucositis, drug- or stress-induced upper gastro-intestinal ulceration or infections may be followed by bleeding. In addition, patients may have clinically silent lesions such as gastric erosions or haemorrhoids, which become clinically more significant with thrombo-cytopenia. Management includes platelet transfusion followed by appropriate investigation and management including endoscopy.

Hepatic complications.

Veno-occlusive disease (VOD). VOD is a serious complication of high-dose cytotoxic therapy, usually occurring within the first 3 weeks after HSCT.[64] The diagnosis is based on a clinical syndrome of jaundice, weight gain, ascites and tender hepatomegaly. Severe VOD is associated with multi-organ failure and high mortality. The pathogenesis is considered to be endothelial damage in hepatic venules that leads to thrombotic obstruction and damage to zone 3 of the liver acinus. Treatment is largely supportive with strict fluid balance, diuretics and pain control. Use of systemic anticoagulants such as heparin and defibrotide may reduce the thrombotic element.

Infections. Fungal infections of the liver may reactivate during and after HSCT and present with liver dysfunction, liver tenderness and antibiotic-resistant fever. Candida species is the most common cause. The diagnosis may be established using a variety of approaches including ultrasound and CT scanning and ultimately liver biopsy. In practice, the diagnosis is often presumptive and empirical treatment with the broad-spectrum antifungal, amphotericin, is instituted. The widespread use of fluconazole prophylaxis has made candidal liver infection relatively rare in current practice. CMV and other viral infections tend to occur later in HSCT, but may complicate the early course of HSCT.

Drugs and therapeutics. The list of drugs and therapeutic agents that cause liver dysfunction is exhaustive, but conditioning regimens, cyclosporin A, methotrexate, antifungals, antibiotics and parenteral nutrition are commonly incriminated. Lipid-containing parenteral nutrition is contraindicated in patients with severe cholestasis.

Complications beyond 2–3 weeks

Later gastrointestinal complications of HSCT are largely restricted to those patients who have undergone allogeneic transplantation. Such patients are immunosuppressed and their slower immune reconstitution predisposes them to infection and reactivation of opportunistic agents. They are also at risk of acute and chronic GVHD.

Infective problems. A variety of cellular and humoral mechanisms of immunity are reduced following HSCT. Following autologous HSCT, immune reconstitution takes place relatively quickly with a return to near normality within 12–18 months. The process of immune reconstitution following allogeneic HSCT is prolonged and complex and is dependent on donor–recipient compatibility, the age of the patient, and the presence and degree of GVHD. In addition, measures such as T-cell depletion of the graft and drugs used to prevent and treat GVHD may reduce immune recovery. Perturbed immune reconstitution following

HSCT predisposes patients to the long-term risk of both standard and opportunistic gastrointestinal infections.[65–67] A 'clean food diet', incorporating cooked as opposed to raw or reheated foods, is recommended for the first 6 months after allogeneic HSCT (Table 5.2).

In the first several months, the allogeneic HSCT recipient is predisposed to cytomegalovirus infection (CMV), especially if the patient or donor is serologically positive for CMV. CMV infection may have a variety of presentations, but commonly involves the oesophagus, stomach, small intestine and colon, causing pain, fever, protein-losing enteropathy, ulceration, bleeding and occasionally perforation. CMV infection may also cause hepatitis. Other infections include herpes simplex, adenovirus, enterovirus, Cryptosporium and Candida. Endoscopic biopsies are often important to differentiate these infections from GVHD, particularly as the treatments are diametrically opposed. Treatment requires use of specific antibiotic agents, if available, along with supportive measures.

Acute GVHD. Acute GVHD principally affects three organ systems: the skin, the liver and the gastrointestinal tract.[68] Its onset is usually within 2–3 weeks of the allogeneic transplant. Biopsies show lymphocytic infiltration in the crypts with pyknotic stem cells in the epithelial layer. The severity may range from scattered cell necrosis to complete denudation of gut epithelium. Negative nitrogen balance may result from exudative diarrhoea and is compounded by the catabolic effects of large doses of steroids used to treat GVHD.

Acute GVHD rarely involves the mouth and oesophagus, but may be responsible for stomatitis, glossitis and dysphagia. Upper gastrointestinal acute GVHD causes nausea, vomiting, anorexia, dyspepsia and food intolerance due to involvement of the stomach and duodenum, which may be confirmed with endoscopic biopsy. Acute GVHD of the bowel presents with diarrhoea, which is characteristically watery green in nature. The severity varies from stage 1 (<500 ml diarrhoea/24 h), stage 2 (500–1000 ml diarrhoea/24 h), to stage 3 (1000–1500 ml diarrhoea/ 24 h) stage 4 (ileus or acute abdominal pain). Bleeding may be a significant problem and usually portends a poor prognosis. The diagnosis may be made clinically in the context of acute GVHD at other sites, although ideally it should be confirmed with endoscopic biopsies; infective causes of colitis such as CMV should be excluded. The liver is commonly involved with acute GVHD, and destruction of small bile ducts may lead to severe cholestasis. Bilirubin concentration and alkaline phosphatase levels are most commonly elevated, and there is impairment of other liver function tests. The clinical presentation ranges from asymptomatic to fulminant liver failure.

Treatment of acute GVHD usually involves resting the gut, traditionally by giving parenteral nutrition, and appropriate use of immunosuppression depending on the overall stage and other organ involvement. Food is poorly absorbed, drives the diarrhoea, may be associated with atypical infection (CMV), and gives a false sense of security. Upper gastrointestinal GVHD is often sensitive to low doses of prednisolone or methylprednisolone, e.g. 1 mg/kg. Lower gut GVHD may respond to similar doses but severe disease usually requires escalation to 2 mg/kg. Oral budesonide has been used as a topical steroid-sparing agent. Refractory disease may be treated with pulsed methylprednisolone 10–15 mg/kg and the addition of antibody-based anti-T-cell therapies such as anti-lymphocyte globulin, anti-CD52 ('Campath®') and IL-2 receptor antibody. In view of the unpredictable absorption, drugs often have to be given intravenously. As the symptoms settle, immunosuppression and parenteral nutrition are gradually reduced, and eventually the introduction of a bland diet may be appropriate.

Chronic GVHD. Chronic GVHD is defined as GVHD that presents after post-transplant day 100.[68] It may evolve from acute GVHD or present *de novo*. It is a complex multisystem disorder with many features of autoimmune disorders such as scleroderma. Treatment often involves continued systemic immunosuppression combined with local or topical treatment where possible.

In the gastrointestinal tract, chronic GVHD may result in a number of problems. The mouth is commonly affected with xerostomia and painful stomatitis and glossitis, with characteristic white plaques. Dysphagia may lead to weight loss, and dental decay may be a problem. In the oesophagus, chronic GVHD may result in dysmotility, dysphagia and reflux. Chronic GVHD of the gut is characterised by mucosal atrophy, malabsorption and fibrosis, which may cause strictures and bacterial overgrowth. Chronic GVHD of the liver causes a range of problems from asymptomatic elevation of liver function tests to fulminant liver failure.

Treatment of chronic GVHD of the gut depends on whether the disease is limited to the gut or is more extensive. There is often a response to systemic immunosuppression, but in the long term the benefits have to be weighed against the risks. Topical immuno-suppression includes prednisolone mouthwash, the use of steroid inhalers in the mouth, and oral budesonide. Symptomatic measures include the use of artificial saliva, regular dental assessment, and dilatation or surgical resection of strictures. Specialised input may be required to investigate and treat malabsorption. Antibiotic treatment may be indicated for bacterial overgrowth. Specialised diets along with bile salt and pancreatic replacement may be indicated in certain patients.[66]

Other late effects. High-dose cytotoxic therapy and HSCT may have a number of other effects on the gastrointestinal tract. Chronic use of total parenteral nutrition is associated with gallbladder sludge, causing nausea and upper abdominal pain after the patient resumes eating. Iron overload from multiple transfusions may be a cause of persistently abnormal liver function tests. Iron overload is managed with venesection with the aim of normal-ising the serum ferritin level.[69] In cases where anaemia persists, the use of erythropoietin may be necessary to permit venesection, although iron chelation with desferrioxamine is an alternative. Epstein–Barr virus lymphoproliferative disease tends to occur in patients with mismatched or T-cell-depleted allografts or after prolonged immuno-suppression and may present with gastrointestinal or hepatosplenic disease, often with fever. The prognosis is usually poor but treatment may be attempted with steroids, chemotherapy, monoclonal antibodies or EBV-specific cytotoxic T-cells.

Nutrition support during HSCT

Nutrition support aims to prevent the occurrence of undernutrition and, if undernutrition has already occurred, to treat it. Matters to be addressed include why, when, via what route, what amount and what to give.

Why and when is nutrition support needed?

With its associated gastrointestinal complications, the process of HSCT is inevitably associated with varying degrees of nutritional depletion.[70] Most patients are well nourished at the start of therapy and the goal of nutrition support is to maintain nutritional status rather than to achieve nutritional repletion. Some patients may be malnourished, usually as a result of recent chemotherapy and sepsis. Nutritional problems arise from reduced food intake and absorption, increased losses of nutritional substrates and increased requirements. The process of HSCT causes significant abnormalities in metabolism of protein, energy and micronutrients. Negative nitrogen balance is com-monly caused by intestinal losses and the catabolic effects on skeletal muscle exerted initially by chemo-therapy and then by sepsis and GVHD. Vitamin deficiency may arise secondary to poor intake and malabsorption of both water- and lipid-soluble vitamins.

In a prospective randomised clinical trial, Weisdorf *et al.* compared outcome in 71 patients supported with parenteral nutrition (1.1–1.5 × calculated basal energy expenditure/day for 5 weeks, starting 1 week before the transplant) compared with 66 controls who received intravenous hydration. A significantly lower mortality at 2 years (50% vs. 65%) and an increased time to relapse and disease-free survival were reported.[71]

Consideration should be given to nutritional matters, including referral to a dietitian/nutrition support team, early in the course of the transplant. As discussed in previous sections, a 'clean food diet' may be given to all neutropenic patients and continued for 6 months in patients receiving allogeneic HSCT (Table 5.2). Long-term dietetic input is often neces-sary in patients with chronic nutritional problems such as GVHD.

By what route should nutrition support be given?

Policies on supplementary nutrition vary between centres. In many centres, patients undergoing HSCT have routinely been fed by PN. PN is reasonably easy to administer as patients usually have a central line; it also offers a number of possible advantages including reliable delivery of nutrients where enteral absorption may be impaired and easier modulation of fluid and electrolyte balance. However, there is now a tendency towards increasing use of enteral nutrition (EN) because of recent advances in HSCT, such as the use of peripheral blood stem cells and mini-allografting, which have resulted in reduced duration of neutropenia and mucosal toxicity.

Table 5.2 – Example of a 'clean diet'

Type of food	Suitable	Unsuitable
Water	Boiled tap water/bottled	Plain tap water
Milk	Fresh pasteurised milk	Unpasteurised milk
	Tinned milk/cream	Powdered milk
Meat	Any hot meat dish	Any cold meat dish
	Freshly opened tinned/vacuum-packed meat from small packs	Pate
		Takeaways
Fish	Any hot fish dish	Any cold fish
	Freshly opened tinned/vacuum-packed Fish from small packs	Shellfish
		Takeaways
Eggs	Hard boiled or firmly cooked eggs	Raw, poached or softly boiled eggs
Cheese	Any hot cooked cheese dish	Any cold cooked cheese dishes
	Individually wrapped cheese	Blue cheese
		Camembert cheese
Butter/margarine	Individually wrapped portions	Any other
Vegetables	All hot cooked vegetables	Raw vegetables/salad
Fruit	Tinned fruit, freshly opened	Dried fruit
	Hot stewed fruit	Cold stewed fruit
	Fresh washed and peeled fruit	
Puddings	All hot cooked puddings and custards	All cold puddings, cakes, mousses, blancmanges,
	UHT puddings	ice cream from parlours
	Yogurts/fromage frais	
	Individually packed ice cream/lollies	
Dried foods	Individual packs of breakfast cereals. Biscuits, cream crackers	Large packets
Bread	Fresh bread taken from the centre of newly opened packet	Any bread not freshly opened
Drinks	Canned or small individual bottles or cartons	Drinks from large bottles
Miscellaneous	Salt, sauces sachets, double-wrapped confectionery and crisps	Nuts, sauces from large bottles, pepper

Clean diet is copyright to Leicester Nutrition and Dietetic Service.

The criteria for starting PN differ between centres: this probably represents the less well-defined aspect of nutrition support in HSCT. For example, well-defined criteria at the University of Minnesota (USA) in adult patients include less than 50% caloric intake for 5 days and weight loss of 5% baseline, patient's weight being less than 95% ideal body weight, and deterioration in clinical condition.[72] However, many centres use less specific criteria or none at all, and a decision to start PN may be based on the patient's general condition along with suboptimal nutrition, degree of mucositis and loss of body weight. Effective treatment of GVHD of the bowel in many cases will require PN to rest the bowel.

Several studies have been published that compare the use of PN and EN in HSCT. When parenteral nutrition, given to 27 patients undergoing HSCT, was compared to oral/enteral feeding in 30 controls in a prospective randomised controlled trial, there was no significant difference between the two groups in terms of rate of haematopoietic recovery, length of hospital stay or survival. Parenteral nutrition was more expensive and associated with more days of diuretic use, more hyperglycaemia, and more frequent catheter-related problems (e.g. sepsis), but less frequent problems of hypomagnesaemia.[73] In a Birmingham study, children who had received bone marrow transplant were commenced on PN (*n*=19) and EN (*n*=20). The duration of enteral feeding correlated with improvements in nutritional status whereas PN was associated with more frequent exocrine pancreatic insufficiency than EN. Bone marrow engraftment, hospital stay and positive blood cultures were similar in both groups. Hypomagnesaemia, hypophosphataemia and biochemical zinc deficiency were common in both groups, although hypoalbuminaemia and biochemical selenium deficiency were more common in the patients receiving PN.[74] The Seattle (USA) group have reported a double-blind randomised controlled trial of outpatient PN (n=128) against intravenous hydration solution (n=138) given for the first 28 days after transplant. Although weight loss was greater in the group given intravenous hydration, PN provided no significant improvement in the hospital readmission rate, relapse rate or survival. Moreover, there was a delay in the resumption of oral intake in the patients receiving PN.[75]

Administration of PN requires a central venous line with its attendant risk of infections and thrombosis, which may be increased if it is used for PN. Hepatic dysfunction is common with HSCT, and PN may result in both elevation of transaminases and evidence of cholestasis. PN may also be associated with hyper-glycaemia, hyperlipidaemia and, rarely, hyperammon-aemia. Long-term use of PN, which is rare in HSCT patients, may result in hepatic steatosis and cirrhosis. PN may also be associated with cytopenias caused by haemophagocytosis in the bone marrow.

Enteral nutrition has several potential advantages including stimulation of intestinal recovery and reduction of cholestasis by stimulation of gallbladder function; bacteraemia may also be reduced by maintaining gastrointestinal function.[76] Gastric stasis commonly accompanies HSCT and a nasojejunal tube may be preferable to a nasogastric tube, although it is more complicated to insert. Enteral feeding tubes should be inserted early in the course of the transplant and a rigorous anti-emetic policy should be instituted to prevent displacement. Enteric tubes are often diffi-cult to insert later on when mucositis is established. Diarrhoea may be associated with EN and may be reduced with the use of peptide or semi-elemental feeds. Clinicians should be aware that vomiting and tube displacement while EN is being administered may be complicated by aspiration.

Enteral feeding may also be administered through percutaneous endoscopic gastrostomy (PEG) or gastrojejunostomy (PEGJ) tubes during and after HSCT, especially if long-term nutritional support is necessary. Clearly, these require insertion several weeks before HSCT to allow time for healing. One study in children, including some bone marrow transplant patients, suggests that this route of feeding is cosmetic-ally acceptable and cheaper than PN, and free of major complications. Minor complications included gastric juice leakage, bleeding and superficial wound infections, mainly during neutropenia, but no docu-mented bacteraemia.[77]

How much should be given?

Mean resting energy expenditure is not very different from normal: Cogoluenhes *et al.* found an increase of 11.5 ± 10.8% after autologous transplant and a reduction of 7.3 ± 8.9% after allogeneic transplant.[78] Energy requirements are generally calculated using Schofield's formula for basal metabolic rate, with additional requirements for stress using Elia's formula.[79] The 'clean food diet' may be supplemented with high-calorie, high-protein drinks that are usually easy for patients to ingest. In a typical enteral feed, protein requirements are met by 0.2 g of nitrogen/kg, except where the body mass index is greater than 30 when requirements are reduced to 75%. When PN is used, increased protein requirements are generally met by 1.4–1.5 g/kg/d of a standard amino acid solution. Lipids (LCT or LCT/MCT) may be administered and can provide 30–40% of non-protein calories; they may achieve the caloric target if hyper-glycaemia develops because of steroid treatment. Many units give prophylactic B_{12}, folic acid and vitamin K supplements. Routine monitoring of nutrition support should include daily weight, urinalysis, food intake, renal function, glucose and thrice-weekly liver function, albumin, calcium, phos-phate and magnesium. Lipids may be measured weekly in patients receiving PN.

Special nutritional issues

Two issues concerning the composition of the feed have been addressed: the use of lipid and the addition of glutamine. Intravenous lipid (especially long-chain fatty acids) is immunosuppressive (partly by affecting the synthesis of cytokines, prostaglandins and leuko-trienes) and its administration may be expected to result in more infectious complications. This has been shown to be the case in trauma patients,[80] but not in patients after a bone marrow transplant when 25–30% of the total daily energy was given as lipid.[81] The added immunosuppression of lipid may be beneficial follow-ing a transplant, particularly in preventing rejection. In a randomised trial, the mortality from acute GVHD was significantly less in 29 patients given lipid-based PN compared with 31 patients given glucose-based PN (n=31). There was a non-significant trend towards increased survival at 18 months in the group receiving the lipid-based feed, but no difference in engraftment times, sepsis, fungal infections, incidence of acute GVHD or relapse. The authors proposed that the immunomodulatory effects of the lipid infusion may have influenced the incidence of severe GVHD.[82]

Glutamine, a primary fuel for the enterocyte and gut-associated lymphoid tissue, may reduce gut mucosal permeability and hence bacterial translocation.[83] Patients treated with parenteral nutrition with added glutamine (0.57 g/kg body weight/day) showed a significantly improved nitrogen balance, fewer infections and a reduced hospital stay compared with patients given a similar amount of energy with parenteral nutrition and no added glutamine.[84] Subsequent studies have been disappointing: one showed only a shorter hospital stay after parenteral glutamine[85] and another no benefit.[86] Although oral glutamine (1 g/m^2) four times a day helped oropharyngeal mucositis after an autologous bone marrow transplant,[87] oral glutamine supplementation (30 g) was not significantly different from placebo as assessed by total days of PN, days until oral intake resumed, length of hospitalisation, and degree of mucositis and diarrhoea (total $n=58$).[88] From a practical point of view, glutamine is usually contained in enteral feeds, whereas it has to be added separately to PN.

In conclusion, nutrition support must be individualised for HSCT patients, and its composition may need to change substantially following HSCT. The involvement of the nutrition team is important at every stage of HSCT (Box 5.5). Based on current evidence, it is difficult to make generalised statements; trials are necessary to answer questions in the context of modern transplant methods (e.g. insertion of a PEG, PEGJ or NJ tube at the time of conditioning treatment). At present, it seems reasonable to adopt a pragmatic approach and identify patients who need additional nutrition support early in the course of the transplant. Such patients might include those with reduced intake early in the course of HSCT, and those with significant weight loss, marked mucositis or GVHD. As an example, Figure 5.3 summarises the institutional protocol in operation at Leicester Royal Infirmary, United Kingdom. The decision also has to incorporate a prediction of the speed of intestinal recovery, which will be more rapid in autologous than in allogeneic HSCT. The possibility that specific nutritional substrates such as lipids or glutamine following HSCT may influence outcome also warrants further investigation.

Box 5.5 – The role of the nutrition team in patients undergoing HSCT

Maintenance of nutritional state from diagnosis, through and after transplantation

Before transplant
Assessment of nutritional status of patient prior to transplant
Assessment of route of feeding
Counselling patient about options
Assessment for intervention, i.e. NG, NJ, PEG or PN
Placing feeding tube
Liaison with hospital kitchen to obtain suitable food

Conditioning
Maintenance of nutritional status to reduce cellular toxicity (glutamine supplementation)
Control emesis

Post transplant
Immediate
Maintenance of oral/enteral or parenteral input
Assessment for further intervention, e.g. PN
Ensure vitamin supplementation, e.g. vitamin K

Long-term
Re-establish normal feeding pattern
Advise about eating when food has no taste and saliva production is low
Assist with chronically poor appetite caused by gastrointestinal GVHD
Night-time enteral feeding
Set targets at which intervention will occur

GENERAL SUMMARY

Gastrointestinal toxicity of chemotherapy and radiotherapy is common and some effect on nutritional balance is almost universal. Most oncologists are unfortunately unaware of the potential importance of this toxicity as a contributory factor to the reduced quality of life and, potentially, to the survival of their patients. There have been clear demonstrations of alterations in major metabolic pathways as a result of neoplasia and its treatment but surprisingly few clinical trials have addressed the potential to provide dietary supplementation in an attempt to correct this. There is a suggestion from the results of randomised studies using enteral and parenteral nutritional support that there may be a benefit to patients receiving these in terms of response rates and survival. It is imperative that large, well-designed randomised trials be undertaken to clarify the role of nutrition support. The composition of solutions used for support must be carefully

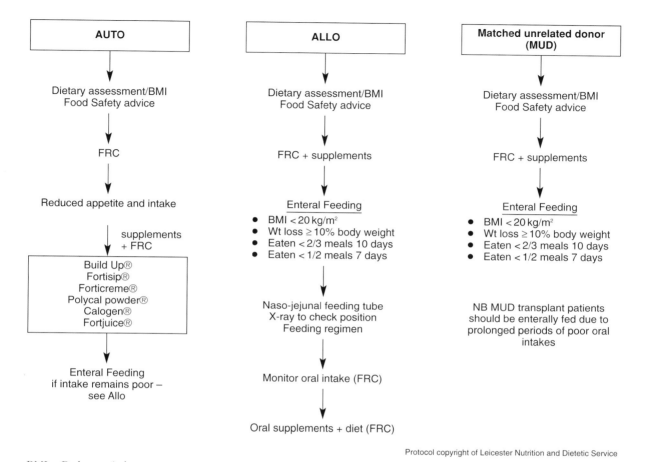

Figure 5.3 – Example of nutrition protocol for patients undergoing HSCT.

BMI = Body mass index.
FRC = Food record chart.

considered, particularly since interesting results suggest a benefit in terms of a reduction of gut toxicity by incorporating glutamine. It is possible that significant benefits for patients with malignancy might accrue if large collaborative groups could conduct further well-designed trials.

REFERENCES

1. Ries LAG, Miller B, Hankey BF (Eds) *SEER Cancer Statistics Review, 1973–1991: Tables and graphs.* National Cancer Institute, Bethesda, MD, 1994.

2. Denekamp J. Cell kinetics and radiation biology. *Int J Radiat Biol* 1986; **49:** 381–387.

3. Tannock IF. Experimental chemotherapy and concepts related to the cell cycle. *Int J Radiat Biol* 1986; **49:** 335–355.

4. Bezwoda WR, Seymour L, Dansey RD. High-dose chemotherapy with hematopoietic rescue as primary treatment for metastatic breast cancer: a randomised trial. *J Clin Oncol* 1995; **13:** 2483–2489.

5. American Society of Clinical Oncology. Update of recommendations for the use of hematopoietic colony-stimulating factors: evidence-based clinical practise guidelines. *J Clin Oncol* 1996; **14:** 1957–1960.

6. Bradford K. A practical application of nutrition for the patient with head and neck cancer. *Cancer Bull* 1977; **29:** 35–41.

7. Schein PS, Macdonald JS, Waters C. Nutritional complications of cancer and its treatment. *Semin Oncol* 1977; **2**: 337–347.

8. Deschner E, Lipkin M. Proliferation and differentiation of gastrointestinal cells in relation to therapy. *Med Clin North Am* 1971; **55**: 601–612.

9. Trier JS. Morphologic alterations induced by methotrexate in the mucosa of human proximal intestine. *Gastroenterology* 1962; **43**: 407–424.

10. Borison HL, Wang WC. Physiology and pharmacology of vomiting. *Pharmacol Rev* 1953; **5**: 193–230.

11. Coates A, Abraham S, Kaye SB, Sowerbutts T, Frewin C, Fox RM, Tattersall MH. On the receiving end – patient perception of the side-effects of cancer chemotherapy. *Eur J Cancer Clin Oncol* 1983; **19**: 203–208.

12. McMurray A, Steward WP. Treatment of vomiting induced by cytotoxic agents. *Prescribers Journal* 1992; **32**: 177–78.

13. Horton J, Olson KB, Sullivan J. 5-Fluorouracil in cancer: an improved regimen. *Ann Intern Med* 1970; **73**: 897–900.

14. Cubeddu L, Hoffman IS, Fuenmayor NT. Antagonism of serotonin S_3 receptors with ondansetron prevents nausea and emesis induced by cyclophosphamide-containing chemotherapy regimens. *J Clin Oncol* 1990; **8**: 1721–1727.

15. Bleyer WA. The clinical pharmacology of methotrexate. *Cancer* 1978; **41**: 36–51.

16. Stroller RG, Hande KR, Jacobs SA, Rosenburg SA, Chabner BA. Use of plasma pharmacokinetics to predict and prevent methotrexate toxicity. *N Engl J Med* 1977; **297**: 630–634.

17. Ansfield FS, Ramirez G. The clinical results of 5-fluorouracil intrahepatic arterial infusion in 528 patients with metastatic cancer to the liver. In: Ariel IM (Ed.) *Progress in clinical cancer.* Vol 7. Grune & Stratton, New York, 1978, pp 201–206.

18. Kennedy JB, Theologides A. The role of 5-fluorouracil in malignant disease. *Ann Intern Med* 1961; **55**: 719–730.

19. Eras P, Goldstein MJ, Sherlock P. Candida infections of the gastrointestinal tract. *Medicine (Baltimore)* 1972; **51**: 367–379.

20. Weiss H, Walker M, Wiernik P. Neurotoxicity of commonly used antineoplastic agents. *N Engl J Med* 1974; **291**: 75–81, 127–133,

21. Rosenthal S, Kaufman S. Vincristine neuotoxicity. *Ann Intern Med* 1975; **80**: 733–737.

22. Holland JF, Scharlau C, Gailani S. Vincristine treatment of advanced cancer: cooperative study of 392 cases. *Cancer Res* 1973; **33**: 1258–1264.

23. Hartwich G, Domschke W, Matzkies F. Disaccharidases of the intestinal mucosa of the rat after cytostatic combined therapy with vincristine sulfate and ifosfamide. *Arzneimittelforschung* 1976; **26**: 350–352.

24. Smith FP, Kisner D, Widerlite L, Schein PS. Chemotherapeutic alterations of small intestinal morphology and function: a progress report. *Clin Gastroenterol* 1979; **1**: 203–207.

25. Ohnuma T, Holland JF, Nagel G. Effects of L-asparaginase in acute myelocytic leukemia. *JAMA* 1969; **210**: 1919–1921.

26. Slavin RE, Dias MA, Sarol R. Cytosine arabinoside induced gastrointestinal toxic alterations in sequential chemotherapeutic protocols. *Cancer* 1978; **42**: 1747–1759.

27. Smith FP, Kisner D, Schein PL. Nutrition and cancer prospects for clinical research. *Nutr Cancer* 1980; **2**: 34–39.

28. Donaldson SS, Jundt S, Ricour C, Sarragin D, Lemerle J, Schweisguth O. Radiation enteritis in children: a retrospective review, clinicopathologic correlation and dietary management. *Cancer* 1975; **35**: 1167–1178.

29. Donaldson SS, Castro JR, Wilbur JR. Rhabdomyosarcoma of head and neck in children: combination treatment by surgery, irradiation and chemotherapy. *Cancer* 1973; **31**: 26–35.

30. Donaldson SS, Lenon RA. Alteration of nutritional status: the impact of chemotherapy and radiation therapy. *Cancer* 1979; **43**: 2036–2052.

31. Knox LS, Crosby LO, Feurer ID, Buzby GP, Miller CL, Mullen JL. Energy expenditure in malnourished cancer patients. *Ann Surg* 1983; **197**: 152–162.

32. Michie HR, Sherman ML, Spriggs DR, Rounds J, Christie M, Wilmore DW. Chronic TNF infusion causes anorexia but not accelerated nitrogen loss. *Ann Surg* 1989; **209**: 19–24.

33. Fearon KC, Hansell DT, Preston T *et al.* Influence of whole body protein turnover on resting energy expenditure in patients with cancer. *Cancer Res* 1988; **48**: 2590–2595.

34. Baron PL, Lawrence W, Chan WM, White FK, Banks WL. Effects of parenteral nutrition on cell cycle kinetics of head and neck cancer. *Arch Surg* 1986; **121**: 1282–1286.

35. Holter AR, Fischer JE. The effects of perioperative hyperalimentation complications in patients with carcinoma and weight loss. *J Surg Res* 1977; **23**: 31–34.

36. Heatley RV, Williams RH, Lewis MH. Pre-operative intravenous feeding: a controlled trial. *Postgrad Med J* 1979; **55**: 541–545.

37. Yamada N, Koyama H, Hioki K, Yamada T, Yamamoto M. Effect of postoperative total parenteral nutrition (TPN) as an adjunct to gastrectomy for advanced gastric carcinoma. *Br J Surg* 1983; **70:** 267–274.

38. Shamberger RC, Brennan MF, Goodgame JT, Lowry SF, Maker MM, Wesley RA, Pizzo PA. A prospective randomised study of adjuvant parenteral nutrition in the treatment of sarcoma: results of metabolic and survival studies. *Surgery* 1984; **96:** 1–13.

39. Jeevanandam M, Horowitz GD, Lowry SF, Brennan MF. Cancer cachexia and protein metabolism. *Lancet* 1984; **1:** 1423–1426.

40. Wasa M, Bode B, Abcouwer S, Collins CL, Tanabe KK, Souba WW. Glutamine as a regulator of DNA and protein biosynthesis in human solid tumor cell lines. *Ann Surg* 1996; **224:** 189–197.

41. Souba WW. Glutamine and cancer. *Ann Surg* 1993; **218:** 715–728.

42. Samuels ML, Selig DE, Ogden S, Grant C, Brown B. IV hyperalimentation and chemotherapy for stage II testicular cancer: a randomised study. *Cancer Treat Rep* 1981; **65:** 615–627.

43. Tandon SP, Gupta SC, Sinha SN, Naithani YP. Nutritional support as an adjunct therapy of advanced cancer patients. *Indian J Med Res* 1984; **80:** 180–188.

44. Valdivieso M, Frankmann C, Murphy WK *et al.* Long-term effects of intravenous hyperalimentation administered during intensive chemotherapy for small cell bronchogenic carcinoma. *Cancer* 1987; **59:** 362–369.

45. Fan ST, Lo CM, Lai EC, Chu KM, Liu CL, Wong J. Perioperative nutritional support in patients undergoing hepatectomy for hepatocellular carcinoma. *N Engl J Med* 1994; **331:** 1547–1552.

46. Blijlevens NM, Donnelly JP, De Pauw BE. Mucosal barrier injury: biology, pathology, clinical counterparts and consequences of intensive treatment for haematological malignancy: an overview. *Bone Marrow Transplant* 2000; **25:** 1269–1278.

47. Klein S, Simes J, Blackburn GL. Total parenteral nutrition and cancer clinical trials. *Cancer* 1986; **58:** 1378–1386.

48. Lesser GT, Bruno MS, Enselberg K. Chylous ascites. Newer insights and many remaining enigmas. *Arch Intern Med* 1970; **125:** 1073–1077.

49. Press OW, Press NO, Kaufman SD. Evaluation and management of chylous ascites. *Ann Intern Med* 1982; **96:** 358–364.

50. Lentz SS, Schray MF, Wilson TO. Chylous ascites after whole-abdomen irradiation for gynaecological malignancy. *Int J Radiat Oncol Biol Phys* 1990; **19:** 435–438.

51. Pabst TS III, McIntyre KE, Schilling JD, Hunter GC, Bernard VM. Management of chyloperitoneum after abdominal aortic surgery. *Am J Surg* 1993; **166:** 194–199.

52. DeHart MM, Lauerman WC, Conely AH, Roettger RH, West JL, Cain JE. Management of retroperitoneal chylous leakage. *Spine* 1994; **19:** 716–718.

53. Jensen GL, Mascioli EA, Meyer LP *et al.* Dietary modification of chyle composition in chylothorax. *Gastroenterology* 1989; **97:** 761–765.

54. Shapiro AM, Bain VG, Sigalet DL, Kneteman NM. Rapid resolution of chylous ascites after liver transplantation using somatostatin analog and total parenteral nutrition. *Transplantation* 1996; **61:** 1410–1411.

55. Guillem P, Billeret V, Houcke ML, Triboulet JP. Successful management of post-esophagectomy chylothorax/chyloperitoneum by etilefrine. *Dis Esophagus* 1999; **12:** 155–156.

56. Cope C. Diagnosis and treatment of postoperative chyle leakage via percutaneous transabdominal catheterisation of the cisterna chyli: a preliminary study. *J Vasc Interv Radiol* 1998; **9:** 727–734.

57. Thomas ED, Blume KG, Forman SJ. *Hematopoietic cell transplantation*. Blackwell Science, Oxford, 1998.

58. Atkinson K. *Clinical bone marrow and blood stem cell transplantation*. Cambridge University Press, 2000.

59. Lennard AL, Jackson GH. Stem cell transplantation. *Br Med J* 2000; **321:** 433–437.

60. Blijlevens NM, Donnelly JP, De Pauw BE. Mucosal barrier injury: biology, pathology, clinical counterparts and consequences of intensive treatment for haematological malignancy: an overview. *Bone Marrow Transplant* 2000; **25:** 1269–1278.

61. Capelli D, Santini G, De Souza D *et al.* Amifostine can reduce mucosal damage after high-dose melphalan conditioning for peripheral blood progenitor cell auto-transplant: a retrospective study. *Br J Haematol* 2000; **110:** 300–307.

62. Hill GR, Ferrara JLM. The primacy of the gastrointestinal tract as a target organ of acute graft-versus-host disease: rationale for the use of cytokine shields in allogeneic bone marrow transplantation. *Blood* 2000; **95:** 2754–2759.

63. Kunkel JM, Rosenthal D. Management of the ileocaecal syndrome: neutropenic enterocolitis. *Dis Colon Rectum* 1986; **29:** 196–199.

64. Bearman SI. The syndrome of hepatic veno-occlusive disease after marrow transplantation. *Blood* 1995; **85:** 3005–3020.

65. Yolken RH, Bishop CA, Townsend TR, Bolyard EA, Bartlett J, Santos GW, Saral R. Infectious gastroenteritis in bone marrow transplant recipients. *N Engl J Med* 1982; **306:** 1010–1012.

66. Van Kraaij MF, Dekker AW, Verdonck LF, van Loon AM, Vinje J, Koopmans MPG, Rozenberg-Arska M. Infectious gastro-enteritis: an uncommon cause of diarrhoea in adult allogeneic and autologous stem cell transplant recipients. *Bone Marrow Transplant* 2000; **26:** 299–303.

67. Snover DC. Mucosal damage simulating acute graft versus host reaction in cytomegalovirus colitis. *Transplantation* 1985; **39:** 669–670.

68. Flowers ME, Kansu E, Sullivan KM. Pathophysiology and treatment of graft-versus-host disease. *Hematol Oncol Clin North Am* 1999; **13:** 1091–112.

69. McKay PJ, Murphy JA, Cameron S, Burnett AK, Campbell M, Tansey P, Franklin IM. Iron overload and liver dysfunction after allogeneic or autologous bone marrow transplantation. *Bone Marrow Transplant* 1996; **17:** 63–66.

70. Papadopoulou A, Lloyd DR, Williams MD, Darbyshire PJ, Booth IW. Gastrointestinal and nutritional sequelae of bone marrow transplantation. *Arch Dis Child* 1996; **75:** 208–213.

71. Weisdorf SA, Lysne J, Wind D et al. Positive effect of prophylactic total parenteral nutrition on long-term outcome of bone marrow transplantation. *Transplantation* 1987; **43:** 833–838.

72. Weisdorf SS, Schwarzenberg SJ. Nutritional aspects of hematopoietic stem cell recipients. In: Thomas ED, Blume KG, Forman SJ (Eds) *Hematopoietic cell transplantation*. Blackwell Science, Oxford, 1998, pp 723–732.

73. Szeluga DJ, Stuart RK, Brookmeyer R, Utermohlen V, Santos GW. Nutritional support of bone marrow transplant recipients: a prospective, randomised clinical trial comparing total parenteral nutrition to an enteral feeding program. *Cancer Res* 1987; **47:** 3309–3316.

74. Papadopoulou A, Williams MD, Darbyshire PJ, Booth IW. Nutritional support in children undergoing bone marrow transplantation. *Clin Nutr* 1998; **17:** 57–63.

75. Charuhas PM, Fosberg KL, Bruemmer B, Akers N, Leisenring W, Seidel K, Sullivan KM. A double blind randomized trial comparing outpatient parenteral nutrition with intravenous hydration: effect of oral intake following marrow transplantation. *J Parenter Enteral Nutr* 1997; **21:** 157–161.

76. Papadopoulou A, MacDonald A, Williams MD, Darbyshire PJ, Booth IW. Enteral nutrition after bone marrow transplantation. *Arch Dis Child* 1997; **77:** 131–136.

77. Pedersen AM, Kok K, Petersen G, Nielsen OH, Michaelsen KF, Schmiegelow K. Percutaneous gastrostomy in children with cancer. *Acta Paediatr* 1999; **88:** 849–852.

78. Cogoluenhes VC, Chambrier C, Michallet M et al. Energy expenditure during allogeneic and autologous bone marrow transplantation. *Clin Nutr* 1998; **17:** 253–257.

79. Elia M, Jebb SA. Assessment of energy expenditure and body composition. *Medicine International* 1990; **82:** 3407–3411.

80. Battistella FD, Widergren JT, Anderson JT, Siepler JK, Weber JC, MacColl K. A prospective, randomized trial of intravenous fat emulsion administration in trauma victims requiring total parenteral nutrition. *J Trauma* 1997; **43:** 52–60.

81. Lenssen P, Bruemmer BA, Bowden RA, Gooley T, Aker SN, Mattson D. Intravenous lipid dose and incidence of bacteremia and fungemia in patients undergoing bone marrow transplantation. *Am J Clin Nutr* 1998; **67:** 927–933.

82. Muscaritoli M, Conversano L, Torelli GF et al. Clinical and metabolic effects of different parenteral nutrition regimens in patients undergoing allogeneic bone marrow transplantation. *Transplantation* 1998; **66:** 610–616.

83. Van der Hulst RRWJ, van Kreel BK, von Meyenfeldt MF, Brummer RJ, Avends JW, Deutz NE, Soeters PB. Glutamine and the preservation of gut integrity. *Lancet* 1993; **341:** 1363.

84. Ziegler TR, Young LS, Benfell K et al. Clinical and metabolic efficacy of glutamine-supplemented parenteral nutrition after bone marrow transplantation. A randomized, double-blind, controlled study. *Ann Intern Med* 1992; **116:** 821–828.

85. Schloerb PR, Amare M. Total parenteral nutrition with glutamine in bone marrow transplantation and other clinical applications (a randomized double-blind study). *J Parenter Enteral Nutr* 1993; **17:** 407–413.

86. Schloerb PR, Skikne BS. Oral and parenteral glutamine in bone marrow transplantation: a randomized, double-blind study. *J Parenter Enteral Nutr* 1999; **23:** 117–122.

87. Anderson PM, Ramsay NK, Shu XO et al. Effect of low-dose oral glutamine on painful stomatitis during bone marrow transplantation. *Bone Marrow Transplant* 1998; **22:** 339–344.

88. Coghlin Dickson TM, Wong RM, Negrin RS et al. Effect of oral glutamine supplementation during bone marrow transplantation. *J Parenter Enteral Nutr* 2000; **24:** 61–66.

6

Human immunodeficiency virus infection

Christine Blanshard and Alastair Forbes

*I*n the early 1980s the first reports began to appear of illnesses in American homosexual men indicating an acquired deficiency of immune function.[1-4] These included an unexpected outbreak of *Pneumocystis carinii* pneumonia, and a large number of cases of cutaneous Kaposi's sarcoma. Soon afterwards a similar illness was found to affect Haitians, intravenous drug abusers, haemophiliacs, transfusion recipients and Africans,[5-7] and epidemiological studies suggested that a blood-borne or sexually transmissible infectious agent was responsible.[8,9] In 1983, the retrovirus responsible for acquired immunodeficiency syndrome (AIDS) was isolated.[10,11] This virus, now known as human immunodeficiency virus (HIV) is prevalent throughout the world, and the World Health Organization estimates that by the year 2000 between 30 and 40 million people will have been infected.

The striking immunological feature of HIV infection is the progressive loss of CD4 T-helper cells, which precedes clinical symptoms and predicts the course of the disease.[12,13] Not only are CD4 cell numbers progressively depleted as the disease progresses, but also the function of the remaining cells is impaired, with abnormal mitogen responses and failure to activate with stimuli such as antigen presentation. In addition natural killer cell function, macrophage function, CD8 cytotoxicity and B-cell response to antigenic stimuli are also impaired. Not all of these abnormalities are corrected by the presence of T-cell-derived cytokines.[14] Some monocytes also exhibit CD4 receptors and may be directly infected by HIV, resulting in the elaboration of cytokines associated with weight loss, and in blood vessel proliferation and fibrosis, which may be responsible for some of the manifestations of HIV infection.

The cellular immune system of the gut (gut-associated lymphoid tissue, GALT) forms part of the common mucosal defence system (Chapter 2). Many of the premonitory features of AIDS such as oral candidiasis, and many AIDS-defining opportunistic infections such as chronic cryptosporidiosis, are due to failures of this system. Other opportunists such as *Mycobacterium avium intracellulare* may gain access to the body due to a breakdown of this barrier. In the organized lymphoid tissue of the tonsils, Peyer's patches and lymphoid follicles there are large numbers of CD4 cells, B-cells expressing surface IgA, IgM or IgG and activated T-cells, macrophages and dendritic/interdigitating cells. In the lamina propria of the gut there are abundant CD4 T-cells, small B-cells and many plasma cells secreting IgA. The intra-epithelial lymphocytes are mainly CD8 cells and probably have a mainly inhibitory or immuno-regulatory phenotype.[15]

Gut CD4 cells become infected with HIV through haematogenous spread, and in the case of the rectal mucosa, possibly by direct inoculation during anal intercourse. The effect of the infection on the gastrointestinal cellular immune system is controversial. It is likely that the number of intra-epithelial lymphocytes remains normal in those without gut pathogens.[16,17] CD4 cells and CD3 cells are probably depleted in the later stages of HIV infection,[18,19] but whether the loss of CD4 cells is mainly of lymphocytes or macrophages is unclear. It is also unclear whether these changes represent an immunodeficiency specific to the gastrointestinal tract, a local response to infection, or merely reflect the systemic immune dysfunction. However, studies of gut biopsies, including those from patients with early HIV infection suggest that CD4 lamina propria lymphocytes are depleted early in HIV infection, before the peripheral blood CD4 count falls significantly, and that CD8 cells initially increase but fall as the disease progresses.[20,21]

Antibody-mediated immune function in the gut is also impaired as demonstrated by a reduction in IgA-secreting plasma cells in the lamina propria,[22] with a specific reduction in IgA subclass 2 in some individuals.[23] Although serum levels of IgA increase as the disease progresses this is less true of secretory IgA, most of which is in particulate form (perhaps because it is complexed with antigen) and therefore nonfunctional.

Non-specific mechanisms of host resistance to gut infections are also impaired. Hypochlorhydria is common and may allow small bowel bacterial overgrowth as well as reducing resistance to many pathogens.[24] The normal gut microflora may be affected by treatment with broad-spectrum antibiotics (e.g. cotrimoxazole prophylaxis against *Pneumocystis carinii* pneumonia). Intestinal motility and sodium and water transport may be impaired by an autonomic neuropathy.[16,25,26]

GASTROINTESTINAL MANIFESTATIONS OF HIV INFECTION

Given the effects of HIV on gastrointestinal immunity and the frequent exposure of the gut to environmental pathogens it is not surprising that gastrointestinal infections are prominent manifestations of HIV infection. These include oropharyngeal and oesophageal candidiasis, oral and oesophageal ulceration from herpes simplex and cytomegalovirus infection, cryptosporidiosis, microsporidiosis and enteric bacterial infections.

Wasting

A wasting syndrome, defined as unintentional weight loss of more than 10% body weight, involves marked loss of lean body mass and fat tissue and is a prominent feature of AIDS. In Africa, AIDS is widely known as 'slim' disease because of the marked weight loss that precedes death.[27] There is a relationship between wasting and survival. If multiple measurements of body cell mass (as assessed by total body potassium) are plotted against time they fit a linear model, with death occurring at 54% of normal body cell mass or 66% of ideal body weight.[28] Rapid weight loss usually indicates secondary infection. Wasting syndrome frequently, but not inevitably, occurs in patients with gastrointestinal disease. A variety of mechanisms are involved (Table 6.1), including decreased nutrient intake and nutrient malabsorption, probably aggravated by elevated levels of tumour necrosis factor (TNF) and other cytokines.[29] Although clinically stable AIDS patients may have a normal or reduced total energy expenditure, resting energy expenditure is increased by opportunistic infections, and food intake is often not increased adequately to compensate.[30]

An early report suggested generally high levels of TNF (or cachectin) in AIDS patients.[31] Although there is evidence for the importance of this cytokine

in the wasting and hypertriglyceridaemia which accompanies infections, there was no relationship between the TNF level and the degree of weight loss in AIDS,[31] and later studies showed no difference between TNF levels in stable AIDS patients and controls.[32,33] An interaction between TNF and other cytokines in the production of anorexia, protein breakdown and accelerated energy expenditure during infections is not, however, excluded.[34]

For reasons that are not yet entirely clear, folate deficiency is common in HIV-infected patients unless oral supplements are taken.[35] However, the ready demonstration of malabsorption of D-xylose in patients with intestinal infections (and in some without a gut pathogen even in the absence of severe small intestinal injury),[36] suggests that there is proximal intestinal dysfunction leading to folate malabsorption also. Ileal dysfunction as demonstrated by vitamin B_{12} malabsorption,[35,37,38] excessive bile salt deconjugation and colonic losses has also been reported, particularly in patients with small intestine pathogens.[39,40]

Diarrhoea

Diarrhoea was recognized as one of the characteristic features of HIV infection early in the epidemic, occurring in 27 of 29 Haitian AIDS patients.[41] It is now known to occur at all stages of disease, and the incidence of diarrhoea has been quoted at between 9% and 93%, depending on the definition of diarrhoea, the population studied and the time period over which they are followed up (Table 6.2).[41–49] In our own study,[50] 322 of 1830 outpatients attended for investigation of diarrhoea over an 18-month study period (18%). Over 90% of those with diarrhoea were homosexual men compared to 81% of all the clinic attendees ($P < 0.0001$), and diarrhoea was significantly more common in patients with a CD4 count $<50/\mu l$ compared with less immunocompromised patients ($P < 0.0001$, Fig. 6.1).

With the advent of highly active antiretroviral therapy it is probable that the incidence, prevalence and severity of gastrointestinal manifestations will diminish though some drugs such as the protease inhibitors may themselves cause diarrhoea. Clear guidance for the clinical management of the gut disease that remains does not yet exist from the literature, but existing, and now relatively historical, data in this area are likely to remain pertinent (if less frequently called upon) in developed countries, and will certainly remain a major issue in Africa for the foreseeable future: they are therefore discussed here.

Table 6.1 – Reasons for wasting and undernutrition in HIV

Problem	Reasons
Reduced energy intake	Anorexia /nausea/vomiting which may be drug related (e.g. protease inhibitors) Depression Oropharyngeal infection
Increased energy expenditure	Opportunistic infections
Malabsorption	HIV-related enteropathy Opportunistic infections Lymphoma/Kaposi's sarcoma Autonomic neuropathy

Table 6.2 – Frequency of diarrhoea in patients with HIV infection

Reference	Population studied	Definition of diarrhoea (if given)	Study period (months, if given)	Prevalence (%)
Malebranche et al., 1983[41]	29 Haitian AIDS patients	–	10	93
Colebunders et al., 1987[42]	243 African AIDS patients	>2 loose stools/day most days	2	40
Girard et al., 1987[43]	87 French AIDS patients	–	–	62
Antony et al., 1988[44]	100 American AIDS patients	–	Retrospective	66
Laughon et al., 1988[45]	77 American homosexuals with AIDS	>3 loose stools in preceding 24 hours	–	64
Heise et al., 1988[46]	200 hospitalized German AIDS patients	–	14	24
Lane et al., 1989[47]	85 Australian AIDS patients	–	38	60
Connolly et al., 1989[48]	1250 UK AIDS and ARC★ patients	>3 stools/day >1 month	16	9
Rolston et al., 1989[49]	250 HIV-positive patients	–	17	27

★ APC: AIDS related complex.

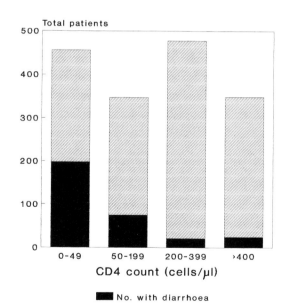

Total patients

CD4 count (cells/µl)

■ No. with diarrhoea

Figure 6.1 – The incidence of diarrhoea in relationship to CD4 count in a cross-sectional study of HIV-positive patients attending a single large London centre (The Kobler Centre, Chelsea and Westminster Hospital). They were mainly outpatients. The total number of patients is given on the y-axis with the number with diarrhoea represented by the filled in area.

Diarrhoea in HIV infection is most commonly caused by opportunistic pathogens such as *Cryptosporidium*, *Microsporidium* and cytomegalovirus (CMV). Non-opportunistic intestinal pathogens such as *Giardia*, *Salmonella* and *Campylobacter* are also identified, and in a variable proportion of cases no cause is found (Table 6.3). Many infections capable of causing diarrhoea (including *Cryptosporidia*, other intestinal protozoa, and some bacteria such as *Shigella*) may be transmitted between homosexual men during oral–anal sex (the 'gay bowel syndrome').[51–54]

The proportion of HIV-infected patients with diarrhoea who are found to have a gut pathogen depends on the CD4 count and the intensity of investigation. In two of our own large studies, a pathogen or gut malignancy was found to account for the diarrhoea in 83% of those with chronic diarrhoea and a CD4 count of <200/µl, and 30% were multiply infected (Table 6.4).[62] In contrast a pathogen was identified in only 57% of episodes of diarrhoea in those with a CD4 count of >200/µl.[50]

The type of pathogen identified also varies with the CD4 count. In the majority of patients with near-normal CD4 counts, no specific cause, or a non-opportunistic pathogen such as *Giardia lamblia* or *Campylobacter jejuni* is found. Perirectal herpes simplex virus infection is common. Patients with CD4 counts above 200/µl are unlikely to have persistent infection with an opportunistic pathogen. Microsporidiosis, *Mycobacterium avium intracellulare* and CMV colitis generally only occur in patients with a CD4 count of less than 200/µl and are rare at CD4 counts greater

Table 6.3 – Percentage prevalence of different pathogens identified in 16 studies of HIV-related diarrhoea

Reference	Cryptosporidium	Microsporidium	Giardia lamblia	Entamoeba histolytica	Isospora belli	CMV	HSV	MAI	Bacteria	>1 pathogen	No pathogen
Malebranche et al., 1983[41]	41	0	0	0	0	15	11	0	0	0	37
Dworkin et al., 1985[55],*	14	0	5	0	0	0	0	14	10	5	54
Colebunders et al., 1987[42]	22	0	0	5	7	0	0	0	4	35	41
Girard et al., 1987[43]	24	0	22	3	3	2	0	0	16	N/A	16
Sewankambo et al., 1987[56]	48	0	4	4	13	0	0	13	13	26	26
Antony et al., 1988[44]	8	0	2	2	2	9	5	14	11	12	45
Colebunders et al., 1988[57]	31	0	5	0	12	6	7	0	2	N/A	50
Laughon et al., 1988[45]	16	0	4	0	2	0	18	2	16	N/A	43
Heise et al., 1988[46]	6	0	4	3	13	13	0	25	10	N/A	N/A
Miró et al., 1988[58],†	23	0	31	0	13	15	0	3	23	23	0
Smith and Janoff, 1988[59]	15	0	15	25	0	45	5	5	35	35	5
Lane et al., 1989[47]	8	0	+	+	0	13	0	13	+	N/A	25
Connolly et al., 1989[48],‡	0	0	11	11	0	7	4	12	15	9	37
Rolston et al., 1989[60]	34	0	6	7	1	18	0	6	9	17	38
Rolston et al., 1989[49]	13	0	7	3	1	6	0	0	9	12	60
Conlon et al., 1990[61]	32	2	2	0	16	0	0	2	0	N/A	N/A

CMV: cytomegalovirus, HSV: herpes simplex virus, MAI: *Mycobacterium avium intracellulare*. ★ not all patients had diarrhoea, † studied only 'infectious gastroenteritis', ‡ patients with cryptosporidiosis were excluded. Bacteria: *Salmonella, Shigella, Campylobacter*. N/A: data not available from the paper. +: pathogen present in some but numbers not given.

Table 6.4 – Pathogens and potential pathogens identified in a cohort of 155 patients in UK after completing an intensive investigation protocol[62]

	Number of patients with pathogen (n)
Cryptosporidium	47
Microsporidium (*Enterocytozoon bieneusi*)	37
Microsporidium (*Encephalitozoon intestinalis*)	1
Mycobacterium avium intracellulare	12
Cytomegalovirus	29★
Giardia	18
Salmonella	2
Shigella	1
Campylobacter	7
Toxigenic *Clostridium difficile*	2
Isospora	1
Adenovirus	10
Rotavirus	2
Coronavirus	3
Small round virus	3
Blastocystis hominis	6
Spirochaetes	7
Entamoeba histolytica	2
Staphylococcus aureus (in duodenal aspirate)	1
Pseudomonas sp. (in duodenal aspirate)	1
Invasive duodenal Candida	1
Non-Infectious causes of diarrhoea	
Radiation proctitis	1
Crohn's disease	1
Extensive small bowel Kaposi's sarcoma	1
Small bowel lymphoma	2

★ In addition, six patients had CMV infection of the oesophagus or stomach only.

The investigation protocol comprised: microscopy and culture of six stool specimens and testing for *Clos. difficile* toxin; electron microscopy of stools for viral pathogens; latex test for rotavirus; upper gastrointestinal endoscopy with light and electron microscopy of duodenal and jejunal biopsies; sigmoidoscopy with light microscopy of rectal biopsies; immunohistochemical staining for CMV and adenovirus; microscopy and culture of duodenal aspirate; and in patients with negative investigations after all of the above, colonoscopy with serial biopsies; small bowel double-contrast radiographs, and repeat duodenal biopsies and stool examinations.

than 100/µl. Cryptosporidiosis occurs across the range of CD4 counts, but the infection is self-limiting in those with a CD4 count above 200–250/µl, and only causes chronic diarrhoea in more immunocompromised patients.[50,63] The clinical features, diagnosis and treatment of opportunistic infections is outlined in Table 6.5.

B-cell non-Hodgkin's lymphoma occurs in 4–10% of patients with AIDS,[64] due to diminished immune surveillance, and the gut is the most common extranodal site. Although the most common gastrointestinal manifestations are obstruction, ulceration or a mass, diarrhoea and malabsorption can occur due to lymphatic obstruction in the small bowel.

Gastrointestinal Kaposi's sarcoma affects 40% of patients with AIDS, or 80% of those with more than 11 skin lesions.[65] It is usually asymptomatic, but we have seen occasional cases of severe intestinal failure due to extensive replacement of the small bowel absorptive surface by tumour.

HIV ENTEROPATHY

The term 'HIV enteropathy' was first used by Kotler and colleagues in 1984 to describe histological abnormalities in the small bowel mucosa occurring in association with diarrhoea and malabsorption.[66] In this influential paper they described their findings in 12 homosexual AIDS patients, including seven with diarrhoea and weight loss, and ten controls, three of whom had diarrhoea. The mean 5-hour urinary xylose excretion was lower in patients with and without diarrhoea than in controls, and those with diarrhoea had more severe malabsorption. Eight patients, including three without diarrhoea, had excess faecal fat excretion. Three patients with diarrhoea had partial villus atrophy in small intestine biopsies, and another two had less severe abnormalities. Three of five biopsies from patients without diarrhoea were also abnormal. These results were interpreted at the time, in the absence of a known alternative intestinal pathogen, as evidence for HIV infection itself causing histological abnormalities and associated intestinal dysfunction. However subsequent review of the biopsies showed the presence of CMV infection in seven cases, and microsporidia in three, casting doubt on this interpretation.[67] In addition the occurrence of similar abnormalities in patients without diarrhoea was perhaps understated.

This paper was followed by a number of studies

Table 6.5 – Treatment of opportunistic gastrointestinal infections

Pathogen	Clinical features	Diagnosis	Treatment
Enteric organisms *Salmonella, Shigella, Campylobacter*	Enteritis/colitis, any CD4 level	Stool microscopy and culture	Ciprofloxacin
Entameoba histolytica	Colitis and cramps, any CD4 level	Stool microscopy	Metronidazole then dilanoxide
Giardiasis	Watery stool, malabsorption any CD4 level	Stool microscopy Duodenal biopsy	Metronidazole Tinidazole
Cryptosporidium	Enteritis, cholangitis, large stool volume CD4 <200	Stool microscopy, modified Ziehl–Neilson stain, biopsy	Paromomycin Azithromycin
Isospora	Watery stool, CD4 <100	Stool electron microscopy	Cotrimoxazole Pyrimethamine
Microsporidia *Enterocytozoan bieneusi Septata intestinalis*	Enteritis, watery stool, malabsorption, CD4 <100	Biopsy and trichrome stain, electron microscopy	Albendazole Metronidazole Atovoquone
Mycobacterium avium intracellulare	Enteritis, watery stool, abdominal pain, CD4 <50	Blood culture, stool Ziehl–Neilson stain and culture, biopsy and histology	Clarithromycin Ethambutol Rifampicin Clofazimine
Cytomegalovirus	Colitis and enteritis, ulceration, perforation, CD4 <50	Biopsy: intranuclear inclusion bodies	Ganciclovir Foscarnet
Idiopathic	Watery diarrhoea, malabsorption	Villous atrophy, all stains and culture negative	Supportive: nutritional supplements/loperamide
Non-infective causes Kaposi's sarcoma Lymphoma	Enteritis and colitis, weight loss, CD4 <100	CT abdomen OGD and colonscopy with biopsy	Radiotherapy Chemotherapy

looking at intestinal absorptive function in patients with AIDS. Gillin and colleagues[68] found abnormal ^{14}C-glycerol-tripalmitin absorption in eight of nine AIDS patients with diarrhoea, and abnormal D-xylose absorption in all nine. Miller *et al.*[69] related jejunal mucosal architectural changes to abnormalities of fat absorption as measured by the ^{14}C triolein breath test. Villus atrophy occurred at all stages of HIV disease and its extent correlated with the ^{14}C triolein breath test result. Nine of 12 patients with abnormal ^{14}C triolein breath tests had diarrhoea. The small bowel morphology in these biopsies was analysed further by the authors in a separate publication[16] and the villus atrophy was found to be associated with crypt hypertrophy.

More detailed studies of small bowel mucosal histology have been performed by Ullrich and his co-workers.[70–72] They demonstrated a reduction in villus length and surface area in HIV-positive patients compared to unmatched, presumably HIV-negative, controls. There was no relationship to intestinal infection or CD4 count. The crypt length was increased in patients with an intestinal infection but normal in those without. Seven of 12 patients tested had an abnormal lactose/hydrogen breath test; 15 out of 25 patients had no detectable lactase activity in the brush border by quantitative enzyme histochemistry. Again the results were not related to the presence of an intestinal infection. In the later study[72] the lactase deficiency but not the villus atrophy correlated with the presence of HIV p24 antigen in the gut mucosa and the absence of zidovudine treatment. More recently, a study of intestinal permeability *in vivo* has indicated that all AIDS patients have a reduced mannitol excretion regardless of the presence of diarrhoea, suggesting a universally reduced mucosal surface area[73] given that this monosaccharide is a relatively good marker of transcellular permeation and that lactulose permeation (intercellular) was normal. Comparative studies employing multiple sugars including those absorbed passively (e.g. xylose) and by active transport (e.g. 3–*O*-methyl glucose) would help to clarify this.

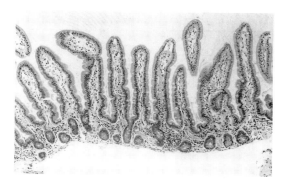

Figure 6.2 – Normal jejunal biopsy.

MECHANISMS OF INTESTINAL FAILURE IN HIV INFECTION

A number of factors are therefore implicated in the origin of the small bowel histological changes and malabsorption seen in patients with HIV infection, including intestinal infections and malignancies, undernutrition and perhaps HIV infection itself.

Small bowel infection

The pathogenesis of diarrhoea and malabsorption in patients with cryptosporidiosis and microsporidiosis remains unclear. Cryptosporidia attach to the surface of enterocytes and produce little apparent cellular damage on light microscopy.[74] However, high volume secretory diarrhoea can occur[41] and it has been postulated that the organism produces an enterotoxin, as cell free supernatants of animal isolates of *C. parvum* produce a secretory response in rabbit jejunum.[75] Microsporidia are intracellular organisms which could potentially disrupt the host cell metabolism and absorptive function. Patients with cryptosporidiosis and microsporidiosis have small bowel villus atrophy.[67,76] Our own data suggest that microsporidia are associated with the most severe villus atrophy, and bacterial infections with the least (Table 6.6, Figs 6.2–6.4). Crypts are longer in the patients with small bowel pathogens than in other HIV-positive patients, suggesting a degree of compensatory crypt hypertrophy in response to enterocyte damage induced by the pathogen, but there is a negative correlation between the height of the villus and the length of the crypt, suggesting that the crypt hypertrophy is impaired in the presence of these pathogens. To account for the fact that villus atrophy also occurs in patients without known enteropathogens, it has been postulated that there is another, as yet undiscovered, small intestine pathogen. However, if this is the case one would have to postulate its virtually universal

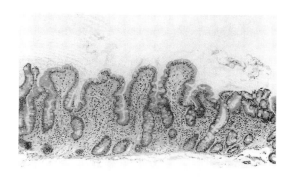

Figure 6.3 – Jejunal biopsy from an AIDS patient with microsporidiosis showing severe villus atrophy and a degree of compensatory crypt hyperplasia.

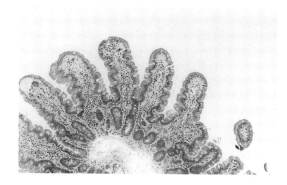

Figure 6.4 – Jejunal biopsy from an AIDS patient who was significantly malnourished (body mass index 19.1 kg/m²) but with no small intestine pathogen. This patient also has villus atrophy and crypt hyperplasia.

Table 6.6 – Jejunal villus heights and crypt depths in HIV-infected patients

	n	Villus height (μ)	Crypt depth (μ)
Normal controls	10	355	77
HIV-positive patients			
Small bowel cryptosporidiosis	15	209	110
Small bowel microsporidiosis	16	156	134
Large bowel pathogen	14	231	109
Pathogen-negative diarrhoea	21	217	107
No diarrhoea	10	192	88

Measurements were obtained from a minimum of eight crypts and villi in well orientated jejunal biopsies, using an image analysis system. All HIV-positive patients had a CD4 count of <200/μl.

occurrence in HIV-positive patients (an argument therefore in favour of the HIV itself being responsible).

Bacterial overgrowth

Villus atrophy occurs in bacterial overgrowth in the blind loop syndrome and in tropical sprue.[77,78] A number of patients with HIV infection develop small bowel bacterial overgrowth in conjunction with hypochlorhydria.[24] This may also contribute to fat malabsorption by bile salt deconjugation.[79] Overgrowth has also been associated with carbohydrate fermentation in the gut lumen and loss of brush border enzymes.[80]

Undernutrition

Protein-energy malnutrition itself has been shown to induce villus atrophy and hypolactasia in children.[81] In adults, disease-related weight loss of more than 30% causes villus atrophy, carbohydrate and fat malabsorption.[82] It is possible that the anorexia and malnutrition associated with both extraintestinal and gut infections cause small bowel villus atrophy. In addition a vicious circle may ensue where malabsorption of essential nutrients results in failure to repair the damaged gut mucosa. For example, in tropical sprue folate deficiency potentiates the villus atrophy, while folate replacement reduces stool volumes and improves mucosal histology.[83,84]

HIV infection of the gut mucosa

HIV-infected patients without known gastrointestinal pathogens have shortened villi compared to age- and sex-matched controls. This led to the hypothesis that pathogen-negative diarrhoea reflected malabsorption resulting from small bowel architectural and functional abnormalities caused directly by HIV acting as an enteric pathogen. Indeed the term 'AIDS enteropathy' has been used to describe chronic pathogen-negative diarrhoea as well as the histological and functional changes in the gut.[56,66,76] However, it is clear from a careful reading of the published studies that histological abnormalities also occur in the bowel of patients without diarrhoea.

Retroviral infection of the small intestine has been shown to occur in a feline immunodeficiency model and viral activation was associated with severe enteropathy[85] A number of workers have reported HIV-infected cells in gut mucosa by in situ hybridization or polymerase chain reaction (PCR).[86,87] The type of cells infected is controversial: some have reported infection of epithelial cells;[86,89,90] others suggest that only intra-epithelial lymphocytes and lamina propria macrophages are infected.[91,70-72] HIV p24 antigen has been identified in jejunal mucosa by immunohistochemical techniques:[70] its expression increases with advancing disease stage and sometimes involves epithelial cells which are PCR-negative and do not contain viral RNA; this may therefore be due to phagocytosis of viral antigen by the epithelial cells.[88] An animal model involving human fetal intestine explants in an immunodeficient mouse did not, however, show evidence of incorporation of cell-free HIV into epithelial or lamina propria cells.[92] Human colonic cancer cell lines, and cultured small intestine mesenchymal and epithelial cells have been infected with HIV in vitro[93,94] but this may have been made possible by the (abnormal) expression of CD4 by these cells,[95,96] there being no evidence that normal entero-cytes express CD4 *in vivo*. Explants of small intestine from aborted 14- to 21-week human fetuses survive in culture for up to 14 days and can be used to study HIV infection of the gut mucosa and its effects on small bowel cell turnover and differentiation.[97] Exposure of such cultures to a variety of strains of HIV results in productive infection of lamina propria lymphocytes and induces crypt epithelial cell proliferation,[98] but the enterocytes themselves are not infected. Any effect of HIV itself in causing an enteropathy therefore is likely to be mediated by cytokine production from infected cells in the GALT. However, in most studies involving human biopsies only about half of the specimens examined are found to contain infected cells and only 1–5 infected cells are found per section. Furthermore, a recent study has suggested that the severity of intestinal injury does not correlate with mucosal HIV infection.[99]

Immunological dysfunction in the gut caused by systemic HIV infection

A number of immunological disorders result in small bowel villus atrophy with or without crypt hyper-plasia, including coeliac disease,[100] graft-versus-host disease,[101,102] allograft rejection[103] and post-infective malabsorption.[104] In coeliac disease the damage to the small bowel villi is thought to be immunologically mediated, involving activation of intra-epithelial lymphocytes and also a humoral reaction. The intra-epithelial lymphocytes in HIV infection also look 'activated' at electron microscopy. In human fetal small intestine explants,[105] experimental small intestine graft-versus-host disease and mouse small intestine allografts undergoing rejection,[101,103,106] villus atrophy without enterocyte damage occurs, and the similarities between the histological changes in these situations and the small intestine in HIV infection have been previously highlighted.[16] The epithelial damage in these experiments is thought to be related to the release of lymphokines from activated T-cells in the lamina propria. Some studies have correlated the presence of HIV antigens in gut mucosa with histological inflammation and an increased tissue content of interleukin-1 beta and TNF.[107,108] Crypt cell hyperplasia and villus atrophy is a T-cell-dependent phenomenon:[105,109] activation of T-cells by pokeweed mitogen or anti-CD3 results in striking villus atrophy and crypt hyperplasia in human fetal small intestine explants. It is possible that HIV infection of gut mucosal T-cells results in altered regulation of small bowel cellular proliferation and maturation. The observation that small intestine morphological changes are partly independent on the occurrence of enteropathogens supports this. It is likely that villus atrophy occurs relatively early in the disease, as in our own studies we observed no differ-ence between patients with a CD4 count above and below 200/µl, and others have reported partial villus atrophy in a patient within 9 months of serocon-version and with a CD4 count within the normal range.[110]

Clinical significance of HIV enteropathy

It appears that villus atrophy and functional changes occur in the small bowel of the majority of patients with AIDS and that these are exacerbated by intestinal infection. How much this contributes to the wasting syndrome is unclear. The villus atrophy and crypt hyperplasia is much less than that seen in coeliac disease.[17] The measurable biochemical malabsorption is relatively modest (for example D-xylose recovery of approximately one-third to half that of normal controls) and could in theory be overcome by increased nutrient intake, particularly of easily absorbed substrates. It seems likely that the major contributions to wasting come from anorexia and the catabolic state that accompanies intercurrent infections.[111] The weight loss is only reversed follow-ing successful treatment of the infection. Thus, most patients show a pattern of accelerated weight loss during infections which may be partially or completely regained during periods of clinical stability.[112]

NUTRITIONAL THERAPY FOR HIV DISEASE

Undernutrition in HIV disease is thus due to a combi-nation of factors including oropharyngeal disease, the increased metabolic demands of infection, mal-absorption, losses from chronic diarrhoea, some drug treatments, and frequently from loss of appetite and depression. A number of nutritional studies have been performed but may now be outdated by the improve-ment in the overall prognosis of HIV infection since the advent of highly active antiretroviral therapy (see below). However, there are no studies as yet to guide the nutritionist in this new era.

Specific nutritional therapy has had a relatively modest impact compared to successful treatment of the underlying immunodeficiency and infections associated with it (e.g. CMV, HIV-related ulcers, tuberculosis, or microsporidiosis[113]). Non-specific therapy, such as the slowing of intestinal transit and other 'short bowel' therapies as covered elsewhere in this book, may also have a role. Many drugs interact with the antiretroviral drugs (e.g. cisapride is contra-indicated with protease inhibitors). It is especially important to recognize depression and treat it when possible, but always to offer support and nutritional encouragement.

Specific nutritional intervention

Recognition that malnutrition is always of potential importance in HIV infection and a principal contri-butor to morbidity has led to a variety of strategies to improve nutritional status. Most studies indicate that inadequate oral intake plays a major role in protein-calorie malnutrition, with or without micronutrient deficiency,[114] so it is logical to look at the influence of specific dietary counselling by a dietician providing support, explanation and advice, to avoid quirky and potentially nutritionally incomplete diets. Typically a high energy density mixed diet with between-meal snacks will be encouraged.

In a retrospective study of 81 HIV-infected out-patients, Burger et al.[115] reported cessation of weight loss by such a strategy in 31 of 54 evaluable patients, and weight gain in a further 18. This contrasts with our experience and it is probable that there was reporting or ascertainment bias in that series. A prospective study of 108 patients who all received standardized dietary counselling (directed towards maintenance of body weight and the prevention of nutritional deficiencies) showed continuing weight loss, largely in line with pre-intervention status, despite apparently successful implementation of the regime.[116] Those with low CD4 counts did least well. Thus, simple nutritional advice, education and counselling is not enough.

The loosely supervised use of dietary supplements might be considered the next increment in intensity of nutritional support. In a careful retrospective clinical review (not a formal controlled trial) of 119 outpatients with HIV infection, 42 had had a dietetic assessment and been advised on the use of supple-ments.[117] It must be assumed that the perceived need for nutritional support was greater in this group than in the 77 patients in whom nutritional intervention

was unrecorded. This assumption is supported by the inclusion of 'all' of those with gastrointestinal and wasting problems within the intervention group. Despite this very clear pointer to a worse expected outcome, the intervention group paradoxically proved able to gain weight (median about 1.3 kg at 6 months), compared to a synchronous weight loss of around 1.7 kg in the controls, alternatively expressed as weight maintenance or weight gain in 63% vs. 42% of patients. Impressive though these data are, it should be remembered that the weight loss of HIV disease is often episodic or cyclical; weight gain is therefore statistically most likely to follow at times that dietetic support is thought indicated, since this is likely to coincide with times at which concern is greatest but at which spontaneous improvement is also most likely.

Appetite stimulants

It is widely considered that appetite stimulants are helpful.[113] A variety of specific agents have been assessed, including progestogens, cannabinoids and octreotide. Megestrol acetate is the most widely employed progestogen.[118] It is clear from placebo-controlled trials that doses of megestrol acetate from 320 to 1600 mg per day are non-toxic and have the potential to improve appetite and food intake in most HIV-infected patients, and to yield weight gain in some. A daily dose of 800 mg should yield at least 2 kg weight gain (of which about half is lean body mass) in two-thirds of treated patients by 12 weeks. This contrasts with a similar gain in less than a quarter of those on placebo.[119] The mechanism of this effect is unclear but may involve changes in food-seeking behaviour.

Cannabis has been advocated by HIV-infected patients to help appetite. While its smoking has not found official favour there are now a number of studies of oral derivatives. A double-blind placebo-controlled crossover trial of dronabinol (delta-9-tetrahydrocannabinol) assessed 12 patients with >5% weight loss, over a 5-week period.[120] Despite a high frequency of drug intolerance and non-compliance, on an intention-to-treat basis there was improved appetite score, reversal of weight loss, and increased pre-albumin. A larger, controlled study supports this,[121] with 88 evaluable patients treated with 2.5 mg dronabinol twice daily showing improved appetite and mood, decreased nausea and no weight loss. Dronabinol may be effective for up to 1 year.[122]

Growth hormone has been reported to be helpful in HIV-associated wasting. In a double-blind, placebo-controlled, multicentre trial involving 178 HIV-infected out-patients with unintentional weight loss of >10%, or to <90% of the lower limit of ideal, recombinant human growth hormone, 0.1 units/kg for 12 weeks produced a sustained and statistically significant increase in weight (1.6 +/− 3.7 kg [P<0.001]) and lean body mass (3.0 +/− 3.0 kg [P<0.001]), with a decrease in body fat (−1.7 +/− 1.7 kg [P<0.001]) and improved treadmill work output.[123] However, quality of life scores, days of disability and use of medical resources were the same for both groups. It remains unclear whether the anthropometric gains will translate into survival advantage or whether this expensive therapy can be justified in the absence of symptomatic benefit.

Octreotide has been quite widely used in therapy for HIV-associated diarrhoea, and there have been suggestions that it is also of nutritional value. However, in a large and careful study (admittedly of only 3 weeks' duration) there was no difference in body weight compared to those on placebo.[124]

Enteral nutrition

In an early, uncontrolled, but prospective study of defined enteral nutrition in AIDS[125] eight patients demonstrated increases in total body potassium, albumin, body cell mass and body fat. Enteral feeding may be particularly helpful in those without severe malabsorption.[113] There is continuing debate as to the most suitable regime. In two studies comparing isocaloric medium-chain triglyceride diets with a long-chain diet and normal solid food,[126,127] patients receiving MCT showed significant reductions in stool volume, stool fat content, improved nitrogen retention and less malabsorption overall. There were no changes in body weight over the 12-day assessment period. Both studies were handicapped by very short intervention and follow-up periods, and it is uncertain how much of the benefit results from inclusion in a therapeutic trial or from the supervized administration of a complete nutritional regime calculated to provide adequate nutrient supply. An alternative approach was taken by Chlebowski et al.[128] who, in a controlled trial of 80 early-stage HIV-infected patients, compared a standard polymeric feed with a peptide-based formula (of somewhat lower energy density: 1.06 kcal/ml vs 1.28 kcal/ml). Unfortunately only 56 patients proved evaluable and the analysis is not fully by intention-to-treat. With these reservations, there appeared to be clear advantage to those receiving the peptide feed, with better maintenance of body weight and skinfold thickness, and more normal nitrogen retention. Especial encouragement was drawn from the observation that the peptide group also had significantly fewer admissions in the 6-month period of evaluation.

Gastrostomy feeding

There are many anecdotal reports, and a few case–control series favouring the use of percutaneous gastrostomy feeding in HIV disease, but no formal controlled trial. Ockenga et al. have described the successful use of PEG feeding in 47 HIV-infected patients in comparison to 15 patients in whom PEG was thought appropriate on the same criteria, but was declined by the patient.[129] Most had a wasting syndrome but neurological causes predominated in 11. Tube insertion and subsequent use were associated with no more complications than in the general non-HIV population, and, over varying times, yielded significant improvements in weight and albumin compared to baseline, and to the 'PEG decliners'. In another study, 14 HIV-infected patients were compared to a well-matched group of controls.[130] Minor complication rates were worse numerically but not statistically in the HIV group (43% vs 19%), but there was an important increase in serious morbidity (stomal cellulitis/gastric bleeding) in four (29%) of the HIV patients. Despite this there was biochemical and anthropometric stability over 3–8 weeks follow-up. Similar gains appear to be achievable in paediatric HIV practice, with probable advantage over nasogastric tube feeding.[131] Given the possibilities of morbidity from the gastrostomy tube and that a few patients may prefer to self-intubate on a nightly basis, a choice should be offered.

Parenteral nutrition

Parenteral nutritional support is unsurprisingly a source of continuing controversy[113] not least since it seems to work best in patients with eating disorders and to a lesser extent in those with malabsorption, but not in those with continuing active infection. As long ago as 1988, Hickey and Weaver had developed screening criteria to help determine the most appropriate form of nutritional support for a given individual.[132] Singer et al. reviewed their first 22 AIDS patients who had received parenteral nutrition at home, and were pleased to be able to record low complication rates (e.g. catheter sepsis in 0.12/100 catheter days) very similar to those in their non–HIV population on this therapy.[133] However, there is an important caution here for those practising in Northern Europe, as this comparison (as well as being uncontrolled) was essentially with patients with terminal malignancy rather than the long-term chronic disease population which predominates in our home parenteral nutrition groups. The OASIS study confirmed this difference in the first analysis of HIV-associated home parenteral nutrition, in which the cancer and HIV patients together formed a short-term survival group with a mean of only 6 months till death, and with a high frequency of complications (4.6 per year: actuarial).[134] Perhaps more importantly only 15% experienced satisfactory rehabilitation for any period of time, questioning further the wisdom of the introduction of intravenous nutrition.

While accepting that nutritional support (whether parenteral or enteral) tended to be given only to the very sickest HIV patients, who are perhaps those least likely to benefit, Brolin et al. were unable to demonstrate any benefit from nutritional intervention in 55 patients treated over a 4-year period in a single institution.[135] Neither survival nor more malleable nutritional characteristics such as albumin or body weight were improved. The worse survival prognosis amongst those treated with parenteral nutrition ($P < 0.03$ compared to those fed enterally) probably reflects selection bias, however. Similar data from Brazil go on to demonstrate not only an absence of survival advantage, but also a substantially greater number of days spent in hospital in those treated with parenteral nutrition (21 vs 7 days).[136] In the absence of controlled data, it is difficult to be sure whether this is generally the case.

If enteral feeding appears to be failing, the existing regimes should always be reviewed and intensified as soon as possible, taking into account the patient's overall prognosis and nutritional status (including gastrointestinal function). If he or she is thought likely to live for more than 2–3 months and has intestinal failure, then long-term intravenous nutrition should be considered and carefully discussed with the patient. It should be remembered also, in addition to the clinical and ethical issues that will be considered prior to commencing intravenous nutrition, that starting this form of treatment incorporates the high probability of necessitating a future decision to stop it.[137] If the decision is in favour of parenteral nutrition, then all standard prerequisites for dedicated line care should be satisfied (including the use of implanted ports ad libitum). The frequent need for long-term central venous access for other purposes (such as antiviral therapy) adds a particular difficulty to line management in HIV patients but not one that cannot be overcome.

ANTIRETROVIRAL THERAPY AND HIV ENTEROPATHY

In 1996 a new class of drugs active against HIV infection became available. These drugs, the protease inhibitors, block the enzyme responsible for post-translational processing of HIV envelope protein precursors, and result in the production of non-infectious virions. The combination of protease inhibitors with nucleoside analogues and non-nucleoside reverse transcriptase inhibitors produces a potent inhibition of HIV replication and allows a dramatic degree of immune reconstitution. Both CD8 and CD4 cells are increased, and their function and that of macrophages improves. In many patients treated with so-called highly active antiretroviral therapy (HAART) HIV RNA levels in serum become nearly undetectable and a prolonged immunological response is seen.

HAART has had a great impact on the course and prognosis of HIV infection.[138] Current UK recommendations are that treatment should start before irreversible damage has occurred to the immune system – for example when the CD4 count is below $350/\mu l$ or in the range $350–500/\mu l$ with high viraemia.[139] The treatment allows CD4 cell counts to remain in the near normal range for prolonged periods, reducing the risk of development of new opportunistic infections, including those associated with HIV enteropathy. As one example, the prevalence of cryptosporidiosis in French HIV-infected patients has more than halved.[140]

In patients already infected with cryptosporidium or microsporidium, treatment with HAART can result in cure of the diarrhoea, weight gain and cessation of oocyst/spore shedding in the stools.[141,142] When small intestinal biopsy specimens have been obtained from patients with cryptosporidiosis and microsporidiosis responding to HAART, the organisms can no longer be seen. In some cases, infection-induced villus atrophy also recovers, but mild inflammation and villus atrophy may persist in post-treatment biopsies.[142] A summary of treatment options for HUV is given in Table 6.7.

***Table 6.7** –* Treatments for HIV infection

Organism	CD4 range	Therapy
HIV	CD4 <350 μl or consider if CD4 350–500 μl with viral load > 30 000 μl	Combination of two nucleoside analogues (NA) and one protease inhibitor (PI) or one non–nucleoside reverse transcriptase inhibitor (NNRTI). Examples: NA: zidovudine, lamivudine, stavudine, didanosine PI: indinavir, ritonavir, saquinavir, nelfinavir NNRTI: efavirenz, nevirapine
Prophylaxis of		
Pneumocystis carnii	CD4 < 200 μl	Cotrimoxazole
Mycobacterium avium intracellulare	CD4 < 50 μl	Azithromycin weekly
Recurrent *Herpes simplex*		Aciclovir
Enteric organisms		Boiled water
Nutritional therapy		Advice and education Oral supplements – high energy diet Gastrostomy feeding Parenteral nutrition Appetite stimulants

Little is known about the effects of HAART on the gut mucosa in patients without pathogens, with as yet (to our knowledge) no published study of the effects of these potent antiretrovirals on the small bowel mucosa. In a small prospective study of patients initiating or changing to HAART, Kotler *et al.* examined rectal biopsies before and after 7 days of treatment.[143] There was a decrease in the amount of HIV detectable in the mucosa by PCR, which paralleled the reduction in viraemia, a rise in the number of lamina propria CD4 cells and a decrease in the number of apoptotic cells.

It is unclear whether the intestinal response to potent antiretroviral therapy is likely to be sustained, but it is known that breakthrough viraemia does occur in patients receiving the new therapies for prolonged periods, either due to non–compliance with therapy or the development of viral resistance. Some patients with cryptosporidiosis and microsporidiosis who have had a clinical and microbiological response to HAART have later relapsed in association with declining CD4 counts and a recurrence of HIV viraemia.[142] It therefore seems likely that gastro-enterologists will continue to see cases of HIV enteropathy for the foreseeable future.

REFERENCES

1. Gottleib MS, Schroff R, Schanker HM, Weisman JD, Fan PT. *Pneumocystis carinii* pneumonia and mucosal candidiasis in previously healthy homosexual men: evidence of a new acquired cellular immunodeficiency. *N Engl J Med* 1981; **305**: 1425–1431.

2. Siegal FP, Lopez C, Hammer GS, *et al.* Severe acquired immunodeficiency syndrome in male homosexuals manifested by chronic perianal ulcerative herpes simplex lesions. *N Engl J Med* 1981; **305**: 1439–1444.

3. Masur H, Michelis MA, Greene JB, *et al. Pneumocystis carinii* pneumonia: initial manifestation of cellular immune dysfunction. *N Engl J Med* 1981; **305**: 1431–1438.

4. Drew WL, Conant MA, Miner RC, *et al.* Cytomegalovirus and Kaposi's sarcoma in young homosexual men. *Lancet* 1982; **2**: 125–127.

5. Ragni MV, Lewis JH, Spero JA, Bontempo FA. Acquired immunodeficiency-like syndrome in two haemophiliacs. *Lancet* 1983; **1**: 213–214.

6. Vieira J, Frank E, Spira TJ, Landesman SH. Acquired immunodeficiency syndrome in Haitians: opportunistic infections in previously healthy Haitian immigrants. *N Engl J Med* 1983; **11**: 403–418.

7. Pitchenik AE, Fischl MA, Dickinson GM, *et al.* Opportunistic infections and Kaposi's sarcoma among Haitians: evidence of an acquired immunodeficiency state. *Ann Intern Med* 1983; **11**: 403–418.

8. Gazzard BG, Shanson DC, Farthing C, *et al.* Clinical findings and serological evidence of HTLV-III infection in homosexual contacts of patients with AIDS and persistent generalised lymphadenopathy in London. *Lancet* 1984; **2**: 480–483.

9. Berkelman RB, Heyward WL, Stehr-Green JK, Curran JW. Epidemiology of human immunodeficiency virus infection and acquired immunodeficiency syndrome. *Am J Med* 1989; **87**: 761–770.

10. Barre-Sinoussi F, Chermann JC, Rey F, *et al*. Isolation of a T-lymphocytotrophic retrovirus from a patient at risk for acquired immunodeficiency syndrome. *Science* 1983; **20**: 868–871.

11. Gallo RC, Salahuddin SZ, Popovic M, *et al*. Frequent detection and isolation of cytopathic retroviruses (HTLV-III) from patients with AIDS and at risk for AIDS. *Science* 1984; **224**: 500–503.

12. Seligmann M, Pinching AJ, Rosen FS, *et al*. Immunology of human immunodeficiency virus infection and the acquired immunodeficiency syndrome. An update. *Ann Intern Med* 1987; **107**: 234–242.

13. Detels R, English PA, Giorgi JV, *et al*. Patterns of CD4+ cell changes after HIV-1 infection indicate the existence of a codeterminant of AIDS. *J Acquir Immune Defic Syndr* 1988; **1**: 390–395.

14. Pinching AJ. Immmunological consequences of human immunodeficiency virus infection. *Rev Med Microbiol* 1990; **1**: 83–91.

15. Cerf-Bensussan N, Guy-Grand D, Griscelli C. Intraepithelial lymphocytes of the human gut: isolation, characterisation and study of natural killer activity. *Gut* 1985; **26**: 81–85.

16. Batman PA, Miller AR, Forster SM, Harris JR, Pinching AJ, Griffin GE. Jejunal enteropathy associated with human immunodeficiency virus infection: quantitative histology. *J Clin Pathol* 1989; **42**: 275–281.

17. Cummins AG, LaBrooy JT, Stanley DP, Rowland R, Shearman DJ. Quantitative histological study of enteropathy associated with HIV infection. *Gut* 1990; **31**: 317–321.

18. Budhraja M, Levendoglu H, Kocka F, Mangkornkanok M, Sherer R. Duodenal mucosal T cell subpopulation and bacterial cultures in acquired immunodeficiency syndrome. *Am J Gastroenterol* 1987; **82**: 427–431.

19. Ellakany S, Whiteside TL, Schade RR, van Thiel DH. Analysis of intestinal lymphocyte subpopulations in patients with acquired immunodeficiency syndrome (AIDS) and AIDS-related complex. *Am J Clin Pathol* 1987; **87**: 356–364.

20. Schrappe-Bacher M, Salzberger B, Fatkenheuer G, Franzen C, Koch B, Krueger GR, Kaufmann W. T-lymphocyte subsets in the duodenal lamina propria of patients with the human immunodeficiency virus type 1 and the influence of high dose immunoglobulin therapy. *J Acq Immun Def Syndr* 1990; **3**: 238–243.

21. Lim SG, Condez A, Lee CA, Johnson MA, Elia C, Poulter LW. Loss of mucosal CD4 lymphocytes is an early feature of HIV infection. *Clin Exp Immunol* 1993; **92**: 448–454.

22. Kotler DP, Scholes JV, Tierney AR. Intestinal plasma cell alterations in acquired immunodeficiency syndrome. *Dig Dis Sci* 1987; **32**: 129–138.

23. Jackson S. Serum and secretory IgA are inversely altered in AIDS patients. In: MacDonald TT, Challacombe SJ, Heatley RV *et al*. (eds). *Advances in Mucosal Immunology*. Kluwer-Academic: Lancaster, UK, 1992.

24. Belitsos PC, Greenson JK, Yardley JH, Sisler JR, Bartlett JG. Association of gastric hypoacidity with opportunistic enteric infections in patients with AIDS. *J Infect Dis* 1992; **166**: 277–284.

25. Griffin GE, Miller A, Batman P, Forster SM, Pinching AJ, Harris JR, Mathan MM. Damage to jejunal intrinsic autonomic nerves in HIV infection. *AIDS* 1988; **2**: 379–382.

26. Barclay GR, Turnberg LA. Effect of cold-induced pain on salt and water transport in the human jejunum. *Gastroenterology* 1988; **94**: 994–998.

27. Serwadda D, Mugerwa RD, Sewankambo NK, *et al*. Slim disease: a new disease in Uganda and its association with HTLV-III infection. *Lancet* 1985; **2**: 849–852.

28. Kotler DP, Tierney AR, Wang J, Pierson RN. Magnitude of body cell mass depletion and the timing of death from wasting in AIDS. *Am J Clin Nutr* 1989; **50**: 444–447.

29. Kotler DP. Cytomegalovirus colitis and wasting. *J Acq Immune Def Syndr* 1991; **4**: S36–41.

30. Kotler DP, Tierney AR, Brenner SK, Couture S, Wang J, Pierson RN. Preservation of short-term energy balance in clinically stable patients with AIDS. *Am J Clin Nutr* 1990; **51**: 7–13.

31. Lahdevirta J, Maury CPJ, Teppo AM, Repo H. Elevated levels of circulating cachectin/tumour necrosis factor in patients with acquired immunodeficiency syndrome. *Am J Med* 1988; **85**: 289–291.

32. Reddy MM, Sorrell SJ, Lange M, Grieko MH. Tumour necrosis factor and HIV p24 antigen in the serum of an HIV-infected population. *J AIDS* 1988; **1**: 436–440.

33. Grunfeld C, Kotler DP, Shigenaga JK, *et al*. Circulating interferon alpha levels and hypertriglyceridaemia in the acquired immunodeficiency syndrome. *Am J Med* 1991; **90**: 154–162.

34. Grunfeld C, Kotler DP. The wasting syndrome and nutritional support in AIDS. *Semin Gastr Dis* 1991; **2**: 25–36.

35. Boudes P, Zittoun J, Sobel A. Folate, vitamin B12 and HIV infection. *Lancet* 1990; **335**: 1401–1402.

36. Ehrenpreis ED, Ganger DR, Kochvar GT, Patterson BK, Craig RM. D-xylose malabsorption: characteristic finding in patients with the AIDS wasting syndrome and chronic diarrhoea. *J Acq Immune Def Synd* 1992; **5**: 1047–1050.

37. Burkes RL, Cohen H, Krailo M, Sinow RM, Carmel R. Low serum cobalamin levels occur frequently in AIDS and related disorders. *Eur J Haematol* 1987; **38**: 141–147.

38. Harriman GR, Smith PD, Horne MK, *et al*. Vitamin B12 malabsorption in patients with acquired immuno-deficiency syndrome. *Arch Intern Med* 1989; **149**: 2039–2041.

39. Kotler DP, Haroutiounian G, Greenberg R, Setchell K, Balistieri WF. Increased bile salt deconjugation in AIDS (abstract). *Gastroenterology* 1985; **88**: 1455A.

40. Kapembwa MS, Bridges C, Joseph AE, Fleming SC, Batman P, Griffin GE. Ileal and jejunal absorptive function in AIDS patients with enterococcidial infection. *J Infect* 1990; **21**: 43–53.

41. Malebranche R, Arnoux E, Guerin JM, *et al*. Acquired immunodeficiency syndrome with severe gastro-intestinal manifestations in Haiti. *Lancet* 1983; **2**: 873–877.

42. Colebunders R, Francis H, Mann JM, *et al*. Persistent diarrhoea strongly associated with HIV infection in Kinshasa, Zaire. *Am J Gastroenterol* 1987; **82**: 859–864.

43. Girard PM, Marche C, Maslo C, *et al*. Digestive mani-festations in acquired immunodeficiency disease (in French). *Ann Med Interne Paris* 1987; **138**: 411–415.

44. Antony MA, Brandt LJ, Klein RS, Bernstein LH. Infectious diarrhoea in patients with AIDS. *Dig Dis Sci* 1988; **33**: 1141–1146.

45. Laughon BE, Druckman DA, Vernon A, Quinn TC, Polk BF, Modlin JF. Prevalence of enteric pathogens in homosexual men with and without the acquired immune deficiency syndrome. *Gastroenterology* 1988; **94**: 984–993.

46. Heise W, Mostertz P, Arasteh K, Skörde J, L'age M. Gastrointestinal findings in human immunodeficiency virus infection. Clinical aspects, microbiological find-ings and endoscopic picture (in German). *Dtsch Med Wochenschr* 1988; **113**: 1588–1593.

47. Lane GP, Lucas CR, Smallwood RA. The gastro-intestinal and hepatic manifestations of the acquired immunodeficiency syndrome. *Med J Aust* 1989; **150**: 139–143.

48. Connolly GM, Shanson DC, Hawkins DA, Harcourt Webster JN, Gazzard BG. Non-cryptosporidial diarrhoea in human immunodeficiency virus (HIV) infected patients. *Gut* 1989; **30**: 195–200.

49. Rolston KV, Rodriguez S, Hernandez M, Bodey GP. Diarrhoea in patients infected with the human immunodeficiency virus. *Am J Med* 1989; **86**: 137–138.

50. Blanshard C, Gazzard BG. The incidence and cause of transient and persisting diarrhoea in relation to CD4 lymphocyte count in HIV infected individuals. *Eur J Gastro Hepatol* 1993; **5**: 823–828.

51. Kazal HL, Sohn N, Carrasco JI, Robilotti JG, Delaney WE. The gay bowel syndrome. Clinicopathologic correlation in 260 cases. *Ann Clin Lab Sci* 1976; **6**: 184–192.

52. Sohn N, Robilotti JG. The gay bowel syndrome. A review of colonic and rectal conditions in 200 male homosexuals. *Am J Gastroenterol* 1977; **67**: 478–484.

53. Quinn TC, Corey L, Chaffee RG, Schuffler MD, Brancato FF, Nolmes KK. The etiology of anorectal infections in homosexual men. *Am J Med* 1981; **71**: 385–406.

54. Quinn TC, Stamm WE, Goodell SE, *et al*. The polymicrobial origin of intestinal infections in homo-sexual men. *New Engl J Med* 1983; **309**: 576–582.

55. Dworkin B, Wormser GP, Rosenthal WS, *et al*. Gastrointestinal manifestations of the acquired immunodeficiency syndrome: a review of 22 cases. *Am J Gastroenterol* 1985; **80**: 774–778.

56. Sewankambo N, Mugerwa RD, Goodgame R, Carswell JW, Moody A, Lloyd G, Lucas SB. Enteropathic AIDS in Uganda. An endoscopic, histo-logical and microbiological study. *AIDS* 1987; **1**: 9–13.

57. Colebunders R, Lusakumuni K, Nelson AM, *et al*. Persistent diarrhoea in Zairian AIDS patients: an endo-scopic and histological study. *Gut* 1988; **29**: 1687–1691.

58. Miró JM, Mallolas J, Moreno A, Gatell JM, Valls ME. Infectious gastroenteritis with the acquired immuno-deficiency (AIDS)(letter). *Ann Intern Med* 1988; **109**: 342.

59. Smith PD, Janoff EN. Infectious diarrhoea in human immunodeficiency virus infection. *Gastroenterol Clin N Am* 1988; **17**: 587–598.

60. Rolston KV, Rodriguez S, Hernandez M, Bodey GP. Diarrhoea in patients infected with the human immunodeficiency virus. *Am J Med* 1989; **86**: 137–138.

61. Conlon CP, Pinching AJ, Perera CU, Moody A, Luo NP, Lucas SB. HIV-related enteropathy in Zambia: clinical, microbiological and histological study. *Am J Trop Med Hyg* 1990; **42**: 83–88.

62. Blanshard C, Francis N, Gazzard BG. Investigation of chronic diarrhoea in acquired immunodeficiency syndrome; a prospective study of 155 patients. *Gut* 1996; **39**: 824–832.

63. Flanigan T, Whalen C, Turner J, Soave R, Toerner J, Havlir D, Kotler D. *Cryptosporidium* infection and CD4 counts. *Ann Int Med* 1992; **116**: 840–842.

64. Levine AM. Non-Hodgkin's lymphoma and other malignancies in the acquired immunodeficiency syndrome. *Semin Oncol* 1987; **14(suppl 3)**: 34–39.

65. Friedman SL, Wright TL, Altman DF. Gastrointestinal Kaposi's sarcoma in patients with acquired immunodeficiency syndrome. Endoscopic and autopsy findings. *Gastroenterology* 1985; **89**: 102–108.

66. Kotler DP, Gaetz HP, Lange M, Klein EB, Holt PR. Enteropathy associated with the acquired immunodeficiency syndrome. *Ann Int Med* 1984; **101**: 421–428.

67. Kotler DP, Francisco A, Clayton F, Scholes JV, Orenstein JM. Small intestinal injury and parasitic diseases in AIDS. *Ann Intern Med* 1990; **113**: 444–449.

68. Gillin JS, Shike M, Alcock N, *et al*. Malabsorption and mucosal abnormalities of the small intestine in patients with the acquired immunodeficiency syndrome. *Ann Intern Med* 1985; **102**: 619–622.

69. Miller AR, Griffin GE, Batman P, Farquar C, Forster SM, Pinching AJ, Harris JRW. Jejunal mucosal architecture and fat absorption in male homosexuals infected with human immunodeficiency virus. *Q J Med* 1988; **69**: 1009–1019.

70. Ullrich R, Zeitz M, Heise W, L'age M, Höffken G, Riecken EO. Small intestinal structure and function in patients infected with human immunodeficiency virus (HIV): evidence for HIV-induced enteropathy. *Ann Intern Med* 1989; **111**: 15–21.

71. Ullrich R, Zeitz M, Heise W, L'Age M, Ziegler K, Bergs C, Riecken EO. Mucosal atrophy is associated with loss of activated T cells in the duodenal mucosa of human immunodeficiency virus (HIV) infected patients. *Digestion* 1990; **46(suppl 2)**: 302–307.

72. Ullrich R, Heise W, Bergs C, L'Age M, Riecken EO, Zeitz M. Effects of zidovudine treatment on the small intestinal mucosa in patients infected with the human immunodeficiency virus. *Gastroenterology* 1992; **102**: 1483–1492.

73. Tepper RE, Simon D, Brandt LJ, Nutovits R, Lee MJ. Intestinal permeability in patients infected with the human immunodeficiency virus. *Am J Gastroenterol* 1994; **89**: 878–882.

74. Gobel E, Brandler U. Ultrastructure of microgameteogenesis, microgametes, and gametogeny of *Cryptosporidium* species in the small intestine of mice. *Parasitologica* 1982; **18**: 331–344.

75. Guarino A, Canani RB, Pozio E, Terracciano L, Albano F, Mazzeo M. Enterotoxic effect of stool supernatant of cryptosporidium-infected calves on human jejunum. *Gastroenterology* 1994; **106**: 28–34.

76. Greenson JK, Belitsos PC, Yardley JH, Bartlett JG. AIDS enteropathy: occult enteric infections and duodenal mucosal alterations in chronic diarrhoea. *Ann Intern Med* 1991; **114**: 366–372.

77. Swanson VL, Thomassen RW. Pathology of the jejunal mucosa in tropical sprue. *Am J Pathol* 1965; **46**: 511–551.

78. Ament ME, Shimoda SS, Saunders DR, Rubin CE. Pathogenesis of steatorrhoea in three cases of small intestinal stasis syndrome. *Gastroenterology* 1972; **63**: 728–736.

79. Tabaqchali S, Hatzioanouu J, Booth CC. Bile-salt deconjugation and steatorrhoea in patients with the stagnant loop syndrome. *Gastroenterology* 1975; **68**: 1193–1203.

80. Kirsch M. Bacterial overgrowth. *Am J Gastroenterology* 1990; **85**: 231–237.

81. Nichols BL, Dudley MA, Nichols VN, *et al*. Effects of malnutrition on the expression and activity of lactase in children. *Gastroenterology* 1997; **112**: 742–745.

82. O'Keefe SJ. Nutrition and gastrointestinal disease. *Scand J Gastroenterol* 1996; **31(S220)**: 52–59.

83. Spies TD, Milanes F, Menendez A, Koch MB, Minnich V. Observations on the treatment of tropical sprue with folic acid. *J Lab Clin Med* 1946; **31**: 227–241.

84. Swanson VL, Wheby MS, Bayless TM. Morphologic effects of folic acid and vitamin B12 on the jejunal lesion of tropical sprue. *Am J Pathol* 1966; **49**: 167–191.

85. Hoover EA, Mullin JI, Quackenbush SL, Gasper PW. Experimental transmission and pathogenesis of immunodeficiency syndrome in cats. *Blood* 1987; **70**: 1880–1892.

86. Nelson JA, Wiley CA, Reynolds-Kohler C, Reese CE, Margaretten W, Levy JA. Human immunodeficiency virus detected in bowel epithelium from patients with gastrointestinal symptoms. *Lancet* 1988; **1**: 259–262.

87. Levy JA, Margaretten W, Nelson J. Detection of HIV in enterochromaffin cells in the rectal mucosa of an AIDS patient. *Am J Gastroenterol* 1989; **84**: 787–789.

88. Kotler DP, Reka S, Borcich A, Cronin WJ. Detection, localisation and quantitation of HIV-associated antigens in intestinal biopsies from patients with HIV. *Am J Pathol* 1991; **139**: 823–830.

89. Mathijs JM, Hing M, Grierson J, Dwyer DE, Goldschmidt C, Cooper DA, Cunningham AL. HIV infection of rectal mucosa (letter). *Lancet* 1988; **i**: 1111.

90. Heise C, Dandekar S, Kumar P, Duplantier R, Donovan RM, Halstead CH. Human immunodeficiency virus infection of enterocytes and mononuclear cells in human jejunal mucosa. *Gastroenterology* 1991; **100**: 1521–1527.

91. Fox CH, Kotler D, Tierney AR, Wilson CS, Fauci AS. Detection of HIV-1 RNA in intestinal lamina propria of patients with AIDS and gastrointestinal disease. *J Infect Dis* 1989; **159**: 467–471.

92. Winter HS, Fox CH, Hendren RB, Isselbacher KJ, Folkman J, Letvin NL. Use of an animal model for the study of the role of human immunodeficiency virus 1 in the human intestine. *Gastroenterology* 1992; **102**: 834–839.

93. Adachi A, Koenig S, Gendelman HE, *et al*. Productive, persistent infection of human colorectal cell lines with human immunodeficiency virus. *J Virol* 1987; **61**: 209–213.

94. Moyer MP, Gendelman HE. HIV replication and persistence in human gastrointestinal cells cultured in vitro. *J Leukoc Biol* 1991; 49: 499–504.

95. Rabenandrasana C, Baghdiguin S, Marvaldi J, Fantini J. CD4 molecules are restricted to the basolateral membrane domain of in vitro differentiated human colon cancer cells (HT29-D4). *FEBS Letters* 1990; **265**: 75–79.

96. Wideman DA, Ramirez A Jr, Xu YL, Moyer MP. Detection of CD4 related protein in human gastro-intestinal epithelial cells cultured in vitro (abstract). In vitro 1990; **26**: 52A.

97. Fleming SC, Kapembwa MS, MacDonald TT, Griffin GE. Direct in vitro infection of human intestine with HIV-1. *AIDS* 1992; 6: 1099–1104.

98. Batman PA, Fleming SC, Sedgwick PM, MacDonald TT, Griffin GE. HIV infection of human fetal intestinal explant cultures induces epithelial cell proliferation. *AIDS* 1994; **8**: 161–167.

99. Kotler DP, Reka S, Chow K, Orenstein JM. Effect of enteric parasitoses and HIV infection upon small intestinal structure and function in patients with AIDS. *J Clin Gastroenterol* 1993; **16**: 10–15.

100. Bramble MG, Zucoloto S, Wright NA, Record CO. Acute gluten challenge in treated adult coeliac disease: a morphometric and enzymatic study. *Gut* 1985; **26**: 169–174.

101. Mowat AM, Felstein MV, Borland A, Parrot DM. Experimental studies of immunologically mediated enteropathy. Development of cell-mediated immunity and intestinal pathology during graft-versus-host reaction in irradiated mice. *Gut* 1988; **29**: 949–956.

102. Sloane JP, Dilly SA. Pathogenesis of graft versus host disease. *Histopathology* 1988; **12**: 105–110.

103. MacDonald TT, Ferguson A. Hypersensitivity reactions in the small intestine III. The effects of allograft rejection and of graft-versus-host reaction on epithelial cell kinetics. *Cell Tissue Kinet* 1977; **10**: 301–312.

104. Sullivan PB, Lunn PG, Northop-Clewes C, Crowe PT, Marsh MN, Neale G. Persistent diarrhoea and malnutrition – the impact of treatment on small bowel structure and permeability. *J Paediatr Gastroent Nutr* 1992; **14**: 208–215.

105. MacDonald TT, Spencer J. Evidence that activated mucosal T cells play a role in the pathogenesis of enteropathy in human small intestine. *J Exp Med* 1988; **167**: 1341–1349.

106. Elson CO, Reilley RW, Rosenberg IH. Small intestine injury in graft–versus–host reaction: an innocent bystander phenomenon. *Gastroenterology* 1977; **72**: 886–889.

107. Reka S, Borchich A, Cronin W, Kotler DP. Diarrhoea associated with intestinal HIV infection in ARC (abstract). *Clin Res* 1989; **37**: A371.

108. Kotler DP, Reka S. Intestinal mucosal inflammation associated with HIV infection. *Dig Dis Sci* 1993; **38**: 1119–1127.

109. Ferguson A, Jarett EE. Hypersensitivity reactions in the small intestine. I. Thymus dependency of experimental 'partial villus atrophy'. *Gut* 1975; **16**: 114–117.

110. Hing M, Oliver C, Melville R. Zidovudine for HIV enteropathy (letter). *Lancet* 1991; **338**: 1086–1087.

111. Kotler DP. Cytomegalovirus colitis and wasting. *J Acq Immune Defic Syndr* 1991; **4 (suppl 1)**: S36–41.

112. Summerbell CD, Perrett JP, Gazzard BG. Causes of weight loss in human immunodeficiency virus infection. *Int J STD AIDS* 1993; **4**: 234–236.

113. Kotler DP. Nutritional effects and support in the patient with acquired immunodeficiency syndrome. *J Nutr* 1992; **122(suppl)**: 723–727.

114. Abrams B, Duncan D, Hertz-Picciotto I. A prospective study of dietary intake and acquired immune deficiency syndrome in HIV-seropositive homosexual men. *J Acquir Immune Defic Syndr* 1993; **6**: 949–958.

115. Burger B, Ollenschlager G, Schrappe M, *et al*. Nutrition behavior of malnourished HIV-infected patients and intensified oral nutritional intervention. *Nutrition* 1993; **9**: 43–44.

116. Chlebowski RT, Grosvenor M, Lillington L, Sayre J, Beall G. Dietary intake and counseling, weight maintenance, and the course of HIV infection. *J Am Diet Assoc* 1995; **95**: 428–432.

117. McKinley MJ, Goodman-Block J, Lesser ML, Salbe AD. Improved body weight status as a result of nutrition intervention in adult, HIV-positive outpatients. *J Am Diet Assoc* 1994; **94**: 1014–1017.

118. Tchekmedyian NS, Hickman M, Heber D. Treatment of anorexia and weight loss with megestrol acetate in patients with cancer or acquired immunodeficiency syndrome. *Semin Oncol* 1991; **18**: 35–42.

119. Von-Roenn JH. Randomized trials of megestrol acetate for AIDS-associated anorexia and cachexia. *Oncology* 1994; **51 (Suppl 1)**: 19–24.

120. Struwe M, Kaempfer SH, Geiger CJ, *et al.* Effect of dronabinol on nutritional status in HIV infection. *Ann Pharmacother* 1993; **27**: 827–831.

121. Beal JE, Olson R, Laubenstein L, *et al.* Dronabinol as a treatment for anorexia associated with weight loss in patients with AIDS. *J Pain Symptom Man* 1995; **10**: 89–97.

122. Beal JE, Olson R, Lefkowitz L, *et al.* Long-term efficacy and safety of dronabinol for acquired immunodeficiency syndrome-associated anorexia. *J Pain Symptom Man* 1997; **14**: 7–14.

123. Serostim Study Group. Recombinant human growth hormone in patients with HIV-associated wasting. A randomised, placebo-controlled trial. *Ann Intern Med.* 1996; **125**: 873–882.

124. Simon DM, Cello JP, Valenzuela J, *et al.* Multicenter trial of octreotide in patients with refractory acquired immunodeficiency syndrome-associated diarrhea [published erratum appears in *Gastroenterology* 1995; **109**: 1024]. *Gastroenterology* 1995; **108**: 1753–1760.

125. Kotler DP, Tierney AR, Ferraro R, Cuff P, Wang J, Pierson RN Jr, Heymsfield SB. Enteral alimentation and repletion of body cell mass in malnourished patients with acquired immunodeficiency syndrome. *Am J Clin Nutr* 1991; **53**: 149–154.

126. Wanke CA, Pleskow D, Degirolami PC, Lambl BB, Merkel K, Akrabawi S. A medium chain triglyceride-based diet in patients with HIV and chronic diarrhea reduces diarrhea and malabsorption: a prospective, controlled trial. *Nutrition* 1996; **12**: 766–771.

127. Craig GB, Darnell BE, Weinsier RL, *et al.* Decreased fat and nitrogen losses in patients with AIDS receiving medium-chain-triglyceride-enriched formula vs those receiving long-chain-triglyceride-containing formula. *J Am Diet Assoc* 1997; **97**: 605–611.

128. Chlebowski RT, Beall G, Grosvenor M, *et al.* Long-term effects of early nutritional support with new enterotropic peptide-based formula vs. standard enteral formula in HIV-infected patients: randomized prospective trial. *Nutrition* 1993; **9**: 507–512.

129. Ockenga J, Suttmann U, Selberg O, *et al.* Percutaneous endoscopic gastrostomy in AIDS and control patients: risks and outcome. *Am J Gastroenterol* 1996; **91**: 1817–1822.

130. Cappell MS, Godil A. A multicenter case–control study of percutaneous endoscopic gastrostomy in HIV-seropositive patients. *Am J Gastroenterol* 1993; **88**: 2059–2066.

131. Miller TL, Awnetwant EL, Evans S, Morris VM, Vazquez IM, McIntosh K. Gastrostomy tube supplementation for HIV-infected children. *Pediatrics* 1995; **96**: 696–702.

132. Hickey MS, Weaver KE. Nutritional management of patients with ARC or AIDS. *Gastroenterol Clin N Am* 1988; **17**: 545–561.

133. Singer P, Rothkopf MM, Kvetan V, Kirvela O, Gaare J, Askanazi J. Risks and benefits of home parenteral nutrition in the acquired immunodeficiency syndrome. *J Parenter Enteral Nutr* 1991; **15**: 75–79.

134. Howard L, Heaphey L, Fleming CR, Lininger L, Steiger E. Four years of North American registry home parenteral nutrition outcome data and their implications for patient management. *J Parenter Enteral Nutr* 1991; **15**: 384–393.

135. Brolin RE, Gorma RC, Milgrim LM, Abbott JM, George S, Gocke DJ. Use of nutrition support in patients with AIDS: a four-year retrospective review. *Nutrition* 1991; **7**: 19–22.

136. Ferrini MT, Waitzberg DL, Pasternak J, Coppini LZ, da-Silva M de L, Gama-Rodrigues J. [Effect of nutritional support on survival of AIDS-IV C patients]. Efeito do suporte nutricional na sobrevida dos pacientes com AIDS-IV C. *Rev Hosp Clin-Fac Med Sao Paulo* 1993; **48**: 161–166.

137. Knowles JB, Gilmore N. Discontinuation of total parenteral nutrition in a patient with acquired immunodeficiency syndrome: a Canadian perspective. *Nutr Rev* 1994; **52**: 271–274.

138. Palella FJ, Delaney KM, Moorman AC, *et al.* Declining morbidity and mortality among patients with advanced human immunodeficiency virus infection. *N Engl J Med* 1998; **338**: 853–860.

139. Gazzard B, Moyle G, on behalf of the BHIVA Guidelines Writing Committee. 1998 Revision of the British HIV Association Guidelines for Antiretroviral Treatment of HIV Seropositive Individuals. *Lancet* 1998; **352**: 314–316.

140. Le Moing V, Bissuel F, Costagliola D, *et al.* Decreased prevalence of HIV-associated cryptosporidiosis in HIV-infected patients concomitant to the widespread use of protease inhibitors. *AIDS* 1998; **12**: 1395–1397.

141. Goguel J, Katlama C, Sarfati C, Maslo C, Leport C, Molina J-M. Remission of AIDS-associated intestinal microsporidiosis with highly active antiretroviral therapy. *AIDS* 1997; **11**: 1658–1659.

142. Carr A, Marriott D, Field A, Vasak E, Cooper DA. Treatment of HIV-associated cryptosporidiosis with combination antiretroviral therapy. *Lancet* 1998; **351**: 256–261.

143. Kotler DP, Shimada T, Snow G, *et al.* Effect of combination antiretroviral therapy upon rectal mucosa HIV RNA burden and mononuclear cell apoptosis. *AIDS* 1998; **12**: 597–604.

Section 3

Chronic intestinal failure

7

Intestinal failure in children

Peter J. Milla

The child is particularly vulnerable to the consequences of intestinal failure which in its chronic form results in protracted diarrhoea, failure to thrive and grow and, in its most severe form, death. The most common type of acute intestinal failure is that associated with gastroenteric infection and it has been estimated that in children under the age of 5 years, 20 million episodes of diarrhoea occur throughout the world per year. Chronic intestinal failure on the other hand has an incidence of approximately 1 in 90 000 per head of total population per annum, and this results in about 500 affected children in England and Wales each year.

While chronic intestinal failure in adults is dominated by acquired diseases, particularly patients with a short bowel complicating Crohn's disease, in children, congenital or early onset disorders are the predominant causes. Of children with severe intestinal failure requiring parenteral nutrition for more than a month, about 75% have congenital diseases affecting the gut, heart or the hepatobiliary system, and these often require major corrective surgery.[1,2] About 50% of children who start on parenteral nutrition do so before the age of 6 months. The majority of intestinal failure in children therefore occurs in the nutritionally most vulnerable group, in whom management is particularly challenging as a result of their limited nutritional reserves, and in whom accurate diagnosis often requires sophisticated techniques.

The natural history of intestinal failure in children is extremely variable and is largely that of the underlying disorder. Virtually all children with acute intestinal failure can be expected to recover with appropriate treatment. Most children with a short bowel have it as a consequence of a disorder in the neonatal period following treatment of congenital anomalies or necrotizing enterocolitis[3] and they do well, partly because their colon is usually preserved. Ninety-five per cent of infants with such conditions are cared for in large experienced centres and will eventually stop parenteral nutrition. It may, however, take as long as 5 years for the intestine to fully adapt. At the other end of the spectrum of chronic intestinal failure are diseases, which without long-term parenteral nutrition or small intestinal transplantation are invariably fatal. Such disorders mainly present at birth or in the first few weeks of life and include mucosal diseases (e.g. congenital microvillus atrophy) and severe neuromuscular diseases (chronic intestinal pseudo-obstruction).

ACUTE INTESTINAL FAILURE

Acute intestinal failure may be due to a variety of insults upon the gut including infection, chemotherapy, radiation damage or postoperative paralytic ileus. Due to the rapid turnover of gut mucosal epithelial cells together with the large mass of mucosal associated lymphoid tissue underneath the epithelial layer, the majority of cases of acute intestinal failure in children are due to mucosal diseases rather than disorders of the neuromuscular layers. The largest and potentially the most important group are the infective gastroenterocolitides.

Mucosal disease

Infectious gastroenterocolitis

Infectious diarrhoea causes more than 5 million deaths each year world-wide, most of whom occur in young children under the age of 5 years.[4] Although numerous public health factors help to explain this situation, it is also the increased susceptibility that small children have to infectious agents by virtue of their immature intestinal host defences. Infectious agents may have their effects on specific regions of the gut; for example *Helicobacter pylori* on the stomach and duodenum, *Shigella* and *Salmonella* largely on the colon. Bacteria have their effects either by producing toxins, which either effect the function of the epithelial cells or are cytotoxic to them, or the organisms directly invade the epithelial cells.[5] The mechanisms of action whereby viruses cause diarrhoea is less well understood and originally was thought to be by producing cell death; however it is becoming clear that rotavirus, in particular, produces an agent that may be directly toxic to the epithelial cells.[6] The mechanism by which *Giardia lamblia* infestation causes diarrhoea is poorly understood.

The three commonest forms of acute infectious diarrhoea in the world are *Vibrio cholera*, enterotoxigenic *Escherichia coli* (ETEC) and rotavirus. Each induces a large secretory component to the diarrhoea. Both the *Vibrio cholera* and ETEC produce secretory diarrhoea by elaborating toxins in the intestinal lumen which attach to the intestinal epithelium.[7] The toxins from each have two components: a binding component and an active component. The active component enters the cell and activates the basolateral enzyme adenylate cyclase, which results in an increase in the intracellular concentration of a cyclic

AMP. Then cyclic adenosine monophosphate (AMP), acting through a protein kinase cascade, results in the phosphorylation of ion channels in the apical brush border membrane of the enterocytes. As a consequence of these events there is inhibition of sodium chloride absorption, and by opening chloride-specific apical channels on the epithelial cells, there is secretion of chloride into the intestinal lumen. The sodium organic solute co-transporters remain intact and it is these transport mechanisms which are utilized for oral rehydration therapy. Many ETEC elaborate and secrete a large molecular weight toxin called the heat-labile toxin, which is very similar to cholera toxin. Other strains of *E. coli* secrete a smaller molecular weight heat-stable toxin which causes luminal secretion by a different mechanism, in which guanylate cyclase is activated and secretion is caused via cyclic guanosine monophosphate (GMP).[8] The effects of this toxin are less marked than of the heat-labile toxin or the cholera toxin.

The pathophysiology of rotaviral diarrhoea is less clear. Davidson *et al.* studied human rotavirus infection in piglets and thought that carbohydrate malabsorption played a significant role due to inhibition of the sodium-glucose co-transporter.[9] Collins and Starkey used a murine rotavirus model and showed marked secretion of electrolyte and water by the infected small intestine at the height of the diarrhoea.[10] Other studies have shown that oral rehydration solution reverses the water secretion and it is likely that rotavirus elaborates a toxin which induces the secretory process.[11]

Emergent infectious diarrhoeas

While the above forms of infectious diarrhoea are most common world-wide, there are a large number of pathogenic organisms which may result in infectious diarrhoea. These are listed on Table 7.1. Over recent years some new agents have emerged, which are likely to prove important gastroenteric pathogens in children.

Bacteria Vibrio cholerae 0139 About 5 years ago a new cholera organism sera group 0139 emerged and caused epidemic diarrhoea in the Indian sub-continent.[12] Studies of this organism led to the recognition that *Vibrio cholerae* harbours additional virulence factors, which may contribute to diarrhoeal disease. Two newly recognized toxins are the zona occludins toxin (ZOT)[13] and the accessory cholera enterotoxin ACE.

Entero aggregative E. coli (EAggEC) EAggEC are characterized by their pattern of bacterial adhesion to tissue culture cells. EAggEC produce enterotoxins that are both heat-labile and heat-stable.[14] This organism may cause persistent diarrhoea in young children.

Diffusely adherent E. coli (DAEC) DAEC are organisms that bind evenly over the surface of tissue culture cells. Epidemiological studies have shown DAEC to be associated with both acute and chronic diarrhoea.

Entero haemorrhagic E coli (EHEC) EHEC cause haemorrhagic colitis with systemic complications including the haemolytic uraemic syndrome and thrombotic thrombocytopaenic purpura. Only a limited number of *E. coli*, including sero types 0157:H7 and 026:H11, cause this disorder. Recent years have shown the large morbidity and mortality together with the financial implications of this type of food-borne infection. All forms of EHEC are characterized by the production of one or more phage-encoded cytotoxins referred to as vero toxin or shiga-like toxin.[15] This is an area that is actively being

Table 7.1 – Less usual enteropathogenic organisms

Bacteria	Viruses	Protozoans and Helminths	Fungi
Helicobacter pylori	Cytomegalovirus	Dientamoeba fragilis	*Candida albicans*
Helicobacter heilmannii	Astrovirus	Blastocystis	*Histoplasma capsulatum*
Vibrio cholerae 0139	Calicivirus	Microsporidium	
Enteroaggregative *E. coli*	Torovirus	Isopora belli	
Diffusely adherent *E. coli*			
Enterotoxogenic *Bacteroidis fragilis*			
Enterohaemoragic *E. coli*			
Brochyspira aalborgi			
Campylobacter upsaliensis			

researched and, although a distinct pattern of attaching and effacing adhesion is produced on the surface of infected epithelial cells, the pathophysiology of the systemic disease remains unclear.

Viruses

Rotavirus is the best known cause of diarrhoea in children. In addition adenovirus, astrovirus and calicivirus are important. Particles, known as torovirus, which resemble the Breda virus of calves, have been found in the stools of children with diarrhoea. These particles are similar to the previously reported coronovirus-like agents.

Treatment of infectious gastroenterocolitis

The development of oral rehydration therapy has had an enormous impact on the survival of young children from acute diarrhoeal disease. It has been hailed as potentially the most important achievement of the century since the discovery of penicillin.[16] The scientific basis of oral rehydration therapy lies in the observation by Fisher and Parsons that glucose enhances water absorption in the rat small intestine[17] and in the description of the sodium glucose co-transporter mechanism by Schultz and Zalusky.[18]

The composition of oral rehydration solutions (ORS) has been widely studied. The original World Health Organization (WHO) solution produced for patients with cholera contained 90 mmol/L sodium, 80 mmol/L chloride, 20 mmol/L potassium, 10 mmol/L citrate (or 30 mmol bicarbonate) and 111 mmol/L glucose.[19] Many studies have shown this to be effective and safe even in small children. However, the high sodium concentration may be unnecessary to treat the mainly viral diarrhoea of the Western world. As a consequence, the European Society of Paediatric Gastroenterology and Nutrition (ESPGHAN) recommended the use of a single 60 mmol/L sodium containing solution for both rehydration and maintenance treatment.[20]

Just as there has been modification of the original sodium content of oral rehydration solution there has been much work to develop alternative substrates to glucose in order to improve the efficacy of ORS. At present it is only polymeric substrates, such as rice, which have been shown to be more effective than glucose. Rice-based oral rehydration solutions appear to be superior to the WHO ORS in rehydration and reduction of stool volume.[21]

Over the last 20 years a body of clinical and epidemiological studies have made clear a number of therapeutic recommendations (Table 7.2).

Table 7.2 – Principles of treating gastroenterocolitis

1. Oral rehydration should be used in all cases. In well-nourished children in Western countries an ORS with a sodium concentration of 60 mmol/L is safe. If an ORS with a sodium concentration of 90 mmol/L is used additional free water must be used in a ratio of 2:1.

2. Anti-diarrhoeal agents should not be used.

3. Antibiotics are only useful where there is evidence of infectious aetiology particularly with an invasive organism such as *Shigella, Salmonella,* enteropathogenic *E. coli,* or giardiasis.

4. Infants should be re-fed as soon as rehydration has been achieved.

Neuromuscular disease

In recent years it has become apparent that, in addition to the direct invasion of epithelial cells by infecting organisms, a very important mechanism of the production of the diarrhoea is mediated through the enteric nervous system and immunocytes. Increasingly a complex interaction of nerves, muscle, mast cell, T-cells and B-cells, together with the host epithelium, is recognized to ultimately modulate the host reponse to the infecting organisms and their toxins.[22] As a consequence the neuromusculature of the gut plays an important role in the host's response to an infection and results in worsening of diarrhoea by rapid transit and vomiting due to activation of the emetic reflex.

Fast transit diarrhoea is predominantly due to the production of giant migrating complexes produced as a direct action of bacterial toxins on the enteric neuromusculature and results in extremely rapid transit of the luminal contents. Studies in the rabbit have shown this to be the case for both invasive organisms such as *Shigella* and *Salmonella* and toxin producing organisms such as *E. coli.*[23]

Alteration of the environment in which the neuromusculature is operating may also be caused by non-infectious agents, such as hypokalaemia and hypochloraemia, which can cause acute paralytic ileus. In chronic renal failure a disturbance of polypeptide hormone metabolism may result in gastroesophageal reflux and impaired gastric emptying.[24] In some patients with a ganglioneuroblastoma, the secretion of large quantities of vasoactive intestinal polypeptide may, in addition to diarrhoea, cause an ileus.[25]

CHRONIC INTESTINAL FAILURE

Conditions, which cause chronic intestinal failure, may result in maldigestion, malabsorption, together with some secretion of fluid by the intestine and failure of salvage of water electrolyte and short-chain fatty acids in the colon. Diarrhoea is caused when the salvage capacity of the colon to absorb water and electrolytes is exceeded either due to disease of the colon itself, or to an increased effluent from the small intestine which overwhelms its reabsorptive capacity. There are two major types of diarrhoea: osmotic and secretory.

Osmotic diarrhoea

Osmotically active molecules in both the small intestine and colon cause water secretion. This can be demonstrated by measuring stool osmolality and comparing it to the stool calculated osmolarity (2 × (sodium + potassium concentration)). If other osmotically active molecules are present, the osmolality will be much higher than the calculated osmolarity due to the presence of other osmotically active molecules (e.g. unabsorbed sugars, laxatives). Osmotic diarrhoea will reduce when nothing is taken orally.

Undigested nutrients, such as sucrose in the case of sucrose-isomaltose deficiency, are fermented by luminal bacteria to monosaccharides and then to short-chain fatty acids, which increase the intraluminal osmotic load and draw water into the lumen of the bowel. Osmotic diarrhoea might occur in motility disorders when there is very rapid transit of intestinal contents, thus partially digested food is dumped into the colon and fermented to osmotically active molecules.

Secretory diarrhoea

This occurs when the intestinal epithelium secretes fluid. Stool osmolality and calculated osmolarity will be nearly the same and fasting may not reduce the stool volume. This may be due to a bacterial toxin,[7] which causes active chloride secretion. It can be due to normal crypt secretion with no/little villus absorption as in the case of an extensive enteropathy. Chloride secretion may also be mediated through the enteric nervous system and by immunocytes. There is a complex interaction of nerves, muscles, mast cells, T-cells and B-cells with the intestinal epithelium that controls the secretion of fluid by the intestine.[22] Consequently inflammatory processes of the bowel such as Crohn's disease, eosinophilic gastroenteropathy and autoimmune disease of the bowel can all cause secretory diarrhoea. Motility disturbances, which result in ileus or slow gastrointestinal transit, may result in bacterial overgrowth; this in turn may result in a secretory diarrhoea or an enterocolitis such as seen in Hirshsprung's disease. In addition inflammatory disorders of the bowel may interact with nerve and muscle and cause motility disturbances as well as effecting the intestinal epithelium.[26] In situations where extensive amounts of small intestine have been resected for either congenital or inflammatory disease there may be insufficient absorptive surface left to reabsorb the salivary, gastric, biliary, pancreatic and intestinal secretions that occur quite normally each day.[3]

In many of the malabsorptive states encountered, regardless of the specific cause, more than one of the above major pathophysiological mechanisms may be operating. In addition, whenever malabsorption is apparent its consequences will unfavourably affect the exocrine pancreatic and intestinal function which in turn worsens the diarrhoea and malabsorption and creates a vicious cycle.

The differential diagnosis of chronic intestinal failure is very extensive, though in paediatric practice most cases of chronic malabsorptive diarrhoea can be attributed to a limited group of conditions. The majority of these are enteropathic processes of which over 60% are due to either coeliac disease or a food-sensitive enteropathy such as cow's milk or soya protein enteropathy. Postinfectious enteropathy with persisting lactase deficiency seems much less common now than formerly. In susceptible populations lactase deficiency occurs in most older children as a consequence of their genetic make-up.

The investigation of patients with chronic intestinal failure can be extremely difficult, and at times, even after the most sophisticated of investigations, the exact diagnosis cannot be reached. In childhood such patients are treated symptomatically to enable them to grow and develop normally and wherever possible to overcome the ill effects of maldigestion and malabsorption secondary to the disease process. In the remainder of this chapter conditions specific to children are discussed together with their investigation and treatment.

Mucosal disorders

Congenital mucosal defects

A variety of congenital defects occur in infants most usually affecting individual functional molecules (e.g. the sodium glucose link transporter (SGLTI)) or structural abnormalities such as that of the brush border in congenital microvillus atrophy or of mucosal lymphatics in intestinal lymphangectasia.

Functional defects

Disacharidase deficiency, most commonly lactase deficiency, may occur secondary to an enteropathy and due to maldigested carbohydrate (e.g. lactose) a fermentative diarrhoea occurs. The degree of secondary disacharidase deficiency is directly related to the extent and severity of the mucosal damage. Failure of digestion of disacharides may also occur in congenital defects of brush border hydrolases, of which congenital sucrase-isomaltase deficiency is most common.

Congenital sucrase-isomaltase deficiency Congenital sucrase-isomaltase deficiency is inherited as an autosomal recessive trait. The gene coding for the human sucrase-isomaltase enzyme has been mapped to chromosome 3 and elegant cell biosynthesis, and trafficking studies by Naim *et al.*[27] have shown that genetic mutation may result in a variety of abnormalities of the sucrase-isomaltase molecule. These are such that either the molecule does not undergo post-translational processing and is not exported to the cell's surface, or it is exported to the wrong domain of the cell's surface (basolateral rather than apical border) or that the active site of the molecule is non-functional. Whatever the molecular nature of the defect, symptoms begin following the introduction of sucrose to the diet. This fermentative diarrhoea can be totally alleviated by the removal of sucrose and the reduction of starch in the diet.

Congenital lactase deficiency Unlike sucrase-isomaltase deficiency, congenital lactase deficiency is extremely rare.[28] The gene for lactase has been mapped to chromosome 2, but due to its extreme rarity the details of the molecular defect in congenital lactase deficiency are not as well understood. The pathogenesis of the diarrhoea is similar to that of sucrase-isomaltase deficiency, the symptoms begin-ning as soon as milk-containing lactose is introduced into the diet. Treatment very simply involves the removal of lactose from the diet.

Congenital glucose-galactose deficiency Congenital glucose-galactose malabsorption is one of a number of congenital transport defects. Other defects may affect amino acid transport, chloride–bicarbonate exchange in congenital chloridorrhoea and sodium absorption in congenital sodium–proton exchange deficiency. The gene coding for the SGLTI is found on chromosome 22 and mutations of the gene have been shown to have similar effects as to those that cause sucrose-isomaltase deficiency;[29] that is, abnormalities of different parts of the molecule may have an effect on the cellular processing of the molecule, its insertion into the brush border and the function of its active site. Like congenital enzyme defects, an osmotic diarrhoea starts as soon as glucose- and galactose-containing foods are consumed. Consequently, as infants are milk fed, symptoms start within the first few days of life and do not cease until glucose- and galactose-containing foods are removed from the diet. Treatment with milk formulae with fructose is the carbohydrate source, and a diet free of glucose and galactose is extremely satisfactory but very difficult to adhere to. Provided the condition is recognized early, normal growth and development can be anticipated. However, dehydration from the massive osmotic diarrhoea in very early infancy can have a high morbidity with thrombotic episodes being well-described.[30]

Other congenital defects

A number of other congenital defects to the mucosa also occur and these include: congenital chloride-losing diarrhoea,[31] congenital sodium diarrhoea,[32] microvillus atrophy[33] and tufting enteropathy.[34]

Congenital chloride-losing diarrhoea Congenital chloridorrhoea or chloride-losing diarrhoea is an inherited defect of chloride absorption in the ileum and colon. The defect is due to abnormality of the chloride–bicarbonate exchange transporter protein found in the apical membrane of ileal enterocytes and colonocytes. The condition usually presents at birth with abdominal distension and watery diarrhoea, or antenatally with intrauterine diarrhoea as shown by dilated loops of fluid-filled gut on an ultrasound scan during the last trimester. In the neonatal period the infants become dehydrated and alkalotic. After the first month of life the diagnosis is easily made by measuring stool electrolytes when the concentration of chloride in stool water will exceed the sum of both sodium and potassium concentration. In addition, the infants are systemically alkalotic. During the first months of life the chloride concentration may not exceed the sum of sodium and potassium concentrations. The condition occurs most commonly in Finland, eastern Europe and the Arabian Gulf states. There is no curative treatment known but the condition may be controlled by the provision of adequate sodium and potassium supplements to prevent the effects of electrolyte loss. As the upper small intestine is completely normal, absorption will readily take place here even though patients continue to have diarrhoea due to their congenital transport defect. Electrolyte supplements commonly need to be in the region of sodium 10–20 mmol/kg/day. Potassium 10 mmol/kg/day. If the patient becomes dehydrated, paradoxically the diarrhoea may slow and even normal stools may be passed suggesting to the unwary that the condition has ameliorated. Such a situation will, however, only lead to persistent hyper-aldosteronism and ultimately renal failure. The affected patients always have diarrhoea if there is good electrolyte and fluid balance.

Congenital sodium diarrhoea This condition presents in a similar way to congenital chloride-losing diarrhoea.[32] However, as might be expected, the key findings are those of sodium depletion without evidence of chloride loss or alkalosis in the circulating blood. The gastrointestinal mucosa throughout the gastrointestinal tract is morphologically and structurally normal and the diarrhoea similarly appears to be lifelong. The condition is thought to be due to an abnormality of the sodium–proton exchanger in the apical brush border membrane of enterocytes and colonocytes. The diagnostic criteria are: presence of massive watery diarrhoea from birth or antenatally; a structurally normal gastrointestinal mucosa; and a hyponatremic acidosis. There is no known curative treatment but the effects of the disorder can be ameliorated with electrolyte supplements, in particular the use of citrate-containing oral electrolyte solutions.

Structural defects

Microvillus atrophy Microvillus atrophy (microvillus inclusion disease) is the most severe of these disorders and almost invariably results in infant death within 1–2 years even with nutritional support.[35] Microvillus atrophy is a familial disorder characterized by massive watery diarrhoea and presents in two clinical forms.

Diarrhoea may occur within the first week of life and persists even when oral feeding is stopped, or later after the neonatal period often at 2 or 3 months of age. There are characteristic morphological abnormalities of the small intestinal mucosa of which the microvillus inclusion in the apical cytoplasm is characteristic. Treatment consists of long-term total parenteral nutrition as attempts at oral feeding with any kind of nutrients have always failed. A variety of other treatments have been tried, including epidermal growth factor and corticosteroids, but all have proved ineffective in the long term. Death nearly always occurs from accelerated cholestasis. A few have undergone combined liver and small bowel transplantation and only two of four known to the author have survived the procedure.

Tufting enteropathy Tufting enteropathy is similar in presentation to microvillus atrophy but is histologically different with a surface epithelium that shows epithelial tufts of lightly packed enterocytes.

Acquired mucosal defects

Necrotizing enterocolitis

Neonatal necrotizing enterocolitis occurs primarily in premature infants (median 29 weeks) and causes diffuse or patchy transmural areas of necrosis in the small and large bowel, which may perforate.[36] It has a 20% mortality and 25–35% of survivors will have intestinal strictures. The exact aetiology is still obscure, but may occur when the immature gut mucosa has blood shunted elsewhere as may occur after asphyxia, hypovolaemia, hypothermia or sepsis. It commonly occurs following the introduction of enteral feeding, especially of high osmolality feeds. Postulated pathogenetic mechanisms include the invasion of the mucosa with intestinal bacteria.

In the typical case, an infant in the second week of life develops abdominal distension, bilious vomiting and bloody stools; the infant is hypoxic and acidotic with a high white cell and low platelet count. Characteristically pneumatosis intestinalis is seen on abdominal radiographs. Treatment consists of resting the gut by withholding oral/enteral feeding, nasogastric suction and oral and parenteral antibiotics. Total parenteral nutrition is often necessary before oral feeding can be resumed. Surgery may be needed for intestinal decompression, to resect necrotic bowel and/or to divert the faecal stream. A variable amount of bowel may be affected and in its most severe forms will result in large amounts of small and large intestine being resected causing a shortened bowel.

Another type of necrotizing enterocolitis can occur in up to 10% of older children undergoing chemotherapy for leukaemia (neutropenic typhlitis). It has a 40–50% mortality mainly due to perforation of the caecum, which is predominantly affected.

Neuromuscular disorders

The vast majority of intestinal pseudo-obstructive disorders and very severe constipating disorders in children are congenital. The commonest of these is Hirschsprung's disease, which accounts for 1 in 4500 live births compared to visceral myopathies and neuropathies which occur in about 1 in 40 000 live births.

Hirschsprung's disease

Hirschsprung's disease is the most common cause of lower intestinal obstruction in neonates and is due to the absence of normal enteric ganglionic neurons. The aganglionosis begins at the anus and extends proximally for a variable distance. It is limited to the rectum and sigmoid in approximately 75% of cases but includes the total colon in about 8–10% and occasionally may affect the whole intestine (total intestinal aganglionosis). It is sometimes associated with other anomalies such as Down's syndrome, Wardenberg syndrome and congenital heart disorders. The condition presents in one of three ways: with complete intestinal obstruction, delayed passage of meconium or constipation starting on the first day of life, or enterocolitis. In children with Hirschsprung's disease 94% fail to pass meconium within the first 24 hours of life and therefore any term infant who does not pass meconium within 48 hours of life should be suspected of having Hirschsprung's disease.[37] Enterocolitis most often occurs during the 2nd to 4th weeks and results as a consequence of delayed diagnosis. It is characterized by fever, explosive foul-smelling diarrhoea and abdominal distension. The diagnostic method of choice is a suction rectal biopsy with acetylcholinesterase staining which shows the presence of thick acetylcholinesterase-positive nerve fibres in the muscularis mucosa together with an absence of ganglion cells from the submucosa.

Management consists of definitive surgery though if enterocolitis occurs treatment consists of fluid resuscitation, broad-spectrum antibiotics, saline rectal washouts and a decompression stoma. Four definitive surgical approaches have been used: the Swenson, Duhamel, Soave and Boley procedures.[38] All involve resection of the aganglionic bowel and reanastomosis of the proximal normal bowel to the normal anal canal; they differ in methods of reconstructing the bowel. A number of complications may occur following operation, including stricture and leakage at the anastomotic site, faecal incontinence and some will have problems with constipation postoperatively.

Visceral neuropathies and myopathies

A variety of disorders may affect the submucous and myenteric plexuses of the gut and these may be limited to one area of the gut or be more widespread throughout the gastrointestinal tract. These disorders may present in a pseudo-Hirschsprung manner or as intestinal pseudo-obstruction. Nutritional support in the form of parenteral nutrition or enteral feeding may be required during obstructive episodes. A very recent review outlines successful forms of treatment in these conditions.[39]

Short bowel

The causes for a short bowel are different in infants and older children (Table 7.3). During embryonic development the mid-gut herniates into a loop in the umbilical cord and from the 6th intrauterine week the mid-gut undergoes an anticlockwise rotation around the superior mesenteric artery and returns to the abdominal cavity. Developmental problems can occur if this process does not occur normally.

Gastroschisis occurs in 1 in 10 000 births and is more common in mothers under the age of 20. The bowel has not returned to the abdominal cavity and herniates through a lateral abdominal wall defect of less than 4 cm, and unlike an omphalocele it does not have a membranous sac surrounding it, thus bowel necrosis and perforation are common and result in large resections of small intestine. Twenty per cent of such

Table 7.3 – Causes of a short bowel

Infants	Older children >3
Necrotizing enterocolitis	Mesenteric infarction
Intestinal atresia	Crohn's disease
Malrotation of volvulus	Radiation enteritis
Intestinal aganglionosis	Tumours
Gastroschisis	Trauma

patients have additional problems (e.g. renal or gall-bladder agenesis).

Malrotation or volvulus can result in the gut cutting off its own blood supply from the superior mesenteric artery, so causing large amounts of gut to become necrotic and need to be resected.

Intestinal atresia occurs in every 330–1500 births, 50% are in the duodenum, 36% in jejunum and 14% in ileum. This distribution is slightly different to intestinal stenosis, which affects mainly the duodenum (75%), but the ileum (20%) is more commonly involved than the jejunum (5%).

Functionally the small intestine has large functional reserve and up to 50% can be resected without major metabolic or nutritional sequele. However, if more than 75% is lost, nutritional status and growth can only usually be maintained with parenteral nutrition. Even when less than 40 cm of small intestine and a functioning colon is present, long-term survival without parenteral nutrition ultimately occurs in 94% of infants.

The management aims in patients with a short bowel are to: maintain growth and development, promote intestinal adaptation, prevent complications and establish enteral nutrition.[3] In the early days after massive small bowel resection, massive intestinal fluid and electrolyte loss occurs and this slowly falls as intestinal adaptation takes place. The success of intestinal adaptation depends on whether jejunum, ileum and/or colon are resected. Humoral drive for adaptation involves polypeptide hormones that are secreted by the ileum and ascending colon and include glucagon–like peptide-2, peptide YY and neurotensin.

The management of children with a short bowel classically follows four phases.

I: During the immediate postoperative period fluid and electrolyte balance is maintained despite large losses and parenteral nutrition is started to maintain nutritional status.

II: Parenteral nutrition maintains nutritional status and enteral nutrition is introduced.

III: Intestinal adaptation is promoted and enteral nutrition is tolerated.

IV: Enteral nutrition is fully established and oral feeds are introduced together with the withdrawal of parenteral nutrition.

A number of complications may occur, of which parenteral nutrition associated cholestasis is the major complicating factor. Its cause is multifactorial and pre-maturity, catheter-related sepsis and toxic components of parenteral nutrition appear to be the most important factors.

The single most important aspect of the surgical management of patients with a short bowel is prevention. Secondary surgical intervention may be required in established patients, where either there is insufficient bowel when a lengthening procedure may be considered, or where the bowel is exceptionally dilated and tapering may help to prevent bacterial overgrowth (Chapter 33). More recently intestinal transplantation has been considered and since the advent of tacrolimus to control graft rejection, transplantation is becoming a real option. However, as parenteral nutrition is generally well tolerated, at present transplantation is reserved for those with failure of venous access or end-stage liver failure.

Enteropathic disorders

Transient food-sensitive enteropathies

In infancy a variety of delayed hypersensitivity reactions to individual food antigens may result in an enteropathy. Under the age of 3 years this is nearly always transient and most commonly a reaction to cow's milk protein. They usually occur in children who have a minor immunodeficiency and/or are atopic. Intolerance may also occur to soya protein, gluten, eggs, chicken, ground rice and fish. The evidence that the enteropathy is directly related to ingestion of a particular food is based upon small intestinal biopsy and studies of dietary elimination and challenge (e.g. coeliac disease). The enteropathy is not usually as severe as that seen in coeliac disease though a flat mucosa is occasionally seen. These disorders usually resolve by the age of 18 months to 2 years.[40]

The underlying causes of temporary food intolerances of infancy relate to transient sensitization of a child to dietary antigens, which may occur following an enteric infection or a breach of the mucosal barrier. The precise mechanisms, which cause the enteropathy, remain unclear though T-lymphocyte activation occurs in all cases.[41]

Clinical features The onset of symptoms may be acute with sudden onset of vomiting and diarrhoea, and with the diarrhoea persisting and becoming chronic. Alternatively the onset is insidious and the presentation very similar to coeliac disease. In most cases the onset is with acute symptoms commencing before the age of 6 months and there is usually a latent interval between the introduction of cow's milk and the onset of symptoms. Clinically the onset may be indistinguishable from acute gastroenteritis. In addition to cow's milk protein intolerance, lactose intolerance may also be present. Whatever the mode of onset of symptoms, at the time of diagnosis the infants almost invariably have intestinal failure which may be associated with a protein-losing enteropathy and iron-deficiency anaemia.

Diagnosis Because of their transient nature it may be difficult to fulfil all the diagnostic criteria for food-sensitive enteropathy. Nevertheless accurate diagnosis is important. Diagnosis is based upon the response to withdrawal and reintroduction of the offending protein with serial biopsies after elimination and rechallenge.

Management Treatment involves the removal of the offending protein from the infant's diet and the use of a milk substitute. The most successful milk substitutes are protein hydrolyates such as Pregestimil® or Nutramigen® or amino acid-based formulae such as Neocate®. By the age of 3 years the infant is usually once again tolerant of the food that caused the enteropathy and it may be reintroduced into the diet.

Permanent food-sensitive enteropathies

Coeliac disease is the permanent intestinal intolerance to a particular component of wheat protein, gluten.[42] The development of various aetiological tests, especially the IgA endomysial antibody, has resulted in increased information regarding the epidemiology of the condition which probably occurs in as many as 1 in 200 of the population.[43] The diagnostic procedure is similar to that of other food-sensitive enteropathies and the latest European Society of Paediatric Gastroenterology, Hepatology and Nutrition (ESPGHAN) diagnostic criteria consist of finding crypt hyperplastic villous atrophy while the patient is eating adequate amounts of gluten and a full clinical remission after withdrawal of gluten from the diet.[44] The finding of circulating IgA antibodies to gliadin, reticulin and endomysium at the time of diagnosis and the disappearance on a gluten-free diet confirm the diagnosis. A control biopsy and a gluten challenge are only considered mandatory when there is an equivocal clinical response or it is necessary to exclude other causes of a subtotal villous atrophy such as a cow's milk-sensitive enteropathy or a post-enteritis syndrome.

Treatment Since the identification of gluten as an aetiological factor in coeliac disease a strict gluten-free diet has become the cornerstone of the management of such patients. Their diet should exclude wheat, rye and barley, though oats may be allowed, as it does not contain the toxic protein. Current understanding would suggest that the treatment should be lifelong. Amongst other long-term problems is an increased risk of intestinal lymphoma in patients on a normal gluten-containing diet.[45]

Autoimmune enteropathy

Autoimmune enteropathy is defined by severe protracted watery diarrhoea starting early in life. In its most severe form circulating antibodies to enterocytes are present and it may be associated with inflammatory disorders of the liver and in other endocrine glands such as the pancreatic islets, thyroid and parathyroids glands.[46] The duodenal mucosa shows subtotal villus atrophy with an inflammatory cell infiltrate consisting of plasma cells and lymphocytes. The inflammatory response may also extend into the colon.[47] In addition to the enterocyte antibodies there may be other organ-specific antibodies such as thyroid and islet cell antibodies and non-organ-specific antibodies including smooth muscle, mitochondrial and nuclear antibodies. Treatment consists of parenteral nutrition with immunosuppressive treatment in the form of prednisolone, azathioprine and cyclosporin.[48] A less severe form occurs when there are non-organ-specific antibodies present, and the disorder may respond to a cow's milk protein-, egg- and gluten-free diet.[48]

SUMMARY

Intestinal failure in children is frequently dominated by congenital or early onset disorders. The failure is often severe and requires parenteral nutrition for a prolonged period of time. The natural history of intestinal failure in children is extremely variable and is entirely due to ability to treat the underlying disorder. Virtually all children can be expected to recover with appropriate treatment and most children with a short bowel do very well; as their colon and/or some ileum often remains. They usually show evidence of intestinal adaptation, though this may take several years. Severe chronic intestinal failure is due to diseases, which are difficult to treat and without long-term parenteral nutrition or perhaps small intestinal transplantation, are invariably fatal. These disorders include conditions affecting the intestinal mucosa and the deeper neuromuscular layers of the bowel.

REFERENCES

1. Larcher VF, Shepherd R, Francis DEM, Harries JT. Protracted diarrhoea in infancy. Analysis of 82 cases with particular reference to diagnosis and management. *Arch Dis Child* 1977; **52**: 597–605.

2. Beath SV, Booth IW, Murphy MS, Buckles JAC, Mayer AD, McKiernan PJ, Kelly DA. Nutritional care and candidates for small bowel transplantation. *Arch Dis Child* 1995; **73**: 348–350.

3. Booth IW, Lander AD. Short bowel syndrome. *Baillière's Clin Gastro Ent* 1998; **12**: 739–774.

4. Cheney CP, Wong RK. Acute infectious diarrhoea. *Med Clin N Am* 1993; **77**: 1169–1196.

5. Jocklik WK. Host parasite relationship. In: *Zinsser Microbiology*. Appleton & Large: Norwalk, CT, 1992, pp. 387–392.

6. Salim AFM. Characterisation of rota virus infection in neonatal rats and its use in the evaluation of oral rehydration solutions. PhD Thesis, University of London, 1990.

7. Field M, Fromm D, al-Awqati Q, Greenough WB. Effects of cholera enterotoxin on ion transport across isolated ileal mucosa. *J Clin Invest* 1972; **51**: 796–804.

8. Guandalini S, Field M. In vitro effects of heat-stable *Escherichia coli* enterotoxin (ST) on intestinal ion transport. *Gastroenterology* 1979; **76**: 1146.

9. Davidson GP, Gall DG, Petric M, Butler DG, Hamilton JR. Human rotavirus enteritis induced in conventional piglets. Intestinal structure and transport. *J Clin Invest* 1977; **60**: 1402–1409.

10. Starkey WG, Collins J, Candy DCA, Spencer AJ, Osborne MP, Stephen J. Transport of water and electrolytes by rotavirus infected mouse intestine: a time course study. *J Pediatr Gastroenterol Nutr* 1990; **11**: 254–260.

11. Hunt JB, Thillainayagam AV, Salim AF, Carnaby S, Elliott EJ, Farthing MJ. Water and solute absorption from a new hypotonic oral rehydration solution evaluation in human and animal perfusion models. *Gut* 1992; **33**: 1652–1659.

12. Levine MM, Levine OS. Changes in human ecology and behaviour in relation to the emergence of diarrheal diseases, including cholera. *Proc Natl Acad Sci USA* 1994; **91**: 2390–2394.

13. Fasano A, Baudry B, Pumplin DW, Wasserman SS, Tall BD, Ketley JM, Kaper JB. Vibrio cholerae produces a second entrotoxin which affects intestinal tight junctions. *Proc Natl Acad Sci USA* 1991; **88**: 5242–5246.

14. Savarino SJ, Fasano A, Watson J, Martin BM, Levine MM, Guandalani S, Guerry P. Enteroaggregative *E. coli* heat stable enterotoxin represents another sub family of *E. coli* heat-stable toxins. *Proc Nat Acad Sci USA* 1993; **90**: 3093–3097.

15. Levine MM. *Escherichia coli* that caused diarrhoea: enterotoxigenic, enteropathogenic, enteroenvasive, enterohemorrhagic and enteroadherent. *J Infect Dis* 1987; **155**: 377–389.

16. Editorial. Oral therapy for acute diarrhoea. *Lancet* 1981; **ii**: 615–617.

17. Fisher RB, Parsons DS. Glucose movements across the wall of the rat small intestine. *J Physiol* 1953; **119**: 210–223.

18. Schultz SG, Zalusky R. Ion transport in isolation rabbit ileum II. The interaction between active sodium and active sugar transport. *J Gen Physiol* 1964; **47**: 1043–1059.

19. Seas C, DuPont H, Valdez LM, Gotuzzo E. Practical guidelines for the treatment of cholera. *Drugs* 1996; **51**: 966–973.

20. Booth IW, Cunha Ferreira R, Desjeux JF. Recommendations for composition of oral rehydration solutions for the children of Europe. Report of an ESPGAN Working Group. *J Pediatr Gastroenterol Nutr* 1992; **14**: 113–115.

21. Pizarro DD, Possada G, Sandi L, Moran JR. Rice-based oral electrolyte solutions for the management of infantile diarrhoea. *N Engl J Med* 1991; **324**: 517–521.

22. Guerrant RL. Lessons from diarrhoeal diseases: demography to molecular pharmacology. *J Infect Dis* 1994; **169**: 1206–1218.

23. Mathias JR, Carson GM, DiMarino AJ, Bertiger G, Morton HE, Cohen S. Intestinal myolectric activity in response to live Vibrio cholerae and cholera enterotoxin. *J Clin Invest* 1976; **58**: 91–96.

24. Ravelli AM, Lederman SE, Bisset WN, Trompeter RS, Barratt TM, Milla PJ. Foregut motor function in chronic renal failure. *Arch Dis Child* 1992; **67**: 1343–1347.

25. Booth IW, Fenton TR, Milla PJ, Harries JT. A pathophysiological study of the intestinal manifestations of a vasoactive intestinal peptide, calcitonin and catecholamine secreting tumour. *Gut* 1983; **24**: 954–959.

26. Collins SM. The immunomodulation of enteric neuromuscular function: implication for motility and inflammatory disorders. *Gastroenterology* 1996; **111**: 1683–1699.

27. Naim HY, Sterchi EE, Lentze M, Milla P, Schmitz J, Hauri HP. Sucrase-isomaltase deficiency in human. Different mutations disrupt intracellular transport, processing and function of an intestinal brush border enzyme. *J Clin Invest* 1988; **82**: 667–679.

28. Holzel A, Schwarz V, Sutcliffe KW. Defective lactose absorption causing malnutrition in infancy. *Lancet* 1959; **i**: 1126–1128.

29. Turk E, Zabel B, Mundlos S, Dyer J, Wright EM. Glucose/galactose malabsorption caused by a defect in the Na⁺/glucose cotransporter. *Nature* 1991; **350**: 354–356.

30. Meeuwisse GW, Melin K. Glucose-galactose malabsorption. A clinical study of 6 cases. *Acta Paediatr Scand* 1969; **Suppl 118**: 3–18.

31. Holmberg C, Perheentupa J. Congenital chloride diarrhoea. *Ergeb Inn Med Kinderheilkd* 1982; **49**: 138–172.

32. Booth IW, Stange G, Murer H, Fenton TR, Milla PJ. Defective jejunal brush-border Na⁺/H⁺ exchange: a cause of congenital secretory diarrhoea. *Lancet* 1985; **1**: 1066–1069.

33. Phillips AD, Schmitz J. Familial microvillus atrophy: a clinicopathological survey of 23 cases. *J Pediatr Gastroenterol Nutr* 1992; **14**: 380–396.

34. Reifen RM, Cutz E, Griffiths AM, Ngan BY, Sherman PM. Tufting enteropathy: a newly recognised clinicopathological entity associated with refractory diarrhoea in infants. *J Pediatr Gastroenterol Nutr* 1994; **18**: 379–385.

35. Phillips AD, Jenkins P, Raafat F, Walker-Smith JA. Congenital microvillus atrophy: Specific diagnostic features. *Arch Dis Child* 1985; **60**: 135–140.

36. Polim RA, Pollock PF, Barlow B, Wigger HJ, Slovis TL, Santulli TV, Heird WC. Necrotizing enterocolitis in term infants. *J Pediatr* 1976; **89**: 460–462.

37. Milla PJ. Hirschsprung's disease and other neuropathies. In: Rudolph AM, Hoffman J, Rudolph CD (eds) *Rudolphs' Paediatrics*. Appleton & Lange: Stamford, CT, 1996, pp. 115–118.

38. Kleinhaus S, Boley SJ, Sheran M, Sieber WK. Hirschsprung's disease – a survey of members of the Surgical Section of the American Academy of Paediatrics. *J Pediatr Surg* 1979; **14**: 588–597.

39. Heneyke S, Smith VV, Spitz L, Milla PJ. Chronic intestinal pseudo obstruction: Treatment and long-term follow up of 44 patients. *Arch Dis Child* 1999; **81**: 21–27.

40. Walker-Smith JA. Food sensitive enteropathies. *Clin Gastroenterol* 1986; **15**: 55–69.

41. MacDonald TT, Spencer J. Evidence that activated mucosal T cells play a role in the pathogenesis of enteropathy in human small intestine. *J Exp Med* 1988; **167**: 1341–1349.

42. Troncone R, Greco L, Auricchio S. Gluten-sensitive enteropathy. *Pediatr Clin North Am* 1996; **43**: 355–373.

43. Greco L, Maki M, Di Donato F. Epidemiology of coaelic disease in Europe and the Mediterranean area: a summary report on the multi-centred study by the European Society of Paediatric Gastroenterology and Nutrition. In: Auricchio S, Visakorpi JK (eds) *Common Food Intolerances. 1. Epidemiology of Coaelic Disease. Dynamics of Nutritional Research*. Karger: Basel, 1992, pp. 14–28.

44. Walker-Smith JA, Guandalini S, Schmitz J, Shmerling DH, Visakorpi JK. Revised criteria for the diagnosis of coeliac disease. Report of Working Group of European Society of Paediatric Gastroenterology and Nutrition. *Arch Dis Child* 1990; **65**: 909–911.

45. Logan RF, Rifkind EA, Turner ID, Ferguson A. Mortality in coeliac disease. *Gastroenterology* 1989; **97**: 265–271.

46. Mirakian R, Richardson A, Milla PJ, Walker-Smith AJ, Unsworth J, Savage MO, Bottazzo GF. Protracted diarrhoea of infancy: evidence in support of an auto-immune variant. *Br Med J* 1986; **293**: 1132–1136.

47. Hill SM, Milla PJ, Bottazzo GF, Mirakian R. Auto-immune enteropathy and colitis. Is there a generalised autoimmune gut disorder? *Gut* 1991; **32**: 36–42.

48. Milla PJ. Autoimmune enteropathy. *GI Futures* 1987; **2**: 32–37.

8

Intestinal Pseudo-obstruction

Jeremy Powell-Tuck, Joanne Martin, Paola Domizio and David Wingate

The normal motility of the gastrointestinal tract depends on an intact enteric nervous system and effective coordinated contractions of the intestinal smooth muscle. Motility disorders of the gastro-intestinal tract encompass areas of gastroenterology where knowledge is fragmentary but slowly accumulating, and the terminology is dubious. The clinical picture of pseudo-obstruction (functional intestinal obstruction) with the signs and symptoms of intestinal obstruction (pain, nausea, distension and a dilated bowel) in the absence of mechanical blockage of the intestinal lumen is generally accepted, but such episodes are usually intermittent, and it is by no means clear whether the term 'pseudo-obstruction' is applicable to such patients during periods of relative remission. Moreover, there are many patients with propulsive disorders that are not sufficiently severe to lead to frank intestinal obstruction; many patients with chronic intractable constipation fall into this category. The fact remains that, at the time of writing, there are no accepted diagnostic terms to cover the grey zone between 'pseudo-obstruction' and 'irritable bowel syndrome'. 'Enteric dysmotility' has been proposed as an umbrella term that is applicable to such patients, but it is not widely used or accepted.

Abnormal motility and failure of intestinal peristalsis are the consequence of a wide variety of nerve and muscle diseases. Most commonly it is an acute response to surgery, trauma or sepsis when gastric motility and small bowel movement are reduced or absent; this self-limiting condition is termed paralytic ileus. Chronic conditions leading to intestinal pseudo-obstruction are relatively uncommon, but they may cause significant morbidity, often ending with intestinal failure. It is these chronic myopathic and neuropathic conditions that will be discussed in this chapter.

PATHOPHYSIOLOGY

The propulsive failure of pseudo-obstruction is usually a consequence of either temporary dysfunction or irreversible damage to enteric neural networks (neuropathy), or less frequently, to disease of the effector system (myopathy). The pathophysiological basis of pseudo-obstruction is propulsive failure. In this context, the term 'motility' is confusing, because it refers to both transit and to the contractile activity of the gut. Clearly when there is reduced transit, there is, in one sense, 'reduced motility'. In the small bowel, however, the most common motor abnormality, in impaired propulsion, is an overall increase in the incidence of contractions; this can be regarded as 'increased motility'. The increased activity, probably due to a reduction in the inhibitory neural input, is obstructive rather than propulsive. This explains why 'prokinetic' drugs, which are designed to increase contractile activity, are usually ineffective in treating propulsive failure.

In the small bowel, the abnormal contractile activity results in distortion of the fasting migrating myo-electric complex (MMC) pattern. This is most easily seen during nocturnal sleep, when fasting activity is always present and consists largely, in health, of alternating sequences of quiescence and the 'migrating' contractions of phase III. In propulsive failure, the nocturnal motor quiescence is replaced by intermittent single or clustered contractions. Phase III episodes are prolonged in duration, and 'migrate' more slowly; phase III may even be altogether absent.

In the colon, the high amplitude propagated contractions (HAPC) that usually occur 2–6 times daily are reduced in chronic constipation.[1]

CLINICAL FEATURES

Symptoms of pseudo-obstruction include chronic abdominal pain, abdominal distension and bloating, early satiety, recurrent nausea and vomiting and alternating diarrhoea and constipation. Without treatment, weight loss and protein–energy malnutrition eventually ensues.[2–5]

The vomiting is faeculent and often of high volume giving rise to serious risk of pulmonary aspiration. The constipation may be so severe that relieving ileostomy becomes necessary, but following the surgery diarrhoea or continuing episodes of obstruction may remain a problem. The severity of the abdominal pain may demand long-term opiates. Abnormalities of swallowing are common. The presence of digital arches on fingerprint, mitral valve prolapse, joint laxity and constipation before age 10 all favour the diagnosis.[6]

Associated symptoms may reflect the underlying condition. Urological complaints including bladder-emptying dysfunction often accompany myopathies.[7–9] The resulting syndrome has been termed hollow visceral myopathy (HVM). Children with HVM present at or before birth with hydronephrosis, mega-ureters and megacystis, or in the first year of life with constipation and episodes of intestinal pseudo-obstruction.[3,9–11] HVM in adults may present at any age, but early to mid adult onset is most common.[3,8,10] Signs of autoimmune disease (arthropathy, Raynauds, proteinuria, etc.) may suggest a secondary myopathy, or the pseudo-obstructive syndrome associated with scleroderma may be declared by the cutaneous manifestations of this disease.

Neuropathies are not usually limited to the intestinal plexuses. Thus autonomic neuropathy, either primary or secondary to diabetes,[12] spinal cord syndromes, mononeuritis multiplex or conditions like Parkinson's disease may coexist with and dominate the intestinal problem.[13]

Though psychosis has been associated with chronic intestinal pseudo-obstruction, psychological problems, which may be severe, are usually secondary to the underlying condition. There is commonly frustration and anxiety produced not only by the severe symptoms of the pseudo-obstructive process but also by the difficulty in being taken seriously by sceptical medical advisors. This can result in a situation where the patient becomes reluctant to discuss the psychological effects of their disease because of past experiences when their condition has been dismissed as being 'all in the mind'.

INVESTIGATIONS

The diagnosis is usually first suspected after plain abdominal radiographs have been performed. In general, patients with a myopathy have a dilated inactive bowel and a dilated duodenal loop may be one of the earliest signs.[14] A patient with a neuropathy has a normal diameter gut but it may be hyperactive with many in-coordinate contractions.

The key to understanding the clinical problem is the recognition that the underlying pathophysiology is disordered motor activity of the small bowel and/or colon leading to relative or total propulsive failure. It is the latter situation that is manifest as frank pseudo-obstruction', when some form of nutritional support is mandatory. In reality, patients often present for diagnosis during periods of relative remission, with a history of an episode of pseudo-obstruction, or with the suspicion that they have a propulsive disorder that may eventually result in an obstructive episode.

The logical sequence in the diagnosis of such patients is:

- The confirmation that there is abnormally impaired transit of luminal content
- The identification of the region of the bowel that is affected

- The identification of the propulsive abnormality
- The identification of specific pathology.

Investigations help establish the presence of intestinal pseudo-obstruction and may delineate an underlying cause. In practice, the diagnosis is often only considered after several laparotomies have excluded a physical obstructive lesion.

Impaired transit and region of bowel affected

The measurement of transit along the gastrointestinal tract is complicated by a number of factors. The luminal contents are invisible, and must be detected by indirect methods. Marker substances such as barium sulphate lack the physical and chemical characteristics of food, and their transit does not necessarily resemble the transit of nutrients. The convoluted and variable geometry of the gut complicates imaging that is sufficiently precise for quantitative measurement. Finally, measurement of the slow and discontinuous movement through the stomach and the colon by fluoroscopy involves unacceptable exposure to ionizing radiations. Many techniques have been proposed to avoid these problems, but, so far, few have proved to be sufficiently robust for diagnostic use.

Whole gut transit

The measurement of mouth to anus transit is, because of wide variation, of little value. Moreover, in patients with no faecal output it is impossible. It can (theoretically) be achieved by subdivision into orocaecal transit and total colonic transit. But, while orocaecal transit can be measured using the rise in breath hydrogen due to the degradation of ingested polysaccharides (e.g. lactulose) by caecal bacteria as a marker of transit, this is of little value in patients with propulsive failure. The reason for this is that bacterial overgrowth of the small bowel is common in such patients, and the test is therefore unreliable.

Colonic transit

Transit through the colon is measured by serial X-rays of ingested radio-opaque solids, usually small lengths of barium-impregnated polyvinyl tubing. In health, there should be 100% excretion of all material after 5 days. The advantage of this technique is that where excretion is impaired, the area of the colon where propulsion has failed can be deduced from the distribution of the markers.

Small bowel transit

Surprising as it may seem, there is no reliable test for measuring small bowel transit. A barium follow–up examination will usually give some indication of accelerated or delayed transit, but the anatomical convolution of the bowel and the hazards of X-ray scrutiny do not allow the acquisition of sufficient data for precise measurement. The propulsion of a meal is determined by the motor, secretory and absorptive response to the presence of nutrients; an inert material such as barium sulphate does not evoke these responses. Labelled nutrients cannot be used to determine small bowel transit since they are digested and absorbed.

Gastric emptying

Measurement of gastric emptying may seem irrelevant to the diagnosis of transit disorders of the bowel, but this is not the case. It is important to distinguish between slow transit along the bowel, and slow delivery of material into the bowel. It may also be important to determine whether the stomach is involved in a generalized disorder of propulsion; in Chagas' disease, for example, the stomach may be the only section of the gut that retains normal function.

The standard technique for measuring gastric emptying is the use of gamma scintigraphy to obtain serial images of a labelled solid (scrambled eggs, liver or pancake), semi–solid (thick soup) or liquid (orange juice) meal in the stomach. Quantitative measurement of the images permits the calculation of the time to empty half the meal (T½).

Oesophageal transit

Assessment of oesophageal propulsion is, like the measurement of gastric emptying, an adjunct to the assessment of propulsive failure. For most purposes, a barium swallow is adequate.

Propulsive abnormalities

Intraluminal pressure sensors incorporated into a catheter can detect the patterns of contractile events that determine propulsion. However, such measurements are only reliable in regions of the gut where contractions normally occlude the lumen – the oesophagus and the small bowel. Likewise, measurements of pressures within occlusive sphincter zones (oesophageal, pyloric, biliary, ileocaecal or anorectal) are possible, but present technical problems arising from the difficulty of retaining a sensor within the sphincter zone.

For the diagnosis of pseudo-obstruction, the logical investigations are manometry of the small bowel and colon. A number of techniques for colonic manometry have been devised, but none have so far been shown to be capable of discriminating abnormal from normal function with any degree of certainty.

Small bowel manometry

Initially, small bowel motor activity was studied using multi–lumen perfused tube systems, with a pump and strain gauge transducers external to the patient.[15] This provides detailed information on motor activity at a number of points in the antrum and proximal duodenum, and has been extensively in the diagnosis of abnormal motility[16] and pseudo-obstruction.[17] The drawback of this technique is that it requires the patient to remain under supervision, attached to a machine, in a laboratory setting; more than 6 h of recording challenges the endurance of the subject, but is less than adequate for recording both fasting and postprandial activity.[18]

The diagnostic technique of choice in many centres is prolonged ambulatory small bowel manometry.[19] With this technique, a catheter with built–in miniature strain gauge transducers is used,[20] with data being recorded on a solid–state digital recorder.[21] The digital encoding of pressure data simplifies the analysis of continuous 24-h recordings by computer software.[22,23] This technique has proved useful in a number of pathologies[24,25] as well as in patients with suspected pseudo-obstruction. A major advantage of this technique is that patients are ambulant and can sleep normally, if possible at home, during a study. It is during the nocturnal sleep that normal stereotypic MMC activity is clearly evident.[26]

Manometry of patients with frank pseudo-obstruction can be difficult, because the peristaltic activity required to propel a manometry catheter into position in the proximal jejunum is lacking, and endoscopic assistance may be needed. In such patients, however, the diagnosis is usually clear and manometric evidence may be superfluous. The investigation assumes greater importance for patients who are in relative remission, or who are less severely affected.

The investigations outlined above should be sufficient to determine whether a pseudo-obstructive syndrome is due to propulsive failure of either the small bowel or the colon, or to a generalized disorder.

If the latter is the case, surgery is usually contra-indicated.

Specific pathology

Biopsy material is not often available and few laboratories have neuropathologists with experience in this field. Good histological samples are needed to make a firm diagnosis. Close liaison between surgeon and pathologist is crucial so that a full-thickness specimen of bowel is taken and immediately processed appropriately. The samples should be divided – some snap-frozen in liquid nitrogen and some fixed for routine histology and electron microscopy. The immediate processing of samples is important if a detailed examination of the nerves, ganglia and muscle tissue is to be carried out. A full-thickness rectal biopsy is needed to exclude Hirschsprung's disease in a child or young adult.

MYOPATHIES

The classification of gastrointestinal myopathies is listed in Table 8.1. Primary myopathies are due to an innate abnormality in enteric muscle while secondary myopathies occur as part of a multi-system disease such as progressive systemic sclerosis.[2,27] In adults, secondary myopathies are more common than primary, while in children the converse is true. Most primary myopathies in children are either congenital or of early onset.[28]

Pathological changes reported in intestinal myopathies include hypertrophy, atrophy or vacuolation of myocytes, replacement of muscle by fibrous tissue,[3,7,29–46] the presence of intracellular inclusion bodies,[44,45,47] abnormal layering of the muscle[28,48–51] and abnormal staining pattern of myocyte contractile proteins.[52]

PRIMARY MYOPATHIES

These disorders can be congenital, of early onset or of late onset. Two main groups of congenital or early onset myopathies are recognized: those resulting from developmental (morphogenic) abnormalities in the intestinal musculature and specific phenotypes in which no developmental abnormality is apparent. A third group of fibrosing myopathies is similar to that occurring in older children and adults.

Primary myopathies can be sporadic or familial. The familial varieties can show any pattern of inheritance;

Table 8.1 – Classification of enteric myopathies

Primary myopathies

Congenital/early onset
- Abnormal muscular development (morphogenic phenotypes)
  Focal absence of enteric muscle coats
  Segmental fusion of enteric muscle coats
  Presence of additional muscle coats
- Other phenotypes
  Myopathy with autophagic activity
  Pink blush myopathy with nuclear crowding
  Contractile protein abnormality
- Myopathies with atrophy and fibrosis

Late onset
- Myopathies with atrophy and fibrosis
  Hollow visceral myopathies: sporadic or familial
  Degenerative leiomyopathy
- Autoimmune myopathy
- Inclusion body myopathies
  Polyglucosan body myopathy
  Mitochondrial leiomyopathy

Secondary myopathies

Systemic disorders
- Progressive systemic sclerosis
- Amyloidosis
- Desmin myopathy
  Muscular dystrophies
  Mitochondrial cytopathies
  Metabolic storage disorders
- Collagen vascular disorders

Acquired disorders
- Irradiation

Adapted from Martin JE, Smith VV, Domizio P. Myopathies of the gastrointestinal tract. In: *Recent Advances in Histopathology 18*, Churchill Livingstone, London, 1999.

autosomal dominant,[10,29,42] autosomal recessive[28] or X-linked.

Congenital/early onset myopathies:

Abnormal muscular development (morphogenic phenotypes)

The number of reported patients with developmental phenotypes is so far small, but there is an increasing awareness of these patients. Reported abnormalities include focal absence of enteric muscle coats,[48,49,51] segmental fusion of enteric muscle coats[28,53] and presence of additional muscle coats.[28,53]

Other phenotypes

Myopathy with autophagic activity   This entity[28] affects the entire gut diffusely and is characterized by profound atrophy and fibrosis of myocytes in the muscularis propria. The circular layer shows a diffuse increase in acetyl cholinesterase activity and a number of myocytes exhibit punctate acid phosphatase activity. Neurofilament-positive small tangled fibres are present in increased numbers in the circular layer.[54] On ultrastructural examination smooth muscle cells may contain lysosomes containing electron-dense degradation products.

Pink blush myopathy with nuclear crowding   In this phenotype described by Smith and Milla in 1997,[28] the myocyte nuclei in the circular layer are abnormally distributed. Some areas show nuclear crowding while others show absence of nuclei associated with a diffuse excess of connective tissue appearing as 'pink blush' on picrosirius stain. Ultrastructurally, myocytes are separated from each other by accumulations of granular proteinacious material and collagen fibres.

Contractile protein abnormality   An abnormal pattern of immunostaining for alpha smooth muscle actin, and sometimes a complete lack of staining, can be seen in gut motility disorders in the absence of any other muscle abnormality.[52] The abnormal staining is seen only in the outer circular muscle layer of the muscularis propria, which is embryologically distinct from the other layers. No abnormality is observed in immunostaining for other contractile proteins.

Myopathies with atrophy and fibrosis

Non-specific pathological findings such as muscular atrophy and fibrosis are seen in about 50% of children with congenital or early onset myopathies. These changes are similar to those described in adults with hollow visceral myopathy (see below).

Late onset gastrointestinal myopathies

Myopathies with atrophy and fibrosis

Hollow visceral myopathies (Fig. 8.1) Familial and sporadic forms of this group of disorders are recog-

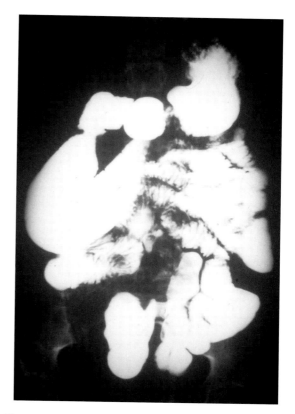

Figure 8.1 – Plain abdominal radiograph of a patient with visceral myopathy. Note huge duodenal loop. Kindly supplied by M A Kamm.

nized and the pathological findings are similar in both types. By light microscopy smooth muscle fibres show varying degrees of atrophy, vacuolation and fibrosis. Ultra-structural changes include perinuclear vacuolation, fragmentation of myofilaments and swelling of mitochondria.[55]

The development of fibrosis in enteric myopathies is not well understood, but it is unlikely to be due to fibroblastic proliferation. Smooth muscle cells of the gut have been reported as showing ultra-structural changes consistent with myofibroblastic differentiation.[56] Myofibroblasts have been implicated in many fibrosing pathological conditions including some in the large intestine.[57,58] The changes seen in intestinal myocytes in some varieties of the fibrosing enteric myopathies may be adaptive rather than a primary pathological mechanism since myofibroblastic changes have been observed in response to a range of stimuli including inflammation.[56,59]

Degenerative leiomyopathy A syndrome of degenerative leiomyopathy has been reported in young Africans with intestinal and bladder dysfunction.[46] The underlying aetiology may be a smooth muscle toxin, possibly derived from herbal medicines.[46] Pathological changes include vacuolar change, muscular atrophy and fibrosis.

Autoimmune myopathy

Inflammatory myopathies with dense T-cell infiltration of the muscularis propria may have an autoimmune aetiology.[28,60–62] Circulating IgG-class auto-antibodies against smooth muscle have been reported in two children with diffuse T-cell myositis and fibrosis.[28] Davies *et al.* reported similar findings in an adult presenting without circulating smooth muscle antibodies.[61] In these acquired autoimmune myopathies, it is the inflammatory infiltrate that causes myocyte damage and dysfunction, perhaps analogous to that occurring in autoimmune enteric ganglionitis.[63] It is possible that this group of disorders may represent the underlying process in a number of fibrosing myopathic conditions affecting the small bowel, but diagnosis is often difficult to establish because of the transient and sometimes focal nature of the inflammation and the relatively late stage in the disease at which biopsies are taken.

Inclusion body myopathies

Polyglucosan body myopathies There have been several reports of a familial myopathy affecting the smooth muscle of the internal anal sphincter.[44,45,64] Women are affected more commonly than men, and proctalgia fugax is the typical presenting feature. Clinical examination and imaging show distinctive hypertrophy of the internal anal sphincter. Histologically, there is hypertrophy and vacuolation of myocytes, but the characteristic feature is the presence of PAS-positive, diastase-resistant ovoid inclusion bodies. These inclusion bodies, which measure up to $200\,\mu m$ in length and have a fibrillary structure by electron microscopy, are virtually identical to corpora amylacea, polyglucosan bodies that are commonly found in the aging brain. Similar inclusions have been seen in the muscularis propria of a man with a gastric and jejunal motility disorder in the absence of other clinical or pathological findings (unpublished data). Fogel *et al.* have reported two cases of sporadic visceral myopathy in which ovoid inclusions bodies staining with PAS were present, in these cases associated with muscle fibre loss and fibrosis, and they suggested that these may be a similar entity to the polyglucosan bodies previously described.[47]

Amphophilic inclusion body myopathy We have noted intracellular inclusion bodies in myocytes of the muscularis propria in up to 40% of adults with a gastrointestinal motility disorder affecting mainly the large bowel. Inclusion bodies apart, the bowel is histologically normal. The inclusion bodies are round, measure up to $150\,\mu$ in diameter and are most easily seen in the longitudinal muscle layer. On haematoxylin and eosin they have an amphophilic-staining pattern but they do not stain with histochemical stains such as periodic acid-Schiff, and fail to express anti-cytoskeletal and stress protein antibodies on immuno-histochemistry. Ultra-structural examination has in some cases shown abnormally convoluted and giant mitochondria clustered at the periphery of the inclusion bodies. Abnormal mitochondria have been described in so-called mitochondrial myopathies in many organs and it is possible that the gastrointestinal tract might be selectively involved in such a disorder. Conversely, it is possible that the inclusion bodies are occurring secondary to the motility disorder rather than being a primary pathological feature.

SECONDARY MYOPATHIES

The pathological features in this group of disorders reflect those of the underlying disease, namely fibrosis, inclusion body formation or amyloid deposition. Except for oesophageal involvement in progressive systemic sclerosis, clinically significant gastrointestinal involvement is uncommon in most systemic disorders.

Systemic disorders

Progressive systemic sclerosis

Although patients with connective tissue disorders (e.g. systemic lupus erythematosis and Sjögren's syndrome) can have associated intestinal pseudo-obstruction, it is more common in patients with progressive systemic sclerosis. The gastrointestinal muscle changes include atrophy of the inner circular muscle layer and relatively dense fibrosis between myocytes and in the subserosa.[2,65] Vacuolation of muscle fibres is not generally regarded as a feature of progressive systemic sclerosis. Whilst some authors have suggested that the histological features are distinct from changes seen in the visceral myopathies,[2,66] others have suggested that there may be an overlap of features, including the presence of inclusion bodies.[27]

Amyloid

Amyloid, an extracellular fibrillar glycoprotein, can be deposited in the muscle layers of the gut and blood vessel walls. Amyloid deposition can be congenital – as in primary familial amyloidosis or familial mediterranean fever – or, more commonly, secondary to multiple myeloma, rheumatoid arthritis or conditions causing chronic sepsis such as bronchiectasis or osteomyelitis.

Desmin myopathy

This is a rare condition in which muscle cells contain cytoplasmic inclusions comprising aggregates of the intermediate filament desmin.[67] Most cases of desmin myopathy have skeletal or cardiac muscle involvement only. However, desmin smooth muscle myopathy has been reported in a patient with intestinal pseudo-obstruction, in association with typical changes in skeletal and cardiac muscle.[67]

Others

Muscular dystrophies, mitochondrial cytopathies, metabolic storage disorders and collagen vascular disorders can all be associated with a myopathy.

Acquired disorders

Irradiation damage

This may cause atrophy and fibrosis and may affect any part of the gastrointestinal tract, but the rectum and internal anal sphincter are particularly susceptible to damage during the course of radiotherapy for cervical and other pelvic neoplasia.[68]

NEUROPATHIES

The embryonic development of the enteric nervous system is becoming increasingly well understood, and some of the cellular mechanisms underlying the co-ordinated neural control of the gastrointestinal tract are also becoming apparent.[69–71] A range of neuropathies has been associated with disorders of gastrointestinal motility, but the ability to diagnose neuropathies clinically using electrophysiological and other modalities has not been accompanied by great advances in the understanding of the pathological processes underlying the clinical syndromes. The classification of enteric neuropathies is listed in Table 8.2.

Table 8.2 – Classification of enteric neuropathies

Generalized neurological disorder
    Parkinson's disease
    Multiple sclerosis
    Spinal cord injury
    Diabetes
    Amyloidosis
    Drugs/toxins
    Chagas' disease

Paraneoplastic syndromes

Developmental abnormalities
    Hirschprung's disease
    Neuronal dysplasia

Visceral neuropathy
    Primary visceral neuropathy
        Familial
        Sporadic
    Associated with inflammation

Generalized neurological disorder

Neurogenic disorders of gastrointestinal motility may be found as part of a relatively pure gastrointestinal disorder, or may be part of a generalized neurological disorder.[72,73] Examples of the latter category include Parkinson's disease, multiple sclerosis, spinal cord injury, diabetes, amyloidosis, drug and toxin effects, Chagas' disease and paraneoplastic syndromes. Paraneoplastic neuropathic syndromes are characterized by a reduction in neuron number and a chronic inflammatory cell infiltrate in the myenteric plexus. It is likely that there is an underlying autoimmune disorder elicited by cross-reactivity between neuronal and tumour antigens.[73]

Developmental abnormalities

Developmental abnormalities associated with diffuse or segmental neuronal maldevelopment such as Hirschprung's disease and so called neuronal dysplasia most commonly affect the colon, though Hirschprung's disease may affect the small bowel in severe cases. Gangliocytic or neuronal intestinal dysplasia is a diagnosis, which is made more commonly in some centres than others. There are currently no firm diagnostic criteria for this entity in widespread use, though some countries have attempted to produce consensus criteria.[74,75] The reported features of the disorder include the presence of coarse, prominent nerve fibres and an 'immature' appearance of ganglion cells.

Visceral neuropathy

Disorders in which the primary pathology is a visceral neuropathy are less well reported in the literature than the visceral myopathies and the range of reported abnormalities is more limited. Diagnosis may be difficult in conventionally orientated and stained sections of gut, and Schuffler and colleagues have advocated the use of whole mount plexus preparations to assess the morphology and distribution of neurons (Fig. 8.2). This technique is not widely available, however, and it is not suitable for small biopsy specimens.

Primary visceral neuropathy

The primary visceral neuropathies can be subdivided into familial and sporadic groups. The chief pathological features of both these groups of disorders are the loss and degeneration of enteric neurons, often accompanied by glial cell proliferation. Subgroups of visceral neuropathies have been reported, some showing associated basal ganglia calcification, leukoencephalopathy or other neurological abnormalities, suggesting that they may be part of a generalized disorder rather than a primary gastrointestinal neuronal disorder.[76] Another subgroup of visceral neuropathy is that bearing intraneuronal intranuclear inclusion bodies. The precise composition of these inclusion bodies is not clear, but association with viral infections, including cytomegalovirus and herpes viruses, has been suggested.[73,77]

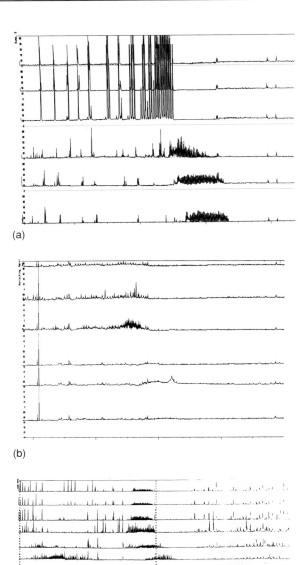

(a)

(b)

(c)

Figure 8.2 – (a) Fasting Antro-Duodenal Motor Activity from a control subject. Simultaneous recording of antral (top 3 channels) and duodenal (lower 3 channels) motor activity demonstrates the sequential phases of the Migrating Motor Complex (MMC). The sequence begins, on the left, with phase II, irregular activity, is followed by phase III a period of uninterrupted phasic activity which migrates along the intestine and finishes with phase I, motor quiescence. (b) Recording from a patient with a visceral myopathy, at a similar moment in an MMC cycle as in (a); in this instance, however, the amplitude of individual contractions in the antrum (top 2 channels) and the duodenum (bottom 4 channels) is markedly reduced through the organization of motor events is preserved. (c) Recording from a patient with a visceral neuropathy, again taken at a similar moment in the MMC cycle. The tracing features intense but apparently uncoordinated motor activity. In this example the phase III seen in the middle of the trace appears bi-directional in propagation and is not followed by the expected quiescence of phase I; the tracing also contains a phase III-like burst during what should be phase II and repeated bursts of intense contractile activity.

Visceral neuropathy associated with inflammation

A further subgroup of visceral neuropathies is that associated with inflammation. The association of an inflammatory neuropathy with neoplasia has been mentioned above, but an inflammatory component to visceral neuropathy has also been described in sporadic cases unassociated with neoplasia. The aetiology of such inflammatory neuropathy is not clear, but viruses have been implicated in sporadic idiopathic intestinal pseudo-obstruction associated with both inflammatory and non-inflammatory visceral neuropathy.[73,77] The presence of antineuronal antibodies in an autoimmune disorder similar to those stimulated by the presence of tumour cross-reactive antibodies may also explain some cases of inflammatory disorder, and ganglionitis has been described without associated neoplasia, particularly in children. These cases were reported to have acquired aganglionosis in the presence of circulating anti-enteric neuronal antibodies.[63] By analogy with the visceral myopathies, a proportion of the apparently non-inflammatory visceral neuropathic disorders may have an undetected autoimmune component that is quiescent at the time of histopathological study, or is focal and therefore missed.

Other physiological tests

In children with congenital disease and adults with suspected HVM, micturating cystourethrography or cystometric studies can be useful. Defecography may be useful in isolated rectal evacuatory defects. It is important to clarify the extent of disease, as surgery is helpful in segmental and focal conditions but is of limited use in diffuse disorders.

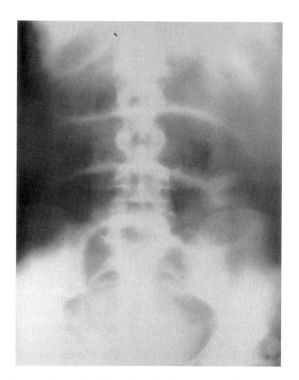

Figure 8.3 – Abdominal radiograph of a patient with progressive systemic sclerosis. Kindly supplied by E A Quigley.

Studies of autonomic function are usually abnormal in patients with pseudo-obstruction secondary to conditions such as diabetes mellitus, previous gastric surgery and other neurological conditions. In about a fifth of patients with idiopathic neuropathic pseudo-obstruction autonomic neuropathy (mainly vagal) is also found.[12]

TREATMENTS

Underlying condition

Treatment of the underlying condition, be it collagen vascular disorder, gut myositis, diabetes, neoplastic disease or myotonic dystrophy is beyond the scope of this chapter except to stress the important impact of steroids and immunosuppressants on gut symptoms in some situations. Immunosuppressive treatment with prednisolone and cyclosporin has been reported to be of particular benefit in autoimmune myopathy.[9,60] Treatment or prevention of any metabolic abnormality, whether electrolyte, mineral or endocrine, is important. For example the postural hypotension associated with an autonomic neuropathy may be exacerbated by saline depletion resulting from the gut neuropathy. Major efforts must be made to exclude or remedy such problems early in the patient's presentation.

Specific treatments

No treatment is ideal and even though some help to correct physiological abnormalities they may not affect symptoms. Some treatment options are charted in Figure 8.4

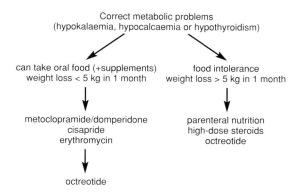

Figure 8.4 – Treatment options for chronic intestinal pseudo-obstruction in patients with connective tissue disease (based on reference[80]).

Constipation

In the early stages of these diseases constipation may be managed by lactulose, senna preparations, or magnesium salts. The anthraquinone laxatives are converted in the intestine to active sennosides, which may function by stimulating the myenteric plexus in the colon and also by inhibiting colonic water absorption. Their principal effect is in the descending and sigmoid colon. Their effect is largely local and depends therefore on sufficient intestinal motility to present them to the colon for bacterial degradation to their active form. Sennosides can, with prolonged use, cause damage to the intestinal smooth muscle and myenteric plexus. Bisacodyl and phenolphthalein are poorly absorbed diphenylmethane derivatives, which stimulate sensory nerves in the proximal colon. They also increase net flux of sodium and water into the colonic lumen. Castor oil can have a place with its principal effect on small bowel fluid secretion. Dioctyl, an anionic detergent, can be used to break down hard stools.

Constipation may need regular enemas initially using low volume phosphate preparations progressing to high volume saline washouts. It is at this stage that colectomy with ileorectal anastomosis or ileostomy may be necessary though non-segmental disease risks ileostomy dysfunction – either constipation or diarrhoea.

Pain

Pain may be managed with antispasmodic agents such as peppermint oil, mebeverine, or alverine citrate. Persistent abdominal pain may be a major problem and its chronicity can result in central nervous system embedding making it very difficult to manage. If antispasmodic agents prove ineffective, opiates and their close derivatives may be the best treatment though they themselves have pro-absorptive/antisecretory effects and cause slowing of intestinal transit through modulation of acetylcholine release influenced by 5-hydroxytryptamine receptors. Oral liquid preparations may be used but sublingual buprenorphine has the advantage of bypassing the abnormal gut function. The transdermal route may be helpful and patches releasing fentanyl have been convenient in this context. There may, in extreme circumstances, be of value in giving the patient a 'pain holiday' in hospital during which sedation and continuous subcutaneous opiates, or even a period of epidural anaesthesia, may reduce the pain threshold allowing reduction of maintenance analgesic dosage. Psychological support from nurses, physicians and psychologists becomes most important and the patient needs to feel that there is strong cohesion between these groups.

Octreotide, though given by a relatively painful subcutaneous injection, may be dramatically beneficial, especially in systemic sclerosis when other treatments have failed.[78-80] It can improve vomiting and pain possibly because octreotide in normal subjects reduces the perception of volume distension due to inhibition of sensory afferent pathways.[78] Octreotide causes low amplitude MMCs to return.[80] Octreotide may have a beneficial effect when cisapride or erythromycin have been unsuccessful, its effect (50–100 µg once or twice a day) is apparent within 48 h and lasts for more than 2 years.[80] It may be more effective when combined with erythromycin.[81] Naloxone 1.6 mg given subcutaneously each day has been reported to be more beneficial than placebo in one patient.[82]

Vomiting

Vomiting is managed with prokinetic agents. Metoclopramide antagonizes D_2 dopamine receptors and also increases the release of acetyl choline from intestinal nerves. In the vomiting related to chemotherapy very large doses up to 10 mg/kg-body weight over a day in divided doses are used and under these circumstances some of the effects are mediated by antagonism of 5-HT$_3$ receptors. Antagonism of dopamine receptors in the basal ganglia may result in dystonia and similar central side-effects. Domperidone is a selective antagonist of peripheral D_2 dopamine receptors, which does not have the acetylcholine-like effect of metoclopramide. It has little effect centrally. Cisapride, a 5-HT$_4$ agonist, enhances acetylcholine release in the myenteric plexus without having anti-dopaminergic effects. Cisapride may be of particular benefit if migrating moter complexes are present on small intestinal manometry. Of 49 children with chronic idiopathic intestinal pseudo-obstruction evaluated, cisapride improved symptoms to a 'fair degree' in 17 and to an 'excellent degree' in seven, with no improvement in 25.[83] It is possible that drugs with mixed 5-HT$_4$ agonist/5-HT$_3$ antagonist activity may combine the anti-emetic qualities of the latter with the prokinetic effects of the former 5-HT$_3$ antagonists like ondansetron which are effective anti-emetics can result in colonic constipation. Erythromycin can be useful[84] if there are absent or impaired antroduodenal migrating complexes. Doses of 900 mg/day have been recommended.[85] In 20 patients reported in a recent series there was a dramatic and sustained response to erythromycin in one patient with a myopathy.[14]

Diarrhoea

As the disease progresses, bacterial overgrowth can result in diarrhoea. This can be reduced with oral metronidazole, tinidazole, cephalosporin, tetracycline or amoxycillin–claevulinic acid combination. They may be used as necessary or in repeated courses with a different antibiotic (chosen from 3–4) being used every 6 weeks (as used to be done to treat patients with bronchiectasis). If metronidazole is used in the long-term, the patient must be warned to stop if they develop numbness or tingling in their feet as an early sign of reversible peripheral neuropathy. Breath tests to diagnose bacterial overgrowth may be misleading and produce false-negative results compared to culture of small bowel aspirate.[86]

Undernutrition

With appropriate therapy, many patients with chronic intestinal pseudo-obstruction manage to maintain their nutritional status.

Gastric motility may be far less deranged for liquids than for solids with the result that many patients tolerate liquid feeds better than solid meals. If liquid feeds are given, any excess can be aspirated by enteric tube or gastrostomy before the start of the next meal to ensure that excess volumes do not accumulate in the stomach. Gastrostomies can be used, therefore, to aspirate liquid gastric contents as well as a conduit for feeding, particularly when there is a need to bypass a malfunctioning oesophagus. Pulmonary aspiration of large volume vomits can be a very serious complication that may be hard to prevent.

Bacterial overgrowth is virtually inevitable and can cause severe cachexia without necessarily causing diarrhoea, thus antibiotics, as suggested above, may be needed often in rotating courses.

Care is needed to ensure that micronutrient deficiencies particularly of iron, vitamin B_{12} and the fat-soluble vitamins, especially vitamin D, do not occur. If nutritional status cannot be maintained or the patient becomes afraid to eat because of pain, then home parenteral nutrition (HPN) may be required. One caveat of this approach is that these patients tend to have more problems with HPN than do patients with a short bowel, particularly problems with line infections, septicaemia and venous thrombosis. The reasons for this are not entirely clear. Procoagulation states sometimes exist and it is possible that there is increased bacterial translocation from the gut. Opiate medication may reduce the care taken by the patient in the management of their infusions at home. The use of feeding lines to administer drugs, especially opiates is to be strongly discouraged. Such patients test the capabilities of the best-organized nutrition teams to the full and should be managed in centres with a large experience. There is real benefit to be gained from the mutual support patients can give to each other in these situations.

Surgical options

When constipation is severe, a colectomy with ileo-rectal anastomosis or temporary ileostomy or colostomy can be carried out. Various drainage procedures have been used when the gut is very dilated (Fig 8.5). If gastric surgery is being performed, a vagotomy must be avoided, as this will further retard gastrointestinal transit.

OUTCOME, QUALITY OF LIFE AND PROGNOSIS

Outcome can vary from minor symptoms consistent with irritable bowel syndrome to problems requiring home parenteral feeding, major analgesics and frequent

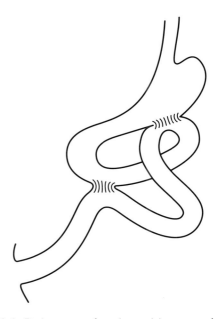

Figure 8.5 – Drainage procedures (gastro-jejunostomy, duodeno-jejunostomy, and ileostomy) occasionally performed in patients with visceral myopathy (after P. Hawley, St Mark's Hospital, London).

hospitalization. Howard *et al.*[87] have emphasized that clinical outcome on home parenteral feeding, like mortality risk, is to a large extent a reflection of the underlying condition. While about 70% of patients with Crohn's disease or ischaemic bowel conditions are fully rehabilitated after the first year on HPN, only a third of those with chronic intestinal dysmotility are similarly rehabilitated. Impairment of strength and of well-being as a result of undernutrition and fluid and electrolyte imbalance will be corrected by HPN but if the patient continues to experience vomiting, diarrhoea or abdominal pain from the underlying condition quality of life will remain suboptimal. The annual risk of catheter-related sepsis among HPN patients is consistently around 0.5 but tend to be higher among those with chronic pseudo-obstruction especially if they remain on opiate analgesia.[88]

Causes of death in these patients include pulmonary aspiration, pulmonary embolism, cardiac failure and suicide. Cardiac failure may be the terminal event in hollow visceral myopathy. The relationship between 'megaduodenum' and upper gastrointestinal tract cancer[89] seems tenuous if it exists. Death will often be related to the underlying condition – obviously so in the case of pseudo-obstruction occurring as a para-neoplastic phenomenon, and also particularly in the degenerative neuropathies, collagen vascular disorders and infiltrative conditons such as amyloid.

REFERENCES

1. Bassotti G, Gaburri M, Imbimbo BP, Rossi L, Farroni F, Pelli MA, Morelli A. Colonic mass movements in idiopathic chronic constipation. *Gut* 1988; **29**: 1173–1179.

2. Schuffler MD, Beegle RG. Progressive systemic sclerosis of the gastrointestinal tract and hereditary hollow visceral myopathy. Two distinguishable disorders of intestinal smooth muscle. *Gastroenterology* 1979; **77**: 664–671.

3. Schuffler MD, Lowe MC, Bill AH. Studies of idiopathic intestinal pseudo-obstruction. 1. Hereditary hollow visceral myopathy: clinical and pathological studies. *Gastroenterology* 1977; **73**: 327–338.

4. Christensen J, *et al.* Pseudo-obstruction. *Gastroenterol Int* 1990; **3**: 107–119.

5. Schuffler MD, Rohrmann CA, Chaffee RG, Brand DL, Delaney JH, Young JH. Chronic intestinal pseudo-obstruction. A report of 27 cases and review of the literature. *Medicine* 1981; **60**: 173–196.

6. Pulliam TJ, Schuster MM. Congenital markers for chronic intestinal pseudoobstruction. *Am J Gastroenterol* 1995; **90**: 922–926.

7. Schuffler MD, Pagon RA, Schwartz R, Bill AH. Visceral myopathy of the gastrointestinal and genitourinary tracts in infants. *Gastroenterology* 1988; **94**: 892–898.

8. Higman D, Peters P, Stewart M. Familial hollow visceral myopathy with varying urological manifestations. *Br J Urol* 1992; **70**: 435–438.

9. Knafelz D, Smith VV, PJ. M. The natural history and treatment of hollow visceral myopathy. *J Pediatr Gastroenterol Nutr* 1996; **22**: 415.

10. Fitzgibbons PL, Chandrasoma PT. Familial visceral myopathy. Evidence of diffuse involvement of intestinal smooth muscle. *Am J Surg Pathol* 1987; **11**: 846–854.

11. Milla PJ. Clinical features of intestinal pseudo-obstruction in children. In: Kamm MA, Lennard-Jones JE (eds) *Constipation.* Wrightson, Petersfield, 1994, pp. 251–258.

12. Camilleri M, Balm RK, Low PA. Autonomic dysfunction in patients with chronic intestinal pseudo-obstruction. *Clin Auton Res* 1993; **3**: 95–100.

13. Ionasescu V, Christensen J, Hart M. Intestinal pseudo-obstruction in adult spinal muscular atrophy. *Muscle Nerve* 1994; **17**: 946–948.

14. Mann SD, Debinski HS, Kamm MA. Clinical characteristics of chronic idiopathic intestinal pseudo-obstruction in adults. *Gut* 1997; **41**: 675–681.

15. Vantrappen G, Janssens J, Hellemans J, Ghoos Y. The interdigestive motor complex of normal subjects and patients with bacterial overgrowth of the small intestine. *J Clin Invest* 1977; **59**: 1158–1166.

16. Oliveira RB, Meneghelli UG, de Godoy RA, Dantas RO, Padovan W. Abnormalities of interdigestive motility of the small intestine in patients with Chagas' disease. *Dig Dis Sci* 1983; **28**: 294–299.

17. Stanghellini V, Camilleri M, Malagelada JR. Chronic idiopathic intestinal pseudo-obstruction: clinical and intestinal manometric findings. *Gut* 1987; **28**: 5–12.

18. Quigley EM, Donovan JP, Lane MJ, Gallagher TF. Antroduodenal manometry. Usefulness and limitations as an outpatient study [see comments]. *Dig Dis Sci* 1992; **37**: 20–28.

19. Quigley EM, Deprez PH, Hellstrom P, *et al.* Ambulatory intestinal manometry: a consensus report on its clinical role. *Dig Dis Sci* 1997; **42**: 2395–2400.

20. Gill RC, Kellow JE, Browning C, Wingate DL. The use of intraluminal strain gauges for recording ambulant small bowel motility. *Am J Physiol* 1990; **258(4 Pt 1)**: G610–615.

21. Lindberg G, Iwarzon M, Stal P, Seensalu R. Digital ambulatory monitoring of small-bowel motility. *Scand J Gastroenterol* 1990; **25**: 216–224.

22. Waldron B, Storey BE, Smith D, Cullen PT, Campbell FC. Computerised method for acquisition and display of gastrointestinal motility data. *Med Biol Eng Comput* 1991; **29**: 304–308.

23. Benson MJ, Castillo FD, Wingate DL, Demetrakopoulos J, Spyrou NM. The computer as referee in the analysis of human small bowel motility. *Am J Physiol* 1993; **264(4 Pt 1)**: G645–654.

24. Oliveira RB, Wingate DL, Castillo FD, *et al.* Prolonged small bowel manometry in Chagas' disease: a model for the diagnosis of enteric dysmotility. *Gastroenterology* 1997; **112**: A800.

25. Hackelsberger N, Schmidt T, Renner R, Widmer R, Pfeiffer A, Kaess H. Ambulatory long-term jejunal manometry in diabetic patients with cardiac autonomic neuropathy. *Neurogastroenterol Motil* 1997; **9**: 77–83.

26. Kellow JE, Gill RC, Wingate DL. Prolonged ambulant recordings of small bowel motility demonstrate abnormalities in the irritable bowel syndrome. *Gastroenterology* 1990; **98**: 1208–1218.

27. Venizelos ID, Shousha S, Bull TB, Parkins RA. Chronic intestinal pseudo-obstruction in two patients. Overlap of features of systemic sclerosis and visceral myopathy. *Histopathology* 1988; **12**: 533–540.

28. Smith VV, Milla PJ. Histological phenotypes of enteric smooth muscle disease causing functional intestinal obstruction in childhood. *Histopathology* 1997; **31**: 112–122.

29. Schuffler MD, Pope CE. Studies of idiopathic intestinal pseudo-obstruction. 2. Hereditary hollow visceral myopathy: family studies. *Gastroenterology* 1977; **73**: 339–348.

30. Faulk DL, Anuras S, Gardner GD, Mitros FA, Summers RW, Christensen J. A familial visceral myopathy. *Ann Intern Med* 1978; **89**: 600–606.

31. Jacobs E, Ardichvili D, Perissino A, Gottignies P, Hanssens J-F. A case of familial visceral myopathy with atrophy and fibrosis of the longitudinal muscle layer of the entire small bowel. *Gastroenterology* 1979; **77**: 745–750.

32. Smith JA, Hauser SC, Madara JI. Hollow visceral myopathy. A light- and electron microscopic study. *Am J Surg Pathol* 1982; **6**: 269–275.

33. Anuras S, Mitros FA, Nowak TV, Ionasescu VV, Gurll NJ, Christensen J, Green JB. Familial visceral myopathy with external opthalmoplegia and autosomal recessive transmission. *Gastroenterology* 1983; **84**: 346–353.

34. Puri P, Lake BD, Gorman F, O'Donnell B, Nixon HH. Megacystis-microcolon-hypoperistalsis syndrome: a visceral myopathy. *J Pediatr Surg* 1983; **18**: 64–69.

35. Milla PJ, Lake BD, Spitz L, Nixon HH, Harries JT, Fenton TR. Chronic idiopathic intestinal pseudo-obstruction in infancy: a smooth muscle disease. In: Labo GBM (ed) *Gastrointestinal Motility*. Cortinal International, Verona, 1983, pp. 125–131.

36. Bagwell CE, Filler RM, Cutz E, *et al.* Neonatal intestinal pseudo-obstruction. *J Pediatr Surg* 1984; **19**: 732–739.

37. Smout AJPM, de Wilde K, Kooyman CD, Ten Thije OJ. Chronic idiopathic intestinal pseudo-obstruction. Coexistence of smooth muscle and neuronal abnormalities. *Dig Dis Sci* 1985; **30**: 282–287.

38. Anuras S, Mitros FA, Soper RT, *et al.* Chronic intestinal pseudo-obstruction in young children. *Gastroenterology* 1986; **91**: 62–70.

39. Kaschula ROC, Cywes S, Katz A, Louw JH. Degenerative leiomyopathy with massive megacolon. Myopathic form of chronic idiopathic intestinal pseudo-obstruction occurring in indigenous Africans. *Perspect Pediatr Pathol* 1987; **11**: 193–213.

40. Vargas JH, Sachs P, Ament ME. Chronic intestinal pseudo-obstruction syndrome in pediatrics. Results of national survey by members of the North American Society of Pediatric Gastroenterology and Nutrition. *J Pediatr Gastroenterol Nutr* 1988; **7**: 323–332.

41. Alstead EM MM, Flanagan AM, Bishop AE, Hodgson HJF. Familial autonomic visceral myopathy with degeneration of muscularis mucosae. *J Clin Pathol* 1988; **41**: 424–429.

42. Rodrigues CA, Shepherd NA, Lennard-Jones JE, Hawley PR, Thompson HH. Familial visceral myopathy: a family with at least 6 involved members. *Gut* 1989; **30**: 1285–1292.

43. Nonaka M, Goulet O, Arahan P, Fekete C, Ricour C, Nezelof C. Primary intestinal myopathy, a cause of chronic idiopathic intestinal pseudo-obstruction syndrome (CIPS): clinicopathological studies of seven cases in children. *Pediatr Pathol* 1989; **9**: 409–424.

44. Martin JE, Swash M, Kamm MA, Marher K, Cox EL, Gray A. Myopathy of internal anal sphincter with polyglucosan inclusions. *J Pathol* 1990; **161**: 221–226.

45. Guy RJ, Kamm MA, Martin JE. Internal anal sphincter myopathy causing proctalgia fugax and constipation: further clinical and and radiological characterisation in a patient. *Eur J Gastroenterol Hepatol* 1997; **9**: 221–224.

46. Rode H, Moore SW, Kaschula ROC, Brown RA, Cywes S. Degenerative leiomyopathy in children. A clinico-pathological study. *Pediatr Surg Int* 1992; **7**: 23–29.

47. Fogel SP, DeTar MW, Shimada H, Chandrasoma PT. Sporadic visceral myopathy with inclusion bodies. *Am J Surg Pathol* 1993; **17**: 473–481.

48. Emanuel B, Gault J, Sanson J. Neonatal intestinal obstruction due to absence of intestinal musculature: a new entity. *J Pediatr Surg* 1967; **2**: 332–335.

49. Humphry A, Mancer K, Stephens CA. Obstructive circular-muscle defect in the small bowel in a 1-year-old child. *J Pediatr Surg* 1980; **15**: 197–199.

50. Yamagiwa I, Ohta M, Obata K, Washio M. Intestinal pseudo-obstruction in a neonate caused by idiopathic muscular hypertrophy of the entire small intestine. *J Pediatr Surg* 1988; **23**: 866–869.

51. Husain AN, Hong HY, Gooneratne S, Muraskas J, Black PR. Segmental absence of small intestinal musculature. *Pediatr Pathol* 1992; **12**: 407–415.

52. Smith VV, Lake BD, Kamm MA, Nicholls JR. Intestinal pseudo-obstruction with deficient smooth muscle alpha actin. *Histopathology* 1992; **21**: 535–542.

53. Hitchcock R, Birthistle K, Carrington D, Calvert SA, Holmes K. Colonic atresia and spinal cord atrophy associated with a case of fetal varicella syndrome. *J Pediatr Surg* 1995; **30**: 1344–1347.

54. Smith VV. Neurofilament antibodies will differentiate muscle and nerve disorders of chronic idiopathic intestinal pseudo-obstruction. *Proc Roy Micr Soc* 1990; **25**: 52.

55. Adler KB, Low RB, Leslie KO, Mitchell J, JN. E. Contractile cells in normal and fibrotic lung. *Lab Invest* 1989; **60**: 473–485.

56. Martin JE, Benson M, Swash M, Salih V, Gray A. Myofibroblasts in hollow visceral myopathy: the origin of gastrointestinal fibrosis. *Gut* 1993; **34**: 999–1001.

57. Balazs M, Kovacs A. The 'transitional' mucosa adjacent to large bowel carcinoma – electron microscopic features and myofibroblast reaction. *Histopathology* 1982; **6**: 617–629.

58. Hwang WS, Kally JK, Shaffer EA, Hershfield NB. Collagenous colitis: a disease of pericryptal fibroblast sheath? *J Pathol* 1986; **149**: 33–40.

59. McHugh KM. Molecular analysis of smooth muscle development in the mouse. *Dev Dyn* 1995; **204**: 278–290.

60. Ginies JL, Francois H, Joseph MG, Champion G, Coupris L, Limal JM. A curable cause of chronic idiopathic intestinal pseudo-obstruction in children: idiopathic myositis of the small intestine. *J Pediatr Gastroenterol Nutr* 1996; **23**: 426–429.

61. Davies SE, Domizio P, Norton AJ. A Case of the impossible – inflamatory myopathy presenting as pseudo-obstruction of the small intestine with bowel loop enlargement. *J Pathol* 1994; **172 (suppl)**: 110A.

62. Schuffler MD, Leon SH, Krishnamurthy S. Intestinal pseudoobstruction caused by a new form of visceral neuropathy: palliation by radical small bowel resection. *Gastroenterology* 1985; **89**: 1152–1156.

63. Smith VV, Gregson N, Foggensteiner L, Neale G, Milla PJ. Acquired intestinal aganglionosis and circulating autoantibodies without neoplasia or other neural involvement. *Gastroenterology* 1997; **112**: 1366–1371.

64. Kamm MA, Hoyle CH, Burleigh DE, *et al*. Hereditary internal anal sphincter myopathy causing proctalgia fugax and constipation; a newly identified condition. *Gastroenterology* 1991; **100**: 805–810.

65. Bevans M. Pathology of scleroderma, with special reference to the changes in the gastrointestinal tract. *Am J Pathol* 1945; **21**: 25–51.

66. Lewin KJ, Riddell RH, Weinstein WM. In: Igaku-Shoin, (ed) *Gastrointestinal Pathology and its Clinical Implications*. New York, 1989, pp. 270.

67. Ariza A, Coll J, Fernandez-Figueras MT, *et al*. Desmin myopathy: a multisystem disorder involving skeletal, cardiac and smooth muscle. *Hum Pathol* 1995; **26**: 1032–1037.

68. Kamm MA. Faecal incontinence. *Br Med J* 1998; **316**: 528–531.

69. Murthy KS, Grider JR, Jin JG, GM. Interplay of VIP and nitric oxide in the regulation of neuromuscular function in the gut. *Ann NY Acad Sci* 1996; **805**: 355–362.

70. Sanders KM. A case for interstitial cells of Cajal as pacemakers and mediators of neurotransmission in the gastrointestinal tract. *Gastroenterology* 1996; **111**: 492–515.

71. Goyal RK, Hirano I. Mechanisms of disease: the enteric nervous system. *N Engl J Med* 1996; **334**: 1106–1115.

72. Chokhavatia S, Anuras S. Neuromuscular disease of the gastrointestinal tract. *Am J Med Sci* 1991; **301**: 201–214.

73. Krishnamurthy S, Schuffler MD. Pathology of neuromuscular disorders of the small intestine and colon. *Gastroenterology* 1987; **93**: 610–639.

74. Lake BD. Intestinal neuronal dysplasia. Why does it only occur in parts of Europe? *Virchows Arch* 1995; **426**: 537–539.

75. Puri P. Variant Hirschprung's disease. *J Paediatr Surg* 1997; **32**: 149–157.

76. Matulis SR, McJunkin B, Chang HH. Familial gastrointestinal neuropathy as part of a diffuse neuronal syndrome: four fatal cases in one sibship. *Am J Gastroenterol* 1994; **89**: 792–796.

77. Debinski HS, Kamm MA, Talbot IC, Khan G, Kangro HO, DJ. DNA viruses in the pathogenesis of sporadic chronic idiopathic intestinal pseudo-obstruction. *Gut* 1997; **41**: 100–106.

78. Soudah HC, Hasler WL, Owyang C. Effect of octreotide on intestinal motility and bacterial overgrowth in scleroderma. *N Engl J Med* 1991; **325**: 1461–1467.

79. Owyang C, . Octreotide in gastrointestinal motility disoders. *Gut* 1994; **35(3 suppl)**: S11–14.

80. Perlemuter G, Cacoub P, Chaussade S, Wechsler B, Couturier D, Piette J-C. Octreotide treatment of chronic intestinal pseudo-obstruction secondary to connective tissue diseases. *Arthritis Rheum* 1999; **42**: 1545–1549.

81. Verne GN, Eaker EY, Hardy E, CA. S. Effect of octreotide and erythromycin on idiopathic and scleroderma-associated intestinal pseudo-obstruction. *Dig Dis Sci* 1995; **40**: 1892–1901.

82. Schang JC, Devroede G. Beneficial effects of naloxone in a patient with intestinal pseudo-obstruction. *Am J Gastroenterol* 1985; **80**: 407–411.

83. Hyman PE, DiLorenzo C, McAdams L, Flores AF, Tomomasa T, Garvey TQ III. Predicting th clinical response to cisapride in children with chronic intestinal pseudo-obstruction. *Am J Gastroenterol* 1993; **88**: 832–836.

84. Surrenti E, Camilleri M, Kammer PP, Prather CM, Schei AJ, RB. H. Antral axial forces postprandially and after erythromycin in organic and functional dysmotilities. *Dig Dis Sci* 1996; **41**: 697–704.

85. Minami T, Nishibayashi H, Shinomura Y, Matsuzawa Y. Effects of erythromycin in chronic idiopathic intestinal pseudo-obstruction. *J Gastroenterol* 1996; **31**: 855–859.

86. Valdovinos MA, Camilleri M, Thomforde GM, Frie C. Reduced accuracy of 14C-D-xylose breath test for detecting bacterial overgrowth in gastrointestinal motility disorders. *Scand J Gastroenterol* 1993; **28**: 963–968.

87. Howard L, Heaphy L, Fleming R, Lininger L, Steiger E. Four years of North American registry home parenteral nutrition outcome data and their implications for patient management. *J Parenter Enteral Nutr* 1991; **15**: 384–393.

88. Richards DM, Scott NA, Shaffer JL, Irving M. Opiate and sedative dependence predicts a poor outcome for patients receiving home parenteral nutrition. *J Parenter Enteral Nutr* 1997; **21**: 336–338.

89. Basilisco G, Hereditary megaduodenum. *Am J Gastroenterol* 1997; **92**: 150–153.

9

Radiation enteritis

Alastair Forbes

Acute radiation enteritis commonly results from the therapeutic use of radiation in cancer therapy, and usually presents within a few days of exposure of the intestine to the radiation field. Although this may be responsible for distressing diarrhoea and bleeding, it is usually rapidly self-limiting, and does not normally involve a gastroenterologist or others involved with managing patients with chronic intestinal failure. This article describes the features and management of chronic radiation enteritis.

PATHOLOGY

While acute radiation enteritis is associated predominantly with reversible damage to the intestinal mucosa, chronic disease affects the whole bowel wall. There is cell depletion, collagen fibrosis, obliterative vascular injury, end-arteritis or vascular degeneration and enteritis cystica profunda.[1,2] Increases in gut endocrine cells have also been reported[3] which could have a bearing on the exaggerated secretory response often seen. Chronic radiation enteritis is not reversible and tends to be progressive with time.

In animal models of radiation enteritis,[4] even with study times of as little as 1 month, increases in collagen deposition in the submucosa, muscularis and serosa can be demonstrated which are dependent on both time and the administered radiation dose. Progressive increases in capillary congestion and lamina propria inflammation do occur with time but are relatively independent of the dose given.

Findings at laparotomy in patients who have previously had abdominal or pelvic radiotherapy[1,2] include ulcerative stricturing, serosal adhesion and sclerosis of the intestinal wall. Serosal adhesion appears to be one of the earliest features of chronic radiation enteritis, and probably contributes to the high frequency of intestinal fistula (18% in the report by Oya *et al*.[2]).

FREQUENCY OF CHRONIC RADIATION DAMAGE

The true frequency of chronic radiation enteritis is not known, but it probably affects in the region of 5% of patients receiving pelvic radiotherapy. There are inevitable reporting biases in a condition that tends to present late, and often to a tertiary referral unit rather than to the unit responsible for giving the radio-

therapy. It is therefore understandable that some authors[5-7] quote frequencies between 0.5 and 15%. The reported rate of 7.2% in 398 patients with abdomino-pelvic Hodgkin's disease followed over 20 years may be especially informative as it reflects a carefully monitored and relatively homogenous group both of patients and therapy given.[8]

CONDITIONS POSING RISK OF RADIATION DAMAGE

The most frequent underlying pathology (Table 9.1), is cervical carcinoma, and this contributes up to 75% of female cases in some series.[9] Genitourinary tumours and their treatment prove responsible for the huge majority of all cases of radiation enteritis. Other underlying diagnoses include Hodgkin's disease and other lymphomas, carcinoma of the colon, and rare tumours such as sarcomas. Pelvic radiation most commonly incriminates the ileocaecal area and recto-sigmoid colon.

Table 9.1 – Patients most commonly affected by chronic radiation damage to the intestine

Genitourinary tumours (>90% of all cases)
Carcinoma of cervix (30–70% of female cases)
Ovarian carcinoma (10–30% of female cases)
Endometrial carcinoma (10–20% of female cases)
Carcinoma of the bladder (most male cases and 10–30% of female cases)
Prostatic carcinoma (currently rare but ? rising most rapidly)
Hodgkin's disease (about 5%)
Carcinoma of colon (about 2% but increasing)
Other lymphomas
Other tumours including sarcomas/seminomas

Pooled data from various references quoted in the text.

RISK FACTORS FOR RADIATION DAMAGE

The patient at particular risk of chronic radiation enteritis is difficult to identify, but the key factor is the radiation exposure:[10] high doses and high dose per radiation fraction are particularly implicated. Radiation enteritis is unusual if less than 40 Gy (4000 rads) have been given. Typically it is associated with doses in excess of 45 Gy, with a median in most reports in the region of 50 Gy.[9] Concomitant,

Table 9.2 – Risk factors for radiation damage

High dose more than 45 Gy (4500 rads)
High dose per radiation fraction
Concomitant chemotherapy
Fixed bowel from previous surgery
Undernutrition
Genetic predisposition (anomalously reactive fibroblasts)

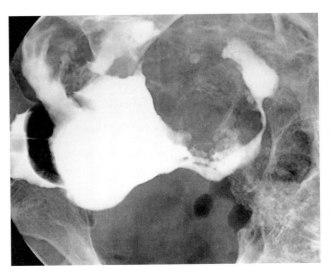

Figure 9.1 – Fistulogram demonstrating a communication between the skin (through which radiographic contrast has been introduced) and the small bowel (upper left) which also demonstrates radiation damage.

previous or subsequent chemotherapy add significantly to the risk,[8,11] as does previous or subsequent intestinal ischaemia.[12] Additional chemotherapy may have had a bearing on the high morbidity rates in one study of rectal cancer.[13] Patients who have had previous abdominal/pelvic surgery resulting in 'bowel-fixing' adhesions are at higher risk, but there does not appear to be an association with the nature of the malignant disease except as a determinant of the site of radiation.

TIME RADIATION DAMAGE PRESENTS

Although experimental data indicate that chronic radiation enteritis begins at time of treatment, it is rarely clinically apparent before 12 months.[7] The timing of presentation may be bimodal with peaks before 2 years and after 8 years, but the overall median lies between 18 and 39 months.[6,9] Some patients may present for first time more than 15 years after therapy and a few after more than 20 years.[14]

CLINICAL FEATURES OF RADIATION DAMAGE

The clinical features of chronic radiation enteritis are typically those of diarrhoea with blood, mucus and urgency, and a sigmoidoscopy showing proctitis. Complicating fistulae – especially to the vagina – are common. In one series no less than 58% of those with chronic proctitis had a rectovaginal fistula[15] (Fig. 9.1).

In a prospective study, Yeoh *et al.* examined 27 patients undergoing potentially curative therapy for abdominal and/or pelvic disease (17 pelvic, 10 abdomino-pelvic) in comparison to 18 healthy controls.[16] Symptoms, stool weights, absorption of bile

acids, vitamin B_{12}, lactose and fat were recorded, together with measurement of intestinal permeability, gastric emptying, small-intestinal and whole-gut transit. Assessments were performed before treatment and then during, at 6–8 weeks, at 12–16 weeks and at 1–2 years. All 27 patients had at least two series of investigations and 18 had all five series. During radiation treatment there was an increased stool frequency ($P < 0.001$), decreased bile acid and vitamin B_{12} absorption ($P < 0.001$), increased faecal fat ($P < 0.05$), more pronounced lactose malabsorption ($P < 0.01$), and more rapid small intestinal ($P < 0.01$) and whole gut ($P < 0.05$) transit. There was a general improvement with time after treatment, but at 1–2 years there was increased bowel frequency ($P < 0.001$), reduced bile acid absorption ($P < 0.05$) and more rapid small-intestinal transit ($P < 0.01$) compared to baseline and to controls. At least one functional parameter remained abnormal in 16 of the 18 patients studied comprehensively. There was a tendency for worse results in the abdomino-pelvic group, and there were statistically worse results in those who had undergone surgery before radiation. It may thus be considered normal for a degree of chronic radiation enteritis to occur after abdominal and pelvic radiotherapy.

In another prospective study of 80 patients who had received radiotherapy for gynaecological malignancy at least 2 years previously, no fewer than 35 had gastro-intestinal symptoms potentially attributable to chronic radiation enteritis.[17] In only three to eight of these were the abnormalities thought to be of clinical significance.

A study of patients with rectal carcinoma has provided comparative data between those with early-stage disease who were treated surgically, and those with more advanced (Astler-Coller B2 or C) tumours who also received adjuvant chemo-radiotherapy.[13] One hundred patients were available for telephone interview 2–5 years after therapy, 41 of whom had received chemo-radiotherapy. Although there are many reasons why this group might be expected to have done less well, the authors of the paper try to diminish these influences in their analysis. They found a significantly higher daily bowel frequency (7 vs 2), regular need for nocturnal defaecation (46% vs 14%) and incontinence rate (39% vs 7%). They attributed these findings to the presence of moderate radiation enteritis.

INVESTIGATIONS

In general, chronic radiation enteritis is diagnosed largely on the basis of a known past history of radiotherapy. Even then it can be difficult to make the distinction from recurrent malignancy in the gastro-intestinal tract, or intestinal ischaemia as the clinical features and the results of investigations may appear to be the same. Barium studies[18] (Fig. 9.2) and computed tomography (CT) scanning[19] are usually helpful, but CT scanning can prove misleadingly normal.[20] CT scanning appears particularly likely to fail in the differ-entiation of radiation enteritis from adhesions and internal herniae.

Sigmoidoscopic and colonoscopic assessment com-monly provides macroscopic evidence for an enteritis involving the mucosa which may appear oedematous, friable spontaneously bleeding or frankly ulcerated. As endoscopic biopsies rarely include intestinal muscle or serosa they do not always give a definitive diagnosis. The histological assessment of surgically derived full-thickness samples may only suggest rather than confirm a diagnosis of radiation enteritis. Biopsies do have a critical role in excluding further neoplasia.[21] Enteritis cystica profunda, which is commonly found on histological sections in radiation enteritis (73% in one series[2]), was once thought to be pathognemonic. However, this is not the case and there are reports in which it is found to mimic adenocarcinoma[14] or to be associated with adenocarcinoma.[22]

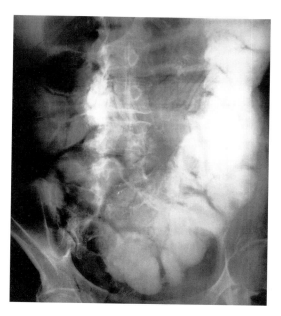

Figure 9.2 – Barium enema showing relatively normal colon but a fistula (lower central part of image) which runs from the sigmoid to communicate with the small bowel and freely within the peritoneal and retroperitoneal spaces.

CLINICAL COURSE

The clinical course of chronic radiation enteritis is very variable, but the presence of some degree of intestinal failure at its presentation is common,[23] intestinal obstruction and fistula being the main indications for surgical referral. In a surgical series by Joyeux *et al.*[24] of 46 patients, 39 had intestinal obstruction, seven had major fistulae and three had free intra-abdominal perforation. Martel *et al.*, report-ing from another Paris institution, give virtually identical figures.[9] These bald statistics disguise major clinical problems. The nature of radiation-related fistulae and the frequent more generalized involve-ment of the surrounding tissues often lead to the surgical description of a 'frozen pelvis' within which satisfactory dissection is almost impossible. Such fistulae may be almost untreatable and continue to discharge faecal material and/or urine from multiple sites for many years.

Physiological changes

Patient may have problems with the consequences of major disturbance of the motility of the apparently unaffected proximal small intestine. In a series of 41 patients with chronic abdominal complaints after gynaecological radiotherapy, Husebye et al. found significantly altered migrating motor complexes in 29%, and abnormal response to a liquid/solid meal in 24%.[25] These disturbances of function were associated with demonstrable malabsorption and correlated with clinical features of pseudo-obstruction. A canine model suggests that these effects may result from direct radiation damage to muscle cells and/or gut neurones.[26]

Relationship of radiation damage with original tumour

Fortunately it seems that radiation-induced cancer is rare in those with radiation enteritis – with no cases in most series of radiation enteritis. This suggests that the processes responsible for the two sequelae are distinct but there are two caveats. There may be an unrecognized association, which is missed through the incorrect attribution of some cases simply to recurrence of the original tumour. Potentially of greater concern is the recognition that premalignant features are common in biopsies from radiation damaged intestinal tissues. Oya et al. found dysplasia in 64%,[2] and Pearson et al. documented aneuploidy in 33%.[27] These observations should heighten the clinician's awareness and perhaps encourage regular histological surveillance of accessible radiation-damaged bowel.

Prognosis

The prognosis of chronic radiation enteritis is influenced by the site of the involved intestine. In multivariate analysis of data from a surgical series, Covens et al. followed 57 patients to a median follow-up of 62 months or death when this occurred sooner.[28] The large and small bowel were variously affected, with more than one contiguous site in nine patients. The actuarial 2- and 5-year survivals were 76 and 74%, but with a median of only 4 months from surgery for radiation enteritis to death from complications. Better outcomes were recorded if there was a single site of radiation damage which avoided ileal involvement. In those with ileal disease the 2-year survival was accordingly only 56%, falling to 46% in those with multiple affected sites. An overall 5-year mortality of around 15% may be expected from the time of diagnosis of chronic radiation enteritis.[24] The main determinant of outcome is recurrent malignancy; if this has been excluded a patient can expect a 94% 5-year survival.[24] Undernutrition at the time of

radiotherapy or later, worsens the outcome from subsequent radiation enteritis.[23] This study considered 100 patients with chronic radiation enteritis and found a global impairment of nutritional and anthropometric parameters in comparison even with 80 in-patient controls with digestive disorders. At 6 months there was a significantly worse outcome in those with the worst nutritional status at the time of initial study, regardless of neoplastic status or magnitude of small bowel resection. Although the latter finding is probably unique to this study, the importance of seeking to establish nutritional adequacy in patients with chronic radiation enteritis should not be underestimated.

Psycho-social consequences

The foregoing illustrates the potentially great relevance of morbidity to patients with chronic radiation enteritis – symptoms of the enteritis can be debilitating, can be expected to worsen with time, and although potentially leading to further surgery are relatively unlikely to lead to death. Psychological issues are important in all patients with chronic and progressive diseases and especially so when the problem is perceived as of iatrogenic origin. The case of chronic radiation enteritis is particularly fraught since it is necessarily preceded by potentially fatal malignancy. The patient must already have dealt with the possibility of death and disability, but by the time that radiation enteritis declares itself, will usually have become reassured by successful oncological treatment and be beginning to think of cure. Radiation enteritis is therefore an especially trying diagnosis from the emotional view-point, linked as it often is with symptoms reminiscent of the patient's own symptoms of malignancy or simply symptoms that are not easily discussed in society. A relatively limited 'at-a-distance' survey of quality of life issues in 101 patients from four centres revealed important psychological dysfunction in 44%;[29] in half of these, gastrointestinal symptoms were held specifically responsible. It would be interesting to learn more of the patients' perceptions of their symptoms in studies such as that of Moschoutis et al. where gastrointestinal symptoms were largely discounted by the investigators as of little clinical import.[17] The tendency of chronic disease to progress with time, but unpredictably so, and the continuing possibility of substantial morbidity pose particular problems. Anger frequently results. Multi-disciplinary psycho-social support should routinely be made available to these patients, with the options for counselling and more formal psychiatric assistance as needed. These techniques may even be of specific value in the patient with post-radiation anorexia and food avoidance states.[30]

PREVENTION OF RADIATION DAMAGE

It is probable that certain patients are inherently predisposed to radiation enteritis – perhaps in consequence of anomalously reactive fibroblasts – but no means of identifying them has yet been established. Strategies to prevent radiation enteritis should therefore be employed whenever possible. Modern multiple plane radiotherapy defined by better, CT image-based planning, can be expected to help. The virtually complete avoidance of the historic parallel opposed fields technique should go a long way to reduce the volume of non-tumour tissue that is unintentionally irradiated. As an example for a centrally sited pelvic tumour, parallel opposed fields applied antero-posterior and postero-anterior with a diameter

of 15 cm would produce a virtually cylindrical radiation volume in excess of 2500 ml (Fig. 9.3A). Even if with better diagnostic imaging, fields of a similar diameter now prove necessary, the use of three non-opposing fields in different planes permits the reduction of the total irradiated volume to somewhere in the region of one-quarter of this, yet with better targeting of radiation to the intended site (Fig. 9.3B).

When possible on oncological grounds, pretreatment surgery should be avoided. This is unfortunately of no benefit to patients who have already developed adhesions from previous unrelated pelvic or low abdominal surgery. Similarly pre-radiation chemotherapy should be restricted to situations where there are well established oncological criteria for this sequence.

A number of animal models for chemo-prevention of radiation enteritis have been explored, and there are some human data. Each of alkali, steroids, bile salt neutralization, antioxidants/vitamin E, sucralfate, non-steroidals (but not 5-ASA preparations[31]), lazaroid and smectite has been lauded, but there are few

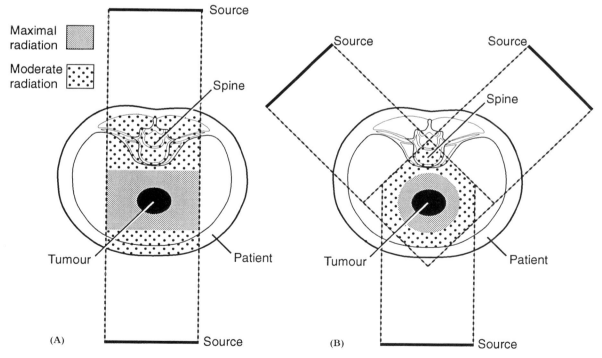

Figure 9.3 – **(A)** Schematic representation of the parallel opposed fields technique to address a tumour fixed centrally in the pelvis indicating the areas of highest and moderately high radiation exposure. **(B)** Schematic representation of the multiple non-opposed fields technique for an equivalent tumour; note that further reduction in maximal radiation exposure of the non-malignant tissues is achieved by the use of the third dimension which is not so easily demonstrated in a flat image as here.

corroborative human data. Prophylactic oral sucralfate may be of value in ameliorating acute radiation enteritis in man, but the significant delay reported between the radiation and the time of first need for gastrointestinal therapy might even indicate a paradoxical increase in the risk of late intestinal damage.[32] Elemental diet and glutamine supplementation do not appear valuable in a canine model.[33] At present, careful planning of radiotherapy for carefully selected patients, treated at the optimal time, with the lowest effective dose, and with the largest feasible number of fractions, is the best strategy.

It is, however, possible to engineer some degree of mechanical protection of the ileum when surgery perforce precedes radiotherapy. The omentum has been utilized to keep the bowel out of the radiation field using the pedicled omentoplasty, omentopexy, or by its transposition. The peritoneum is used in a form of pelvic reconstruction, and there are a variety of slings described using meshes of Dexon or Vicryl, silicon implants (which may be inflatable), and the wonderfully named 'bellyboard' in which the bowel is forced upwards by extra-abdominal compression during therapy sessions, and which does not necessitate pre-therapy laparotomy like the other techniques.[34] Each of these has its advocates and is claimed to reduce acute radiation enteritis. It is reasonable extrapolation to suppose that such techniques should also reduce the frequency of later chronic radiation enteritis, but there are very scanty longer term data. None of these strategies helps to protect the rectum.

TREATMENT FOR RADIATION DAMAGE

Chronic radiation enteritis has been tackled therapeutically by a wide range of methods, their breadth perhaps emphasizing the generally disappointing results. The options can be grouped into those that are essentially medical, interventional, surgical or nutritional. Many of these are extensions of strategies that have been thought helpful in acute disease.

Medical

There are positive data for topical sucralfate (2 g in 20 ml water twice daily),[35] topical and systemic steroids (as Colifoam® once daily or oral prednisolone

Table 9.3 – Treatment options for radiation enteritis

Sucralfate (2-g enema daily)
Formaldehyde by direct application
Topical steroids (e.g. hydrocortisone acetate foam 125 mg or prednisolone metasulphobenzoate foam 20 mg daily)
Oral steroids (e.g. prednisolone 0.5 mg/kg daily)
Loperamide-*N*-oxide (3 mg orally twice daily)
Oral or parenteral glutamine (dose uncertain)
Nutritional support
Hyperbaric oxygen
Surgery

None is supported by controlled trial data apart from loperamide-*N*-oxide, which is currently unavailable.

0.5 mg/kg).[23,36] Formaldehyde-soaked cotton-wool pledgets applied directly to affected areas at rigid sigmoidoscopy for a matter of minutes have also been found helpful.[37] However, none of these strategies are supported by the stringent trial criteria that would be required for their acceptance in therapy of (say) ulcerative colitis or Crohn's disease. Interestingly 5-ASA (given as a daily 4 g enema) proved no better than placebo.[38] In a rare placebo-controlled cross-over study, 18 patients with chronic radiation enteritis were exposed to loperamide-*N*-oxide.[39] The drug (3 mg twice daily) reduced bowel frequency and improved most aspects of gastrointestinal function studied to a significant degree. It is not clear that there is advantage over conventional forms of loperamide. There is a case report of a patient with radiation-induced renal and intestinal fibrosis who appeared to benefit from glutamine supplemented intravenous nutrition – a phenomenon attributed to improved intestinal integrity.[40] The combination of total parenteral nutrition and octreotide in the management of unselected chronic enterocutaneous fistula was least helpful in those in whom radiation enteritis was responsible for the fistula.[41]

Interventional treatments

Interventional options explored – predominantly for uncontrolled lower gastrointestinal bleeding – include hyperbaric oxygen,[42,43] and use of the endoscopically introduced heater probe and laser.[44,45] Topical formaldehyde is also advocated in this context.[37] Although frank bleeding may be ameliorated, the underlying enteritis is little affected. The endoscopic techniques also pose a risk of intestinal perforation. Results and interpretation are limited mainly to the reports of single cases.

Surgical treatment

Surgical therapy of chronic radiation enteritis is wisely avoided by most surgeons, given the difficulties of identifying normal bowel for anastomosis (or stoma creation), the fragility of the overtly diseased bowel (and the risk of iatrogenic perforation) and the frequency of the 'frozen pelvis' within which any dissection is laborious, hazardous and time-consuming. Once a surgical course has been decided upon, a wide resection of involved bowel is to be preferred if at all possible. Despite careful selection and meticulous operative technique the complication rates are high. The perioperative mortality frequently exceeds 10% (e.g. 16% in Fenner's series[46]), and the morbidity is borne out by a 67% requirement for intravenous nutrition in another series.[24]

Some radiation-induced fistulae may prove almost untreatable and continue to discharge faecal material and/or urine from potentially multiple sites on the abdominal wall, via the vagina or directly from the perineum. Early experience with a seromuscular intestinal patch graft showed promise in a preliminary series of four patients with vesico- and recto-vaginal fistulae[47] but necrosis of interposition grafts has often been a problem in other series and the long-term results are not yet known. Spontaneous resolution is most unusual and if surgical resection or satisfactory upstream diversion of the faecal and/or urinary stream is not possible, the patient can expect to have to deal with a complex regime of pads, dressings and stoma appliances for many years.

Nutritional therapy

Radiation enteritis may be associated with intestinal failure as a result of extensive damage to the bowel or due to surgical resections, or most commonly a combination of both these factors. The principles of management are the same as for other forms of intestinal failure with an emphasis on utilization of the enteric route for nutrition whenever possible. Artificial nutritional support is most likely to be required when radiation and its sequelae have left a high output stoma or fistula. The central tenets of supplementing ordinary food with nutrient preparations given by mouth, nasogastric or gastrostomy tube, with fluid restriction, and oral rehydration solution for those with a high output state, apply no less in radiation enteritis-related intestinal failure (Fig. 9.4). Only when enteral nutrition proves inadequate, or when diarrhoea or fistula output severely limit the quality of life, is parenteral nutrition considered. The outcome for

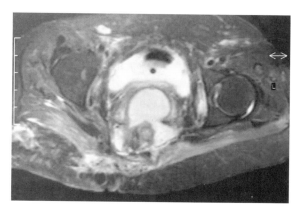

Figure 9.4 – MRI scan of pelvic sepsis in a patient with severe radiation enteritis, in whom fistulation from a rectosigmoid focus has reached the skin posteriorally and has led to free perforation into the pelvis anteriorly. The imaging sequence shown here highlights inflammatory tissue as white in strong distinction from surrounding normal tissues.

patients needing parenteral nutrition for radiation damage is often poor, mainly due to other organ systems being involved (e.g. ureteric obstruction causing renal failure). As for radiation enteritis in general, the prognosis depends most on the continuing absence of recurrent malignancy.

The outcomes of home nutritional support were examined in a wide-ranging study of patients with intestinal failure, including 123 on intravenous nutrition for radiation enteritis who were considered cured from their prior malignancy.[48] They were compared with 1672 patients with active cancer on parenteral nutrition, 1296 cancer patients on enteral nutrition, 480 on parenteral nutrition for Crohn's disease and 918 patients on home enteral nutrition for non-malignant dysphagia. After starting home parenteral or enteral nutrition, patients with active cancer survived a mean of 6 months, with little difference between those treated enterally and parenterally. Almost all of the Crohn's patients survived more than a year, as did 80% of those with radiation enteritis, and 60% of those with non-cancer dysphagia.

A smaller but informative study[49] tried to identify prognostic factors relevant to the radiation enteritis patient, once a need for intravenous nutrition has become apparent. Thirty-one patients were considered of whom – perhaps a little atypically – only 13 had previously undergone extensive intestinal resection. They were followed for a median of 2.5 years (range 0.1–12) after the implementation of intravenous nutrition. There were 18 deaths, 13 from radiation enteritis, four from cancer and one that was unrelated. The overall survival was 58% at 1 year and 36% at 5 years. The outlook was worse if the patient was older, had pre-existing vascular disease or diabetes, and if there was an enterocutaneous fistula and/or perforation. The high prevalence of these parameters probably explains the unusually high mortality in this series.

THE FUTURE

It is to be expected that gynaecological malignancy will continue to require the deployment of radio-therapy for the foreseeable future. There is increasing confidence in the North American and Scandinavian data in favour of the more novel use of radiotherapy in rectal carcinoma,[13,50,51] prostatic carcinoma is increasingly recognized and felt worthy of radiation treatment, and there will continue to be a range of other neoplastic conditions for which radiation of intestinal sites is an unfortunate hazard of optimal therapy. Although, as has been indicated, improved planning and radiation technology should permit the better localization of therapy to tumour, we can anticipate needing to care for a continuing and perhaps enlarging cohort of patients in whom radiation enteritis is the unfortunate result. These patients need an especially proficient and supportive team approach as the aetiology of their intestinal failure is extremely traumatizing.

REFERENCES

1. Mann WJ. Surgical management of radiation enteropathy. *Surg Clin N Am* 1991; **71**: 977–990.

2. Oya M, Yao T, Tsuneyoshi M. Chronic irradiation enteritis: its correlation with the elapsed time interval and morphological changes. *Hum Pathol* 1996; **27**: 774–781.

3. Pietroletti R, Blaauwgeers JL, Taat CW, Simi M, Brummelkamp WH, Becker AE. Intestinal endocrine cells in radiation enteritis. *Surg Gynecol Obstet* 1989; **169**: 127–130.

4. Rubio CA, Jalnas M. Dose–time-dependent histological changes following irradiation of the small intestine of rats. *Dig Dis Sci* 1996; **41**: 392–401.

5. Letschert JG. The prevention of radiation-induced small bowel complications. *Eur J Cancer* 1995; **31A**: 1361–1365.

6. Libotte F, Autier P, Delmelle M, et al. Survival of patients with radiation enteritis of the small and the large intestine. *Acta Chir Belg* 1995; **95**: 190–194.

7. Touboul E, Balosso J, Schlienger M, Laugier A. Grele radique. Aspects radiobiologiques et radiopathologiques; facteurs de risque et prevention. *Ann Chir* 1996; **50**: 58–71.

8. Olver IN, Pearl P, Wiernik PH, Aisner J. Small bowel obstruction as a late complication of the treatment of Hodgkin's disease. *Aust NZ J Surg* 1990; **60**: 585–588.

9. Martel P, Deslandes M, Dugue L, et al. Lesions radiques de l'intestin grele. Traitement chirugical. *Ann Chir* 1996; **50**: 312–317.

10. Rodier JF. Radiation enteropathy – incidence, aetiology, risk factors, pathology and symptoms. *Tumori* 1995; **81**: 122–125.

11. Zilling TL, Ahren B. Ischaemic pancolitis: a serious complication of chemotherapy in a previously irradiated patient. Case report. *Acta Chir Scand* 1989; **155**: 77–78.

12. Israeli D, Dardik H, Wolodiger F, Silvestri F, Scherl B, Chessler R. Pelvic radiation therapy as a risk factor for ischemic colitis complicating abdominal aortic reconstruction. *J Vasc Surg* 1996; 23: 706–709.

13. Kollmorgen CF, Meagher AP, Wolff BG, et al. The long-term effect of adjuvant postoperative chemo-radiotherapy for rectal carcinoma on bowel function. *Ann Surg* 1994; **220**: 676–682.

14. Ng WK, Chan KW. Postirradiation colitis cystica profunda. Case report and literature review. *Arch Pathol Lab Med* 1995; **119**: 1170–1173.

15. Bannura G. Tratamiento quirurgico de las complicaciones intestinales de la radioterapia pelvica. *Rev Med Child* 1995; **123**: 991–996.

16. Yeoh E, Horowitz M, Russo A, et al. Effect of pelvic irradiation on gastrointestinal function: a prospective longitudinal study. *Am J Med* 1993; **95**: 397–406.

17. Moschoutis P, Labib A, Le Quintrec Y, Fenton J, Mathieu G. Etude prospective de l'atteinte radique chronique de l'intestin grele apres radiotherapie pour cancer gynecologique. *Ann Gastroenterol Hepatol Paris* 1992; **28**: 1–6.

18. Weijers RE, van-der-Jagt EJ, Jansen W. Radiation enteritis: an overview. *Rofo Fortschr Geb Rontgenstr Neuen Bildgeb Verfahr* 1990; **152**: 453–459.

19. Solduga C, Torrents C, Comet R, Salvador J, Palmer J, Alvarez-Moro J. El CT en la enteritis radica. *Rev Esp Enferm Dig* 1991; **80**: 243–246.

20. Taourel PG, Fabre JM, Pradel JA, Seneterre EJ, Megibow AJ, Bruel JM. Value of CT in the diagnosis and management of patients with suspected acute small-bowel obstruction. *Am J Roentgenol* 1995; **165**: 1187–1192.

21. Marshall JB, Singh R, Diaz-Arias AA. Chronic, un-explained diarrhea: are biopsies necessary if colon-oscopy is normal? *Am J Gastroenterol* 1995; **90**: 372–376.

22. Struyf NJ, Verbist LM, Colemont LJ, Vallaeys J, Van-Moer EM. Colitis cystica profunda. *Ned Tijdschr Geneeskd* 1995; **139**: 238–240.

23. Cosnes J, Laurent-Puig P, Baumer P, Bellanger J, Gendre JP, Le-Quintrec Y. La denutrition de l'enterite radique chronique. Etude de cent malades. *Ann Gastroenterol Hepatol Paris* 1988; **24**: 7–12.

24. Joyeux H, Matias J, Gouttebel MC, *et al.* Strategie therapeutique dans 46 cas d'intestin radique. *Chirurgie* 1994–95; **120**: 129–133.

25. Husebye E, Hauer-Jensen M, Kjorstad K, Skar V. Severe late radiation enteropathy is characterized by impaired motility of proximal small intestine. *Dig Dis Sci* 1994; **39**: 2341–2349.

26. Summers RW, Glenn CE, Flatt AJ, Elahmady A. Does irradiation produce irreversible changes in canine jejunal myoelectric activity? *Dig Dis Sci* 1992; **37**: 716–722.

27. Pearson JM, Kumar S, Butterworth DM, Schofield PF, Haboubi NY. Flow cytometric DNA characteristics of radiation colitis – a preliminary study. *Anticancer Res* 1992; **12**: 1647–1649.

28. Covens A, Thomas G, De Petrillo A, Jamieson C, Myhr T. The prognostic importance of site and type of radiation-induced bowel injury in patients requiring surgical management. *Gynecol Oncol* 1991; **43**: 270–274.

29. Padilla GV. Gastrointestinal side effects and quality of life in patients receiving radiation therapy. *Nutrition* 1990; **6**: 367–370.

30. Lesko LM. Psychosocial issues in the diagnosis and management of cancer cachexia and anorexia. *Nutrition* 1989; **5**: 114–116.

31. Baughan CA, Canney PA, Buchanan RB, Pickering RM. A randomized trial to assess the efficacy of 5-aminosalicylic acid for the prevention of radiation enteritis. *Clin Oncol R Coll Radiol* 1993; **5**: 19–24.

32. Valls A, Algara M, Domenech M, Llado A, Ferrer E, Marin S. Eficacia del sucralfato en la profilaxis de la diarrea secundaria a la enteritis aguda inducida por radiacion. Resultados preliminares de un ensayo aleatorizado a doble ciego. *Med Clin Barc* 1991; **96**: 449–452.

33. McArdle AH. Protection from radiation injury by elemental diet: does added glutamine change the effect? *Gut* 1994; **35**: S60–64.

34. Bertelrud K, Mehta M, Shanahan T, Utrie P, Gehring M. Bellyboard device reduces small bowel displace-ment. *Radiol Technol* 1991; **62**: 284–287.

35. Kochhar R, Mehta SK, Aggarwal R, Dhar A, Patel F. Sucralfate enema in ulcerative rectosigmoid lesions. *Dis Colon Rectum* 1990; **33**: 49–51.

36. Szepesi S, Jacobi V, Vecsei P, Bottcher HD. Die Therapie der radiogenen Kolitis mit einem cortisol-haltigen Rektalschaum. Klinische und pharmako-logische Daten. *Strahlenther Onkol* 1990; 166: 271–274.

37. Heilmann HP. Konservative Therapie der Strahlenkolitis. *Dtsch-Med-Wochenschr* 1989; **114**: 1466.

38. Baum CA, Biddle WL, Miner JB Jr. Failure of 5-aminosalicylic acid enemas to improve chronic radiation proctitis. *Dig Dis Sci* 1989; **34**: 758–760.

39. Yeoh EK, Horowitz M, Russo A, Muecke T, Robb T, Chatterton BE. Gastrointestinal function in chronic radiation enteritis – effects of loperamide-N-oxide. *Gut* 1993; **34**: 476–482.

40. Wicke C, Gottwald T, Becker HD. Brief clinical report: glutamine-enriched total parenteral nutrition in a patient with radiation-induced renal and intestinal fibrosis. *Nutrition* 1996; **12**: S85–86.

41. Spiliotis J, Briand D, Gouttebel MC, *et al.* Treatment of fistulas of the gastrointestinal tract with total parenteral nutrition and octreotide in patients with carcinoma. *Surg Gynecol Obstet* 1993; **176**: 575–580.

42. Nakada T, Kubota Y, Sasagawa I, *et al.* Therapeutic experience of hyperbaric oxygenation in radiation colitis. Report of a case. *Dis Colon Rectum* 1993; **36**: 962–965.

43. Neurath MF, Branbrink A, Meyer-zum-Buschenfelde KH, Lohse AW. A new treatment for severe mal-absorption due to radiation enteritis [see comments]. *Lancet* 1996; **347**: 1302.

44. Fuentes D, Monserat R, Isern AM, *et al.* Colitis por radiacion: manejo endoscopico con sonda caliente. *GEN* 1993; **47**: 165–167.

45. Alexander TJ, Dwyer RM. Endoscopic Nd:YAG laser treatment of severe radiation injury of the lower gastro-intestinal tract: long-term follow-up. *Gastrointest Endosc* 1988; **34**: 407–411.

46. Fenner MN, Sheehan P, Nanavati PJ, Ross DS. Chronic radiation enteritis: a community hospital experience. *J Surg Oncol* 1989; **41**: 246–249.

47. Mraz JP, Sutory M. An alternative in surgical treatment of post-irradiation vesicovaginal and rectovaginal fistulas: the seromuscular intestinal graft (patch). *J Urol* 1994; **151**: 357–359.

48. Howard L. Home parenteral and enteral nutrition in cancer patients. *Cancer* 1993; **72**: 3531–3541.

49. Silvain C, Besson I, Ingrand P, *et al*. Long-term outcome of severe radiation enteritis treated by total parenteral nutrition. *Dig Dis Sci* 1992; **37**: 1065–1071.

50. Cedermark B, Johansson H, Rutqvist LE, Wilking N for the Stockholm Colorectal Cancer Study Group. The Stockholm I trial of preoperative short term radio-therapy in operable rectal carcinoma. A prospective randomized trial. *Cancer* 1995; **75**: 2269–2275.

51. Swedish Rectal Cancer Trial Group. Local recurrence rate in a randomised multicentre trial of preoperative radiotherapy compared with operation alone in resectable rectal carcinoma. *Eur J Surg* 1996; **162**: 397–402.

10

Gastric surgery

Alistair S. McIntyre

Operations have been performed on the stomach to treat cancer and peptic ulcer disease since Billroth's first partial gastrectomy in 1881. These operations disrupted normal gastrointestinal physiology to a marked degree. As surgical techniques developed, morbidity and mortality was reduced but some patients fared badly following surgery with a variety of symptoms subsequently grouped under the term 'post-gastrectomy syndrome'. These can be attributed to alterations in gastric, intestinal and pancreatic physiology and may result directly or indirectly in mal-absorption or nutritional deficiencies. Elective surgery for peptic ulcer disease has become much less common since the 1950s because of the natural decline in the incidence of ulcers and the success of acid suppression therapy (H_2-antagonists and proton pump inhibitors). Most recently the recognition of the role of *Helicobacter pylori* and development of successful eradication regimes has further reduced the requirement for surgical treatment of peptic ulcers. Emergency surgery for the complications of bleeding and perforation are still required but seldom disrupt gastric physiology. In contrast there is a continued and increasing need for subtotal and total gastrectomy in the treatment of gastric carcinoma and so the post-gastrectomy syndromes remain important to the patient and medical personnel who are subsequently involved in the patient's care.

UNDERNUTRITION FOLLOWING GASTRIC SURGERY

Post-gastrectomy syndromes comprise a wide spectrum of conditions, many of which have detrimental nutritional consequences because of reducing nutrient intake or causing malabsorption so resulting in weight loss. The different facets of post-gastrectomy symptoms overlap in individual patients. Malnutrition and malabsorption are often multi-factorial in origin.

Inadequate nutritional intake can result from early satiety due to the small volume of the gastric remnant or lack of compliance. Operations, which alter gastric motor function without an adequate drainage procedure being performed, can lead to delayed gastric emptying with post-prandial fullness and early satiety. Alterations in gastric motility resulting in inadequate mixing and a surgically induced reduction of acid, pepsin and intrinsic factor probably contribute in variable amounts to malabsorption. The inappropriate delivery of large particles of food, large volumes of gastric contents of high osmolality or high energy content to the small intestine result in disturbances of intestinal digestive function. The problem is compounded by sub-optimal pancreatic function due to a reduction in pancreatic exocrine output as well as pancreatico-cibal asynchrony if pancreatic secretions drain into an afferent loop before mixing with food. In addition the digestive processes have limited time to act because of rapid intestinal transit and may be further disrupted by bacterial overgrowth. Despite these major disturbances in physiology, the small intestinal mucosa appears to function virtually normally as regards its absorptive processes. Patients can dramatically reduce food and liquid intake in an attempt to avoid distressing post-prandial symptoms such as dumping syndrome, afferent loop syndrome, or diarrhoea.

EFFECTS OF SURGERY

The disruptions in physiological processes observed in patients depends on the operation performed as well as the individual's response to surgery. The major elements of gastric surgery which disrupt physiology comprise vagotomy, selective vagotomy, antrectomy or partial gastrectomy, the drainage procedures of pyloroplasty and gastroenterostomy and Roux-en-Y anastomosis (Figs 10.1 and 10.2). Vagotomy reduces acid secretion by removing vagal stimulation of the gastric parietal cells. Highly selective vagotomy has little effect on gastric function except in reducing acid secretion. In contrast, truncal vagotomy has a profound effect on gastric motor function with changes in gastric emptying processes, compliance and more subtle effects on pancreatic function. Resection of part of the stomach (antrectomy or partial gastrectomy) reduces gastric volume (reduces acid secretion in the case of antrectomy), alters compliance and changes the stomach's mixing and sieving function. Drainage procedures such as pyloroplasty or gastroenterostomy were in part developed to overcome the delayed and at times almost absent gastric emptying which can occur following some gastric surgery but can lead to precipitate gastric emptying and rapid intestinal transit. Finally, reconstruction to allow continuity of the gut for pancreaticobiliary secretions (e.g. Roux-en-Y) results in an afferent loop which brings with it its own disruption in physiological function. These procedures contribute to malnutrition, malabsorption and haematological abnormalities following gastric surgery and will be discussed below. Other aspects of post-gastrectomy syndrome such as alkaline reflux gastritis

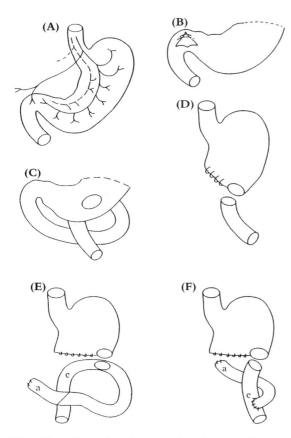

Figure 10.1 – Types of gastric surgery done for peptic ulceration. **(A)** The vagus nerve which supplies the stomach may be divided proximally (a truncal vagotomy), or more distally (selective or highly selective vagotomy). **(B)** Pyloroplasty (frequently used with truncal vagotomy to prevent delay in gastric emptying). **(C)** Gastroenterostomy (which enhances emptying by bypassing the pylorus). **(D)** Billroth I partial gastrectomy. **(E)** Billroth II (or Polya) gastrectomy with afferent (a) and efferent (e) small intestinal limbs. **(F)** Roux-en-Y reconstruction with afferent (a) and efferent (e) small intestinal limbs.

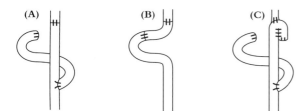

Figure 10.2 – Types of total gastrectomy. **(A)** Roux-en-Y oesophago-jejunostomy. **(B)** Interposition of jejunal, ileal or colonic loop. **(C)** Small bowel pouch and Roux-en-Y oesophago-jejunostomy.

and oesophagitis, gastric remnant carcinoma and surgical complications following gastric surgery are not covered in this chapter.

WEIGHT LOSS AND DIETARY RESTRICTION

Loss of weight following gastric surgery is common and may be substantial.[1] The studies that have been performed are difficult to evaluate because of the heterogeneous mix of patients included, the lack of baseline body weights (many studies start using pre-operative body weight which by the nature of the disease is usually sub-optimal), and failure to compare with adequate control populations. Thus, for example, although significant weight loss may not occur (related to immediately preoperative weight), failure to gain weight appropriate to a comparable middle aged population may be lacking.[2] Overall some 50% of patients following gastric surgery are underweight.[3–5] In general, patients with no post-cibal symptoms tend to eat normally whilst those with symptoms induced by eating reduce intake roughly in proportion to the severity of their symptoms.[6] Weight loss correlates best with reduction in food intake[5–7] and perhaps speed of orocaecal transit.[8,9] Patients who are underweight following partial gastrectomy eat less than half the nutritional intake of normal subjects or patients who have had similar surgery but have maintained their weight.[10] In those who can be induced to eat normal amounts of food, weight gain usually occurs. Although some of the reduction in intake is caused by a desire to reduce post-prandial symptoms other factors also probably play a role including inappropriate satiety (Table 10.1). The increased intake of food in response to starvation and weight loss appears blunted in patients following Billroth gastrectomy possibly due to an abnormal feeling of satiety.[1]

MALABSORPTION

Gastric emptying

Following gastric surgery the stomach's role in food mixing and sieving, and in optimizing duodenal entry to maximize digestion, are disrupted. Under normal circumstances the stomach regulates entry of nutrients into the duodenum titrating against osmolality and calorie load so as not to overwhelm the luminal digestive or mucosal absorptive processes.[11] Surgery

Table 10.1 – Nutritional effects of total gastrectomy

Problem			Treatment
Reduced food intake			Eat little and often
Malabsorption	Pancreatic insufficiency		Pancreatic enzymes
	Blind loops		Antibiotics
	Food not broken down by stomach		Eat puréed, iso-osmolar diet
Early and late dumping syndromes			Eat little and often or octreotide
Iron and B_{12} deficiency			Give iron and B_{12}

can result in profoundly accelerated gastric emptying with precipitate dumping of nutrients into the small intestine.[12] Liquid meals empty abnormally rapidly following vagotomy and pyloroplasty, antrectomy or gastroenterostomy.[13] Many patients have particular problems when oils (liquid fats) are ingested and this is probably because their rapid gastric efflux overwhelms the pancreas' digestive abilities.[1] The emptying of solid food following gastric surgery is much more variable – the initial phase often results in rather rapid emptying of some solids but after 30–60 minutes emptying of solids may either become very slow or continue at rapid rates depending on the individual. Following truncal vagotomy and pyloroplasty, emptying of solids is delayed[14] whilst after subtotal and total gastrectomy emptying is almost always abnormally rapid.[13] The upper intestinal absorptive capacity can be exceeded and if the reserve intestinal length is not sufficient to accommodate the digestive process nutrients are dumped into the colon. In some patients colonic salvage of fat and carbohydrate prevents diarrhoea.[15] Gastric emptying using a two-phase (liquid and solid) radio-isotopic method can give clinically useful information on the rate of emptying. Pharmacological agents can slow emptying and transit (see below).

Gastric sieving

The normal stomach only allows entry into the duodenum of particles less than 1 mm in size.[14] Defective sieving allows entry of particles greater than 1 mm into the small bowel following vagotomy and antrectomy or vagotomy and pyloroplasty[16,17] but following proximal gastric vagotomy alone gastric sieving appears normal.[17] Seven of nine patients who had had a vagotomy and antrectomy emptied abnormally large meat particles into the small intestine with more than a third (37%) of the meat particles failing to be retained in the stomach until they were less than 1 mm in size.[16] The effect on gastric emptying in individuals is quite variable since two of nine patients

studied had normal sieving; in one patient only 2% of the particles reaching the small intestine were greater than 1 mm in size whilst in the worst affected patients 75% of particles were > 2 mm in size. In a similar study following vagotomy and pyloroplasty only two of seven patients were detected as having abnormal sieving.[17]

When large particles are emptied into the small intestine they have a low surface to mass ratio which results in slow hydrolysis, digestion and absorption.[18,19] In a controlled experiment on dogs absorption of ^{14}C triolein from margarine in the liquid phase was almost complete by the mid-gut in control animals and those who had had Billroth I gastrectomies. When the ^{14}C triolein was incorporated in steak and liver more than 50% was recovered unabsorbed in the mid small intestine in dogs that had Billroth gastrectomies because the fat was shielded from the digestive processes in meat particles which were observed to exceed 0.5 mm in size. In the control dogs less than 2% of meat particles were larger than 0.5 mm in diameter and less than 20% of ^{14}C triolein was recovered from the mid small intestine.[18,19] Similar studies have not been performed on humans but studies looking at iron absorption imply that similar processes are acting.[20] Under normal circumstances absorption of ^{55}Fe in aqueous solution is similar to the absorption of ^{55}Fe bound in the solid phase of muscle myoglobin. Following both Billroth I and Billroth II gastrectomies there is a markedly reduced absorption of ^{55}Fe from the solid phase component suggesting that it is not available for absorption. This is presumed to be due to failure of mixing and sieving by the stomach, and also to the lack of availability of the iron to the small bowel digestive processes due to its inclusion in abnormally large particles.

Small intestine

Following gastric surgery the intestinal mucosa is normal histologically and as judged by absorption of salt, water, soluble iron, glucose and [131]labelled fatty acids.[21] The dominant problem in small intestinal function is the limited time available for absorption because of the rapid transit (see below). The transit effects of surgery are ameliorated to a certain extent by intestinal length (supplemented by colonic salvage mechanisms) since there is reserve capacity in most patients.[15]

Pancreatic function

The effect of gastric operations on pancreatic enzyme secretion is more complex. Pancreatic enzyme secretion appears normal following proximal gastric vagotomy[22] but is reduced by 30–50% following truncal vagotomy and pyloroplasty.[13,17] Truncal vagotomy with antrectomy reduced total pancreatic enzyme secretion more profoundly (50–70%).[16,17]

Similarly following total gastrectomy there is evidence for primary exocrine pancreatic insufficiency with reduction in output of trypsin, chymotrypsin and amylase after secretin–cerulein stimulation tests and abnormal glucose tolerance tests. Baseline and post-prandial pancreatic polypeptide (PPP) and gastrin levels are low whilst meal-stimulated cholecystokinin is significantly increased.[23]

The reductions in pancreatic enzyme secretion with resultant slower digestion of fat, carbohydrate and protein are compounded following certain operations by asynchronous delivery of pancreatic secretions to the point where digestion needs to occur. In the initial phase of gastric emptying the synchronous delivery of food from the stomach with maximum delivery of pancreatic enzymes optimizes digestion. A negative feedback loop inhibits gastric emptying ensuring this relationship is maintained in normal subjects but is lost following many gastric surgical procedures. The coordination of the gastric emptying with pancreatic secretion is less critical in later phases of emptying. Following a Billroth II gastrectomy (and total gastrectomy) pancreatic secretions are sequestered in the afferent loop of the small intestine and do not mix with gastric effluent until relatively late.[8,13] The mechanism that leads to pancreatic enzymes leaving the afferent loop has not been well studied but a combination of passive filling and overflow with post-prandial motor function must contribute. Thus it may be that reductions in total pancreatic enzyme secretion are less important than the synchronous timing of peak enzyme contact with food. After a Billroth I gastrectomy total post-cibal pancreatic enzyme secretion does not appear to be affected, but fat mal-absorption still occurs. There is evidence that the early post-cibal peak in enzyme secretion is lost resulting in malabsorption of the early phase of the meal.[13] Some authors have suggested (though no trial results have been reported) utilizing this asynchrony in treatment by recommending that patients with partial or total gastrectomies ingest a small quantity of fat or oil 60 minutes before ingestion of a meal.[24] This stimulates pancreatic secretion, fills the afferent loop so priming the system for the meal that is about to be ingested. More conventionally ingestion of oils is reduced and pancreatic enzyme supplementation is given in sufficient dose with a meal and these measures will greatly ameliorate any effect of pancreatic dys-function.[1,8] When pancreatic enzymes are given it is important to give non-coated preparations as these do not depend on an acidic pH in order to release their contents.

Occasionally it will be necessary to use a naso-jejunal or percutaneously placed jejunostomy tube to give nutrients at times when the gut is not normally used (e.g. late at night). A peptide-based feed may be most appropriate.

Effect on protein, fat and carbohydrate absorption

Despite all these abnormalities it is remarkable that so little malabsorption of protein, fat or carbohydrate usually occur. Significant failure to absorb protein (with its loss in the stool – azotorrhoea) rarely occurs in patients who have undergone total or subtotal gastrectomy and does not appear to occur at all in patients who have undergone vagotomy with pyloro-plasty or gastroenterostomy.[1]

Carbohydrate malabsorption undoubtedly does occur but is difficult to quantify accurately. It results in flatulence, bloating, cramps and diarrhoea. The intestine's ability to absorb carbohydrate is directly related to speed of transit. In normal subjects even fructose can be malabsorbed if the ingested dose exceeds a threshold dictated by the intrinsic speed of intestinal transit.[25] In patients following gastric surgery transit is faster and any propensity to carbohydrate mal-absorption is therefore expressed. Thus starch and disaccharide, including lactose, malabsorption may occur[26] and subclinical lactose intolerance may be un-masked.[27] Rarely, even glucose may be malabsorbed.[28]

Fat malabsorption (steatorrhoea) does not occur following vagotomy alone[29] and is seldom present in patients following vagotomy and pyloroplasty or Billroth I gastrectomies.[1] Under normal circumstances less than 6% of ingested fat is lost in faeces but following Billroth II gastrectomy and vagotomy with gastroenterostomy greater than 8% (mean) can be detected. Following total gastrectomy a mean of 15–19% of fat is typically malassimulated.[1,8] Considering the multiplicity and complexity of changes in nutrient processing that occur following gastric surgery it is perhaps not surprising that neither weight loss nor nutritional status correlate well with any individual component of the malfunctioning physiological process, even the degree of steatorrhoea.[7]

Bacterial overgrowth

Bacterial overgrowth is common with and increased number of organisms identified in the small intestine following subtotal and total gastrectomy.[30] Colonization ($> 10^5$ organisms per ml aspirate) with faecal type organisms occurs in up to 40% of patients.[31] Although bacterial overgrowth can cause diarrhoea, steatorrhoea and malabsorption its contribution following gastrectomy is unclear. Browning *et al* found that colonization was as common in 24 patients who did not have diarrhoea following truncal vagotomy as in 32 patients who had diarrhoea following surgery.[31] Anecdotal reports of cessation of steatorrhoea and a resolution of B_{12} deficiency after antibacterial therapy suggest overgrowth may on occasion have a role in postgastrectomy symptomatology. If overgrowth is suspected as a cause for symptoms a trial of antibiotic treatment is the simplest test since breath hydrogen based tests have to be interpreted with caution due to rapid orocaecal transit.[28]

Dumping syndrome

Early dumping syndrome, first reported by Hertz in 1913[12] and termed 'dumping' by Mix in 1922[31] is typified by weakness, faintness or syncope, palpitations, sweating with nausea and vomiting, pallor, abdominal pain (colicky) and diarrhoea occurring 30 minutes after eating. Rapid early gastric emptying (particularly of the liquid phase) with resultant delivery of hypertonic fluid into the duodenum causes a reduction in vascular volume and a neural and/or hormonal (vasoactive intestinal peptide (VIP), serotonin, neurotensin, enteroglucagon, peptide YY (PYY) and kinins) response to duodenal stimulation and distension.[34,35] These changes lead to the vasomotor changes, which cause the distressing symptoms. In late dumping syndrome faintness, palpitations, perspiration and confusion occur 1–3 hours post-prandially and are due to the rapid transit of food causing excessive release of gastric inhibitory peptide (GIP) and insulin which results in reactive hypoglycaemia.[36,37]

Undernutrition can occasionally result from dumping syndrome because the patient's desire to reduce symptoms leads to avoidance of food. Attempts should be made to encourage the eating of small frequent meals with reduction in rapidly assimilated carbohydrate (rice or potatoes as a source of carbohydrate should be preferred to drinks containing monosaccharides for example). Liquid ingestion should be limited to just before or with meals. Measures to slow gastric emptying with pectin, glucomannan, acarbose or loperamide are useful in some patients.[37] In the few patients where these measures fail, octreotide (50–100 μg) given subcutaneously 15–60 minutes before meals has been shown to control symptoms successfully in the majority of patients.[37] Octreotide slows gastric emptying of liquids and solids, slows orocaecal transit and reduces the plasma levels of several of the vasoactive hormones incriminated in symptom generation.

POST-VAGOTOMY DIARRHOEA

In patients with post-vagotomy diarrhoea, avoidance of food to reduce symptoms is probably common a reason for weight loss as malabsorption. Diarrhoea following truncal vagotomy occurs frequently. Depending on the definition for diarrhoea it occurs in 2%[38] to 53%.[39] Of 102 patients studied 13 years after vagotomy and pyloroplasty, 53% complained of diarrhoea attacks (7% in a control group); 11% had continuous diarrhoea and 22% had at least one attack of diarrhoea per week.[39] In 8% of patients the diarrhoea had been a serious problem particularly because the diarrhoea can be sudden and unpredictable in onset; sufficient at times to lead to incontinence. The diarrhoea in this syndrome does not appear to be limited to patients who had pyloroplasty since most series also include some patients who have had a gastroenterotomy as a drainage procedure following truncal vagotomy. Treatment with Lomotil (diphenoxylate hydrochloride and atropine sulphate) reduces stool frequency to a significant degree but was not useful in the prophylaxis of the more severe or episode attacks of diarrhoea.[40] In an attempt to reduce the rapid efflux of food from the stomach to the small bowel, reducing the liquid content of meals was investigated. McKelvey demonstrated that low fluid meals gave complete control of diarrhoea in two patients, improved the diarrhoea in 12 patients, all of whom had less frequency and nine of whom had less urgency, in 16 patients studied.[12] In patients with more resistant diarrhoea, however, such manipulation of meal content is less successful.

Following Ayulo's report (1972) that 11 of 13 patients with post-vagotomy diarrhoea responded to cholestyramine it was postulated that the diarrhoea may be mediated by the cathartic action of bile acid reaching the colon.[41] A controlled study[42] demonstrated increased faecal content of total bile acids, in particular chenodeoxycholic acid, in patients with post-vagotomy diarrhoea compared with controls. Patients who had undergone a vagotomy but did not have diarrhoea lay intermediate between the two groups. In subsequent trials cholestyramine has been shown to improve control of the diarrhoea in this group of patients, though it does not work in all patients.[43]

The major factor in post-vagotomy diarrhoea appears to be rapid gastric emptying and rapid upper gastrointestinal transit which results in reduced digestion and absorption in the small intestine and delivery of an osmotic load to the colon as shown by intubation studies.[44] Transit is so fast that it even overwhelms the gut's ability to absorb glucose.[28,44] In patients with post-vagotomy diarrhoea there is a rapid rise in breath hydrogen (concurrently with arrival of barium in the caecum) resulting in mean transit time of 25 minutes. Codeine (60 mg) and loperamide (12–24 mg) delayed transit by 58 minutes and 63 minutes respectively and improved symptoms dramatically in most patients.[28] It is probably critical that such drugs are given in sufficient dose and well before a meal is ingested to allow absorption since ingestion immediately prior to or with food probably results in colonic dumping before the drug has a chance to work. Presumably many patients do not get post-vagotomy diarrhoea because they have an efficient mechanism for colonic salvage.[15]

HAEMATOLOGICAL ABNORMALITIES FOLLOWING GASTRIC SURGERY

General features

Specific nutritional deficiencies, which may result in anaemia, are common following gastric operations.

The reported incidence of anaemia following gastric resections ranges from 3 to 77%.[45–47] In the largest report comprising some 7000 patients the overall incidence was about 30%.[48] Anaemia is more common following operations for gastric ulcer (30%) than duodenal ulcer (9%).[49,50] Patients with Billroth II anastomoses tend to become anaemic more commonly than patients with Billroth I anastomoses.[45,49,51] Anaemia following gastroenterostomy is unusual, but tends to be iron-deficient in type when it occurs, and anaemia following a vagotomy and pyloroplasty is very rare.[11,12]

Deficiencies of iron and B_{12} make approximately equal contributions to the incidence of anaemia following partial gastrectomy, with folate deficiency being less common.[51] The relative contributions are typified by Shafer et al.'s study of 142 male patients, 33 of whom had Billroth I and 109 Billroth II gastrectomies an average of 8.3 years after surgery.[53] Anaemia was present in 69 of the 142 patients, 32% of whom were found to have iron deficiency (low serum iron) with 42% being B_{12}-deficient (low serum B_{12}) and deficiency of red cell folate occurring in 25%. Analysis of anaemic patients showed that in 23% the cause was isolated iron deficiency, in 20% isolated B_{12} deficiency and isolated folate deficiency in only 9%. Mixed deficiencies were present in the remaining 48%.

Following total gastrectomy a similar frequency of anaemia and spectrum of deficiency is found. Anaemia is present in 49% of cases, with evidence of iron deficiency (low ferritin) in 27%, though it is likely that haematological abnormalities will increase the longer patients survive following operation.[54]

Iron deficiency

Iron deficiency occurs in 30–50% of patients following partial gastrectomy.[45,50,51] The causes of iron deficiency are multifactorial. It has been suggested that males with anaemia following partial gastrectomy consume less iron in their diet,[52] though it was acknowledged in the study that other factors also contributed. Other studies have found dietary iron intake to be adequate.[50] Chronic faecal blood loss, as measured by chromium-labelled red cell studies, is typically 3.2–6.5 ml/day and must contribute to the anaemia.[55] It has been suggested that there is an inability to up-regulate absorption in the iron-deficient state.[56] Reduced absorption of inorganic iron is also a result of reduced acid secretion by the stomach and possibly high mucosal cell turnover. Rapid intestinal transit through the upper gut and bypass of the duodenum, which is the preferential site for iron absorption, almost certainly also contributes.[57] Replacement with oral iron is usually sufficient treatment when iron deficiency is found, provided other causes have been adequately excluded.

B$_{12}$ deficiency

The incidence of B$_{12}$ deficiency following gastric resection is typically reported as ranging from 1 to 20%.[45,50] In one series of 351 patients[58] with Billroth II anastomoses, 36% of patients had low (20% serum B$_{12}$ levels below 150 pg/ml) or borderline low (16% B$_{12}$ levels between 150 and 250 pg/ml) B$_{12}$ levels reflecting some measure of deficiency, though some authors using measures such as red cell B$_{12}$ and the presence of hypersegmented polymorphocytes suggest that minor deficiency may be present in as many as 68–100% of patients.[51] The incidence of B$_{12}$ deficiency appears to increase with time from surgery.

Lack of intrinsic factor contributes to the deficiency in between 30 and 70% of patients,[50,58] though elective assessment of B$_{12}$ absorption shortly after surgery suggests it is usually normal.[59] It may be that, although B$_{12}$ absorption is normal when measured by conventional absorption tests, e.g. the Schilling test,[60] the abnormal emptying of food particles of stomach and their subsequent disintegration may reduce B$_{12}$ availability on a normal diet.[61] In the small intestine the role of bacterial overgrowth in contributing to B$_{12}$ deficiency is unclear but bacteria have the ability to compete for dietary B$_{12}$. In some patients with a Billroth II anastomosis, treatment with a broad-spectrum antibiotic has been shown to correct B$_{12}$ deficiency.[62] Similarly pancreatic insufficiency is a compounding factor in patients with Billroth anastomoses and may reduce the absorption of B$_{12}$. The relative contributions of these causes of deficiency are unclear but modern treatment with parenteral B$_{12}$ administration in patients with deficiencies is so reliable that it should be the preferred method of treatment when B$_{12}$ deficiency is identified.

Folate deficiency

Although serum folate levels are low in 40% of patients following gastric resection and dietary inadequacy is extremely common,[50] Pryor et al. found little evidence of clinical folate deficiency.[49] As detailed above it is a relatively unusual cause for the anaemia following gastric surgery though it should be sought in any patient who is anaemic. Replacement should be given orally when levels are low and should probably also be given in the short-term prophylactically in patients receiving iron or B$_{12}$ for deficiencies of these haematinics to prevent the unmasking of borderline folate deficiency during rapid haemopoesis induced with treatment.

METABOLIC BONE DISEASE

Reports of metabolic bone disease (osteoporosis and/or osteomalacia) following gastric surgery suggest the incidence varies from 1 to 25%.[1] Bone pain and tenderness is reported when sought by up to 26% of patients following surgery compared with 4% of controls.[63] Serum calcium levels are lower in patients than controls though seldom to the point of falling outside the normal range. Similarly, inorganic phosphate levels are low in 5% of patients and serum alkaline phosphatase tends to be elevated. X-ray evidence of osteopenia can be found in 24% (controls 4%). It has been suggested that vitamin D levels and calcium loss may be proportional to loss of faecal fat which would be consistent with the findings that bone disease seems to affect patients following Billroth II rather than Billroth I gastrectomies.[63] Dietary deficiency of vitamin D may contribute. Affected patients should try and increase vitamin D and calcium intake (though milk being liquid and containing lactose may have to be taken cautiously)[1] and monitoring of bone density should be considered. Despite the frequency of metabolic bone disease when sought in patients who have had gastric surgery there is no persuasive evidence of increase in fracture rate or its reduction by increased calcium intake or therapeutic intervention with hormone treatment or biphosphonates.

SUMMARY

Subtotal and total gastrectomy frequently leads to symptoms resulting in a change in eating habit and more rarely results in malnutrition, malabsorption or specific nutritional deficiencies. The causes are often multifactorial and a knowledge of the likely problems and an understanding of the pathophysiological mechanisms help organize an approach for the individual patient. A combination of dietary changes, drug therapy to slow transit, bind bile salts or enzyme supplementation and addition of dietary supplements usually leads to successful control of the problem though many remain underweight in the long-term.

REFERENCES

1. Meyer JH. Nutritional outcomes of gastric operations. *Gastroenterol Clin North Am* 1994; **23(2)**: 227–260.

2. Glober GA, Rhoads GC, Liu F, Kagan A. Long-term results of gastrectomy with respect to blood lipids, blood pressure, weight and living habits. *Ann Surg* 1979; **179**: 896–901.

3. Fischer AB. Twenty-five years after Billroth II gastrectomy for duodenal ulcer. *World J Surg* 1984; **8**: 293–302.

4. Ivy AC, Grossman MI, Bachrach WH. Surgical therapy for peptic ulcer. In: *Peptic Ulcer*. Churchill: London 1950, pp 964–1080.

5. Wastell C. Long-term clinical and metabolic effects of vagotomy with either gastrojejunostomy or pyloroplasty. *Ann R Coll Surg Eng* 1969; **45**: 193–211.

6. Johnston IDA, Welbourn R, Acheson K. Gastrectomy and loss of weight. *Lancet* 1958; **1**: 1242–1245.

7. Robins RE, Robertson R, McIntosh HW. Fecal fat and nitrogen studies in postgastrectomy patients: The relationship of fat and nitrogen assimilation to weight loss and a comparison between Billroth I and Billroth II subtotal gastrectomies. *Surgery* 1957; **41**: 248–253.

8. Bradley EL, Isaacs JT, Hersh T, Chey WY. Pathophysiology and significance of malabsorption after Roux-en-Y reconstruction. *Surgery* 1977; **81**: 684–691.

9. Armbrecht U, Lundell L, Lindstedt G, Stockbruegger RW. Causes of malabsorption after total gastrectomy with Roux-en-Y reconstruction. *Acta Chir Scand* 1988; **154**: 37–41.

10. Tovey F. A comparison of Polya gastrectomy, total and selective vagotomy and of pyloroplasty and gastrojejunostomy. *Br J Surg* 1969; **56**: 281–286.

11. McIntyre AS. Studies on the adrenergic control of upper gastrointestinal function in man. MD Thesis, University of London, 1990.

12. McKelvey STD. Gastric incontinence and postvagotomy diarrhoea. *Br J Surg* 1970; **57**: 741–747.

13. MacGregor IL, Parent J, Meyer JH. Gastric emptying of liquid meals and pancreatic and biliary secretion after subtotal gastrectomy or truncal vagotomy and pyloroplasty in man. *Gastroenterology* 1977; **72**: 195–205.

14. Kumar D. Gastric motor physiology and pathophysiology. In: Gustavsson S, Kumar D, Graham DY (eds) *The Stomach*. Churchill Livingstone: Edinburgh, 1992, pp. 129–142.

15. Read NW. Diarrhoea the failure of colonic salvage. *Lancet* 1982; **I**: 481–483.

16. Mayer EA, Thomson JB, Jehn D, Reedy T, Elashoff J, Meyer JH. Gastric emptying and sieving of solid food and pancreatic and biliary secretion after solid meals in patients with truncal vagotomy and antrectomy. *Gastroenterology* 1982; **83**: 184–192.

17. Mayer EA, Thomson JB, Jehn D, Reedy T, Elashoff J, Deveny C, Meyer JH. Gastric emptying and sieving of solid food and pancreatic and biliary secretion after solid meals in patients with nonresective ulcer surgery. *Gastroenterology* 1984; **87**: 1264–1271.

18. Doty JE, Meyer JH. Vagotomy and antrectomy impairs intracellular but not extracellular fat absorption in the dog. *Gastroenterology* 1988; **94**: 50–56.

19. Doty JE, Gu YG, Meyer JH. Vagotomy and antrectomy with gastrojejunostomy impairs fat absorption from liquid and solid food. *Gastroenterology* 1989; **96**: A128.

20. Meyer JH, Porter-Fink V, Crott R, Figeuroa W. Absorption of heme iron after truncal vagotomy with antrectomy. *Gastroenterology* 1987; **92**: 1534.

21. Johnson JH, Horswell RR, Tyor MP, Owen EE, Ruffin JM. Effect of intestinal hormones on 131-I-triolein absorption in subtotal gastrectomy patients and intubated normal persons. *Gastroenterology* 1961; **41**: 215–219.

22. Lavigne ME, Wiley ZD, Martin P, Way LW, Meyer JH, Sleisenger MH, MacGregor IL. Gastric pancreatic, and biliary secretion and the rate of emptying after parietal cell vagotomy (PCV). *Am J Surg* 1979; **138**: 644–651.

23. Freiss H, Bohm J, Muller MW, Glasbrenner B, Riepl RL, Malferdieiner P, Buchler MW. Maldigestion after total gastrectomy is associated with pancreatic insufficiency. *Am J Gastroenterol* 1996; **91**: 341–347.

24. Tyor MP, Ruffin JM. The effect of prefeeding of fat on 131-I-triolein absorption in subtotal gastrectomy patients. *Proc Soc Exp Biol Med* 1958; **99**: 61–64.

25. McIntyre AS, Thompson DG, Burnham WR, Walker ER. The effect of beta-adrenoreceptor agonists and antagonists on fructose absorption in man. *Aliment Pharmacol Ther* 1993; **7**: 267–274.

26. Bond JH, Levitt MD. Use of pulmonary hydrogen measurements to quantitate carbohydrate absorption: Study of partially gastrectomized patients. *J Clin Invest* 1972; **51**: 1219–1225.

27. Condon JE, Westerholm P, Tanner NC. Lactose malabsorption and postgastrectomy milk intolerance. *Gut* 1964; **10**: 311–314.

28. O'Brien JD, Thompson DG, McIntyre A, Burnham VJR, Walker E. Effect of codeine and loperamide on upper intestinal transit and absorption in normal subjects and patients with postvagotomy diarrhoea. *Gut* 1988; **29**: 312–318.

29. Edwards JP, Lyndon PJ, Smith RB, Johnston D. Faecal fat excretion after truncal, selective, and highly selective vagotomy. *Gut* 1974; **15**: 521–525.

30. Greenlee HB, Vivit R, Paez J, Dietz A. Bacterial flora of the jejunum following peptic ulcer surgery. *Arch Surg* 1971; **102**: 260–265.

31. Browning GG, Buchan KA, MacKay C. Clinical and laboratory study of postvagotomy diarrhoea. *Gut* 1974; **15**: 644–653.

32. Hertz AF. The cause and treatment of certain unfavourable after-effects of gastroenterostomy. *Ann Surg* 1913; **58**: 466–472.

33. Mix CL. 'Dumping stomach' following gastrojejunostomy. *Surg Clin N Am* 1922; **2**: 617–622.

34. Woodward ER. The early postprandial dumping syndrome: clinical manifestations and pathogenesis. In: Bushkin FL, Woodward ER (eds) *Postgastrectomy Syndromes*. WB Saunders: Philadelphia, 1976.

35. Ralphs DNL, Thomson JP, Haynes S, Lawson-Smith C, Hobsley M, Le Quesne LP. The relationship between the rate of gastric emptying and the dumping syndrome. *Br J Surg* 1978; **65**: 637–641.

36. Woodward ER, Neustein CL. The late postprandial dumping syndrome. In: Bushkin FL, Woodward ER (eds) *Postgastrectomy Syndromes*. WB Saunders: Philadelphia, 1976.

37. Nightingale JMD. Octreotide to treat dumping and short bowel syndrome. *Curr Med Lit Gastroenterol* 1993; **12**: 75–82.

38. Stempien SJ, Dragadi AE, Lee ER, Simonton JH. Status of duodenal ulcer patients ten years or more after vagotomy-pyloroplasty (V-P). *Am J Gastroenterol* 1971; **56**: 99–108.

39. Raimes SA, Smimiotis V, Wheldon EJ, Venables CW, Johnston IDA. Postvagotomy diarrhoea put into perspective. *Lancet* 1986; **ii**: 851–853.

40. Collins CD. Lomotil in treatment of post-vagotomy diarrhoea. *Br Med J* 1966; **2**: 560–561.

41. Ayulo JA. Cholestyramine in postvagotomy diarrhoea. *Am J Gastroenterol* 1972; **57**: 207–225.

42. Allan JG, Gerskowitch VP, Russell RI. The role of bile acids in the pathogenesis of postvagotomy diarrhoea. *Br J Surg* 1974; **61**: 516–518.

43. Duncombe VM, Bolin TD, Davis AE. Double-blind trial of cholestyramine in post-vagotomy diarrhoea. *Gut* 1977; **18**: 531–535.

44. Ladas SD, Isaacs PET, Quereshi Y, Sladen G. Role of the small intestine in postvagotomy diarrhea. *Gastroenterology* 1983; **85**: 1088–1093.

45. Deller DJ, Wits LJ. Changes in the blood after partial gastrectomy with special reference to vitamin B_{12}. *Q J Med* 1962; **31**: 71–88.

46. Bjomeboc E, Farber H, Mikkelsen O, Toleiassen F. Surgical treatment of gastric and duodenal ulcer. *Acta Med Scand* 1951; **141**: 16–26.

47. Wallensten S. Results of surgical treatment of peptic ulcers by partial gastrectomy according to Billroth I and Billroth II methods. *Acta Chir Scand* 1954; **191 (suppl)**: 1–161.

48. Chanarin I. *The Megloblastic Anaemias*. Blackwell: Oxford, 1969.

49. Pryor JP, O'Shea JM, Brooks PL, Datar GK. The long-term metabolic consequences of partial gastrectomy. *Am J Med* 1971; **51**: 5–10.

50. Hines ID, Hoffbrand AV, Mollin DL. The haematologic complications following partial gastrectomy. *Am J Med* 1967; **43**: 555–569.

51. Mahmud K, Ripley D, Swaim WR, Doscherhohnen A. Haematologic complications of partial gastrectomy. *Ann Surg* 1973; **177**: 432–435.

52. Baird IM, Blackbum EK, Wilson GM. The pathogenesis of anaemia after partial gastrectomy, I; development of anaemia in relation to time after operation, blood loss and diet. *Q J Med* 1959; **28**: 21–34.

53. Shafer RB, Ripley D, Swain WR, Mahmud K, Doscherholmen A. Hematologic alterations following partial gastrectomy. *Am J Med Sci* 1973; **266**: 240–248.

54. Bragelmann R, Armbrecht U, Rosemeyer D, Schneider B, Zilly W, Stockbrugger RW. Nutrient malassimilation following total gastrectomy. *Scand J Gastroenterol* 1996; **31 (suppl 218)**: 26–33.

55. Kimber C, Patterson JF, Weintraub AR. The pathogenesis of iron deficiency anaemia following partial gastrectomy. A study of iron balance. *JAMA* 1967; **202**: 935–938.

56. Baird IM, Wilson GM. The pathogenesis of anaemia after partial gastrectomy. II. Iron absorption after partial gastrectomy. *Q J Med* 1959; **28**: 35–40.

57. Wheby MS, Jones LG, Crosby WH. Studies on iron absorption. Intestinal regulatory mechanisms. *J Clin Invest* 1964; **43**: 1433–1442.

58. Rygold O. Hypovitaminosis B_{12} following partial gastrectomy by the Billroth II method. *Scand J Gastroenterol* 1974; **29 (suppl)**: 57–64.

59. Loewenstein F. Absorption of Cobalt [60]-labeled vitamin B_{12} after subtotal gastrectomy. *Blood* 1958; **13**: 339–347.

60. Mahmud K, Ripley D, Dosherholmen A. Vitamin B_{12} absorption tests, their unreliability in post-gastrectomy states. *JAMA* 1971; **216**: 1167–1171.

61. Dosherholmen A, Swaim WR. Impaired assimulation of egg Co^{57} vitamin B$_{12}$ in patients with hypochlorhydria and achlorhydria and after gastric resection. *Gastroenterology* 1973; **64**: 913–919.

62. Toskes PP. Haematologic abnormalities following gastric resection. In: Bushkin FL, Woodward ER (eds) *Postgastrectomy Syndromes*. WB Saunders: Philadelphia, 1976, pp. 119–128.

63. Eddy RL. Metabolic bone disease after gastrectomy. *Am J Med* 1971; **50**: 442–448.

11

Surgery for obesity

Eamonn M. M. Quigley and Jon S. Thompson

Obesity appears to have reached epidemic proportions in the Western world. Defined as a body mass index in excess of 30 kg/m^2,[1] the prevalence of obesity has been estimated at 15% in the UK and between 20 and 25% in the USA.[2]

The medical risks of obesity and morbid obesity (BMI > 40 kg/m^2) are well recognized and include diabetes mellitus, ischaemic heart disease, sleep apnoea, musculoskeletal problems, acid reflux, cholelithiasis, some types of cancer (breast and endometrium in women; colon in men), anxiety and depression. Furthermore, weight loss (0.5–9.0 kg), in the obese, has been shown to ameliorate hypertension, hyperglycaemia and hyperlipidaemia and reduce overall mortality by 20%.[3] A measurement of waist circumference (more than 88 cm in a woman and 102 cm in a man) provides a guide to those at greatest risk of developing associated diseases.[3]

Despite its risks and the well-documented benefits of weight reduction, the medical management of obesity has often proven most challenging. Despite their proliferation, programmes based on dietary restriction, exercise and behaviour modification have been far from universally successful, especially in the morbidly obese. In this group, even the most closely supervised medical regimes rarely prove successful, either because of poor compliance or rebound on completion of the programme. Pharmacological approaches have met with similar frustration. Though modest weight reduction has been described with a number of medical regimes, several have been complicated by serious side effects, and others have failed to provide consistent evidence of efficacy. These approaches have variably attempted to suppress appetite, increase metabolism, or decrease absorption. As an appetite suppressant, flenfluramine showed considerable promise until it was reported to cause valvular heart disease. Increasing metabolism by giving thyroxine or sympathomimetic drugs is potentially dangerous though phentermine is licensed in the UK.[3] The pharmacological induction of a malabsorptive state appears to offer some promise and, in a recent report, the combination of orlistat (a pancreatic lipase inhibitor) and a hypocaloric diet was associated with an approximately 10% loss of original weight over a 12-month period.[4] In comparison, a hypocaloric diet alone resulted in 6.1% weight loss. Olestra, a sucrose polyester, which is an engineered lipid that cannot be digested or absorbed and does not cause any serious physiological problems, is, in effect, a lipid substitute of no energy content that can be used in food and for cooking.[5] In the future, leptin analogues may be manufactured and thus provide a way of reducing appetite.

At present, there remains a need for alternative approaches to the management of the morbidly obese patient. This chapter will review the current status of bariatric (obesity) surgery and, in particular, the gastrointestinal complications related to these procedures.

TYPES OF BARIATRIC SURGERY

The surgical approach to the management of the morbidly obese patient is directed at two objectives, namely, to restrict caloric intake and to induce a malabsorptive state. Procedures such as the various types of gastroplasty, gastric banding and wrapping and the placement of a gastric bubble or balloon all attempt to dramatically reduce the intra-gastric volume available to receive the meal and, thereby, promote early satiety and reduce appetite. In contrast, procedures such as intestinal resection, jejuno-ileal and jejuno-colonic bypasses, and bilio-intestinal bypass aim to induce a malabsorptive state. Some procedures, such as the various types of gastric bypass, though primarily attempting to induce satiety by decreasing available gastric volume, also produce some degree of malabsorption and both factors, therefore, contribute to weight loss following these operations.[6]

Gastric reduction

As a testament to either lack of efficacy or prevalence of complications related to several of these procedures, the literature is literally replete with various variations on these general themes. The first gastric reduction procedures were performed manually, now they are based on the use of a stapler. By a process of trial and error, the ideal requirements for an effective gastroplasty have been defined, over the years, to be as follows: the gastric pouch should be between 15 and 20 ml in capacitance and the outlet from the pouch should be no greater than 12 mm (36 French guage) in diameter. It is crucial to minimize the risk of disruption or dehiscence of the staple line, to ensure that the stoma will not dilate and that distension of the pouch will be minimal. For these reasons, the vertical banded gastroplasty (Fig. 11.1) has emerged as the preferred procedure among the many variations of the gastroplasty. Recently, this procedure has been accomplished by a laparoscopic approach.[7–9] In one

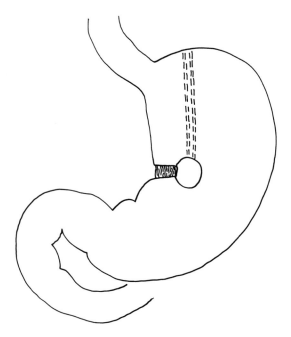

Figure 11.1 – Vertical banded gastroplasty.

gastroplasty in terms of weight loss. The goals of gastric bypass are similar to gastroplasty, i.e. to produce a gastric pouch similar in size to that produced by a gastroplasty that communicates directly with the small intestine.[12] Nowadays, this is most commonly achieved through anastomosis with a 60 cm-long Roux limb. It is thought that the greater efficacy of the bypass in producing weight loss is related to a number of factors: its potential to cause 'dumping' on carbohydrate ingestion, the post-prandial satiety induced, on eating, by distension of the Roux limb, and some degree of malabsorption resulting from bypass of the upper gastrointestinal tract. For these reasons, the gastric bypass with Roux-en-Y gastrojejunostomy has become a popular procedure for the surgical approach to morbid obesity (Fig. 11.2).

series which followed over 300 patients for 2 years, the average weight loss was 35.7% of initial weight.[10] The failure rate was 5.5%, due largely to dietary indiscretion, with a low incidence of staple line disruption. The principle complications were vomiting, usually secondary to stomal narrowing and secondary bezoar formation, with just one incidence each of stomal stricturing and upper gastrointestinal haemorrhage. Naslund and colleagues reported similar efficacy in almost 200 patients followed for up to 7 years, but documented a high re-operation rate.[11] Other approaches to gastric volume reduction, such as banding, wrapping, the intra-gastric (Garren) balloon and the gastric bubble have all been abandoned as ineffective or associated with an unacceptable risk of complications.

There are few, if any, prospective, randomized comparisons of gastric restrictive operations. Most follow-up is short-lived, and long-term efficacy rates are rarely provided. Truly comparative data on morbidity related to these procedures is also scanty.

Gastric bypass

While technically more difficult than a gastroplasty, gastric bypass procedures have achieved considerable popularity because of their apparent superiority over

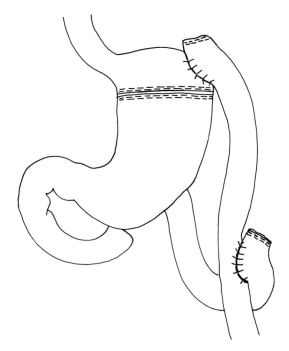

Figure 11.2 – Gastric bypass with Roux-en-Y gastro-jejunostomy.

Jejuno-ileal bypass

For many years, various types of intestinal bypass operation were popular based on their apparent efficacy in producing significant weight reduction.[13] Again, several variations were described, including end-to-side and end-to-end jejuno-ileal bypass procedures, jejuno-colonic bypass and bilio-intestinal bypass. The jejuno-ileal bypass aimed to create a short bowel and disrupt the enterohepatic circulation. In the jejuno-ileal bypass procedure, a 25 cm segment of jejunum was anastamosed to the distal 10 cm of the ileum (Fig. 11.3). The net effect of each of these procedures was to produce malabsorption and, thereby, weight loss. Diarrhoea was common, but of greatest concern was the prevalence of significant liver disease and serious complications of vitamin and trace element deficiency, including neuropathy and encephalopathy. For this reason these procedures were largely abandoned in the late 1970s, though patients will still be encountered in clinical practice with an intact bypass procedure and at-risk for these complications.

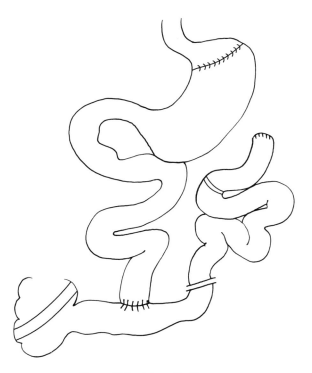

Figure 11.3 – Jejuno-ileal bypass.

Bilio-pancreatic bypass

This procedure, performed by Scopinaro *et al.*,[14] aimed to produce selective malabsorption of macronutrients. It avoided both disrupting the enterohepatic circulation of bile salts and leaving a long blind loop.

Additionally by performing a distal two-thirds gastrectomy it reduced the chance of gastric acid hypersecretion and peptic ulceration. A partial bilio-pancreatic bypass consists of a distal gastrectomy with transection of the small bowel distal to the duodeno-jejunal flexure. The proximal end (containing pancreatico-biliary secretions) is anastomosed to the distal ileum about 50 cm from the ileocaecal junction. The remaining ileum is anastomosed to the stomach. In a total bilio-pancreatic bypass, all the ileum from the gastric remnant (except the distal 50 cm) is anastomosed to the ascending colon. Due to the high post-operative chance of developing gallstones a cholecystectomy is performed at the same time as a bilio-pancreatic bypass operation.[14]

CONSEQUENCES OF BARIATRIC SURGERY

In discussing gastrointestinal complications of obesity surgery, it is important to consider perioperative problems, the consequences of rapid weight loss and specific gastrointestinal complications.

Perioperative complications

The most important perioperative complications of bariatric surgery are anastomotic leak, ateleclasis, pulmonary embolism and wound infection. Intra-abdominal sepsis secondary to a leak is the most important cause of morbidity and may prove difficult to detect clinically and radiologically in these very obese patients. Therefore the surgeon maintains a low threshold for re-exploration of these patients.

Weight loss

The most common and predictable gastrointestinal complication of weight loss is cholelithiasis (see Chapter 14). Mediated through the induction of gall bladder stasis, decreased stimulation of biliary secretions and changes in bile composition, patients undergoing rapid weight loss are prone to the development of gallbladder sludge and stones. The prevalence of gallstones has been estimated at anywhere from 9 to 33% and complications such as cholecystitis, choledocholithiasis and cholangitis have been documented in up to 10% of cases, regardless of the means whereby the weight loss was attained. This has led many surgeons to advocate prophylactic cholecystectomy at the time of bariatric surgery.

Gastrointestinal complications[15]

Gastric restrictive operations and gastric bypass

Systematic reviews of the obesity surgery literature have emphasized the poor quality of most studies in terms of lack of such features as randomization, use of appropriate controls and prospective analysis, but conclude that these operations are effective in the relative short-term and that gastric bypass is, in general, more effective than gastroplasty.[16–19] These procedures have also resulted in an improved quality of life[20] but there is little documentation of their impact on the significant, life-threatening complications of morbid obesity. The importance of careful patient selection has been consistently emphasized.[21]

Buckwalter and Herbst performed a retrospective analysis of perioperative complications of five different gastric restrictive operations performed on 565 patients over an 8-year period.[22] Intra-operative complications occurred in 4%; of these, splenic injury and faulty gastrojejunostomy occurred only among patients who underwent a gastric bypass procedure rather than a gastroplasty (Table 11.1). Seven patients required splenectomy. A total of 4% of the patients had general, postoperative complications that were unrelated to the type of operation. Postoperative complications specific to each procedure occurred in 14% of those undergoing gastric bypass with loop gastrojejunostomy (leaks, afferent limb obstruction, bezoars, bile gastritis and bleeding), 15% with gastric bypass and Roux-en-Y gastrojejunostomy (leaks, stomal obstruction, dumping syndrome, staple separation and stomach ulceration), 23% with greater curvature gastroplasty (stomal obstruction, leak and bezoar), 10% with gastro-gastrostomy (bezoars, stomal obstruction, leak, staple separation, gastritis and bleeding) and 0% with vertical banded gastroplasty. They concluded that the vertical banded gastroplasty is the safest operation and as effective as the alternatives.

Individual symptoms

Vomiting

Gastric restrictive operations, such as gastric bypass or gastroplasty, aim to produce weight loss through the creation of a small gastric pouch with a small outlet. It should come as no surprise, therefore, that vomiting is a common sequel of these procedures and is especially

Table 11.1 – Gastrointestinal complications of bariatric surgical procedures

Gastroplasty
  Vomiting
  Stomal obstruction
  Bezoars
  Gastrointestinal haemorrhage

Gastric bypass
  Vomiting
  Stomal obstruction
  Stomal ulceration
  Bezoars
  Anastomotic leaks
  Dumping syndrome
  Gastrointestinal haemorrhage
  Gastro-oesophageal reflux

Jejuno-ileal bypass

Malabsorption	Steatorrhoea
	Renal stones
	Vitamin and divalent cation deficiencies (e.g. vitamin D and magnesium)
Bacterial overgrowth	Steatohepatitis
	Arthritis and dermatitis
	B_{12} deficiency

Bilio-pancreatic bypass

Malabsorption	Steatorrhoea
	Vitamin and divalent cation deficiencies (e.g. vitamins A, D, E, Mg and Se)

common in relation to the ingestion of large volumes, as well as to certain foods such as meat.

Vomiting may also be a consequence of narrowing of the stoma due to excessive calibration, oedema, ulceration, fibrosis or obstruction by certain food particles or a bezoar.[23] Stomal obstruction will typically lead to chronic vomiting in association with weight loss. In contrast, vomiting due to excessive distension of the pouch by over-filling will occur in the context of weight gain.

Less commonly, vomiting may result from gastroparesis in the distal stomach or obstruction of the small intestine or Roux loop. In these situations, effective vomiting may be difficult to achieve due to the presence of a narrowed stoma and retching may be the dominant feature.

The most useful tools in the evaluation of the post-bariatric surgery patient with vomiting are radiology and endoscopy. These often provide complementary information, with radiology providing a more accurate depiction of anatomy, and endoscopy a better visualization of the mucosa and related pathology.[24,25] Endoscopy may also prove therapeutic by removing obstructing food particles or dilating stenosed stomas.

Stomal ulceration has been associated with staple line perforation and pouch hyperacidity.[26] Staple line dehiscence provides access to the pouch and jejunum for acid from the previously bypassed stomach.[27] In one report, stomal ulceration occurred only in those bypass patients who had suffered a staple line dehiscence. Similarly, gastro-oesophageal reflux (GORD) should only complicate a bypass procedure if staple line dehiscence has occurred. In contrast, reflux and even severe oesophagitis may complicate vertical banded gastroplasty.[28] It has been reported that oesophagitis related to this procedure can be reversed by conversion to a gastric bypass. GORD may also be a consequence of stomal stenosis or gastroparesis.

Dilation has been achieved with the endoscope itself, with Eder-Puestow, Maloney or Savary-type dilators and, most commonly, with Gruntzig, Fogarty, Rigiflex and pneumatic-type latex balloons.[29–33] In performing dilation, the endoscopist must, first, avoid dilation in the presence of stomal ulceration and, second, be mindful of the original size of the stoma. Dilation should attempt to achieve this same diameter, with allowance being made for the thickness of the gastric wall. Sing and colleagues described a 10% incidence of obstruction among 732 patients who underwent a vertical banded gastroplasty.[34] Two factors contributed to obstruction – channel angulation and stenosis. Whereas all but 13% of those with stenosis responded to dilation, 86% of those with angulation required surgical correction.

Less commonly, ulceration may occur within the bypassed stomach and lead to bleeding or pain. In this situation, endoscopic access may present a formidable challenge but can be achieved even in the patient with a Roux-en-Y anastomosis with appropriate equipment and experience.

Bleeding

Bleeding, whether overt or occult (and leading to iron deficiency) may complicate any restrictive operation and is most commonly due to stomal ulceration. Other possible aetiologies include oesophagitis and gastric ulcer within the bypassed stomach. A major challenge in the evaluation and therapy of gastrointestinal bleeding is achieving endoscopic access to the entire upper gastrointestinal tract; due to the anatomical changes that may render the distal stomach inaccessible by the direct approach.[35] Retrograde access may be achieved by using a paediatric colonoscope.

Specific complications of procedures

Gastroplasty

The major gastrointestinal symptoms which may occur following gastroplasty are, primarily, those related to the reduced size of the stomach and to the narrowed outlet. Resultant symptoms may include nausea, vomiting and even symptoms suggestive of gastric outlet obstruction. It has been suggested that GORD may be precipitated or aggravated.[28] However, while reflux symptoms and oesophagitis are common following gastroplasty, prospective endoscopic studies suggest that the creation of a vertical banded gastroplasty does not, per se, promote reflux and have documented little change in prevalence of oesophagitis following gastroplasty. One study also documented a reduction in prevalence of gastritis following gastroplasty.[36] The development of vomiting and reflux usually relate to stomal stenosis. In some instances the narrowing of the outlet may be sufficient to offer an actual obstruction and lead to bezoar formation. Non-steroidal intake may precipitate stomal ulceration and lead to fibrosis. Haemorrhage has also been reported following gastroplasty and may originate as a direct consequence of the surgery or originate from a peptic ulcer disease in the gastric pouch or in the defunctioned stomach. Band erosion may occur, rarely, and usually requires re-operation, which has been associated with an excellent outcome in most instances.[27] Rare instances of encephalopathy have also been reported.[38]

Gastric bypass procedures

A major consequence of a gastric bypass procedure is that the bypassed stomach is no longer accessible by the conventional route and, should problems arise within it, may present diagnostic difficulties.[39] Thompson and colleagues reported on follow-up for at least 6 years on 150 patients following an Alden loop gastrojejunostomy.[40] Overall, mortality was 2%. Early complications occurred in 23% of these patients and included wound problems, atelectasis, stomach tears, gastric perforation (two patients) and bleeding duodenal ulcer (one patient). Late complications were also common, occurring in 40% of the patients. The most common complication was the development of a ventral hernia, which occurred in 18%. Biliary disease developed in 24% of those at risk, leading the authors to propose prophylactic cholecystectomy at the time of the gastric bypass procedure. The ventral hernia rate was threefold that reported in other series and may have been related to the particular closure technique employed. They also recommended that confining the patient to oral liquids for the first 8 weeks could reduce the dehiscence rate. Other complications included stomal enlargement (2.0%), pouch enlargement (1.3%), bile reflux (1.4%), efferent loop obstruction (0.7%), blind loop syndrome (0.7%) and stomal stenosis (0.7%). Overall, weight loss was 36% of initial weight at 12 months and then remained stable, though at least one complication occurred in 82 (55%) of the patients. Mason and colleagues, pioneers in this area, reported on 434 patients.[10] Early mortality was similar, at 3%, with overall mortality of 5%. Wound problems were noted in 8% and stomal ulceration in 2%. Most patients had normal bowel habits, but early vomiting was relatively common. Printen and colleagues documented a 0.3% incidence of significant distal, gastric or duodenal bleeding in over 3000 gastric bypass procedures.[35] Flickinger and colleagues reported on 397 patients with a gastric bypass and Roux-en-Y-type anastomosis.[41] Again, maximum weight loss occurred between 18 and 24 months, to an average 61 % of original weight and 120% of ideal body weight. Mortality was low, at 0.8%; 16% of patients reported early nausea and vomiting and 71% the dumping syndrome. Supporting the concept of a component of malabsorption with this procedure, they documented iron, B_{12}, B_6 and folate deficiency in from 9 to 46% of these patients. Fewer than 2% developed a symptomatic gastric ulcer. These authors went on to describe a technique to examine the bypassed stomach, by advancing a paediatric colonoscope through the Roux limb and in an orad fashion up into the remnant. Using this approach, they documented a reasonably high incidence of gastritis in the remnant; in another study, in contrast, which involved both pre- and postoperative endoscopy, the prevalence of gastritis was actually reduced following bypass.[42] The occurrence of GORD or bleeding (from gastritis or a marginal ulcer) in a patient who has undergone a gastric bypass procedure usually indicates staple line disruption,[43] thereby permitting acid reflux. Others have reported leaks[44] and gastro colonic fistula formation.[45]

A variation of the gastric bypass, the Roux-en-Y gastric bypass, which incorporates a longer efferent Roux limb produces, in effect, a malabsorption state akin to that produced by a jejuno-ileal bypass.

Jejuno-ileal bypass

Malabsorption is an expected consequence of jejuno-ileal bypass. All patients have diarrhoea in the immediate aftermath of these procedures due to bile salt malabsorption and steatorrhoea.[46] This usually resolves with time. Malabsorption, however, persists. Within 1 year, up to 50% of patients have been documented to have developed hypokalaemia and malabsorption of calcium, magnesium, iron, B_{12}, other B vitamins, vitamin D, folic acid and fat-soluble vitamins. In some, severe electrolyte deficiencies and protein-calorie malnutrition may develop.[47] These, no doubt, contribute to the frequency of neuropathy and encephalopathy among these patients. Oxalate urinary stones develop in 12–32% due to excessive colonic absorption of oxalic acid and may lead to pyelo-nephritis and renal failure (Chapter 15).

Other systemic complications may relate to the blind loop of intestine in which bacterial overgrowth may occur. These include arthritis and dermatitis (80%) which are related to enhanced absorption of bacterial products and which, in turn, generate immune complexes. Intestinal complications have included volvulus (of the bypassed small intestine at the ileo-colostomy in patients who have undergone an end-to-side anastomosis), intussusception[48] (of the jejunal end of the bypassed intestine), bypass (diversion), enteritis (in the bypassed intestine and the colon) and acquired megacolon. The latter tends to occur late after surgery and, usually, more than 12 months postoperatively.

Most sinister is the development of liver disease in the form of progressive steatohepatitis, which can lead to decompensated liver disease and may prove fatal. Hepatic steatosis has been reported in up to 90% of liver biopsies obtained at the time of bariatric surgical procedures. Non-alcoholic steato-hepatitis (NASH) is well known to occur in the obese and a recent survey documented the unexpected finding of cirrhosis, at the time of surgery, in 0.14% of 86,500 bariatric operations.[49] Jejuno-ileal bypass surgery has been associated with the development and progression of steato-hepatitis to fibrosis and decompensated liver disease. Several patients have required transplantation for decompensated liver disease following jejuno-ileal bypass.[50–52] To avoid the development of steatosis in the engrafted liver it is important to simultaneously take down the bypass. An instance of precipitation of liver failure following takedown of a bypass has also been described in a patient with cirrhosis.

Several approaches have been recommended for the management of these patients, especially once complications develop. Formal takedown of the jejuno–ileal bypass has been shown to lead to weight gain unless another procedure, such as a gastric bypass or gastroplasty, is performed. An alternative approach, lengthening of the intestine in continuity, will increase the absorptive surface area and has been reported by some to produce an amelioration of the malabsorptive state. Whether this will prevent or reverse liver disease is not clear. Other, poorly validated, approaches have included the creation of anti-reflux valves to prevent reflux into the defunctioned limb, the creation of either a cholecysto-jejunostomy to the blind end of the defunctioned limb or an ileogastrostomy, revision of the end-to-side anastomosis to end-to-end, and small bowel resection. At present, the prudent approach would appear to be a formal takedown with refashioning of another bariatric procedure, if clinically and technically feasible.[53]

Bilio-pancreatic bypass

The bilio-pancreatic bypass, which combined a Roux-en-Y distal jejuno-ileostomy with a subtotal gastrectomy and bypass was also associated with problems due to malabsorption, including hypoproteinemia, osteoporosis, steatorrhoea and deficiencies of the fat-soluble vitamins. No deterioration in liver function tests occurred after the surgery.[14]

REFERENCES

1. National Institutes of Health. Gastrointestinal surgery for severe obesity: NIH consensus development conference statement, 25–27 March 1991. *Am J Clin Nutr* 1992; **55**: 615S–619S.

2. Bray GA. Obesity: a time bomb to be defused. *Lancet* 1998; **352**: 160–161.

3. Editorial. Why and how should adults lose weight? *Drug Ther Bull* 1998; **36**: 89–92.

4. Sjostrom L. Randomized placebo-controlled trial of orlistat for weight loss and prevention of weight regain in obese patients. *Lancet* 1998; **352**: 167–172.

5. Thomson ABR, Hunt RH, Zorich NL. Review article: olestra and its gastrointestinal safety. *Aliment Pharmacol Ther* 1998; **12**: 1185–1200.

6. Linner JH. Overview of surgical techniques for the treatment of morbid obesity. *Gastro Clin N Amer* 1987; **16**: 253–272.

7. Awad W, Loehnert R. Laparoscopic gastroplasty. Technique and preliminary results in patients with morbid obesity. *Rev Esp Enferm Dig* 1997; **89**: 753–758.

8. Watson DI, Game PA. Hand-assisted laparoscopic vertical banded gastroplasty. Initial report. *Surg Endosc* 1997; **11**: 1218–1220.

9. Lonroth H, Dalenback J, Haglind E, Josefsson K, Olbe L, Fagevik-Olsen M, Lundell L. Vertical banded gastroplasty by laparoscopic technique in the treatment of morbid obesity. *Surg Laparosc Endosc* 1996; **6**: 102–107.

10. Willbanks DL. Long-term results of silicone elastomer ring vertical gastroplasty for the treatment of morbid obesity. *Surgery* 1987; **101**: 606–610.

11. Naslund E, Backman L, Granstrom L, Stockeld D. Seven-year results of vertical banded gastroplasty for morbid obesity. *Eur J Surg* 1997; **163**: 281–286.

12. Mason EE, Printen KJ, Hartford CE, Boyd WC. Optimizing results of gastric bypass. *Ann Surg* 1975; **182**: 405–416.

13. Jorgensen S, Olsen M, Gudman-Hoyer E. A review of 20 years of jejunoileal bypass. *Scand J Gastroenterol* 1997; **32**: 334–339.

14. Scopinaro N, Gianetta E, Civalleri D, Bonalumi U, Bachi V. Two years of clinical experience with bilio-pancreatic bypass for obesity. *Am J Clin Nutr* 1980; **33**: 596–514.

15. Khol JA. Management of the problem patient after bariatric surgery. *Gastro Clin N Am* 1994; **23**: 345–369.

16. Brolin RE. Update: NIH consensus conference. Gastrointestinal surgery for severe obesity. *Nutrition* 1996; **12**: 403–404.

17. Glenny AM, O'Meara S, Melville A, Sheldon TA, Wilson C. The treatment and prevention of obesity: a systematic review of the literature. *Int J Obes Relat Metab Disord* 1997; **23**: 715–737.

18. Kolanowski J. Surgical treatment for morbid obesity. *Br Med Bull* 1997; **53**: 433–444.

19. National Institutes of Health. Gastrointestinal surgery for severe obesity: NIH consensus development conference, 25–27 March 1991. *Nutrition* 1996; **12**: 397–404.

20. Isacsson A, Frederiksen SG, Nilsson P, Hedenbro JL. Quality of life after gastroplasty is normal: a controlled study. *Eur J Surg* 1997; **163**: 181–186.

21. Balsiger BM, Luque de Leon E, Sarr MG. Surgical treatment of obesity: who is an appropriate candidate? *Mayo Clin Proc* 1997; **72**: 551–557.

22. Buckwalter JA, Herbst CA Jr. Perioperative complications of gastric restrictive operations. *Am J Surg* 1983; **146**: 613–618.

23. Hocking MP, Bennett RS, Rout R, Woodward ER. Pouch outlet obstruction following vertical ring gastroplasty for morbid obesity. *Am J Surg* 1990; **160**: 496–500.

24. Strodel WE, Khol JA, Eckhauser FE. Endoscopy of the partitioned stomach. *Ann Surg* 1984; **200**: 582–586.

25. Verset D, Houben JJ, Gay F, Elcheroth J, Bourgeois V, Van-Gossum A. The place of upper gastrointestinal tract endoscopy before and after vertical banded gastroplasty for morbid obesity. *Dig Dis Sci* 1997; **42**: 2333–2337.

26. Griffen WO Jr. Stomal ulcer after gastric restrictive operations. *J Am Coll Surg* 1997; **185**: 87–88.

27. MacLean LD, Rhode BM, Nohr C, Katz S, McLean PH. Stomal ulcer after gastric bypass. *J Am Coll Surg* 1997; **185**: 1–7.

28. Kim CH, Sarr MG. Severe reflux esophagitis after vertical banded gastroplasty for treatment of morbid obesity. *Mayo Clin Proc* 1992; **67**: 33–35.

29. Wolper JC, Messmer JM, Turner MA, Sugerman HJ. Endoscopic dilation of late stomal stenosis. *Arch Surg* 1984; **119**: 836–837.

30. Al-Halees ZY, Freeman JB, Burchett H, Braxeau-Gravelle P. Nonoperative management of stomal stenosis after gastroplasty for morbid obesity. *Surg Gynecol Obstet* 1986; **162**: 349–354.

31. Eckhauser FE, Khol JA, Strodel WE, Cho K. Hydrostatic balloon dilation for stomal stenosis after gastric partitioning. *Surg Gastroentrol* 1984; **3**: 43–50.

32. Sapala JA, Sapala MA. Technique for correction of stomal dilation in the failed gastric exclusion procedure. *Dig Surg* 1989; **6**: 66–69.

33. Kretzschmar CS, Hamilton JW, Wissler DW, Yale CE, Morrissey JF. Balloon dilation for the treatment of stomal stenosis complicating gastric surgery for morbid obesity. *Surgery* 1987; **102**: 443–446.

34. Sing RF, Seinige UL, Lieber CP, Sataloff DM. An increase in pouch outlet obstruction as a delayed finding after vertical-banded gastroplasty. *Dig Surg* 1993; **10**: 65–68.

35. Printen KJ, Le Favre J, Alden J. Bleeding from the bypassed stomach following gastric bypass. *Surg Gynecol Obstet* 1983; **156**: 65–66.

36. Naslund E, Granstrom L, Melcher A, Stockeld D, Backman L. Gastro-oesophageal reflux before and after vertical banded gastroplasty in the treatment of obesity. *Eur J Surg* 1996; **162**: 303–306.

37. Moreno P, Alastrue A, Rull M, *et al.* Band erosion in patients who have undergone vertical banded gastroplasty: incidence and technical solutions. *Arch Surg* 1998; **133**: 189–193.

38. Christodoulakis M, Maris T, Plaitakis A, Medlissas J. Wernicke's encephalopathy after vertical banded gastroplasty for morbid obesity. *Eur J Surg* 1997; **163**: 473–474.

39. Anderson OS, Paine GT, Morse EK. An unusual complication of gastric bypass: perforated antral ulcer. *Am J Gastroenterol* 1982; **77**: 93–96.

40. Thompson WR, Amaral JF, Caldwell MD, Martin HF, Randall HT. Complications and weight loss in 150 consecutive gastric exclusion patients. *Am J Surg* 1983; **146**: 602–612.

41. Flickinger EG, Pories WJ, Meelheim HD, Sinar DR, Blose IL, Thomas FT. The Greenville gastric bypass: progress report at 3 years. *Ann Surg* 1984; **199**: 555–560.

42. Papavramidis ST, Theocharidis AJ, Zaraboukas TG, Christoforidou BP, Kessissoglou II, Aidonopoulos AP. Upper gastrointestinal endoscopic and histologic findings before and after vertical banded gastroplasty. *Surg Endosc* 1996; **10**: 825–830.

43. Messmer JM, Wolper JC, Sugerman HJ. Stomal disruption in gastric partition in morbid obesity (Comparison of radiographic and endoscopic diagnosis). *Am J Gastroenterol* 1984; **79**: 603–605.

44. Buckwalter JA, Herbst CA Jr. Leaks occurring after gastric bariatric operations. *Surgery* 1988; **103**: 156–160.

45. Cucchi SGD, Pories WJ, MacDonald KG, Morgan EJ. Gastrogastric fistulas. *Ann Surg* 1995; **221**: 387–391.

46. Steinbach G, Lupton J, Reddy BS, Lee JJ, Kral JG, Holt PR. Calcium carbonate treatment of diarrhoea in intestinal bypass patients. *Eur J Gastroenterol Hepatol* 1996; **8**: 559–562.

47. Ehrenpreis ED, Wieland JM, Cabral J, Estevez V, Zaitman D, Secrest K. Symptomatic hypocalcemia, hypomagnesemia, and hyperphosphatemia secondary to Fleet's Phospho-Soda colonoscopy preparation in a patient with a jejunoileal bypass. *Dig Dis Sci* 1997; **42**: 858–860.

48. Cossu ML, Coppola M, Iannuccelli M, Noya G. Simultaneous ileal intussusception and volvulus after jejunoileal bypass for morbid obesity. *Panminerva Med* 1997; **39**: 141–143.

49. Brolin RE, Bradley LJ, Taliwal RV. Unsuspected cirrhosis discovered during elective obesity operations. *Arch Surg* 1998; **133**: 84–88.

50. Markowitz JS, Seu P, Goss JA, *et al.* Liver transplantation for decompensated cirrhosis after jejunoileal bypass: a strategy for management. *Transplantation* 1998; **65**: 570–572.

51. D'Souza-Gburek SM, Batts, KP, Nikias GA, Wiesner RH, Krom RA. Liver transplantation for jejunoileal bypass-associated cirrhosis: allograft histology in the setting of an intact bypassed limb. *Liver Transpl Surg* 1997; **3**: 23–27.

52. Lowell JA, Shenoy S, Ghalib R, Caldwell C, White FV, Peters M, Howard TK. Liver transplantation after jejunoileal bypass for morbid obesity. *J Am Coll Surg* 1997; **185**: 123–127.

53. Behrns KE, Smith CD, Kelly KA, Sarr MG. Reoperative bariatric surgery. *Ann Surg* 1993; **218**: 646–653.

12

The short bowel

J. M. D. Nightingale

INTRODUCTION

A patient has a short bowel when there is an insufficient length of small bowel remaining to maintain health without the need for macronutrient and/or sodium chloride and water supplements. This is likely to be the case if less than 200 cm small bowel remains.

BACKGROUND

In 1880, Koberle performed the first reported successful small intestinal resection of more than 200 cm on a 22-year-old girl with multiple intestinal strictures.[1] At the beginning of the twentieth century, a resection of more than 200 cm of small intestine, thought to be a third of the total small intestinal length, was referred to as an 'extensive' intestinal resection and was thought to be the maximum length of small intestine that could be removed and for the patient to survive.[2] In 1935, Haymond used the term 'massive' in preference to 'extensive' of intestinal resection when he reviewed the literature of 257 patients, most of whom had had a resection for an intestinal volvulus (Table 12.1); he noted an overall survival of 67%.[3]

Table 12.1 – Reasons for a 'massive' intestinal resection in adults as published in 1935[3]

	n=257
Volvulus	76
Strangulated hernia	45
Mesenteric thrombosis	34
Tuberculosis	16
Mesenteric tumours	14
Uterine perforation	11
Adhesions/bands	7
Other	54

In the 1960s, as an awareness developed that the outcome from an intestinal resection depended upon the length of small bowel remaining rather than the length resected, so the term 'short bowel syndrome' came into use. The syndrome was characterized by 'intractable diarrhoea with impaired absorption of fats, vitamins, and other nutrients, ultimately leading to malnutrition, anaemia, and continued weight loss'.[4] This description implies a slow chronic illness and is adequate to describe most patients who have a short bowel and retained functioning colon, but it does not describe the acute fluid balance problems experienced by patients with a jejunostomy (end-jejunostomy syndrome). The first report of a patient surviving with a jejunostomy, 120 cm from the duodeno-jejunal flexure, was made in 1963.[5]

LENGTH OF SMALL INTESTINE

The length of the adult intestine, measured surgically, radiologically or at autopsy from the duodeno-jejunal flexure, ranges from about 275 to 850 cm and tends to be shorter in women than in men (Ch. 2). Congenital cases of a short bowel have been reported and are usually associated with malrotation of the gut.[6,7] Patients who have a small intestinal length at or below the lower end of the normal range may develop the problems associated with a short bowel after relatively little small intestine has been removed. In a study of 11 patients with Crohn's disease and less than 200 cm small bowel remaining, the median original small bowel length was calculated from the lengths resected and remaining to be 240 cm (range 205–315 cm), indicating a short small bowel length before any resections.[8] The large range of normal human small intestinal length means that it is more important to refer to the length of small bowel remaining rather than to the length removed.

ASSESSMENT OF RESIDUAL SMALL INTESTINE

Anatomical length

The remaining small bowel length is ideally assessed at surgery by measuring 10–30 cm segments of bowel along the antimesenteric border, taking great care not to over-stretch the bowel. If there is no surgical measurement available, the bowel can be measured radiologically using an opisometer, a device used for measuring distances on maps. It traces the long axis of the small bowel on a small bowel meal radiograph. This technique is relatively accurate if the total small intestinal length is less than 200 cm and if the entire small bowel is shown on one film.[9,10]

Functional length

Citrulline is a non-essential amino acid that is synthesized in the enterocyte by pyrolline-5-carboxylase-synthase from glutamine. It is not derived from food or proteolysis and is not incorporated into body proteins. Some of the citrulline made by the enterocyte passes to the liver, where it is an important intermediate in the urea cycle (urea made from ammonia) and some passes into the systemic circulation. All the citrulline in the systemic circulation is derived from small intestinal enterocytes, thus plasma levels of citrulline are related to the length of the remaining functional small bowel.[11]

ANATOMICAL CONSIDERATIONS OF REMAINING BOWEL

Ileum or jejunum

A jejunal resection is better tolerated than an ileal resection. Ileal mucosa, in contrast to the jejunal mucosa, has tight intercellular junctions and thus can concentrate its contents. Gastrointestinal transit is naturally slower in the ileum than jejunum, so allowing more time for absorption.[12,13] The terminal ileum absorbs vitamin B_{12}[14,15] and bile salts. Ileum remaining after a small bowel resection can adapt in both structure and function to increase absorption,[16–18] while the jejunum can only adapt functionally if some distal bowel remains (Ch. 16).

Ileocaecal valve

It is traditionally considered that preservation of the ileocaecal valve is beneficial as it may slow transit and prevent reflux of colonic contents into the small bowel; however, studies of ileocaecal valve excision show no evidence for the former, and small bowel peristalsis probably prevents the latter[12,19] (Ch. 2).

Some reports suggest that conservation of the ileocaecal valve in children is beneficial in terms of survival and the need for parenteral nutrition;[20,21] others show no such benefits.[22,23] The reports proposing benefit of ileocaecal valve preservation in adults may reflect preservation of a significant length of terminal ileum.

Colon

Conservation of the colon is beneficial because it absorbs water, sodium,[24–28] calcium[29] and short- and medium-chain fatty acids;[30–32] it also slows gastro-intestinal transit[33] and stimulates small intestinal hyperplasia.[34] Patients with an entero-colic anastomosis may survive without parenteral support with a very short[35,36] or even no remaining jejunum.[37] Patients with a preserved functioning colon rarely need regular water and sodium supplements.[26–28] In terms of the need for parenteral nutrients, preservation of at least half of the colon after a jejuno-ileal resection is equivalent to about 50 cm of small intestine.[28]

CAUSES OF A SHORT BOWEL

The three most common reasons for patients to have less than 120 or 200 cm of small bowel are superior mesenteric artery thrombosis, Crohn's disease and irradiation damage[10,28,38] (Tables 12.2, 12.3). Resection of an ischaemic small intestine mainly results in colonic preservation (75%) and affects an older age group (median age 57 years).[28] Patients with Crohn's disease and jejunum in continuity with a functioning colon had undergone a median of 3 small intestinal resections (range 2–6) over a median of 14 years (range 0–29), compared with 4 resections (range 1–12) over a median of 11 years (range 1–26) in those with a jejunostomy.[28] The median time from irradiation to having a small intestinal length of less than 200 cm in 8 patients with irradiation damage (5 gynaecological cancers, 2 carcinomas of the colon and 1 seminoma) was 5 years (range 1–16).[28]

A short bowel occurs more commonly in women (67%) than in men;[28] this may be because women start with a shorter length of small intestine than men.

Table 12.2 – Reasons for a short bowel in adults in 1969[38] (less than 120 cm small bowel remaining; almost all patients had a remaining functional colon)

	$n=123$
Superior mesenteric artery thrombosis/embolus	49
Volvulus	24
Superior mesenteric vein thrombosis	10
Tumours	10
Non-occlusive gangrene	10
Strangulated herniae	5
Regional enteritis	1
Other	14

Table 12.3 – Reasons for a short bowel in adults in 1992 (less than 200 cm small bowel remaining)[27]

	Jejunum–colon	Jejunostomy
Total (sex)	38 (26F)★	46 (31F)
Age (range)	46 (7–70)	42 (16–68)
Median jejunal length (cm)	90 (0–190)	115 (20–190)
Diagnosis		
Crohn's disease	16	33
Ischaemia	6	2
Irradiation	5	3
Ulcerative colitis	–	5
Volvulus	5	–
Adhesions	4	1
Diverticular disease	1	1
Desmoid tumour	1	1

★ 7 had an ileocaecal valve and 31 a jejuno-colic anastomosis.

The causes of a short bowel arising in childhood and infancy usually result in colonic preservation and include mid-gut volvulus, necrotizing enterocolitis, multiple jejuno-ileal atresia and gastroschisis[20–23,39–41] (Chs 7, 27). As the management and thus the survival of these children improves,[21–23] they will be cared for as adults.

TYPES OF PATIENT WITH A SHORT BOWEL

There are three types of patient with a short bowel (Fig. 12.1):

1. **Jejunum–colon.** Patients in whom the ileum has been removed, often with the ileocaecal valve, to leave a jejuno-colic anastomosis (jejunum–colon); patients who have less than 10 cm of terminal ileum are included in this group.

2. **Jejunostomy.** Patients in whom some jejunum, the ileum and colon have been removed, so they are left with an end-jejunostomy.

3. **Jejunum–ileum.** Patients who have had a predominantly jejunal resection, and have more than 10 cm of terminal ileum and the colon remaining (jejuno-ileal).[10,28,42] This last group is not common (2 of 86 patients[28]); since the residual ileum can adapt both structurally and functionally, these patients rarely have major problems and they are not specifically discussed in this chapter.

Patients with a jejunostomy can be classified according to the results of balance studies as net 'absorbers' or net 'secretors'. The 'absorbers' in general have more than 100 cm of residual jejunum and absorb more water and sodium from their diet than they take orally (usual daily jejunostomy output about 2 kg); they can therefore be managed

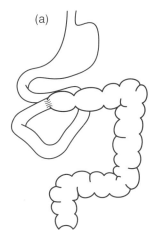
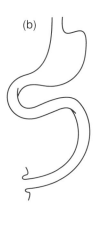
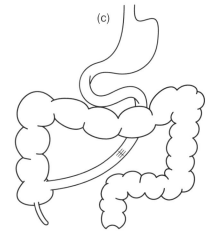

Figure 12.1 – The three types of patient with a short bowel. Patients with a jejuno-colic anastomosis or a jejunostomy are most commonly encountered. (a) Jejuno-colic anastomosis; (b) Jejunostomy; (c) Jejuno-ileal anastomosis.

with oral sodium and water supplements, and parenteral fluids are not needed. The 'secretors' usually have less than 100 cm residual jejunum and lose more water and sodium from their stoma than they take by mouth (the usual daily stomal output may be 4–8 kg). 'Secretors' cannot convert from negative to positive water and sodium balance by taking more orally, and so they need long-term parenteral supplements.[43] These requirements change very little with time.[28] The jejunostomy output from a net 'secretor' increases during the daytime in response to food and decreases at night; any drug therapy that aims to reduce the output is therefore given prior to food. The change from a net secretory state, in terms of water and sodium balance, to a net absorptive state occurs at a jejunal length of about 100 cm (Ch. 24).

BOWEL LENGTH AND FLUID/NUTRITIONAL SUPPORT

Jejunum–colon. While it is possible for a patient with no remaining jejunum to survive without parenteral nutrition, quality of life is poor.[36] A patient with 100–200 cm of jejunum in continuity with a functioning colon may need oral nutrient supplements for a few months but in the long-term would not be expected to need any supplements unless the remaining bowel was diseased. When the jejunal length is between 50 and 100 cm, some patients will need long-term parenteral nutrition (PN), if it is between 30 and 50 cm most will do so, and if it is less than 30 cm almost all patients will need PN[28,42] (Fig. 12.2). Sometimes parenteral nutrition is needed not to maintain nutritional status but to prevent the severe diarrhoea associated with eating.

Jejunostomy. The survival of patients with a jejunostomy has improved since 1963.[5,44] If 100–200 cm jejunum remains, oral sodium supplements (glucose–saline solution or sodium chloride tablets) are likely to be needed, often with oral nutrient solutions to which sodium chloride has been added.[28,42,43] A patient with a jejunostomy and less than 100 cm jejunum remaining would be expected to need long-term parenteral saline. If less than 85 cm jejunum remains, long-term parenteral nutrition is likely to be required in addition to the saline. Patients usually need

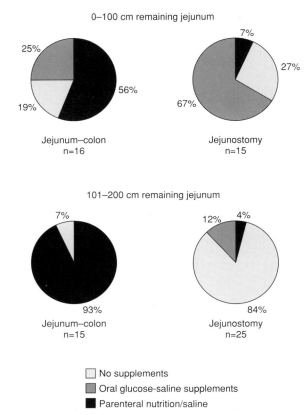

Figure 12.2 – Pie chart showing the need for parenteral and enteral sodium and water supplements in patients with less than 200 cm jejunum remaining. Few patients with a colon needed oral or parenteral sodium and water supplements, but almost all jejunostomy patients did.[28]

long-term parenteral nutrition when they absorb less than a third of their oral energy intake.[43,45]

PHYSIOLOGICAL CHANGES

Of the physiological changes observed after a small intestinal resection, some reflect normal and some altered physiology. Most experimental work in animals involves a predominantly jejunal resection (jejuno–ileal anastomosis); this has a better prognosis but is not a common situation in humans, in whom an ileal resection with or without a colectomy is most common.

Gastrointestinal motility

Gastric emptying

There are mechanisms (brakes) in the jejunum, ileum and colon that slow gastric emptying (Ch. 2). In addition, events external to the bowel can affect gastric emptying; for example, parenteral nutrition delays the gastric emptying of solids.[46] Studies in animals have shown that gastric emptying of liquid is normal after a jejunal resection.[47,48]

Jejunum–colon. Gastric emptying of liquids is normal in patients who have had a distal small intestinal resection that does not result in a short bowel.[49] Studies in which a dual isotope meal (liquid and solid components of the meal are labelled with different isotopes) has been given to patients with a jejuno-colic anastomosis have shown that some liquid leaves the stomach rapidly and travels quickly through the short length of remaining jejunum to reach the colon. In the colon, by a neural or hormonal mechanism, the liquid meal activates a colonic braking mechanism by which subsequent gastric emptying is slowed and overall measurements of liquid and solid gastric emptying are normal.[33] This colonic braking mechanism may be caused by the release of peptide YY from the colon[50] (Fig. 12.3). Infusions of peptide YY that achieve similar levels in normal subjects delay the gastric emptying of liquid.[51]

Jejunostomy. The rate of gastric emptying of solids is normal in patients who do not have a short bowel but have had a proctocolectomy and distal ileal resection.[52] In patients with a jejunostomy, barium taken orally has been observed to pass rapidly into the jejunostomy bag. Dual radio-isotope studies have shown that the early rate of liquid gastric emptying is rapid and that this tends to correlate inversely with the remaining length of jejunum.[33] This is probably caused by the loss of cells secreting peptide YY in the terminal ileum and colon, and the consequent low plasma levels.[50]

Small bowel transit

As there is normally faster transit of chyme through the jejunum than ileum,[12,13,17,52] it is not unexpected that small bowel transit has been shown to be fast after an ileal and slow after a jejunal resection.[47,48,53]

Jejunum–colon. The first part of a liquid meal travels rapidly from the stomach to the colon, reflecting both the normal faster jejunal transit and the short distance it has to travel. The transit rate for

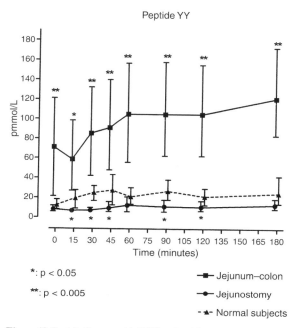

Peptide YY

Figure 12.3 – Median peptide YY levels with interquartile range for 6 jejunum–colon patients, 7 jejunostomy patients and 12 normal subjects after a pancake and orange juice meal.[50]

solid is normal, however, suggesting that jejunal transit has been slowed by the colonic brake already activated by the prior arrival of some liquid in the colon. This effect may have been mediated by peptide YY.

In the fasting state, in patients with a short bowel and a retained colon, the interdigestive migrating motor complex (MMC) occurs more frequently but for a shorter total time than in normal subjects, and phase 2 activity is of a shorter duration.[54,55] The frequency and amplitude of jejunal contraction is unaffected.[55]

Jejunostomy. The rate of liquid and solid small bowel transit is rapid in patients with a jejunostomy. This may be due to low peptide YY levels. Six hours after a meal there is still some meal residue within the stomach, and this may result from a disorder of the MMC.[33]

Gastrointestinal secretions

Salivary secretion

The volume of saliva produced at rest was significantly less in 7 jejunostomy patients (median 0.6 g/5 min, range 0.0–1.4) than in 13 normal subjects (median 2.2 g/5 min, range 0.9–8.7, $p<0.005$). After stimulation of salivary flow by chewing paraffin wax for 5 minutes, the volume of saliva was significantly less in jejunostomy patients (median 4.6 g/5 min, range 2.2–8.2) than in normal subjects (median 9.7 g/5 min, range 7.0–20.5, $p<0.005$). These observations are likely to reflect altered physiology, but a degree of dehydration was not excluded.[56]

Gastric secretion

In 1914, Stassoff[57] performed experiments on six dogs in which he demonstrated that if the distal half of the small intestine was removed, the chyme that emerged from a duodenal fistula was more liquid and had left the stomach more quickly than before the resection. Many studies in dogs with denervated Heidenhain pouches[58–73] and in some with innervated Pavlov pouches[67] have shown hypersecretion of gastric acid. In most studies, the colon has been retained, though in one a colectomy alone caused gastric acid hypersecretion.[74] The larger the intestinal resection, the greater is the postoperative gastric acid hypersecretion.[61,75] The greatest rises in acid output are produced by jejunal rather than ileal resection[66,72,75] (with the exception of one study[63]) and by defunctioning bowel[60,65] rather than resecting it. The increased secretion is prevented by antrectomy[65,70,72,73] but not by a vagotomy and pyloroplasty.[70,73]

Fielding and Cooke showed an 8% incidence of peptic ulcer among 300 patients with Crohn's disease and they noted that resections of 60 cm or more of the small bowel caused an increase in basal and pentagastrin-stimulated acid output.[76] They related this increased gastric acid output to a previous terminal ileal resection rather than to active disease.[77]

In humans, the survival of some patients with a very short bowel has been attributed to their previous gastric surgery.[61,78,79] The evidence for gastric acid hypersecretion in the long term in patients with a retained colon is not good. Miura et al. reported 3 of 7 patients with a short gut and a retained colon who developed duodenal ulcers.[80] Windsor et al. described 19 patients in whom more than 300 cm of small intestine had been resected and noted in 8 patients large postoperative aspirates of gastric juice of more than 1.5 litres daily which lasted for less than 14 days. The volume of aspirate did not correlate with the remaining length of small intestine. In 6 of the 19 patients the increased secretion was attributed to impaired liver function, which these researchers postulated might increase circulating histamine levels.[69]

One patient with a jejunostomy 90 cm from the duodeno-jejunal flexure following surgery for Crohn's disease had an acidic (pH 1–6) jejunostomy output of 4.8 litres daily that was reduced by gastric irradiation.[63] O'Keefe et al. showed normal pentagastrin-stimulated gastric acid secretion in 9 patients with a jejunostomy (jejunal length 25–200 cm) more than a year after surgery.[81]

High gastrin levels have been observed[50,82,83] and may result from a reduced length of small bowel being available to catabolize gastrin.[84,85] However, gastrin may not be of major physiological importance as studies in the Rhesus monkey have shown that, 6 months after a distal small intestinal resection, basal and histamine-induced acid secretion are at their highest levels, yet serum gastrin levels have returned to normal.[86] Another reason for gastric acid hypersecretion may be the loss of a normal inhibitor of gastric acid secretion, such as neurotensin or peptide YY, from the distal small bowel/colon. In an extensive review in 1974, Buxton suggested that stasis in remaining bowel segments allowed bacterial colonization; these bacteria then either deconjugate bile salts or degrade 'protein' which directly or indirectly causes the release of gastrin or a gastrin-like hormone that causes increased gastric acid secretion.[87]

Excess gastric acid in the duodenum, in addition to increasing the incidence of peptic ulceration, causes bile salt precipitation,[88] reduced pancreatic enzyme function and increased jejunal motility; all of which impair nutrient absorption.

The evidence indicates that gastric acid hypersecretion, after a small intestinal resection, occurs in dogs with denervated gastric pouches and colons left in situ. It may be present for the first two weeks after a small bowel resection in humans, but there is no good evidence that it occurs in the long term in patients with a short bowel with or without a colon, even though high gastrin levels are observed.

Pancreatico-biliary secretions

If a person is undernourished,[89] or if no food passes through the gut,[90] pancreatic function is reduced. In 7 well-nourished patients who had had a mean small bowel resection of 164 cm (leaving colon) and were taking an oral diet, the post-prandial secretion of trypsin and bilirubin (measured by jejunal aspiration after a liquid meal) was the same as in normal healthy individuals.[91] However, another study in children showed reduced pancreatic volume and enzyme secretion, after an injection of secretin and cholecystokinin, in 2 of 5 patients; both of these had most of their colon remaining.[92]

After cholecystokinin administration, pancreatic volume and enzyme secretion is increased in patients with a jejunostomy compared with healthy subjects.[78]

When more than 100 cm of terminal ileum has been resected the increased hepatic synthesis of bile salts cannot keep pace with the stool or stomal losses and thus fat malabsorption results.[93] The greatest lipid malabsorption (steatorrhoea) occurs in patients with a jejunostomy: partly because of a very reduced bile salt pool, partly due to rapid transit, and, in a few cases, due to bacterial overgrowth in the remaining bowel.[94] It has not yet been determined if changes occur in the volume of bile produced each day after an intestinal resection.

Gastrointestinal hormones

There are differences in the systemic plasma gastrointestinal hormone profiles after a meal in patients with a short bowel compared to normal subjects. However, it is only as studies are performed in these patients, using the hormones, specific agonists or antagonists, that the physiological importance of the observations can be understood; until then the significance of many observations remains a matter for speculation.

Parenteral nutrition itself does not affect the gastrointestinal hormone response to food.[95] The levels of some plasma hormones (e.g. enteroglucagon, pancreatic polypeptide and somatostatin and gastric inhibitory polypeptide) before and after a meal in patients with a short bowel (with or without a colon) are the same as in normal subjects. Plasma levels of vasoactive intestinal peptide in patients with a colon were normal in one study,[96] but high in another.[97] High plasma gastrin and cholecystokinin levels and low plasma neurotensin, GLP-1 and insulin levels occur in both types of patient. The plasma neurotensin levels correlate with the length of residual jejunum.[50] The high plasma cholecystokinin levels could cause satiety in some patients with a very short gut.[50]

There are differences between the two types of patient, the most significant ones being in the plasma levels of two hormones produced by the terminal ileum and colon, namely peptide YY[50,96] (Fig. 12.3) and GLP-2[98,99] (Fig. 12.4). Peptide YY slows gastrointestinal

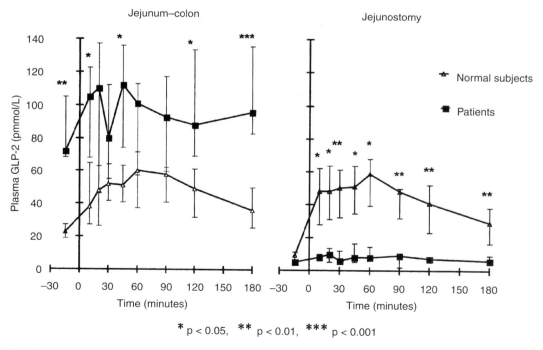

Figure 12.4 – Median GLP-2 levels with interquartile range in 7 jejunum–colon patients, 7 jejunostomy patients and 7 normal subjects after a continental breakfast.[98,99] Courtesy of P Jeppesen and PB Mortensen.

transit and GLP-2 stimulates small bowel villus growth (Ch. 2). Patients with a colon have high fasting plasma peptide YY and GLP-2 levels, and both hormone levels are low in patients with a jejunostomy.[50,98–100] Low plasma peptide YY levels also occur in ileostomy patients who have had a colectomy.[100] High plasma motilin levels occur in patients with a jejunostomy, but this is unlikely to be of physiological importance as the highest levels occur in those with the longest lengths of jejunum remaining who do not have rapid intestinal transit.[50]

Changes in absorption

In addition to absorption of nutrients, there are some specialist functions that are particular to the ileum. The ileum has the unique functions of absorbing vitamin B_{12} and bile salts. Vitamin B_{12} deficiency is likely to occur if more than 60 cm of terminal ileum has been resected.[14,53] If more than 100 cm ileum has been removed, the enterohepatic circulation will be disrupted and diarrhoea is likely to be due to steatorrhoea.[93] If less than 100 cm has been resected, diarrhoea may result from unabsorbed deoxybile salts (secondary bile acids) causing colonic sodium and water secretion.[93]

CLINICAL PROBLEMS AND THEIR TREATMENT

The problems experienced by patients with a short bowel depend upon the type and length of remaining small bowel and the presence or absence of a functioning colon. Most of these problems are dealt with in specific chapters and only a brief summary follows here.

Presentation

The presentation and long-term outcome from a resection can be predicted from knowledge of the remaining small bowel length and the presence or absence of a functioning colon. In both types of patient, treatment is aimed first at maintaining fluid balance. Nutritional supplements are usually started 24–48 hours after the surgery, to prevent loss of lean body mass. This may entail a period of parenteral nutrition, which is gradually reduced as the patient takes more food orally.

Jejunum–colon. These patients are often deceptively well after the resection except for diarrhoea/steatorrhoea, but in the succeeding months they may lose weight and present as severely undernourished (classical 'short bowel syndrome').

Jejunostomy. These patients have immediate problems after surgery due to the large volume of stomal output, which increases with food and drink. This high-volume output results in patients rapidly becoming depleted in water and sodium. Recognition of this high output means that clinicians are often aware that nutritional problems will follow, hence nutritional care is often addressed at a much earlier stage than in patients with a retained colon. Jejunostomy patients are highly dependent on treatments to compensate for water and sodium losses. If they miss their treatment for one day they are likely to become unwell from sodium and water depletion. Their requirements for water and sodium supplements change little with time (Ch. 16).

Undernutrition (protein–energy malnutrition, Ch. 13)

Loss of muscle leads to weakness and early fatigue. Loss of body fat results in feeling cold, a gaunt facial appearance, dry and wrinkled skin, and dull hair. These features, together with a stooped posture, give an impression of premature ageing. Patients may dislike looking in the mirror and weighing themselves, and may avoid company because they are self-conscious about their wasted appearance. Apathy, depression and irritability associated with undernutrition may stop the patient from being motivated to recover. Short bowel patients who can be maintained on an oral diet need to consume more energy than normal subjects because as much as 50% of the energy from the diet may be malabsorbed. Patients can achieve this by eating more high-energy food, having oral sip-feeds, or receiving high-energy enteral feeds at night through a nasogastric or gastrostomy tube. Once weight is regained, the daily energy requirements may decrease, especially in those with a retained colon. Only if these measures fail and the patient continues to lose weight, or fails to regain lost weight, is parenteral nutrition given. Even then, parenteral supplements may be needed for only a limited period of weeks or months, and thereafter oral supplements may be adequate.

In the long term, parenteral nutrition is needed if a patient absorbs less than one-third of the oral energy intake,[43,45] if there are high energy requirements and absorption is about 30–60%, or if increasing the oral/enteral nutrient intake causes a socially unacceptably large volume of stomal output or diarrhoea. In addition to consumption of a high-energy diet, the dietary advice given to the two types of patient is different (Ch. 25).

Jejunum–colon. In order to increase energy absorption and to reduce the risk of renal stones, patients with a retained colon need a large total energy intake with a diet high in carbohydrate (polysaccharides)[31] but not increased in fat (long-chain triglycerides); the diet should also be low in oxalate. D(−) lactic acidosis may occur if a diet is high in monosaccharides.[101] If oxalate is not reduced there is a 25% chance of the patient developing symptomatic calcium oxalate renal stones[28] (see Ch. 15). Long-term parenteral nutrition is likely to be needed if less than 50 cm jejunum remains.[28]

Jejunostomy. Jejunostomy patients need a diet high in energy. It does not matter whether this is as carbohydrate or lipid so long as the osmolality is kept low by using large molecules (polysaccharides, protein and triglycerides)[102,103] and thus allowing extra sodium chloride to be added to give the meal/liquid feed a total sodium concentration of 90–120 mmol/L and an osmolality of about 300 mOsm/kg. An elemental diet has a high osmolality and little sodium and should therefore be avoided as it may increase water and sodium losses. A high-lipid diet may increase stomal calcium and magnesium losses (Ch. 25).

Water and sodium losses

Clinical assessment/monitoring

Deficiencies of water and sodium (most common in those without a retained colon) are common and result in a loss of extracellular fluid volume, hypotension and, if severe, pre-renal failure. Daily body weight and an accurate fluid balance (to include stomal effluent) are essential measurements during the initial stages of management. Acute sodium and water deficiencies are detected by a rapid fall in body weight, postural hypotension, low urine volume and, if very severe, by a rising serum creatinine and urea. A useful guide to sodium depletion is measurement of sodium concentration in a random urine sample: lack of body sodium is suggested by a concentration of only 0–5 mmol/L. It is ideal, though not always possible, to achieve a daily urine volume of at least 800 ml with a sodium concentration greater than 20 mmol/L. In addition to relatively normal haematological and biochemical measurements, it is desirable (though again not always possible with oral medication) to have a plasma magnesium level greater than 0.6 mmol/L (Ch. 17).

Jejunum–colon. The colon has a large capacity to absorb sodium and water; thus patients with a short bowel and a preserved colon are rarely in negative water and sodium balance and rarely need water or sodium supplements.[25,28] If sodium deficiency does develop, a glucose–saline drink can be sipped during the day, as for patients with a jejunostomy. Although the colon secretes potassium, a low serum potassium level is rare.[28] There is an exchange mechanism of chloride absorption/bicarbonate secretion in the colon; thus, if much sodium chloride is consumed, bicarbonate may be lost in the stools and give rise to a metabolic acidosis similar to that occurring in patients who have an ileo-conduit following a cystectomy.

Jejunostomy. Patients with a jejunostomy have a large volume of stomal output that is greater after eating or drinking. Each litre of jejunostomy fluid contains about 100 mmol/L of sodium.[43] This high-volume output is mainly the result of loss of the normal daily secretions produced in response to food and drink (about 4 litres per day) although gastric acid hypersecretion and rapid liquid gastric emptying and small bowel transit may contribute.

The effluent from a jejunostomy or ileostomy contains relatively little potassium (about 15 mmol/L).[26,43] Potassium balance is not often a problem, and net loss through the stoma occurs only when less than 50 cm jejunum remains.[43] A low serum potassium level may be caused by sodium depletion with secondary hyperaldosteronism and thus greater than normal urinary losses of potassium[26] or by magnesium depletion[104] (Ch. 24).

Treatment of water and sodium depletion

Jejunostomy. Intravenous fluid is given initially while the patient takes no oral food or fluid. This will reduce the high output dramatically; food is then gradually reintroduced. Parenteral nutrition/saline is likely to be needed in the long term if less than 100 cm jejunum remains. Oral hypotonic fluids are restricted and a glucose–saline solution (sodium concentration 90–120 mmol/L) is given to sip during the day. Some clinicians suggest that liquid and solids be taken at different times although there is no published evidence that this reduces stool/stomal output.[105] Drugs that reduce gastrointestinal secretions or motility may be used; often both types of drug are administered. In general, patients who are net 'secretors' have the greatest reduction in their stomal output when drugs that predominantly reduce gastrointestinal secretions are given, for example omeprazole 40 mg daily, ranitidine 300 mg twice daily, cimetidine 200 mg every 6 hours or 300 mg continuously over 6 hours or, if there is insufficient gut to absorb these (less than 50 cm), subcutaneous or intravenous octreotide 50 μg twice a day. However, these treatments rarely completely alleviate the need for parenteral supplements. Patients who are net 'absorbers' have the greatest reduction when drugs that predominantly reduce gastrointestinal motility (e.g. loperamide 4 mg four times a day and codeine phosphate 60 mg four times a day) are given half an hour before food (Ch. 24).

Magnesium and other micronutrients

The clinical syndrome of magnesium deficiency in man was described in 1960[106,107] and in the same year was reported as occurring after a massive intestinal resection.[108] It has subsequently been reported after jejuno-ileal bypass for obesity[109] and after ileal resections of more than 75 cm.[110] Its features include fatigue, depression, jerky and weak muscles, ataxia, athetoid movements, cardiac arrhythmias and, if severe, convulsions.[106,107,111,112] Carpopedal spasm and positive Chvostek and Trousseau signs generally occur if there is a concomitant hypocalcaemia.[107,111,113]

Low serum magnesium levels are more common in patients with a jejunostomy than in patients with a retained colon. Of short bowel patients who were not receiving parenteral nutrition, 11 of 27 (41%) of those with a colon were receiving magnesium or had low serum magnesium levels, compared with 19 of 28 (68%) with a jejunostomy.[28] Patients with a preserved colon require less magnesium and have higher serum values than those without a retained colon. This, together with reports that magnesium poisoning can occur after a magnesium sulphate enema, provides further evidence that the colon absorbs magnesium.[114]

Most clinicians use a serum magnesium measurement of less than 0.6 mmol/L as their guide to magnesium depletion; however, urine, skeletal muscle, mononuclear cell or ionized magnesium levels[112] are more sensitive indicators.

There are several reasons for magnesium deficiency. Magnesium is normally absorbed by passive diffusion in the distal small bowel and colon. Bowel resections reduce the absorptive area and may increase stool losses;[115] however, this does not occur in an easily predictable manner and balance studies have shown that magnesium balance does not relate to the length of small bowel remaining.[56] The composition of the diet consumed may be another cause of stool losses of magnesium. Fatty acids, derived either from digestion of dietary fat or from bacterial fermentation of malabsorbed carbohydrate, combine with magnesium, calcium and zinc and prevent their absorption, increasing faecal or stomal losses.[116] A third reason, occurring particularly in patients with a jejunostomy, is stool/stomal loss of salt and water and the consequent secondary hyperaldosteronism. Aldosterone increases renal excretion of magnesium in rats and man and the faecal excretion of magnesium in rats.[117,118]

A low serum magnesium level reduces both the secretion and function of parathormone.[119] Thus parathormone cannot promote magnesium absorption in the ascending limb of the loop of Henle or activate renal 1α-hydroxylase to make 1,25-hydroxycholecalciferol. The failure to make 1,25-hydroxycholecalciferol results in reduced magnesium and calcium absorption from the gut.[120] Na^+/K^+-ATPase activity, which normally keeps potassium within a cell and sodium out, depends upon magnesium. When the serum magnesium level is low, activity of this enzyme is impaired. Potassium is therefore lost from cells and renal potassium excretion is increased, resulting overall in hypokalaemia. This hypokalaemia may not respond to the administration of oral or intravenous potassium, but does to magnesium supplementation.[121]

The treatment of hypomagnesaemia is outlined in Box 12.1. Patient hydration and, thus, secondary hyperaldosteronism must first be corrected. Serum magnesium levels can usually be improved by oral supplements, however the data on magnesium absorp-

---

Box 12.1 – Treatment of hypomagnesaemia

1. Correct water and sodium depletion (and thus secondary hyperaldosteronism).
2. Give oral magnesium preparation (e.g. 12 mmol magnesium oxide at night).
3. Reduce lipid in diet.
4. Give 1α-cholecalciferol (1–9 μg daily).
5. Give intravenous magnesium (occasionally subcutaneous or intramuscular magnesium sulphate).

tion from different preparations are often derived from normal volunteer studies. Tablet dissolution and magnesium availability may be different in patients with a short bowel. Various magnesium salts have been given as oral treatment including magnesium sulphate, chloride, hydroxide, acetate, carbonate, gluconate, lactate, citrate, aspartate, pyroglutamate, oxide (magnesia) and diglycinate. Most magnesium salts are poorly absorbed and may worsen diarrhoea/stomal output. Magnesium acetate causes less diarrhoea than magnesium gluconate.[122] Magnesium oxide is commonly given and contains more elemental magnesium than the other salts. It is insoluble in water and alcohol but soluble in dilute acid. In the stomach it is converted to magnesium chloride. It is given as gelatine capsules of 4 mmol magnesium oxide (160 mg of MgO) to a total of 12–24 mmol daily. Magnesium diglycinate (chelate) is absorbed as well as magnesium oxide as an intact dipeptide in the proximal jejunum and after an ileal resection it results in the passage of fewer stools than magnesium oxide.[123] Oral magnesium treatment is usually given at night when intestinal transit is assumed to be slowest and there is more time for absorption. This regimen does not appear to increase stomal or stool output. A low-fat diet decreases stool/stomal magnesium losses, especially in patients with a retained colon.[116] If oral magnesium supplements, dietary advice and correction of water and sodium depletion do not bring the magnesium level into the normal range, oral 1α-hydroxycholecalciferol in a dose of 1–9 μg daily may improve magnesium balance.[124,125] It may exert its effect by increasing both intestinal and renal magnesium absorption.[125]

Magnesium can occasionally be given as a subcutaneous injection of 4 mmol magnesium sulphate every 2 or more days, but can cause skin ulceration. Intramuscular injection of 10 mmol/L is an alternative, but is painful. Regular intravenous infusions of 12 mmol or more can be given, usually in a litre of saline over 1–2 hours, but can cause flushing.

Selenium

Patients receiving parenteral nutrition are commonly deficient in selenium[126–128] and need larger amounts of selenium than are required in the diet of normal subjects.[128] This suggests a loss of selenium from the gastrointestinal secretions. Patients with a jejunostomy also have a reduction in selenium absorption, the amount by which absorption is reduced correlating with residual jejunal length.[129] The kidney can conserve selenium but often not to a sufficient extent. Selenium deficiency is therefore common and may cause weak muscles and a dilated cardiomyopathy.[130]

Vitamin B$_{12}$ deficiency

Both groups of patients have had more than 60 cm of the terminal ileum removed and need long-term hydroxycobalamin injections, 1 mg every 3 months.[14,53]

Other vitamin and mineral deficiencies

There may be impairment of absorption of the fat-soluble vitamins A, D, E and K and essential fatty acids. Essential fatty acid deficiency may be treated by rubbing sunflower oil into the skin.[131] Zinc deficiency is not common unless stool volumes are large, when 12–15 mg are needed daily.[132] In patients receiving parenteral nutrition the deficiencies depend on the regimen used, but deficiencies of iron, vitamin D and biotin[133–135] may occur.

Diarrhoea (jejunum–colon patients)

The oral intake determines the amount of stool passed. Diarrhoea may severely limit a patient's lifestyle; limiting food intake can reduce diarrhoea but may increase the problems of undernutrition. Rarely, a patient requires parenteral nutrition to allow him or her to eat less and so reduce the diarrhoea.

Diarrhoea may be treated with loperamide, 2–8 mg, given half an hour before food. Loperamide is usually given in preference to codeine phosphate (30–60 mg half an hour before food), as it is non-sedative and non-addictive; occasionally, however, both are needed. If tablets/capsules emerge unchanged in stool/stomal output, they can be crushed, opened, mixed with water or put on food. If less than 100 cm of terminal ileum has been resected, bile salt malabsorption may contribute to the diarrhoea. This may be helped by cholestyramine which has the additional advantage of reducing oxalate absorption but may be detrimental by reducing fat absorption and by further reducing the bile salt pool.[93] Gastric anti-secretory drugs may reduce diarrhoea shortly after surgery but are not usually effective in the long term.

Confusion

In addition to the many common general medical causes of confusion (e.g. hypoxia, hepatic, renal or cardiac failure, sepsis, hypoglycaemia, alcohol or other drugs), other specific causes should be sought in a patient with a short bowel. Hypomagnesaemia may cause mild confusion. In patients with a preserved colon, severe confusion can result from D-lactic acidosis, in which a metabolic acidosis with a high anion gap will be observed (Ch. 25). Hyperammonaemia may cause confusion in both types of patients with a short bowel because ammonia cannot be detoxified. The small amount of intestine remaining cannot manufacture adequate citrulline to detoxify ammonia created in the urea cycle. If there is concomitant renal impairment, the increase in blood ammonia causes a problem as the kidney will not be able to excrete the excess ammonia. Hyperammonaemia can be corrected by giving arginine (an intermediary in the urea cycle).[136,137]

Drug absorption

Omeprazole can be absorbed in the duodenum and upper jejunum; problems are likely to occur only if less than 50 cm jejunum remains. Warfarin[138] and thyroxine may need to be given orally in high doses. Loperamide circulates in the enterohepatic circulation, which is disrupted, and higher doses than usual may need to be given (see Ch. 24).

Adaptation

Intestinal adaptation is the process that attempts to restore the total gut absorption of macronutrients, macrominerals and water to that occurring before the intestinal resection (Ch. 16). In a classical paper in 1959, Pullan described three phases that related to the changing situations in patients after a 'massive intestinal resection' leaving a functioning colon *in situ* (i.e. 'short bowel syndrome').[139] These changes mainly reflect structural and functional adaptation.

Stage 1. As intestinal motility returns in the first few days after the resection, profuse diarrhoea occurs and is maximal for the first 2–3 weeks. During this stage there may be large losses of fluid and electrolytes (up to 10 litres/day). These losses have been attributed to gastric acid hypersecretion.

Large volumes of saline (sometimes with magnesium) may be needed to maintain fluid balance, especially when the patient first starts to eat. A protein pump inhibitor or H_2 antagonist, loperamide and often codeine phosphate are empirically given. If the residual bowel length is less than 100 cm, parenteral nutrition may be started on the second postoperative day. Anal

soreness and excoriations may be a problem. This phase ends as the diarrhoea lessens.

Stage 2. The problem changes from that of fluid and electrolyte balance to that of progressive undernutrition requiring nutrition support. If untreated, the patient may rapidly lose weight and, despite a large oral energy intake, not absorb enough to maintain weight. Fat malabsorption is much more significant than that of carbohydrate and protein. Deficiencies of the fat-soluble vitamins A, D, E and K may occur, causing night blindness, bone pains, ataxia and bleeding respectively. Vitamin B and C deficiencies sometimes occur and cause glossitis, angular stomatitis, pellagra, psychotic changes and bleeding. Anaemia and hypoproteinaemia are rare after an uncomplicated resection.

The patient may complain of abdominal cramps, distension and nausea. During this time the gastrointestinal transit rate slows, although a large volume of fatty stool is still passed. Carbohydrate and protein are better absorbed and a state of equilibrium is reached after 3–6 months.

Stage 3. In the final stage relative equilibrium has been reached and minor adjustments are made. The dietary regimen tries to limit the lipid intake. Long-term parenteral nutrition is unlikely to be needed unless less than 50 cm jejunum remains. The beneficial effects of a proton pump inhibitor may have ceased by the end of the first year and the drug can be stopped.

After a large resection of small intestine, improvement in absorption of macronutrients, macrominerals and water may occur by: (1) the patient eating more food than normal (hyperphagia); (2) the remaining bowel increasing in size and absorptive area (structural adaptation); and (3) reduction in bowel transit rate to allow more time for absorption (functional adaptation). An increased oral intake has been observed.[140] After a jejunal resection in animals, the ileal remnant undergoes structural changes which include elongation of villi, deepening of crypts, and an increase in the number of absorptive cells in a given length of villus. After a jejuno-ileal resection in man to leave a jejuno-colic anastomosis, no structural adaptation (except possibly hyperplasia) has been demonstrated even though high GLP-2 levels are observed.[99] A degree of functional adaptation with slowing of liquid gastric emptying and solid small bowel transit has been demonstrated[50] and is likely to be caused by high peptide YY levels. Functional adaptation does occur, as demonstrated by the findings that there is a small reduction in faecal weight in the 3 months after a small bowel resection,[141] and that there is increased jejunal absorption of water,[142] sodium,[143] glucose[144] and calcium[145] with time. The intestinal calcium absorption may continue to increase for more than 2 years after a resection.[145]

Although adaptation occurs in the months after the creation of an ileostomy, there is no evidence for any structural[81] or functional[28,146] adaptation at any time in patients with a jejunostomy.

Gallstones

Gallstones are common (45%) in both types of patient and are more common in men[28] (Ch. 14). It was originally thought that gallstones in this circumstance resulted from deposition of cholesterol because of a depleted bile-salt pool. However, the gallstones tend to contain calcium bilirubinate. Such stones probably result from gallbladder stasis: biliary sludge develops and this subsequently forms calcium bilirubinate stones which often appear calcified on abdominal radiographs.[147] Calcium bilirubinate crystals within biliary sludge are more commonly found in men than in women.[148] Cholecystokinin injections have been used to prevent gallbladder stasis[149] and there may be a role for prophylactic cholecystectomy.[150]

Social problems

Most long-term patients with a short bowel have a body mass index within the normal range, and most are in full-time work or look after the home and family unaided.[28] Both groups of patients may have diarrhoea, which causes problems, especially if housing conditions are poor. In those with a colon the diarrhoea is malodorous and bulky due to steatorrhoea.

The effluent from a small-bowel stoma, unlike that from a colostomy, is not offensive. The large volume of fluid that emerges, however, may trouble the patient; sometimes 3 or more litres in 24 hours may be passed from the stoma. The bag then has to be emptied frequently and, if it becomes overfull, the adhesive flange may separate from the skin with embarrassing leakage of fluid and with the likelihood of skin soreness.

NEW AND FUTURE TREATMENTS

New treatments are likely to be aimed at increasing the absorptive function of the remaining gut (Ch. 16).

Most are currently directed at inducing structural adaptation, for example GLP-2,[151] epidermal growth factor,[152,153] colostrums or aminoguanidine.[154] Studies using growth hormone, glutamine and fibre have been disappointing.[155,156] Studies that use analogues of peptide YY have yet to be tried.[157] Cholylsarcosine is a synthetic bile acid resistant to bacterial deconjugation and dehydroxylation, that does not itself cause colonic secretion and thus diarrhoea, but does result in a variable improvement in fat and calcium absorption in patients with a short bowel, with or without a retained functioning colon.[158,159] Attempts are being made to replace colonic mucosa with small intestinal mucosa to increase absorption.[160] Another area of importance is the prevention of gallstones after an intestinal resection: trials using prophylactic antibiotics, urso-deoxycholic acid and cholecystokinin are awaited. An oral nutrient solution containing 100 mmol/L sodium and having an osmolality of 300 mOsm/kg has yet to be commercially manufactured as an ideal nutrient solution to give to patients with a jejunostomy or high-output ileostomy.

Small bowel transplantation is becoming safer (Ch. 34) but the outcome is not yet as good as that of prolonged parenteral nutrition (Ch. 26).

PREVENTATIVE MEASURES

Immunosuppressive medical therapy for Crohn's disease (e.g. anti-tumour necrosis factor antibody, azathioprine, 6-mercaptopurine and methotrexate) is improving and is being used at an earlier stage in the disease. This may reduce the need for repeated or major resections of Crohn's disease.

A small bowel embolus/venous infarction may be prevented by identification of risk factors such as atrial fibrillation, a poorly functioning myocardium, recent myocardial infarction, coagulation abnormalities or a period of hypotension. Anticoagulation therapy may be given to a patient in whom a potential source of emboli is identified. Intestinal ischaemia can be treated with nitrates, calcium antagonists or octreotide,[161] thus reducing the chance of a small bowel infarction. Percutaneous transluminal angioplasty or a surgical revascularization procedure can be performed to treat mesenteric angina. The diagnosis of a small bowel infarction can be difficult but needs to be made soon after the event. Clues to the diagnosis include the presence of the risk factors above, pain (usually of sudden onset and continuous), and usually a rise in the white cell count, amylase, phosphate and lactate.

Ideally, an angiogram should be performed within 2–3 hours of the onset of pain if a plain abdominal radiograph has shown no obvious abnormality.[162] If clot is shown in the superior mesenteric artery or vein, a bolus of a vasodilator (e.g. papaverine 60 mg or tolazoline 25 mg, phenoxybenzamine, adenosine triphosphate, glucagon or prostaglandin E) may be given into the superior mesenteric artery. If this is unsuccessful, surgery may be needed but papaverine can continue to be infused at a rate of 30–60 mg/h (1 mg/ml).[162] Thrombolytic drugs, heparin and low molecular weight dextran may all be infused into the superior mesenteric artery or peripherally to halt and/or reverse the progression of the infarction or ischaemia. The outcome is best if there are no signs of peritonitis at the onset of treatment.[162] Experimentally, the most severe problems occur after ischaemic bowel is reperfused as the resultant toxins and cytokines can cause liver and multi-organ failure. Other drugs that may be of benefit include free-radical scavengers (e.g. superoxide dismutase, 5-aminosalicylate) or xanthine oxidase inhibitors (e.g. allopurinol) and antibiotics.[163,164] Prostacyclin analogues may be useful when bowel is reperfused as they produce vasodilatation, reduce white cell and platelet aggregation and protect ischaemic tissues. If bowel is resected, a primary anastomosis is avoided and a temporary stoma created; it is wise to re-explore the abdomen the following day and resect any further ischaemic bowel.[163,165]

The techniques used to deliver abdominal radiotherapy have improved, with avoidance of the parallel opposed fields technique and the administration of glutamine and sucralfate (Ch. 9), so radiation damage should become uncommon.

SUMMARY

There are two common types of patient with a short bowel: those with jejunum in continuity with a functioning colon, and those with a jejunostomy. Both groups potentially have problems with protein–energy malnutrition, but it is a greater problem in those without a colon as they cannot derive energy from the colonic anaerobic bacterial fermentation of carbohydrate to short-chain fatty acids (Ch. 25). Patients with a jejunostomy have major problems from the large volume of stomal output and thus water, sodium and magnesium losses. Both types of patient have lost at least 60 cm of terminal ileum and so need vitamin B_{12} injections every 3 months. Both groups have a high prevalence of gallstones (45%), and patients with a retained colon have a 25% chance of developing calcium oxalate renal stones[28] (Table 12.4). The survival of these patients is good, even if they need long-term parenteral nutrition.[28,166,167]

REFERENCES

1. Koberle E. Resection de deux metres d'intestin grele. *Bull Acad Med* 1881; **4**: 128–131.

2. Flint JM. The effect of extensive resections of the small intestine. *Bull Johns Hopkins Hosp* 1912; **23**: 127–144.

3. Haymond HE. Massive resection of the small intestine. An analysis of 257 collected cases. *Surg Gynecol Obstet* 1935; **61**: 693–705.

4. Conn JH, Chavez CM, Fain WR. The short bowel syndrome. *Ann Surg* 1972; **175**: 803–814.

Table 12.4 – Problems of a short bowel

	Jejunum–colon	Jejunostomy
Presentation	Gradual, diarrhoea and undernutrition	Acute fluid losses
Water, sodium and magnesium depletion	Uncommon (in the long-term)	Common
Nutrient malabsorption	Common★	Very common
D(−) lactic acidosis	Occasionally	None
Renal stones (calcium oxalate)	25%	None
Gallstones (pigment)	45%	45%
Adaptation	Functional adaptation	No evidence
Social problems	Diarrhoea	High stomal output
		Dehydration
		Dependency on treatment

★ Bacterial fermentation of carbohydrate salvages some energy, but D(−) lactic acidosis can occur if the diet is high in mono- and oligosaccharides.

5. Mayo HW Jr., Duggan JJ. Post colectomy enteritis: survival after extensive small bowel resection complicated by magnesium deficiency. Case report. *Ann Surg* 1963; **157**: 92–96.

6. Wu T-J, Teng R-J, Chang M-H, Chen C-C. Congenital short bowel syndrome: report of a case treated with home central parenteral nutrition. *J Formosan Med Assoc* 1992; **91**: 470–472.

7. Schalamon J, Schober PH, Gallippi P, Matthyssens L, Hollwarth ME. Congenital short-bowel; a case study and review of the literature. *Eur J Pediatr Surg* 1999; **9**: 248–250.

8. Nightingale JMD, Lennard-Jones JE. Patients with a short bowel due to Crohn's disease often start with a short normal bowel. *Eur J Gastroenterol Hepatol* 1995; **7**: 989–991.

9. Nightingale JMD, Bartram CI, Lennard-Jones JE. Length of residual small bowel after partial resection: Correlation between radiographic and surgical measurements. *Gastrointest Radiol* 1991; **16**: 305–306.

10. Carbonnel F, Cosnes J, Chevret S *et al.* The role of anatomic factors in nutritional autonomy after extensive small bowel resection. *J Parenter Enteral Nutr* 1996; **20**: 275–280.

11. Crenn P, Coudray-Lucas C, Thullier F, Cynober L, Messing B. Post-absorptive plasma citrulline concentration is a marker of absorptive enterocyte mass and intestinal failure in humans. *Gastroenterology* 2000; **119**: 1496–1505.

12. Singleton AO, Redmond DC, McMurray JE. Ileocecal resection and small bowel transit and absorption. *Ann Surg* 1964; **159**: 690–694.

13. Summers RW, Kent TH, Osbourne JW. Effects of drugs, ileal obstruction and irradiation on rat gastrointestinal propulsion. *Gastroenterology* 1970; **59**: 731–739.

14. Booth CC, Mollin DL. The site of absorption of vitamin B_{12} in man. *Lancet* 1959; **i**: 18–21.

15. Thompson WG, Wrathell E. The relation between ileal resection and vitamin B_{12} absorption. *Can J Surg* 1977; **20**: 461–464.

16. Nygaard K. Resection of the small intestine in rats. III. Morphological changes in the intestinal tract. *Acta Chir Scand* 1967; **133**: 233–348.

17. Nygaard K. Resection of the small intestine in rats. IV. Adaptation of gastrointestinal motility. *Acta Chir Scand* 1967; **133**: 407–416.

18. Dowling RH, Booth CC. Structural and functional changes following small intestinal resection in the rat. *Clin Sci* 1967; **32**: 139–149.

19. Fich A, Steadman CJ, Phillips SF, Camilleri M, Brown ML, Haddad AC, Thomforde GM. Ileocolonic transit does not change after right hemicolectomy. *Gastroenterology* 1992; **103**: 794–799.

20. Wilmore D. Factors correlating with a successful outcome following extensive intestinal resection in newborn infants. *J Pediatr* 1972; **80**: 88–95.

21. Galea MH, Holliday H, Carachi R, Kapila L. Short-bowel syndrome: A collective review. *J Pediatr Surg* 1992; **27**: 592–596.

22. Goulet OJ, Revillon Y, Dominique J *et al.* Neonatal short bowel syndrome. *J Pediatr* 1991; **119**: 18–23.

23. Weber TR, Tracy T Jr., Connors RH. Short-bowel syndrome in children. Quality of life in an era of improved survival. *Arch Surg* 1991; **126**: 841–846.

24. Philips SF, Giller J. The contribution of the colon to electrolyte and water conservation in man. *J Lab Clin Med* 1973; **81**: 733–746.

25. Debongnie JC, Phillips SF. Capacity of the colon to absorb fluid. *Gastroenterology* 1978; **74**: 698–703.

26. Ladefoged K, Ølgaard K. Fluid and electrolyte absorption and renin–angiotensin–aldosterone axis in patients with severe short-bowel syndrome. *Scand J Gastroenterol* 1979; **14**: 729–735.

27. Ladefoged K, Ølgaard K. Sodium homeostasis after small-bowel resection. *Scand J Gastroenterol* 1985; **20**: 361–369.

28. Nightingale JMD, Lennard-Jones JE, Gertner DJ, Wood SR, Bartram CI. Colonic preservation reduces the need for parenteral therapy, increases the incidence of renal stones but does not change the high prevalence of gallstones in patients with a short bowel. *Gut* 1992; **33**: 1493–1497.

29. Hylander E, Ladefoged K, Jarnum S. Calcium absorption after intestinal resection. The importance of a preserved colon. *Scand J Gastroenterol* 1990; **25**: 705–710.

30. Ruppin H, Bar-Meir S, Soergel KH, Wood CM, Schmitt MG Jr. Absorption of short chain fatty acids by the colon. *Gastroenterology* 1980; **78**: 1500–1507.

31. Nordgaard I, Hansen BS, Mortensen PB. Colon as a digestive organ in patients with short bowel. *Lancet* 1994; **343**: 373–376.

32. Jeppesen PB, Mortensen PB. The influence of a preserved colon on the absorption of medium chain fat in patients with small bowel resection. *Gut* 1998; **43**: 478–483.

33. Nightingale JMD, Kamm MA, van der Sijp JRM *et al.* Disturbed gastric emptying in the short bowel syndrome. Evidence for a 'colonic brake'. *Gut* 1993; **34**: 1171–1176.

34. Miazza BM, Al-Mukhtar MYT, Salmeron M *et al.* Hyperenteroglucagonaemia and small intestinal mucosal growth after colonic perfusion of glucose in rats. *Gut* 1985; **26**: 518–524.

35. Jordan PH, Stuart JR, Briggs JD. Radical small bowel resection. Report of two cases. *Am J Dig Dis* 1958; **3**: 823–843.

36. Anderson CM. Long-term survival with six inches of small intestine. *Br Med J* 1965; **1**: 419–422.

37. Kinney JM, Goldwyn RM, Barr JS Jr., Moore FD. Loss of the entire jejunum and ileum, and the ascending colon: Management of a patient. *JAMA* 1962; **179**: 529–532.

38. Simons BE, Jordan GL. Massive bowel resection. *Am J Surg* 1969; **118**: 953–959.

39. Pilling GP, Cresson SL. Massive resection of the small intestine in the neonatal period. *Pediatrics* 1957; **19**: 940–948.

40. Grosfeld JL, Rescoria FJ, West KW. Short bowel syndrome in infancy and childhood. Analysis of survival in 60 patients. *Am J Surg* 1986; **151**: 41–46.

41. Grosfeld JL, Rescoria FJ. Current management of short bowel syndrome in children. *J Arkansas Med Soc* 1987; **84**: 243–249.

42. Gouttebel MC, Saint-Aubert B, Astre C, Joyeux H. Total parenteral nutrition needs in different types of short bowel syndrome. *Dig Dis Sci* 1986; **31**: 718–723.

43. Nightingale JMD, Lennard-Jones JE, Walker ER, Farthing MG. Jejunal efflux in short bowel syndrome. *Lancet* 1990; **336**: 765–768.

44. Simko V, Linscheer WG. Absorption of different elemental diets in a short-bowel syndrome lasting 15 years. *Dig Dis* 1976; **21**: 419–425.

45. Rodrigues CA, Lennard-Jones, Thompson DG, Farthing MJG. Energy absorption as a measure of intestinal failure in the short bowel syndrome. *Gut* 1989; **30**: 176–183.

46. MacGregor IL, Wiley ZD, Lavigne ME, Way LW. Total parenteral nutrition slows gastric emptying of solid food. *Gastroenterology* 1978; **74**: 1059.

47. Nylander G. Gastric evacuation and propulsive intestinal motility following resection of the small intestine in the rat. *Acta Chir Scand* 1967; **133**: 131–138.

48. Reynell PC, Spray GH. Small intestinal function in the rat after massive resections. *Gastroenterology* 1956; **31**: 361–368.

49. Dew MJ, Harries AD, Rhodes M, Rhodes J, Leach KG. Gastric emptying after intestinal resection in Crohn's disease. *Br J Surg* 1983; **70**: 92–93.

50. Nightingale JMD, Kamm MA, van der Sijp JRM, Walker ER, Ghatei MA, Bloom SR, Lennard-Jones JE. Gastrointestinal hormones in the short bowel syndrome. PYY may be the 'colonic brake' to gastric emptying. *Gut* 1996; **39**: 267–272.

51. Savage AP, Adrian TE, Carolan G, Chatterjee VK, Bloom SR. Effects of peptide YY (PYY) on mouth to caecum intestinal transit time and on the rate of gastric emptying in healthy volunteers. *Gut* 1987; **28**: 166–170.

52. Neal DE, Williams NS, Barker MJC, King RFGJ. The effect of resection of the distal ileum on gastric emptying, small bowel transit and absorption after procto-colectomy. *Br J Surg* 1984; **71**: 666–670.

53. Booth CC. The metabolic effects of intestinal resection in man. *Postgrad Med J* 1961; **37**: 725–739.

54. Remington M, Malagelada J-R, Zinsmeister A, Fleming CR. Abnormalities in gastrointestinal motor activity in patients with short bowels: Effect of a synthetic opiate. *Gastroenterology* 1983; **85**: 629–636.

55. Schmidt T, Pfeiffer A, Hackelsberger N, Widmer R, Meisel C, Kaess H. Effect of intestinal resection on human small bowel motility. *Gut* 1996; **38**: 859–863.

56. Nightingale JMD. *Physiological consequences of major small intestinal resection in man and their treatment*. MD Thesis, University of London, 1993, pp 190–195.

57. Stassoff B. Experimentelle Untersuchungen uber die Kompensatorischen Vorgange bei Darmresektionen. *Beitr Klin Chir* 1914; **89**: 527–586.

58. Sabsai BI. The effect of extensive resections of the proximal and distal portions of the small intestine on canine gastric secretion. *Bull Exp Biol Med (Moscow)* 1963; **55**: 387–390.

59. Landor JH, Baker WK. Gastric hypersecretion produced by massive small bowel resection in dogs. *J Surg Res* 1964; **4**: 518–522.

60. Westerheide RL, Elliot DW, Hardacre JM. The potential of the upper small bowel in regulating acid secretion. *Surgery* 1965; **58**: 73–81.

61. Frederick PL, Sizer JS, Osbourne MP. Relation of massive bowel resection to gastric secretion. *N Engl J Med* 1965; **272**: 509–514.

62. Reul GJ, Ellison EH. Effect of 75% distal small bowel resection on gastric secretion. *Am J Surg* 1966; **111**: 772–776.

63. Osbourne MP, Frederick PL, Sizer JS, Blair D, Cole P, Thum W. Mechanism of gastric hypersecretion following massive intestinal resection; clinical and experimental observations. *Ann Surg* 1966; **164**: 622–634.

64. Grundberg AB, Lopez AS, Dragstedt LR. Effect of intestinal reversal and massive resection on gastric secretion. *Arch Surg* 1967; **94**: 326–329.

65. Copeland EM, Miller LD, Smith GP. The complex nature of small bowel control of gastric secretion. *Ann Surg* 1968; **168**: 36–46.

66. Kerr G, Elliot DW, Endahl GL. Effect of antrectomy on gastric acid hypersecretion induced by isolation of the proximal small bowel. *Am J Surg* 1968; **115**: 157–164.

67. Santillana M, Wise L, Schuck M, Ballinger WF. Changes in gastric acid secretion following resection or exclusion of different segments of small intestine. *Surgery* 1969; **65**: 777–782.

68. Yakimets WW, Bondar GF. Hormonal stimulatory mechanism producing gastric hypersecretion following massive small intestinal resection. *Can J Surg* 1969; **12**: 241–244.

69. Windsor CWO, Fejfar J, Woodward DAK. Gastric secretion after massive small bowel resection. *Gut* 1969; **10**: 779–786.

70. Burrington JD, Hamilton JR. Steatorrhea after massive bowel resection: effects of surgical reduction of gastric acid secretion. *Surg Forum* 1969; **20**: 341–343.

71. Landor JH. Intestinal resection and gastric secretion in dogs with antrectomy. *Arch Surg* 1969; **98**: 645–646.

72. Wiens E, Bondar GF. Control of gastric hypersecretion following massive intestinal resection. *Surg Forum* 1970; **21**: 310–312.

73. Saik RP, Copeland EM, Miller LD, Smith GP. Effect of ileal exclusion on the Heidenhain pouch acid response to histamine in dogs. *Ann Surg* 1971; **173**: 67–77.

74. Landor JH, Alancia EY, Fulkerson CC. Effect of colectomy on gastric secretion in dogs. *Am J Surg* 1967; **113**: 32–36.

75. Landor JH, Behringer BR, Wild RA. Post enterectomy gastric hypersecretion in dogs: the relative importance of proximal versus distal resection. *J Surg Res* 1971; **11**: 238–242.

76. Fielding JF, Cooke WT. Peptic ulceration in Crohn's disease (regional enteritis). *Gut* 1970; **11**: 998–1000.

77. Fielding JF, Cooke WT, Williams JA. Gastric acid secretion in Crohn's disease in relation to disease activity and bowel resection. *Lancet* 1971; **i**: 1106–1107.

78. Shelton EL, Blaine MH. Massive small bowel resection in postgastrectomy patients. Report of 2 cases. *Texas J Med* 1954; **50**: 96–101.

79. Craig TV, Stewart WRC. Massive bowel resection in a patient with 75% gastrectomy. *Surgery* 1960; **48**: 678–681.

80. Miura S, Shikata J, Hasebe M, Kobayashi K. Long-term outcome of massive small bowel resection. *Am J Gastroenterol* 1991; **86**: 454–459.

81. O'Keefe SJD, Haymond MW, Bennet WM, Oswald B, Nelson DK, Shorter RG. Long-acting somatostatin analogue therapy and protein metabolism in patients with jejunostomies. *Gastroenterology* 1994; **107**: 379–388.

82. Straus E, Gerson CD, Yalow RS. Hypersecretion of gastrin associated with the short bowel syndrome. *Gastroenterology* 1974; **66**: 175–180.

83. Williams NS, Evans P, King RFGJ. Gastric acid secretion and gastrin production in the short bowel syndrome. *Gut* 1985; **26**: 914–919.

84. Temperley JM, Stagg BH, Wyllie JH. Disappearance of gastrin and pentagastrin in the portal circulation. *Gut* 1971; **12**: 372–376.

85. Becker HD, Reeder DD, Thompson JC. Extraction of circulating endogenous gastrin by the small bowel. *Gastroenterology* 1973; **65**: 903–906.

86. Moossa AR, Hall AW, Skinner DB, Winans CS. Effect of 50% small bowel resection on gastric secretory function in Rhesus monkeys. *Surgery* 1976; **80**: 208–213.

87. Buxton B. Small bowel resection and gastric acid hypersecretion. *Gut* 1974; **15**: 229–238.

88. Fitzpatrick WJF, Zentler-Munro PL, Northfield TC. Ileal resection: effect of cimetidine and taurine on intrajejunal bile acid precipitation and lipid solubilisation. *Gut* 1986; **27**: 66–72.

89. Barbezat GO, Hansen JDL. The exocrine pancreas and protein-calorie malnutrition. *Pediatrics* 1968; **42**: 77–92.

90. Kotler DP, Levine GM. Reversible gastric and pancreatic hyposecretion after long-term total parenteral nutrition. *N Engl J Med* 1979; **300**: 241–242.

91. Remington M, Fleming CR, Malagelada J-R. Inhibition of postprandial pancreatic and biliary secretion by loperamide in patients with short bowel syndrome. *Gut* 1982; **23**: 98–101.

92. Socha J, Ryzko J, Bogoniowska Z, Cichy W, Creutzfeldt W. Exocrine and endocrine pancreatic functions in children with the short bowel syndrome. *Materia Medica Polona* 1987; **3**: 169–173.

93. Hofmann AF, Poley JR. Role of bile acid malabsorption in the pathogenesis of diarrhoea and steatorrhoea in patients with ileal resection. I. Response to cholestyramine or replacement of dietary long chain triglyceride by medium chain triglycerides. *Gastroenterology* 1972; **62**: 918–934.

94. Kristensen M, Lenz K, Nielsen OV, Jarnum S. Short bowel syndrome following resection for Crohn's Disease. *Scand J Gastroenterol* 1974; **9**: 559–565.

95. Greenberg GR, Wolman SL, Christofides ND, Bloom SR, Jeejeebhoy KN. Effect of total parenteral nutrition on gut hormone release in humans. *Gastroenterology* 1981; **80**: 988–993.

96. Andrews NJ, Irving MH. Human gut hormone profiles in patients with short bowel syndrome. *Dig Dis Sci* 1992; **37**: 729–732.

97. Lezoche E, Carlei F, Vagni V, Mora GV, Speranza V. Elevated plasma levels of vasoactive intestinal polypeptide in short bowel syndrome. *Am J Surg* 1983; **145**: 369–370.

98. Jeppesen PB, Hartmann B, Hansen BS, Thulesen J, Holst JJ, Mortensen PB. Impaired stimulated glucagon-like peptide 2 response in ileal resected short bowel patients with intestinal failure. *Gut* 1999; **45:** 559–563.

99. Jeppesen PB, Hartmann B, Thulesen J, Hansen BS, Holst JJ, Poulsen SS, Mortensen PB. Elevated plasma glucagon-like peptide 1 and 2 concentrations in ileum-resected short bowel patients with a preserved colon. *Gut* 2000; **47:** 370–376.

100. Adrian TE, Savage AP, Fuessl HS, Wolfe K, Besterman HS, Bloom SR. Release of peptide YY (PYY) after resection of small bowel, colon or pancreas in man. *Surgery* 1987; **101:** 715–719.

101. Editorial. The colon, the rumen, and D-lactic acidosis. *Lancet* 1990; **336:** 599–600.

102. McIntyre PB, Fitchew M, Lennard-Jones JE. Patients with a high jejunostomy do not need a special diet. *Gastroenterology* 1986; **91:** 25–33.

103. Woolf GM, Miller C, Kurian R, Jeejeebhoy KN. Nutritional absorption in short bowel syndrome. Evaluation of fluid, calorie and divalent cation requirements. *Dig Dis Sci* 1987; **32:** 8–15.

104. Whang R, Whang DD, Ryan MP. Refractory potassium repletion. A consequence of magnesium deficiency. *Arch Intern Med* 1992; **152:** 40–45.

105. Woolf GM, Miller C, Kurian R, Jeejeebhoy KN. Diet for patients with a short bowel: High fat or carbohydrate? *Gastroenterology* 1983; **84:** 823–828.

106. Vallee BL, Wacker WEC, Ulmer DD. The magnesium-deficiency tetany syndrome in man. *N Engl J Med* 1960; **262:** 155–161.

107. Hanna S, Harrison M, MacIntyre I, Fraser R. The syndrome of magnesium deficiency in man. *Lancet* 1960; **ii:** 172–176.

108. Fletcher RF, Henly AA, Sammons HG, Squire JR. A case of magnesium deficiency following massive intestinal resection. *Lancet* 1960; **i:** 522–525.

109. Swenson SA, Lewis JW, Sebby KR. Magnesium metabolism in man with special reference to jejunoileal bypass for obesity. *Am J Surg* 1974; **127:** 250–255.

110. Hessov I, Hasselblad C, Fasth S, Hulten L. Magnesium deficiency after ileal resections for Crohn's disease. *Scand J Gastroenterol* 1983; **18:** 643–649.

111. Booth CC, Hanna S, Babouris N, MacIntyre I. Incidence of hypomagnesaemia in intestinal malabsorption. *Br Med J* 1963; **1:** 141–144.

112. Fleming CR, George L, Stoner GL, Tarrosa VB, Moyer TP. The importance of urinary magnesium values in patients with gut failure. *Mayo Clin Proc* 1996; **71:** 21–24.

113. Rude RK, Singer FR. Magnesium deficiency and excess. *Ann Rev Med* 1981; **32:** 245–259.

114. Fawcett SL, Cousins RJ. Magnesium poisoning following enema of epsom salt solution. *JAMA* 1943; **123:** 1028–1029.

115. Kayne LH, Lee DBN. Intestinal magnesium absorption. *Miner Electrolyte Metab* 1993; **19:** 210–217.

116. Hessov I, Andersson H, Isaksson B. Effects of a low-fat diet on mineral absorption in small-bowel disease. *Scand J Gastroenterol* 1983; **18:** 551–554.

117. Hanna S, MacIntyre I. The influence of aldosterone on magnesium metabolism. *Lancet* 1960; **2:** 348–350.

118. Horton R, Biglieri EG. Effect of aldosterone on the metabolism of magnesium. *J Clin Endocrinol Metab* 1962; **22:** 1187–1192.

119. Fatemi S, Ryzen E, Flores J, Endres DB, Rude RK. Effect of experimental human magnesium depletion on parathyroid hormone secretion and 1,25 dihydroxy-vitamin D metabolism. *J Clin Endocrinol Metab* 1991; **73:** 1067–1072.

120. Zofkova I, Kancheva RL. The relationship between magnesium and calciotropic hormones. *Magnes Res* 1995; **8:** 77–84.

121. Solomon R. The relationship between disorders of K^+ and Mg^+ homeostasis. *Semin Nephrol* 1987; **7:** 253–262.

122. Kaufman SS, Loseke CA, Anderson JB, Murray ND, Vanderhoof JA, Young RJ. Magnesium acetate vs magnesium gluconate supplementation in short bowel syndrome. *J Pediatr Gastroenterol* 1993; **16:** 104–105.

123. Schuette SA, Lashner BA, Janghorbani M. Bioavailability of magnesium diglycinate vs magnesium oxide in patients with ileal resection. *J Parenter Enteral Nutr* 1994; **18:** 430–435.

124. Selby PL, Peacock M, Bambach CP. Hypomagnesaemia after small bowel resection: treatment with 1 alpha-hydroxylated vitamin D metabolites. *Br J Surg* 1984; **71:** 334–337.

125. Fukumoto S, Matsumoto T, Tanaka Y, Harada S, Ogata E. Renal magnesium wasting in a patient with short bowel syndrome with magnesium deficiency: effect of 1 α-hydroxyvitamin D_3 treatment. *J Clin Endocrinol Metab* 1987; **65:** 1301–1304.

126. Davis AT, Franz FP, Courtnay DA, Ullrey DE, Scholten DJ, Dean RE. Plasma and mineral status in home parenteral nutrition patients. *J Parenter Enteral Nutr* 1987; **11:** 480–485.

127. Shenkin A, Fell GS, Halls DJ, Dunbar PM, Holbrook IB, Irving MH. Essential trace element provision to patients receiving home intravenous nutrition in the United Kingdom. *Clin Nutr* 1986; **5:** 91–97.

128. Rannem T, Ladefoged K, Hylander E, Hegnhoj J, Jarnum S. Selenium depletion in patients on home parenteral nutrition. The effect of selenium supplementation. *Biol Trace Element Res* 1993; **39:** 81–90.

129. Rannem T, Hylander E, Ladefoged K, Staun M, Tjellesen L, Jarnum S. The metabolism of [^{75}Se] Selenite in patients with short bowel syndrome. *J Parenter Enteral Nutr* 1996; **20:** 412–416.

130. Arthur JR, Beckett GJ. New metabolic roles for selenium. *Proc Nutr Soc* 1994; **53:** 615–624.

131. Press M, Hartop PJ, Prottey C. Correction of essential fatty-acid deficiency in man by cutaneous application of sunflower-seed oil. *Lancet* 1974; **ii:** 597–599.

132. Wolman SL, Anderspon GH, Marliss EB, Jeejeebhoy KN. Zinc in total parenteral nutrition: requirements and metabolic effects. *Gastroenterology* 1979; **76:** 458–467.

133. Mock DM, DeLorimer AA, Liebman WM, Sweetman L, Baker H. Biotin deficiency: an unusual complication of parenteral alimentation. *N Engl J Med* 1981; **304:** 820–823.

134. Khalidi N, Wesley JR, Thoene JG, Whitehouse WM Jr., Baker WL. Biotin deficiency in a patient with short bowel syndrome during home parenteral nutrition. *J Parenter Enteral Nutr* 1984; **8:** 311–314.

135. Matsusue S, Kashihara S, Takeda H, Koizumi S. Biotin deficiency during total parenteral nutrition: its clinical manifestation and plasma nonesterified fatty acid level. *J Parenter Enteral Nutr* 1985; **9:** 760–763.

136. Yamada E, Wakabayashi Y, Saito A, Yoda K, Tanaka Y, Miyazaki M. Hyperammonaemia caused by essential aminoacid supplements in patient with short bowel. *Lancet* 1993; **341:** 1542–1543.

137. Yokoyama K, Ogura Y, Kawabata M *et al.* Hyperammonemia in a patient with short bowel syndrome and chronic renal failure. *Nephron* 1996; **72:** 693–695.

138. Brophy DF, Ford SL, Crouch MA. Warfarin resistance in a patient with short bowel syndrome. *Pharmacotherapy* 1998; **18:** 646–649.

139. Pullan JM. Massive intestinal resection. *Proc R Soc Med* 1959; **52:** 31–37.

140. Crenn P, Belouicf L, Morin MC, Thuillier F, Messing B. Adaptive hyperphagia and net digestive absorption in short bowel patients. *Gastroenterology* 1997; **112:** A356.

141. Cosnes J, Carbonnel F, Beaugerie L, Ollivier J-M, Parc R, Gendre J-P, Le Quintrec Y. Functional adaptation after extensive small bowel resection in humans. *Eur J Gastroenterol Hepatol* 1994; **6:** 197–202.

142. Weinstein LD, Shoemaker CP, Hersh T, Wright HK. Enhanced intestinal absorption after small bowel resection in man. *Arch Surg* 1969; **99:** 560–562.

143. De Francesco A, Malfi G, Delsedime L *et al.* Histological findings regarding jejunal mucosa in short bowel syndrome. *Transplant Proc* 1994; **26:** 1455–1456.

144. Dowling RH, Booth CC. Functional compensation after small bowel resection in man: Demonstration by direct measurement. *Lancet* 1966; **ii:** 146–147.

145. Gouttebel MC, Saint Aubert B, Colette C, Astre C, Monnier LH, Joyeux H. Intestinal adaptation in patients with short bowel syndrome. Measurement by calcium absorption. *Dig Dis Sci* 1989; **34:** 709–715.

146. Hill GL, Mair WSJ, Goligher JC. Impairment of 'ileostomy adaptation' in patients after ileal resection. *Gut* 1974; **15:** 982–987.

147. Heaton KW, Read AE. Gallstones in patients with disorders of the terminal ileum and disturbed bile salt metabolism. *Br Med J* 1969; **3:** 494–496.

148. Lee SP, Nicholls JF, Park HZ. Biliary sludge as a cause of acute pancreatitis. *N Engl J Med* 1992; **326:** 589–593.

149. Doty JE, Pitt HA, Porter-Fink V, Denbesten L. Cholecystokinin prophylaxis of parenteral nutrition-induced gallbladder disease. *Ann Surg* 1985; **201:** 76–80.

150. Thompson JS. The role of prophylactic cholecystectomy in the short bowel syndrome. *Arch Surg* 1996; **131:** 556–560.

151. Jeppesen PB, Hartmann B, Thulesen J *et al.* Treatment of short bowel patients with glucagon like peptide-2 (GLP-2), a newly discovered intestinotrophic, antisecretory, and transit modulating peptide. *Gastroenterology* 2000; **118:** A178–A179.

152. Walker-Smith JA, Phillips AD, Walford N, Gregory H, Fitzgerald JD, MacCullagh K, Wright NA. Intravenous epidermal growth factor/urogastrone increases small-intestinal cell proliferation in congenital microvillous atrophy. *Lancet* 1985; **ii:** 1239–1240.

153. Sullivan PB, Brueton MJ, Tabara ZB, Goodlad RA, Lee CY, Wright NA. Epidermal growth factor in necrotising enteritis. *Lancet* 1991; **338:** 53–54.

154. Rokkas T, Vaja S, Murphy GM, Dowling RH. Aminoguanidine blocks intestinal diamine oxidase (DAO) activity and enhances the intestinal adaptive response to resection in the rat. *Digestion* 1990; **46(suppl 2):** 447–457.

155. Scolapio JS, Camilleri M, Fleming CR *et al.* Effect of growth hormone, glutamine, and diet on adaptation in short-bowel syndrome: a randomized, controlled study. *Gastroenterology* 1997; **113:** 1074–1081.

156. Szkudlarek J, Jeppesen PB, Mortensen PB. Effect of high dose growth hormone with glutamine and no change in diet on intestinal absorption in short bowel patients: a randomised, double blind, crossover, placebo controlled study. *Gut* 2000; **47:** 199–205.

157. Litvak DA, Iseki H, Evers M *et al.* Characterization of two novel proabsorptive peptide YY analogs, BIM-43073D and BIM-43004C. *Dig Dis Sci* 1999; **44:** 643–648.

158. Gruy-Kapral C, Little KH, Fortran JS, Meziere TL, Hagey LR, Hofmann AF. Conjugated bile acid replacement therapy for short-bowel syndrome. *Gastroenterology* 1999; **116:** 15–21.

159. Heydorn S, Jeppesen PB, Mortensen PB. Bile acid replacement therapy with cholylsarcosine for short-bowel syndrome. *Scand J Gastroenterol* 1999; **34:** 818–823.

160. Campbell FC, Tait IS, Flint N, Evans GS. Transplantation of cultured small bowel enterocytes. *Gut* 1993; **34:** 1153–1155.

161. Anderson SHC, Dalton HR. Use of octreotide in the treatment of mesenteric angina. *Am J Gastroenterol* 1997; **92:** 1222–1223.

162. Boley SJ, Sprayregan S, Siegelman SS, Veith FJ. Initial results from an aggressive roentgenological and surgical approach to acute mesenteric ischaemia. *Surgery* 1977; **82:** 848–855.

163. Marston A. Acute intestinal ischaemia. Resection rather than revascularisation. *Br Med J* 1990; **301:** 1174–1176.

164. Clavien PA. Diagnosis and management of mesenteric infarction. *Br J Surg* 1990; **77:** 601–603.

165. Levy PJ, Krausz MM, Manny J. Acute mesenteric ischaemia: improved results – a retrospective analysis of ninety-two patients. *Surgery* 1990; **107:** 372–380.

166. Messing B, Leman M, Landais P *et al.* Prognosis of patients with nonmalignant chronic intestinal failure receiving long-term home parenteral nutrition. *Gastroenterology* 1995; **108:** 1005–1010.

167. Messing B, Crenn P, Beau P, Boutron-Ruault MC, Rambaud JC, Matuchansky C. Long-term survival and parenteral nutrition dependence in adult patients with the short bowel syndrome. *Gastroenterology* 1999; **117:** 1043–1050.

Section 4

Consequences of intestinal failure

13

Undernutrition

Simon P. Allison

Gastrointestinal disease gives rise to under-nutrition by reduction of appetite, failure of digestion and absorption, or increased metabolic demands. The physical and mental consequences of starvation and undernutrition have been known since ancient times. An ancient Egyptian royal tomb of more than 2000 years BC bears the inscription:

I am mourning on my high throne for the vast misfortune, because the Nile flood in my time has not come for seven years! Light is the grain; there is lack of crops and of all kinds of food. Each man has become a thief to his neighbours. They desire to hasten and cannot walk. The child cries, the youth creeps along as does the old man; their souls are bowed down, their legs are bent together and drag along the ground and their hands rest in their bosoms. The counsel of the great ones in the court is but emptiness. Torn open are the chests of provisions, but instead of contents there is air. Everything is exhausted.

During the twentieth century, a number of studies of normal and obese individuals undergoing prolonged starvation,[1,2] of populations under famine conditions,[3] and of patients suffering from disease-related under-nutrition,[4] have given us a clearer picture of the relationship between weight loss or, more particularly, loss of body cell mass and deteriorating mental and physical function. The relationship between structure and function is not always linear[5] with some functions beginning to deteriorate early in the process of starvation, whereas others are relatively unimpaired until later. In some cases there may be a threshold above, which function is largely maintained but below which it falls rapidly.[6] Much depends upon the initial nutritional state of the subject and also on the rate at which tissue is lost.[7] Total starvation may have different effects from partial starvation, and there may also be a process of adaptation to chronically low intakes, as seen among the lean subsistence farmers of Asia. The relative proportions of energy and protein deficiency, the development of single or multiple deficiencies of minerals, trace elements and vitamins, and the presence of disease may all modify the consequences of partial starvation.

This chapter outlines the consequences of disease-related undernutrition consequent upon intestinal failure, with supportive and relevant evidence from other studies of starvation.

SURVIVAL

The most striking example of total starvation in previously healthy young men without disease was provided by the 30 Irish Republican Army (IRA) hunger strikers of Northern Ireland.[7] In 60–70 days, they lost 38% of their body weight and one-third of them had died, allowing us to conclude that, in the absence of disease, previously normally nourished adults may survive weight loss of 35%, or approximately 60 days of total starvation (Fig. 13.1). Beyond this point mortality rises steeply. This time point is considerably reduced if a patient has already lost weight or has underlying sepsis or malignancy. One of the hunger strikers, who was suffering from a gunshot wound, survived for only 45 days, emphasizing the cumulative effect of illness and starvation. Studley in 1936 showed that if patients had lost more than 20% of their body weight prior to surgery for peptic ulcers, they had a 33% mortality compared with 4% if less than 20% body weight had been lost.[8]

Children are even more vulnerable because of the demands of growth and development and, during infancy, because of their high metabolic rate in relation to body size and high surface to volume ratio. The survival of a totally starved neonate may be no more than a few days. Studies among undernourished Asian children by Pelletier *et al.* suggested that their odds of dying from disease and undernutrition increased by a compound rate of more than 7% for each percentage point deterioration in weight for age.[9] There was also an exponentially increasing probability of morbidity as weight fell below 80% of normal for age.

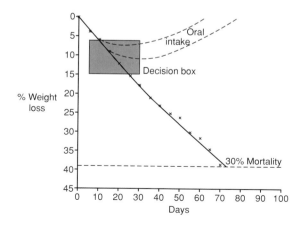

Figure 13.1 – Percentage weight loss and days after starting to starve. The decision box indicates the time when an oral intake will lead to a rapid recovery.

The protective effect of obesity is illustrated by reports of survival by fat adults undergoing periods of starvation of 130–382 days.[2] This protective effect is not only due to greater fuel reserves, but also to the lower daily losses of nitrogen in relation to lean mass, implying a metabolic control mechanism as yet undefined. Whether obesity is similarly protective in the presence of intercurrent illness is unclear.

The extraordinary studies carried out by the Jewish physicians in the Warsaw ghetto in 1942 gives us further insight.[3] Most of the inhabitants had been on 800 kcal a day or less for many months and at the point where they were studied had already lost between 20 and 50% of their pre-war weight and weighed between 30 and 40 kg. One woman, for example, with a height of 1.52 m weighed 24 kg, giving a body mass index (BMI) of 10.3 kg/m². Many were suffering from intercurrent infections and most died within 3 weeks of the studies, although there were clearly some variations in the ability to survive starvation. A review suggests that the lower limit of BMI compatible with survival is approximately 10 kg/m² in women and 12 kg/m² in men.[10] These observations have important implications for clinical work. It is not uncommon to be referred patients for nutritional support who have lost 20–35% of their body weight and in whom not only function but also survival is at stake. It can also be argued that, if parenteral nutrition is required for a total of 60 days or more because of continuing gastro-intestinal dysfunction, such treatment is life-saving in the same sense that dialysis is life-saving in renal failure and ventilation in respiratory failure. The difference between these situations is not one of principle but of time-scale.

CONSEQUENCES OF UNDERNUTRITION

Biochemical

In uncomplicated starvation, hepatic gluceonogenesis maintains blood glucose for use by the brain, blood cells and renal medulla. Muscle, some neural tissue, adrenal cortex and adipose tissue switch from using glucose to using fatty acids and ketones, derived from lipolysis, for energy. Muscle supplies alanine, glycine and lactate for hepatic gluceonogenesis, and glutamine as a source of energy to intestinal and lymphoid tissue. In the presence of sepsis, lipolysis is impaired and so an increase in muscle protein catabolism occurs.

Psychological and neurological

Apathy/depression

The mental changes associated with starvation, noted by the ancient Egyptians, were a striking feature of the studies carried out by the Warsaw physicians.[3] They reported: 'The most striking psychiatric finding is the prevalence of depression, even in young people. There is complete apathy, lack of interest, poor thinking, and even incoherence.'

In his introduction to the *Biology of Human Starvation*,[1] Sir Jack Drummond wrote of the famine in Holland in 1945:

Two impressions dominated: firstly the immense importance of the psychological aspects of inanition; secondly the comparative simplicity of the nutritional and biochemical problem. One of the curious and rather disconcerting psychological manifestations of starvation, seen repeatedly in Western Europe, was the unresponsive and uncooperative attitude of those to whom relief was brought. It disappeared without trace when calorie intakes rose above 1500 to 1800 a day. . . . An outstanding impression gained in Western Holland in 1945 was the importance and significance of the psychological consequences of food shortage. . . . From the grumbling and grousing that are inevitably provoked when the energy intake is deficient to the extent of 15–20%, to the apathy and dissolution of higher human qualities that come with severe starvation, there is a wide variety of psychological reactions to hunger, many of which are almost of themselves diagnostic of the level of calorie intake.

In their study of normal young male volunteers undergoing semi-starvation for 24 weeks, Ancel Keys and his colleagues described not only the diminished physical powers which were associated with a loss of up to 23% of the body weight during that time, but also a rise in a depression score of 30%.[1,11] This was slow to recover during the process of re-feeding. Indeed it took up to 4 months to return to normal. Similar observations have been made in prisoner of war camps, during the Russian famine of 1918–1921 and among undernourished children in the Indian subcontinent and in Africa.

It is important to remember that patients suffering from disease-related undernutrition are often apathetic, depressed and awkward. These difficulties soon dissolve with appropriate nutritional care. The fatigue, which follows illness, may also be prolonged by undernutrition.

Intellectual performance/sleep

Intellectual performance changes little though short-term memory is reduced and sleep-time increased.[1,10,12]

Appetite

Undernutrition causes a reduction in appetite. A vicious circle is thereby created which needs to be broken if normal oral intake is to be resumed. After 1–2 weeks of overnight nasogastric tube feeding, the appetite may be restored so that voluntary oral intake by day is increased.[12] This is sometimes very striking in some cases of inflammatory bowel disease. Once a certain weight has been reached, the appetite appears to be self-perpetuating and nutritional support may be discontinued.

Skeletal muscle function

Protein/energy malnutrition is characterized by muscle wasting with particular loss of the Type II fast-twitch fibres, which are prevalent in the respiratory muscles, including the diaphragm.[14–19] The poor function of skeletal muscle in the chest increases the risk of developing chest infections[20] including tuberculosis[13] and the resulting reduction in mobility increases the risk of deep venous thrombosis, pulmonary emboli and pressure sores.[21–23]

In a study of ten patients with various gastrointestinal disorders, Lopez et al.[14] measured the function of the adductor pollicis muscle by electrical stimulation of the ulnar nerve and found that undernutrition resulted in increased muscle fatiguability and an altered pattern of muscle contraction and relaxation, all of which were reversible by nutritional supplementation. In a study of five morbidly obese female subjects, on a 400 kcal/day carbohydrate diet, Russell et al.[15,16] showed similar changes in muscle function, significant reductions in muscle enzymes and a change in muscle histochemistry with type II fibre atrophy. Comparing the effect of undernutrition with the effects of surgery and sepsis, Brough et al.[17] found abnormal muscle function consequent upon sepsis, but the changes were easily distinguishable from subjects taking an inadequate diet. They found no effect on muscle function following trauma, surgery or steroid administration. They also showed that, following the initiation of parenteral nutritional support, there was a rapid initial improvement in muscle function within days, which occurred before any change in anthropometric variables or plasma proteins. Hill found similar changes in undernourished patients with inflammatory bowel disease.[4,6] Measuring whole body protein by neutron activation techniques, he showed that a 20% reduction in total body protein, reflecting lean mass, was associated with little change in respiratory muscle strength, but beyond this there was a steep deterioration.

Over the first 5 days of nutritional support, both grip strength and peak expiratory flow rate rose from a mean of 65 to 75% of normal.[4,6] This was followed by a much more gradual and sustained improvement over the ensuing weeks as body composition was restored. This again illustrates the two-phase response to refeeding. The first is associated with a rapid improvement in cellular function and the second with the much more gradual process of the restoration of body cell mass. Muscle function may also be seriously impaired with single or multiple electrolyte mineral or micronutrient deficiencies, conditions that are not uncommon in patients with gastrointestinal disease. Hypokalaemia may be responsible for muscle weakness or even paralysis; selenium deficiency causes impairment of both myocardial and skeletal muscle function. Deficiencies of magnesium and of calcium decrease peristalsis but increase skeletal neuromuscular excitability and may cause fits.

Respiratory

Undernutrition impairs respiratory function, chiefly through its effect on respiratory muscles, impairing ventilation and the ability to cough and clear secretions.[24–30] It also reduces respiratory response to hypoxia[31] and the ability to wean from ventilators.[32] In contrast, nutritional support improves ventilatory function and has facilitated weaning from ventilators. Respiratory complications of surgery, trauma or acute illness are one of the major consequences of undernutrition. The terminal event in progressive starvation is nearly always bronchopneumonia.

One corollary of weak respiratory muscles is the inability to cope with the additional respiratory demands imposed by excessive caloric feeding, particularly of carbohydrate. Such patients may be rendered breathless by carbohydrate loads in excess of 5 mg/kg/min or total energy intakes in excess of 40 kcal/kg/day, owing to increased oxygen consumption and CO_2 production.[33,34]

Cardiovascular and sympathetic nervous system

The Warsaw studies of advanced starvation[3] showed that this was associated with lower systolic and

Table 13.1 – Consequences of undernutrition

System with reduced function	Consequence
Psychological/neurological	Apathy/depression
	Increased sleep time
	Reduced recent memory
	Loss of appetite
Muscle	
Skeletal	Chest infections
	Pressure sores
	DVT/pulmonary emboli
Cardiac	Bradycardia/low BP
	Cardiac failure
	Long QT interval
Gastrointestinal	Reduced gastric acid and pancreatic enzymes
	Mucosal atrophy
	Reduced gut associated lymphoid tissue
	Reduced colonic sodium and water absorption
	Diarrhoea
	Sepsis/multi-organ failure
Endocrine (low sex hormones)	Poor growth
	Delayed puberty
	Amenorrhoea
	Infertility
	Reduced bone density
Thermoregulation	Hypothermia
Repair mechanisms	Slow wound healing
	Pressure sores
Immune	Reduced lymphocyte count
	Infections
Fluid and electrolytes	Oedema

diastolic blood pressures at rest and in response to exercise. Bennett *et al.* showed that starvation, with sodium supplementation, for 48 hours in healthy men was associated with a small drop in supine blood pressure, but after 10 minutes standing, there was a fall in systolic blood pressure of 15 mmHg with no change in the non-starved controls.[35] There is a reduction in heart rate, blood pressure[13] and cardiac muscle mass; although this reduction in cardiac muscle is considerably less than that of skeletal muscle,[25] it could predispose to cardiac failure.[36,37] A prolonged QT interval may lead to ventricular arrhythmias.[38]

As sympathetic nervous system function is a major determinant of metabolic rate and as its function is reduced in undernourished patients, it is not surprising to find a markedly reduced resting metabolic expenditure in these patients. This must be borne in mind when estimating the nutritional requirements of depleted patients.

Gastrointestinal

The effects of undernutrition upon the gastrointestinal tract are complex and depend upon its severity. The Warsaw studies[3] demonstrated, in patients with more than 30% weight loss, an impairment of gastric acid secretion. Lack of luminal nutrition during parenteral nutrition, in studies on normal subjects or associated with undernutrition, may result in villous atrophy, impaired small bowel mucosal function and increased intestinal permeability.[39–42] Gut mucosal atrophy may be responsible for bacterial translocation which may gives rise to an endotoxaemia, which in turn may contribute to multi-organ failure.[43] The colon can be affected, losing its ability to reabsorb water and electrolytes, so diarrhoea may result.[44,45] There may be altered intestinal flora with migration of bacteria proximally into the small bowel, thereby exacerbating malabsorption.[46]

These changes may be seen during parenteral feeding when there is a lack of oral/enteral intake, or in segments of bowel that have been by-passed. The introduction of food, by the oral or enteral route, reverses these changes and accelerates adaptation of a retained ileum in patients with a short bowel. Particular substrates may be important. Fibre, giving rise to short-chain fatty acids, may enhance both small and large bowel mucosal growth and function. Glutamine is an essential fuel for the mucosal epithelium and may enhance the protective effect of the gut-associated lymphatic tissue.

Pancreatic function has been studied in undernourished infants and in adults, and been shown to be impaired. Winter and colleagues[47–49] studied a series of patients with a mean BMI of 13.6 kg/m² before treatment and 16.5 kg/m² after nutritional support. They found that before treatment, pancreatic protein synthesis and enzyme production was reduced, so that 70% of gastric and pancreatic secretion was lost with consequent impairment of xylose and fat absorption. All parameters were restored towards normal by refeeding. They confirmed findings of impaired gastric acid secretion, as well as pancreatic amylase and trypsin secretion.

Endocrine and bone

Anorexia nervosa with a BMI below 17 kg/m² is characterized by amenorrhoea with subdued hypothalamic function and secondary effects upon the pituitary and the ovaries or testes. Exactly the same changes are seen in patients who are cachectic as a result of gastrointestinal disease. Low sex hormone levels reduce muscle mass, strength and energy, as well as reducing bone density. We have observed a young patient with Crohn's disease to have a bone density three standard deviations below the mean for his age and a low serum testosterone. These were both restored to normal within 2 years, once his chronic state of undernutrition had been adequately treated. Protein/energy malnutrition may also affect bone structure; osteoporosis is characteristically more prevalent in the undernourished. Malabsorption of fat-soluble vitamins may result in vitamin D deficiency and osteomalacia.

Growth and development

Undernutrition in childhood leads to reduced growth velocity which may be restored by nutritional intervention. However, prolonged undernutrition permanently impairs achievement of genetic potential for height, which cannot be recovered even with optimal nutrition.[50,51] Puberty is also delayed since the pituitary gonadal axis fails to function normally and it is a common experience to find impaired growth and development among adolescents with severe gastrointestinal disease and malabsorption.

Thermoregulation

The Warsaw physicians observed lower than normal body temperatures in their patients, as well as failure to develop a fever in response to typhoid or tuberculosis.[3] Similar changes may be seen among the undernourished and the elderly in routine hospital practice. Bastow et al.[52] observed low core temperatures in winter (< 36°C) among elderly women admitted with fractured femur, whose anthropometric indices were more than two standard deviations below the reference range. In contrast, the normally nourished fractured femur patients had core temperatures in excess of 36°C on admission. When undernourished individuals were put in a cooling suit, Fellows et al.[53] found normal vasoconstriction but no increase in thermogenesis in response to the challenge. Mansell et al.[54] showed, in younger subjects, that the thermogenic response to cooling was restored when body composition was returned to normal by nutritional support. They also showed[55] that the vasoconstrictor response to cooling was impaired in normal subjects who fasted for 48 hours. Both short-term starvation and weight loss, therefore, impair thermoregulation but by different mechanisms.

Thus undernourished patients are prone to hypothermia and the recognition of sepsis/fever may be difficult as their temperature tends to be low.

Wound healing

The metabolic response to injury in which energy and substrates are mobilized from within the body to meet the demands of illness and injury must have a survival value to have evolved at all. The paradox is that, when taken to extremes, it may threaten survival. One of the crucial features of the response is the mobilization of nitrogen from muscle to meet metabolic requirements. This feature was blunted in traumatized rats that had previously been exposed to a low protein diet.[56]

There is an impairment of wound healing.[57–63] Windsor et al.[57] showed in man that a low preoperative food intake impaired wound healing. Haydock and Hill[58] also documented impaired wound healing in undernourished surgical patients and further observed that this can occur with quite modest degrees of undernutrition. Pressure sores are also more likely to develop in undernourished patients and are slower to heal.[59] Nutritional support may contribute to more rapid healing. An adequate supply of minerals and micronutrients is necessary for wound healing, including vitamins A, B, C, D, E and K.[60] Zinc is a cofactor for collagen formation,[60] and zinc deficiency has been associated with failed wound healing which is restored to normal by zinc supplementation.[61,62]

Immunological

In undernutrition, many aspects of immune function, particularly of cell-mediated immunity, are impaired and increased susceptibility to infection is well documented in adults,[3,64–67] children[68,69] and the elderly.[70] Conversely, one of the consistent features of positive trials of nutritional support is a reduction in post-operative and other infections.[68–74] Much of the tissue involved in immune responses lies in the gastro-intestinal tract and the gut-associated lymphatic tissue. The provision of luminal nutrients and special sub-strates such as glutamine may have their beneficial effects partly through providing essential nutrients to this tissue. It is important, however, not to over-simplify the situation, since the relationship between nutritional status and immune competence is a complex one and may vary according to the clinical condition and the nutritional deficiencies involved. As well as protein-energy undernutrition, mineral and micronutrient deficiencies may also impair immunity. Good et al.,[67] for example, found zinc to be an important factor for the maintenance of cell-mediated immunity.

Fluid and electrolytes

Famine and refeeding oedema have been described by a number of authors, including the Physicians of the Warsaw ghetto.[3] Keys et al., studying normal subjects undergoing semi-starvation, showed that, although the fat and lean compartments of the body tissues shrink, the extra-cellular fluid volume remains either at its pre-starvation level or decreases very slowly.[1] Relatively, therefore, the extra-cellular fluid volume occupies an increasing proportion of the body composition as starvation progresses. The degree of oedema may be related to access to salt and is exacerbated by refeeding.

Depleted subjects, therefore, are particularly susceptible to fluid overloading when nutritional support is given in an excessive volume of fluid or with excessive sodium. This inability to excrete an excess sodium and water load is also exacerbated by illness and surgery.[75] It is not uncommon to find depleted postoperative patients with a 10–15 litre fluid overload, gross oedema and dilutional hypoalbuminaemia. Starker et al. showed that many depleted patients given preoperative nutritional support retained fluid.[76] In contrast to those able to maintain normal fluid balance and serum albumin, these patients had more postoperative complications. Similar observations were made by Gil et al. in patients undergoing gastrectomy for malignant disease.[77] In studies on rabbits, this group also demonstrated the effect of nutritional depletion on fluid retention[78] and confirmed the observations of Gamble[79] that carbohydrate administration led to more salt and water retention than when a predominantly fat-based feed was used. Oedema and hypoalbuminaemia may produce secondary effects upon gastrointestinal function, delaying gastric emptying,[80] and possibly impairing bowel function.

In the tropics, childhood protein-energy mal-nutrition has been classified into marasmus in which the child looks very cachectic, and Kwashiorkor in which there is predominantly protein deficiency, hypo-albuminaemia and oedema. Although analogies have been drawn between these and depleted and sick hospital patients, and they have much in common, there are also important differences and I prefer not to use these terms out of context. In patients with intestinal failure the picture may be further modified by losses from diarrhoea, vomiting or fistulae which may cause excessive losses, not only of salt and water, but of potassium, magnesium and selenium with consequent clinical effects. The serum albumin concentration has been much vaunted as a nutritional marker, however, it changes little in pure starvation.[1] It is a good marker of the severity of disease, and moves inversely as the acute phase reactants rise.[81] It is reduced by excessive losses from wounds or the gastrointestinal tract or by dilution from salt and water overload. While undernutrition may not, of itself, cause the serum albumin concentration to fall, it may prevent it recovering to normal following illness. Conversely, nutritional support may accelerate recovery to normal levels.[82]

Careful monitoring of fluid, electrolytes and mineral balance and consideration of the patient's requirements and tolerances are an important part of the nutritional management of patients with intestinal failure.

REFEEDING

Functional improvements in cell function occurs long before any gain in tissue mass. Muscle function may improve rapidly (15% over the first 5 days) with refeeding, but the restoration of muscle mass, unlike that of adipose tissue, is very slow.[1,7]

Sudden death can occur rarely during the early phase of refeeding, sometimes this is due to a rapid cellular uptake of phosphate and a consequent hypophosphataemia[83,84] (Chapter 31). In children death during refeeding has been predicted by a high leucocyte sodium efflux.[85]

SUMMARY

Undernutrition progressively impairs the function of all systems throughout the body, impairing growth, development and quality of life, ultimately leading to death when weight loss is extreme. It also increases susceptibility to disease, increases the complications of illness and of surgery, and delays recovery. These problems result in undernourished patients in hospital requiring high-dependency nursing, having an increased hospital stay with an increased morbidity and mortality compared with patients of normal weight having similar underlying clinical problems.[86–90] Careful restoration of as near normal a nutritional state as possible should be an important part of clinical management, particularly of the patient with intestinal failure.

REFERENCES

1. Keys A, Brozek J, Henschel A, Michelsen O, Taylor HL. *The Biology of Human Starvation*. University of Minnesota Press: Minneapolis, MN, 1950.

2. Elia M. Effect of starvation and very low calorie diets on protein-energy interrelationships in lean and obese subjects. In: Scrimshaw NS, Schürch B (eds) *Protein-energy Interactions*. Nestlé Foundation, PO Box 581, Lausanne, Switzerland, 1992.

3. Winick M (ed) *Hunger Disease: Studies by the Jewish Physicians in the Warsaw Ghetto*. Wiley: New York, 1979.

4. Hill GL. *Disorders of Nutrition and Metabolism in Clinical Surgery*. Churchill Livingstone: Edinburgh, 1993.

5. Kinney JM. The influence of calorie and nitrogen balance on weight loss. *Br J Clin Prac* 1988; **42** (Suppl 63): 114–120.

6. Hill GL. Body composition research: Implications for the practice of clinical nutrition. *J Parenter Enteral Nutr* 1992; **16**: 197–218.

7. Allison SP. The uses and limitations of nutritional support. *Clin Nutr* 1992; **11**: 319–330.

8. Studley HO. Percentage of weight loss. A basic indicator of surgical risk in patients with chronic peptic ulcer. *JAMA* 1936; **106**: 458–460.

9. Pelletier DL, Frongillo EA, Habicht JP. Epidemiological evidences for a potentiating effect of malnutrition on childhood mortality. *Am J Public Health* 1993; **83**: 1130–1133.

10. Henry CJK. Body mass index and the limits of human survival. *Eur J Clin Nutr* 1990; **44**: 329–335.

11. Brozek J. Effects of generalised malnutrition on personality. *Nutrition* 1990; **6**: 389–395.

12. Leyton GB. Effects of slow starvation. *Lancet* 1946; **xx**: 73–79.

13. Bastow MD, Rawlings J, Allison SP. Overnight nasogastric tube feeding. *Clin Nutr* 1985; **4**: 7–11.

14. Lopez J, Russell DM, Whitwell J, Jeejeebhoy KN. Skeletal muscle function in malnutrition. *Am J Clin Nutr* 1982; **36**: 602–610.

15. Russell DM, Leiter LA, Whitwell J, Marliss EB, Jeejeebhoy KN. Skeletal muscle function during hypocaloric dieting and fasting: a comparison with standard nutritional assessment parameters. *Am J Clin Nutr* 1983; **37**: 133–138.

16. Russell DM, Walker PM, Leiter LA, *et al.* Metabolic and structural changes in muscle during hypocaloric dieting. *Am J Clin Nutr* 1984; **39**: 503–513.

17. Brough W, Horne G, Blount A, Irving MH, Jeejeebhoy KN. Effects of nutrient intake, surgery, sepsis, and long term administration of steroids on muscle function. *Br Med J* 1986; **293**: 983–988.

18. Russell DM, Pendergast PJ, Darby PL, Garfinkel PE, Whitwell J, Jeejeebhoy KN. A comparison between muscle function and body composition in anorexia nervosa: the effect of refeeding. *Am J Clin Nutr* 1983; **38**: 229–237.

19. Pichard C, Jeejeebhoy KN. Muscle dysfunction in malnourished patients. *Q J Med* 1988; **260**: 1021–1045.

20. Windsor JA, Hill GL. Risk factors for post-operative pneumonia: the importance of protein depletion. *Ann Surg* 1988; **208**: 209–214.

21. Allman RM, Laprade CA, Noel LB, Walker JM, Moorer CA, Dear MR, Smith CR. Pressure sores among hospitalized patients. *Ann Intern Med* 1986; **105**: 337–342.

22. Pinchcofsky-Devin GD, Kaminski MV. Correlation of pressure sores and nutritional status. *J Am Geriatr Soc* 1986; **34**: 435–440.

23. Holmes R, MacChiano K, Jhangiani SS, Agarwal NR, Savino JA. Combating pressure sores – nutritionally. *Am J Nurs* 1987; **xx**: 1301–1303.

24. Arora NS, Rochester DF. Respiratory muscle strength and maximal voluntary ventilation in undernourished patients. *Am Rev Respir Dis* 1982; **126**: 5–8.

25. Arora NS, Rochester DF. Effect of body weight and muscularity on human diaphragm muscle mass, thickness and area. *J Appl Physiol: Resp Envir Exerc Physiol* 1982; **52**: 64–70.

26. Kelsen SG, Ference M, Kapoor S. Effects of prolonged undernutrition on structure and function of the diaphragm. *J Appl Physiol* 1985; **58**: 1354–1359.

27. Lewis MI, Sieck GC, Fournier M, Belman MJ. Effect of nutritional deprivation on diaphragm contractility and muscle fibre size. *J Appl Physiol* 1986; **60**: 596–603.

28. Lewis MI, Sieck GC. Effect of acute nutritional deprivation on diaphragm structure and function. *J Appl Physiol* 1990; **68**: 1938–1944.

29. Kelly SM, Rosa A, Field S, Coughlin M, Shizgal HM, Macklem PT. Inspiratory muscle strength and body composition in patients receiving total parenteral nutrition therapy. *Am Rev Respir Dis* 1984; **130**: 33–37.

30. Murciano D, Armengaud MH, Rigaud D, Pariente R, Aubier M. Effect of renutrition on respiratory and diaphragmatic function in patients with severe mental anorexia. *Am Rev Resp Dis* 1990; **141**: A547.

31. Doekel RC Jr, Zwillich CW, Scroggin CH. Clinical semi-starvation: depression of hypoxic ventilatory response. *N Engl J Med* 1976; **295**: 358–361.

32. Bassili HR, Deitel M. Effect of nutritional support on weaning patients off mechanical ventilation. *J Parenter Enteral Nutr* 1981; **5**: 161–163.

33. Askanazi J, Carpentier YA, Elwyn DH, *et al.* Influence of total parenteral nutrition on fuel utilisation in injury and sepsis. *Ann Surg* 1980; **191**: 40–46.

34. Burke JF, Wolfe RR, Mullany CJ, Mathews DE, Bier SM. Glucose requirements following burn injury. Parameters of optimal glucose infusion and possible hepatic and respiratory abnormalities following excessive glucose intake. *Ann Surg* 1979; **190**: 274–285.

35. Bennett T, MacDonald IA, Sainsbury R. The influence of acute starvation on the cardiovascular responses to lower body sub-atmospheric pressure or to standing in man. *Clin Sci* 1984; **66**: 141–146.

36. Heymsfield SB, Bethel RA, Ansley JD, Gibbs DM, Felner JM, Nutter DO. Cardiac abnormalities in cachectic patients before and during nutritional repletion. *Am Heart J* 1978; **95**: 584–594.

37. Gottdiener JS, Gross HA, Henry WL, Borer JS, Ebert MH. Effects of self-induced starvation on cardiac size

38. Isner JM, Sours HE, Paris AL, Ferrans VJ, Roberts WC. Sudden, unexpected death in avid dieters using the liquid-protein-modified-fast diet. Observations in 17 patients and the role of the prolonged QT interval. *Circulation* 1979; **60**: 1401–1412.

39. Elia M, Goren A, Behrens R, Barber RW, Neale G. Effect of total starvation and very low calorie diets on intestinal permeability in man. *Clin Sci* 1987; **73**: 205–210.

40. Jackson WD, Grand RJ. The human intestinal response to enteral nutrients: a review. *J Am Coll Nutr* 1991; **10**: 500–509.

41. Buchman AL, Moukarzel AA, Bhuta S, *et al.* Parenteral nutrition is associated with intestinal morphologic and functional changes in humans. *J Parenter Enteral Nutr* 1995; **19**: 453–460.

42. Groos S, Hunefeld G, Luciano L. Parenteral versus enteral nutrition; morphological changes in adult human intestinal mucosa. *J Submicrosc Cytol Pathol* 1996; **28**: 61–74.

43. Deitch E A, Winterton J, Li M, Berg R. The gut as a portal of entry for bacteremia: role of protein malnutrition. *Ann Surg* 1987; **205**: 681–690.

44. Roediger WEW. Famine, fibre, fatty acids and failed colonic absorption: does fibre fermentation ameliorate diarrhoea? *J Parenter Enteral Nutr* 1994; **18**: 4–8.

45. Roediger W E W. Metabolic basis of starvation diarrhoea: implications for treatment. *Lancet* 1986; **I**: 1082–1084.

46. Berg RD. Translocation of indigenous bacteria from the intestinal tract. In: Hentges DJ (ed) *Human Intestinal Microflora in Health and Disease.* Academic Press: New York, 1983.

47. Winter TA, Ogden JM, Lemmer E, Bridger SA, Tigler-Wybrandi NA, Young GO, O'Keefe SJD. Assessment of entero-pancreatic function in normal and malnourished subjects during enteral feed stimulation. *S African Med J* 1994; **84**: 440.

48. Winter TA, De Coito P, O'Keefe SJD, Bridger S, Marks T. Entero-pancreatic function in patients with severe malnutrition due to anorexia. *Gut* 1997; **41** (Suppl 3): A14.

49. Winter TA, Ogden JM, De Coito P, O'Keefe SJD, Marks T. The vicious circle of malnutrition, maldigestion and malabsorption: Response to refeeding. *S African Med J* 1997; **87**: 1245.

50. Widdowson EM. Intra-uterine growth retardation in the pig. 1. Organ size and cellular development at birth and after growth to maturity. *Biol Neonate* 1971; **19**: 329–340.

51. Moy RJD, Smallman S, Booth IW. Malnutrition in a UK children's hospital. *J Hum Nutr Dietet* 1990; **3**: 93–100.

52. Bastow MD, Rawlings J, Allison SP. Undernutrition, hypothermia and injury in elderly women with fractured femur: an injury response to altered metabolism? *Lancet* 1983; **1**: 143–146.

53. Fellows IW, Macdonald IA, Bennett T, Allison SP. The effect of undernutrition on thermoregulation in the elderly. *Clin Sci* 1985; **69**: 525–532.

54. Mansell PI, Fellows IW, Macdonald IA, Allison SP. Defect in thermoregulation in malnutrition reversed by weight gain. Physiological mechanisms and clinical importance. *Q J Med* 1990; **280**: 817–829.

55. Macdonald IA, Bennett T, Sainsbury R. The effect of a 24-hour fast on the thermoregulatory responses to graded cooling in man. *Clin Sci* 1984; **67**: 445–452.

56. Munro HN. In: Munro HN, Allison JB (eds) *Mammalian Protein Metabolism*. Academic Press: New York, 1964.

57. Windsor JA, Knight GS, Hill GL. Wound healing response in surgical patients: recent food intake is more important than nutritional status. *Br J Surg* 1988; **75**: 135–137.

58. Haydock DA, Hill GL. Impaired wound healing in surgical patients with varying degrees of malnutrition. *J Parenter Enteral Nut* 1986; **10**: 550–554.

59. Ek AC, Unosson M, Larsson J, von Schenck H, Bjurulf P. The development and healing of pressure sores related to the nutritional state. *Clin Nutr* 1991; **10**: 245–250.

60. Goodson WH, Hunt TK. Wound healing. In: Kinney JM, Jeejeebhoy KN, Hill GL, Owen OE (eds) *Nutrition and Metabolism in Patient Care*. WB Saunders: Philadelphia, 1988, pp. 635–642.

61. Sandstead HH, Henriksen LK, Greger JL, Prasad AS, Good RA. Zinc nutriture in the elderly in relation to taste activity, immune response and wound healing. *Am J Clin Nutr* 1982; **36**: 1046–1059.

62. Pories WJ, Henzel JH, Rob CG, Strain WH. Acceleration of wound healing in man with zinc sulphate given by mouth. *Lancet* 1967; **1**: 121–124.

63. Shukla VK, Roy SK, Kumar J, Vaidya MP. Correlation of immune and nutritional status with wound complications in patients undergoing abdominal surgery. *Am Surg* 1985; **51**: 442–445.

64. Chandra RK. Immunodeficiency in undernutrition and overnutrition. *Nutr Rev* 1981; **39**: 225–231.

65. Dominioni L, Dionigi R. Immunological function and nutritional assessment. *J Parenter Enteral Nutr* 1987; **11** (suppl): 70S–72S.

66. Brookes GB, Clifford P. Nutritional status and general immune competence in patients with head and neck cancer. *J R Soc Med* 1981; **74**: 132–139.

67. Good RA, Lorenz E. Nutrition and cellular immunity. *Int J Immunopharmacol* 1992; **14**: 361–366.

68. Abbassy AS, el-Din MK, Hassan AI, *et al.* Studies of cell mediated immunity and allergy in protein-energy malnutrition. I: Cell-mediated delayed hypersensitivity. *J Trop Med Hyg* 1974; **77**: 13–17.

69. Abbassy AS, el-Din MK, Hassan AI, Aref GH, Hammad SA, el-Araby II, el-Din AA. Studies of cell mediated immunity and allergy in protein-energy malnutrition: II Immediate hypersensitivity. *J Trop Med Hyg* 1974; **77**: 18–21.

70. Lesourd B. Protein undernutrition as the major cause of decreased immune function in the elderly: clinical and functional implications. *Nutr Rev* 1995; **53**: S86–94.

71. Collins JP, Oxby CB, Hill GL. Intravenous amino acids and intravenous hyperalimentation as protein sparing therapy after major surgery. *Lancet* 1978; **1**: 788–791.

72. Kudsk KA, Minard G, Croce MA, *et al.* A randomized trial of isonitrogenous enteral diets after severe trauma. An immune-enhancing diet reduces septic complications. *Ann Surg* 1996; **224**: 531–543.

73. Beier-Holgersen R, Boesby S. Influence of postoperative enteral nutrition on postsurgical infections. *Gut* 1996; **39**: 833–835.

74. Von Meyenfeldt MF, Meijerink WJHJ, Rouflart MMJ, Buil-Maassen MTHJ, Soeters PB. Perioperative nutritional support: a randomised clinical trial. *Clin Nutr* 1992; **11**: 180–186.

75. Wilkinson AW, Billing BH, Nagy G, Stewart CP. Excretion of chloride and sodium after surgical operations. *Lancet* 1949; **i**: 640–644.

76. Starker PM, LaSala PA, Forse RA, Askanazi J, Elwyn PH, Kinney JM. Response to total parenteral nutrition in the extremely malnourished patient. *J Parenter Enteral Nutr* 1985; **9**: 300–302.

77. Gil MR, Franch G, Guirao X, *et al.* Response to severely malnourished patients to preoperative parenteral nutrition: a randomized clinical trial of water and sodium restriction. *Nutrition* 1997; **13**: 26–31.

78. Sitges-Serra A, Arcas G, Guirao X, Garcia-Dominho M, Gil MJ. Extracellular fluid expansion during parenteral refeeding. *Clin Nutr* 1992; **11**: 63–68.

79. Gamble GL. Physiological information gained from studies on the life raft ration. *Harvey Lectures* 1946–1947; **42**: 247–263.

80. Mecray PM, Barden RP, Ravdin IS. Nutritional edema: its effect on the gastric emptying time before and after gastric operations. *Surgery* 1937; **1**: 53–64.

81. Fleck A. Plasma proteins as nutritional indicators in the peri-operative period. In: Allison SP and Kinney JM (eds) Perioperative Nutrition. *Br J Clin Pract* 1988; **42** (Suppl 63): 20–24.

82. Bastow MD, Rawlings J, Allison SP. Benefits of supplementary tube feeding after fractured neck of femur: a randomised controlled trial. *Br Med J* 1983; **287**: 1589–1592.

83. Weinsier RL, Krumdieck CL. Death resulting from overzealous total parenteral nutrition: the refeeding syndrome revisited. *Am J Clin Nutr* 1981; **34**: 393–399.

84. Solomon SM, Kirby DF. The refeeding syndrome: a review. *J Parent Enteral Nutr* 1990; **14**: 90–97.

85. Patrick J. Death during recovery from severe malnutrition and its possible relationship to sodium pump activity in the leucocyte. *Br Med J* 1977; **1**: 1051–1054.

86. Weinsier RL, Hunker EM, Krumdieck CL, Butterworth CE Jr. A prospective evaluation of general medical patients during the course of hospitalization. *Am J Clin Nutr* 1979; **32**: 418–426.

87. Walesby RK, Goode AW, Spinks TJ, Herring A, Ranicar ASO, Bentall HH. Nutritional status of patients requiring cardiac surgery. *J Thorac Cardiovasc Surg* 1979; **77**: 570–576.

88. Warnold I, Lundholm K. Clinical significance of preoperative nutritional status in 215 noncancer patients. *Ann Surg* 1984; **199**: 299–305.

89. Windsor JA, Hill GL. Weight loss with physiologic impairment: a basic indicator of surgical risk. *Ann Surg* 1988; **207**: 290–296.

90. Sullivan DH, Patch GA, Walls RC, Lipschitz DA. Impact of nutrition status on morbidity and mortality in a select population of geriatric rehabilitation patients. *Am J Clin Nutr* 1990; **51**: 749–758.

14

Gallstones

Michael F. Byrne and Frank E. Murray

Gallstone disease is a major public health issue. Gallstones are present in over 10% of adults in the Western world[1] and are of two main types: cholesterol stones, comprising about 75% of stones, and pigment stones. Cholesterol gallstones are composed of cholesterol, mucin, bile pigments, calcium salts and other compounds, whereas pigment stones are made up of calcium salts including bilirubinates. Mixed stones are intermediate in character.

PATHOGENESIS OF GALLSTONE DISEASE

Three major factors are critically involved in the pathogenesis of cholesterol gallstones, namely, cholesterol supersaturation of bile;[2] accelerated crystallization of cholesterol in bile involving nucleating agents;[3] reduced gallbladder contractility and resultant prolonged bile stasis.[4] All these factors may lead to the formation of biliary sludge.

Cholesterol secretion into bile and supersaturation

In essence, cholesterol gallstones develop from microscopic crystals of cholesterol, which precipitate from bile supersaturated with cholesterol. The process of crystallization may involve a number of nucleating agents. Microscopic crystals thus formed may then grow into macroscopic stones.[5]

Hepatocytes secrete phospholipid molecules as vesicles that bud from their cell membranes. Cholesterol is also secreted into the bile canalicular lumina and subsequently taken up by biliary lipid vesicles with a cholesterol:phospholipid ratio of 0.34:0.38 but the ratio is higher in lithogenic bile.[6,7] Cholesterol, lecithin (the most abundant biliary phospholipid) and bile salts aggregate to produce mixed micelles and vesicles in bile, in which the hydrophilic portions of these lipids are located peripherally with the hydrophobic portions orientated centrally in a hydrophobic domain, thus permitting lipid solubility in an aqueous environment.[8]

Cholesterol solubility in bile has been defined using a triangular coordinate map comprising the three main biliary lipids, namely cholesterol, bile salts and phospholipids.[9] Maximal cholesterol solubility in bile is a function of the relative concentrations of these three biliary lipids. Cholesterol saturation (maximum cholesterol saturation) is defined as the cholesterol/lecithin and bile salt molar ratio.[10] A saturation boundary limit separates unsaturated from supersaturated solutions. At points above this boundary, cholesterol crystals may form by precipitation of cholesterol out of solution.

Thus, cholesterol solubility in bile is very much a function of the relative concentrations of phospholipids, bile salts and cholesterol. Bile supersaturated with cholesterol may be a result of increased cholesterol secretion or decreased phospholipid or bile salt secretion. Cholesterol-rich vesicles play an important part in the formation of cholesterol crystals.[11]

Nucleation and crystallization

During crystallization, nucleation occurs first followed by crystal growth. It is difficult to discriminate bile from patients with cholesterol gallstones from that of controls on the basis of cholesterol saturation. Indeed, most subjects with supersaturated bile do not appear to develop gallstones. Nucleating factors are importantly involved in gallstone formation.

Bile contains both anti-nucleating and pro-nucleating factors, the balance of which is important in determining the likelihood of gallstone formation. Apolipoprotein A–1 and A–2, and a glycoprotein (120 kDa), all found in human bile, have been identified as anti-nucleating factors.[12] Pro-nucleating factors include both mucin glycoproteins[13] and non-mucin glycoproteins.[14] Mucin is thought to play a significant role in crystallization of cholesterol. The evidence for this comes from three main sources. First, mucin glycoproteins have been found in the matrix of cholesterol gallstones.[15] Second, mucin hypersecretion precedes crystallization of cholesterol in animal models[16] and probably humans.[17] Third, mucin has been shown to promote crystal nucleation in cholesterol supersaturated bile *in vitro*. Mucin may act as a nidus for crystal aggregation by entrapping cholesterol crystals or calcium bilirubin on non-glycosylated hydrophobic domains of the peptide chain of the mucin glycoprotein molecule.[18]

In addition to mucin, several other non-mucin pro-nucleating factors have been identified *in vitro* such as amino peptidase N, a low-density lipoprotein particle, and haptoglobins. However, their relative roles in bile and gallstone formation remain unclear.

Crystal growth in bile follows nucleation. Cholesterol monohydrate crystals are composed of bilayers of cholesterol bonded to a water layer. Rapid growth occurs as these crystals pack side-by-side in their long axis, resulting in plate-like monohydrate crystals. Cholesterol also precipitates in other forms such as helical, tubular and filamentous forms of non-hydrated cholesterol.[19]

Gallbladder contractility

As well as cholesterol supersaturation and mucin hypersecretion, reduced gallbladder contractility appears crucially important in cholelithiasis by allowing the cholesterol crystals entrapped in mucin to grow to a sufficient size to allow them to remain in the gallbladder. Early cholesterol crystals are likely to develop into macroscopic stones only if formed in the mucus layer adherent to the epithelium in gallbladders with reduced contractility.

It would appear that all three requirements − cholesterol supersaturation, increased nucleation rate mediated by mucin hypersecretion, and reduced gallbladder contractility − occurring simultaneously allow cholelithiasis to occur. This is referred to as the triple defect of gallstone formation.

Pigment stones have been shown to be largely composed of calcium bilirubinate and other calcium salts. Less is known about the process of pigment stone formation than about cholesterol gallstones, but biliary stasis appears to play a dominant role. Unconjugated bilirubin concentration is higher in gallbladder bile in certain patients with pigment gallstones than in controls and it may be that unconjugated bilirubin forms gallstones by precipitation from bile in a similar fashion to that of cholesterol.[20]

Biliary sludge

Biliary sludge may be an important intermediate factor in the formation of different types of gallstones.[18] Sludge was initially identified by ultrasonography as low amplitude echoes without acoustic shadowing which layered in the most dependent portion of the gallbladder[21] (Fig. 14.1).

Biliary sludge is an amorphous precipitant of mucin glycoproteins, bile pigments, protein and lipids. An ever-present constituent of biliary sludge in humans is calcium bilirubinate or unconjugated bilirubin. Cholesterol monohydrate crystals are also commonly found in sludge.[18] Lee and Nicholls found that there was a marked increase in the amount of mucus in biliary sludge. Mucin is an important constituent of

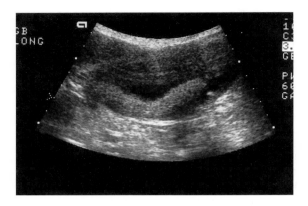

Figure 14.1 − Ultrasound image of the gallbladder in longitudinal section showing layering of sludge without acoustic shadowing (courtesy of Professor M. J. Lee, Radiology Department, Beaumont Hospital, Dublin 9).

mucus. They also noted that the cholesterol and phospholipid concentration in bile from sludge-forming patients was no different to that of normal controls and gallstone patients.

Several possible factors leading to biliary sludge formation are cited in the literature including biliary stasis, use of total parenteral nutrition, mucin hypersecretion, bile infection and acute illness. A definite association between development of biliary sludge and gallbladder stasis has been noted especially in patients receiving total parenteral nutrition (TPN) with no oral intake. Patients receiving TPN frequently develop sludge and may go on to develop gallstones.[22]

The exact mechanism of sludge formation has not yet been elucidated but one theory is that decreased gallbladder contractility leads to bile becoming progressively more concentrated and the cholesterol vesicular carriers becoming enriched in cholesterol content and depleted of lecithin and other phospholipids. Crystals of cholesterol are thus formed, and calcium salts (especially bilirubinate) precipitate secondary to stasis as well. Thus, sludge may form. Prolonged stasis and further growth may lead to the development of gallstones themselves.[23] Biliary sludge may disappear spontaneously or have a fluctuating course but it frequently evolves into gallstones.[24] It would appear from present data that sludge may persist or recur in at least 50% of cases and that gallstones may form in up to 14% of affected subjects over 3 years.[25]

EPIDEMIOLOGY OF GALLSTONES IN INTESTINAL FAILURE

In general, patients with intestinal failure of various aetiologies are at increased risk of developing gall-stones. Gallstones are more prevalent in patients with acute intestinal failure, and in chronic illnesses such as Crohn's disease, after intestinal resections and with the long-term use of total parenteral nutrition (TPN). Increased rates of cholelithiasis and cholecystitis have been shown also following trauma, burns, truncal vagotomy and pregnancy.

Inflammatory bowel disease

Several studies (involving cholecystography and ultra-sonography) have demonstrated an increased prevalence of gallstone formation (average prevalence 30%) in patients with Crohn's ileitis or ileo-colitis.[26,27] This is 4–5 times the expected prevalence of gallstones in the general population.[28] These stones often appear calcified on a plain abdominal radiograph.[26]

The distribution of Crohn's disease may be an important determining factor for gallstone formation. Some evidence suggests that gallstones appear to be more common in patients with ileitis than in those with ileo-colitis or colitis.[29] The likelihood of gallstone development may also be directly related to the extent of ileal resection.[30] Patients with loss of functioning distal ileum due to disease or surgical excision have a disruption to the normal enterohepatic circulation of bile salts. In one review of several studies, the frequency of gallstones in patients with an ileal resection greater than 50 cm in length was 33%, compared to 17% in those who underwent a lesser resection.[30] However, some series suggest that the likelihood of gallstone formation is not related to the site of disease or resection but have suggested that duration of disease and previous surgery were positive risk factors.[31] Thus it is not clear which is more important in the aetiology of gallstones, either ileal dysfunction or reduction in postoperative gallbladder contractility.

There are less data available regarding gallstone formation in ulcerative colitis. Patients with ulcerative colitis (without operation) have on average a 7.5% prevalence of gallstones, essentially the same as controls.[31] One large series showed that patients who had undergone an ileostomy after panprocto-colectomy (during which usually up to 10 cm of terminal ileum is resected) had no significant increased risk of developing gallstones compared to patients with Crohn's disease who had undergone a lesser (less than 10 cm) terminal ileal resection.[27] This may relate to the intact remaining terminal ileum in patients with ulcerative colitis.

Earlier data regarding patients with Crohn's disease and those receiving TPN did not describe the type of gallstones formed after ileal resection or with ileal disease. There is conflict in that some series suggest a predilection for formation of cholesterol gallstones, postulating a supersaturation of bile with cholesterol crystals,[32] whereas more recent studies demonstrate that the majority of patients (children and adults) who undergo ileal resection and require long-term TPN develop pigment gallstones.[33] Similar findings were noted in animal studies.[34] This lends support to the hypothesis that alteration of bilirubin metabolism rather than cholesterol metabolism in ileal resection patients may result in the formation of pigment gallstones.

The high incidence of gallstones in patients who have undergone ileal resection has been demonstrated mainly in patients in whom the colon has been preserved and the jejunum is in continuity with the colon. In some patients with Crohn's disease, the colon is also removed during surgery resulting often in a high jejunostomy or ileostomy. Comparison of patients with a high jejunostomy and those with colonic preservation after small bowel resection showed no significant difference in the high prevalence of gallstones between the two groups.[35] Thus, although preservation of the colon may reduce the need for parenteral nutrition, the incidence of gallstones is similar in both groups.

Total parenteral nutrition

TPN is a life-saving measure.[36] Septic and metabolic problems are less frequent but hepatobiliary compli-cations still occur. Data from studies of gallbladder disease in patients on TPN have contributed much to the understanding of the possible aetiology of gallstone disease in intestinal failure. Considerable evidence suggests that use of TPN increases the risk of biliary sludge formation and thus cholelithiasis.

Patients on long-term parenteral nutrition undergo long periods of limited enteral intake. As a result, they may experience long periods when food-stimulated intestinal hormone secretion is not activated.

Anecdotal reports in the 1970s suggested that TPN might be associated with an increased incidence of both acalculous cholecystitis and cholelithiasis.[37] There were also descriptions of massively dilated gallbladders in patients on TPN.[38]

Several studies since have validated the association between TPN and gallstone formation. In one study of patients receiving TPN for a minimum of 3 months, 23% developed gallbladder disease after commencement of TPN.[39] Patients with ileal disorders (Crohn's or ileal resection) were studied separately because of the known increase in cholelithiasis in these groups. There was a 40% incidence of gallbladder disease in this group receiving TPN, which is significantly greater than that in Crohn's disease or ileal resection patients not receiving TPN. The same researchers also found that the risk of development of gallstones whilst on TPN was greater in patients under 30 years of age and in patients whose ileal resection had been performed less than 15 years previously. Research on a population of children on TPN showed that 43% of children on long-term TPN (mean duration 20 months) developed gallstones.[40]

Biliary sludge in TPN and Crohn's disease

As previously mentioned, sludge formation may well be an important stage in gallstone development. Biliary sludge was shown to be associated with TPN. Messing *et al.* reported a progressive increase in the incidence of biliary sludge from 6% after 3 weeks of TPN to 50% between 4 and 6 weeks, and reaching 100% in patients receiving intravenous nutritional therapy for more than 6 weeks.[22] Gallstone formation was noted in six of 14 patients who developed sludge, while none of the patients without sludge developed gallstones. Five of seven patients who earlier had sludge or gallstones were found to be free of both after a short period of oral refeeding.

The findings suggest that stasis of bile and bowel rest during use of TPN increases the risk of sludge development and subsequent gallstone formation. The content of sludge in this group of patients was found to be very similar to that in previous studies; namely that it consisted of pigment granules, calcium bilirubinate, thick bile, cholesterol crystals and small stones.

There are considerably less data available on the prevalence of sludge in Crohn's disease itself without the concomitant use of TPN but reduced gallbladder

contractility has been demonstrated in patients with Crohn's disease especially in those who have undergone ileal resection,[41] and this reduction in contractility predisposes to sludge formation.

Sludge also commonly develops in patients on intensive care units. In one study, biliary sludge was found to develop frequently and rapidly in intensive care patients. Some of the patients who developed sludge had a previously recognized risk factor such as abdominal surgery or TPN but neurosurgical procedures were also associated with formation of sludge. Thus, the range of patients who develop sludge in an intensive care setting is wider than previously described.[42]

PATHOGENESIS OF GALLSTONES IN INTESTINAL FAILURE

Ileal resection

Disturbance of the enterohepatic circulation of bile salts is accepted as playing an important role in gallstone formation in Crohn's disease, but it is clear now that lithogenic bile alone does not cause cholelithiasis and that other factors contribute significantly to gallstone formation, including increased nucleation rate and gallbladder stasis.

Earlier research suggested that the cholesterol saturation index was increased in patients with Crohn's disease.[43] Since cholesterol solubility in bile is related to bile salt and phospholipid concentration, depletion of the bile salt content of bile subsequent to terminal ileal disease may lead to a decrease in the solubility of cholesterol in bile and predispose to cholesterol crystal formation and thus to gallstone formation.

Animal studies in the 1970s supported this 'lithogenic bile' model. For example, it was found that following major interruption of the bile salt enterohepatic circulation in Rhesus monkeys, either by mechanical means or by ileal resection, secreted bile became supersaturated with cholesterol.[44] A relative increase in cholesterol concentration or a decrease in the concentration of phospholipids or bile salts, or both, could result in an increased saturation with cholesterol.

Another group found that resection of the distal 30% of the small intestine in dogs resulted in an increased cholesterol:phospholipid (C:P) ratio compared to controls.[45] The increased cholelithiasis noted in these animals was attributed to the formation of lithogenic bile due either to this increased C:P ratio or an increase in the ratio of glycine to taurine-conjugated bile salts.

However, more recent data suggest that ileal resection results in alteration of bilirubin rather than cholesterol metabolism resulting in pigment gallstone formation (see Table 14.1). Ileal resection in the prairie dog led to the development of pigment gallstones in 44% of animals compared to none in the control group.[46] Calcium bilirubinate crystals were found in up to 94% of animals who underwent ileal resection and in none of the control groups. It was noted that calcium and total bilirubin concentrations in bile were significantly greater in ileal-resected animals. The previously described increase in cholesterol saturation of bile in Rhesus monkeys after ileal resection was confirmed in later studies but the bile was not supersaturated with cholesterol and was stable with respect to cholesterol solubility.

Data from patients with ileal resection receiving TPN have shown that there is a predisposition to development of pigment gallstones. Analysis of stones from adults and children who have had significant ileal resection necessitating long-term parenteral nutrition shows that pigment rather than cholesterol stones form in the majority of these patients.[33]

More recent research in humans has shown that there is a two- to tenfold increase in bilirubin levels (unconjugated and conjugated) in gallbladder bile in patients with Crohn's disease or ileal resection compared to other patient groups (ulcerative colitis and gallstone patients).[47] This is thought to be due to an increase in the enterohepatic cycling of bilirubin secondary to enhanced uptake of bilirubin in the colon. This may explain the increased risk of pigment gallstone formation in Crohn's disease and after ileal resection.

Impaired fatty-meal-stimulated gallbladder contractility in patients with Crohn's disease has been demonstrated.[41] The impairment of contractility was found to be most marked in patients with both small and large bowel involvement, and in those with a history of prior resection.

There are several proposed mechanisms for reduced gallbladder contractility in Crohn's patients. Reduction in intestinal release of cholecystokinin or other peptides due to proximal small bowel disease may be a factor. The number of argentaffin cells in colonic mucosa in patients with ulcerative colitis is reduced.[48] Reduction in levels of peptide YY concentration in the colonic mucosa of patients with ulcerative colitis and Crohn's disease has also been demonstrated.[49] Thus, changes in peptide secretion by small and large bowel may occur in Crohn's disease and may influence gallbladder contractility. However, other investigators have found no reduction in cholecystokinin levels or other peptides in Crohn's disease, so this mechanism remains debatable.

In contrast to the increased prevalence of gallstones in women compared to men in the general population, female sex does not seem to be a risk factor for gallstones in Crohn's disease.[30] In fact, some data suggest a higher prevalence of gallstones in men

Table 14.1 – Gallstones in Crohn's disease: disturbance of cholesterol or bilirubin metabolism?

Researchers	Year	Subjects	Main findings
Dowling RH, Bell GD, White J[43]	1972	Patients with Crohn's disease	Increased cholesterol saturation index
Dowling RH, Mack E, Small DM[44]	1971	Rhesus monkeys Ileal resection	Cholesterol supersaturation Lithogenic bile model
Kelly TR, Klein RL, Woodford JW[45]	1972	Prairie dogs Ileal resection	Increased cholesterol/phospholipid ratio
Pitt HA, Lewinski MA, Muller EL, Porter-Fink V, Den Besten L[46]	1984	Prairie dogs Ileal resection	Pigment gallstones Increased bilirubin concentration in bile
Brink MA, Slors FM, Keulemans YCA, *et al*[47]	1998	Patients with Crohn's disease or ileal resection	Increased bilirubin levels in bile, probably secondary to enhanced colonic uptake of bilirubin

receiving TPN compared to women.[50] Men with a short bowel with or without a retained colon have a much higher prevalence of gallstones than women.[35]

In summary, the increase in gallstone prevalence in Crohn's disease may well be multi-factorial in origin. Altered bilirubin or cholesterol metabolism, impaired gallbladder contractility and increased nucleation rate appear to be the major factors involved. The nucleation time in the disease group may be abnormally shortened due to the presence of an as yet unidentified nucleation-promoting factor. Increased mucin glycoprotein secretion is a possibility.[13] Of note, some researchers have found normal or even low cholesterol saturation of bile after resection of ileum.[51] Other factors such as use of TPN in Crohn's disease and the prolonged fasting involved will be described later.

Total parenteral nutrition

Prolonged periods of fasting may promote gallbladder stasis. During fasting, there are reduced hormonal and neural stimuli to the biliary tract. Coupled with decreased gallbladder contractility, this leads to stasis of stagnant bile within the gallbladder, promoting lithiasis. The incidence of gallstone formation is also strongly linked to the duration of TPN.

Bile flow is impaired in patients on TPN.[52] Evidence to date suggests that bile is not supersaturated consequent to TPN,[53] but that prolonged stasis may be the key pathogenetic mechanism for increased cholelithiasis. The evidence for the dominant role of stasis in this scenario comes from several sources. Gallbladder contractility measured by ultrasound is reduced in patients receiving parenteral feeding.[54] The cholesterol saturation index in bile in prairie dogs receiving TPN is not increased but gallbladder stasis is noted.[55]

Improved radiological imaging has lent itself to the investigation of gallbladder disease. Radionuclide imaging of the gallbladder revealed biliary tract abnormalities in 92% of patients who received TPN.[56] Ultrasonographic measurements of gallbladder motility during use of TPN showed that, while maximal gallbladder volume was similar in TPN patients and controls, gallbladder emptying was significantly reduced in parenterally fed patients during both continuous and cyclic infusion.[54]

The mechanism underlying impaired gallbladder contractility in patients receiving TPN is unclear. In one animal model using cholesterol-fed ground

squirrels, agents which by-passed receptors and their subsequent interactions with calcium channels in the sarcolemma can restore gallbladder contractility in gallstone disease. This suggested that bile saturated with cholesterol causes excessive integration of cholesterol into the sarcolemma, thus changing its functional characteristics. The primary smooth muscle defect in this animal model would appear to involve the sarcolemmal membrane, rather than the intracellular signal transduction pathways or contractile apparatus.[57]

The finding of biliary sludge and potential for gallstone formation during TPN has also been documented during fasting after surgery. Ultrasound studies have provided evidence of the relationship between prolonged periods of fasting and gallbladder sludge formation in patients who have undergone gastrointestinal surgery.[58]

Is gallbladder stasis alone sufficient to cause gallbladder disease in patients receiving TPN?

In untreated coeliac disease, massive gallbladder enlargement associated with sluggish contractility may be seen. Reduced gallbladder contractility in response to a fatty meal has been noted in coeliac disease. This defect appears to correlate well with decreased cholecystokinin secretion. Furthermore, gallbladder emptying improves after successful treatment with a gluten-free diet. However, no increase in the prevalence of cholelithiasis has been found in patients with coeliac disease despite documented impaired gallbladder contractility.[59] Thus, factors other than gallbladder stasis appear to be important in the development of gallstones but the lack of enteric stimulation of bile flow and impaired gallbladder contractility secondary to absence of significant oral intake may be the primary factors in biliary sludge and gallstone development during TPN use.

Drug treatments

Use of narcotics[60] and anti-cholinergics[61] in patients receiving TPN has led to an increase in gallbladder disease. Narcotics, by reducing bile flow through the sphincter of Oddi, encourage gallbladder stasis, and anti-cholinergics have been shown to antagonize the protective effect of sphincterotomy on gallstone formation – both lending strong support to the idea of gallbladder stasis playing an important role in gallstone formation.

Octreotide, a long-acting somatostatin analogue used in the treatment of a high output jejunostomy, may itself increase the risk of cholelithiasis.[62] This is due to a reduction in gallbladder contractility, decreased post-prandial contractility and the development of altered bile.[63] The bile composition, due to slowed intestinal transit, may favour the formation by intestinal bacteria of secondary bile acids (e.g. deoxycholic acid) which are more lithogenic than the primary bile acids.[64]

Abdominal surgery

Many factors appear to influence development of gallstones in patients with inflammatory bowel disease who undergo surgery including gender, episodes of fasting, TPN and the type of surgery involved. Particular operations such as ileal resection which interfere with the enterohepatic bile salt cycle are more likely to lead to gallstone formation, but major abdominal surgery itself (not involving the biliary system) also appears to accelerate gallstone development in some patients. Indeed, in one retrospective study of gallstone formation after major abdominal surgery, surgery and age were the only statistically significant independent predictors of gallstone development during follow-up.[65]

The possible mechanisms responsible for gallstone formation in patients who have undergone major abdominal surgery outside the biliary tract have been briefly discussed earlier in this chapter. Lee *et al.* found that sludge preceded gallstone formation in six of 14 sludge-forming patients receiving TPN.[25] Gallbladder stasis and bowel rest were felt to be important factors in sludge development. Patients on intensive care units (who undergo periods of fasting) are predisposed to sludge development.

Harrison *et al.* found that patients who underwent valve replacement surgery for rheumatic heart disease had a gallstone prevalence of 39% compared to 12% in a matched control population.[66] No difference in the degree of haemolysis between the two groups was detected, undermining the suggestion that excess haemolysis might be the cause of increased cholelithiasis in the surgical group.

Thus, major surgery per se may well predispose to gallstone formation, probably via sludge formation during fasting. Particular operations, such as ileal resection for inflammatory bowel disease, also

interfere with the enterohepatic circulation and have additional potential to formation of gallstones. This finding has important practical and financial implications, and identification of patients at risk for development of gallstones postoperatively might allow use of prophylactic measures (see later) such as earlier enteral feeding or administration of cholecystokinin.

Weight loss

Other data concerning gallstone formation in intestinal failure come from studies of individuals who experience weight loss by dieting or surgery. Obese individuals have a two to three times increased prevalence of gallstones, usually cholesterol gallstones.[67] It has been shown that up to 40% of morbidly obese patients who present for surgical treatment of obesity have gallstones.[68] There is also a substantive body of evidence demonstrating an increase in gallstone formation in patients who undergo weight reduction surgery or dieting with rapid weight loss.[69] This suggests that the significant weight loss in patients with inflammatory bowel disease or intestinal failure of other aetiology might be an important factor in their propensity to develop gallstones. In one study, 38% of patients who underwent gastric by-pass surgery developed gallstones, and a further 12% developed gallbladder sludge.[70] Gallstones formed during the time of maximal weight loss, although there was no direct correlation between the amount of weight loss and the incidence of gallstone formation noted.

The proposed factors involved in gallstone formation during weight loss include impaired gallbladder motility and modifications in biliary nucleation. Twenty-one obese patients were placed on a low-calorie, low-fat diet for weight reduction purposes.[71] A significant increase in the gallbladder volume after 10 days ingestion of the above diet was noted, and was attributed to poor gallbladder contractility secondary to minimal stimulation of cholecystokinin (CCK) secretion or to excess secretion of gallbladder wall relaxants such as pancreatic polypeptide or somatostatin.[72,73]

Thus, dieting programmes seem to predispose to gallstone formation, probably via increased gallbladder stasis, and this is perhaps of relevance to cholelithiasis in patients with inflammatory bowel disease who also experience significant weight loss.

There is an increased biliary cholesterol secretion and a higher cholesterol saturation index in obese patients. During weight loss, the cholesterol saturation index has been found to increase further.[70] This may also be a factor in the increased cholelithiasis noted during episodes of rapid weight loss, but gallbladder stasis would appear to play an important role.

PREVENTION OF BILIARY SLUDGE AND GALLSTONES

Cholecystokinin

Several investigators have described the critical role of stasis of the gallbladder in the pathogenesis of stone formation. In animal models, daily injections of CCK,[74] or sphincterotomy,[75] prevent gallstone formation. In another study, 4 weeks of oral refeeding led to elimination of TPN-induced biliary sludge after stopping the TPN infusion.[76]

Data from human studies suggest that use of CCK in patients receiving TPN stimulates gallbladder emptying and prevents stasis and subsequent sludge formation.[77] There is a body of evidence to support the prophylactic use of CCK in patients receiving TPN, especially those with ileal resection in whom the incidence of gallstone formation is already known to be increased. The use of periodic pulsed infusions of amino acids or small amounts of enteral feed, by stimulating endogenous cholecystokinin release, causes gallbladder contraction and prevents gallbladder stasis.[78-80]

Prophylactic cholecystectomy?

As several risk factors have been identified for cholelithiasis in patients with a short bowel, namely ileal resection (especially if fewer than 120 cm of intestinal remnant is left), resection of the ileo–colonic junction, long-term TPN and the presence of Crohn's disease itself, a role for prophylactic cholecystectomy in patients with a short bowel has been suggested.[81] In patients with short bowel syndrome, it has been shown that cholelithiasis is usually symptomatic, often complicated by inflammation or bile duct stones, and is associated with significant morbidity and mortality rates postoperatively. On the whole, it is felt that the role of prophylactic cholecystectomy should be determined by the underlying disease and should be considered only in patients with short bowel syndrome when the risk for development of gallstones is over 40% and long-term survival is anticipated.

Aspirin and non-steroidal anti-inflammatory drugs

Studies involving the cholesterol-fed prairie dog showed that use of high-dose aspirin prevented gallstone recurrence after successful dissolution therapy. A decrease in mucin glycoprotein involved in nucleation was found and, as aspirin is an inhibitor of prostaglandin formation, it was suggested that secretion of mucin might be prostaglandin-mediated.[82] However, more recent research in the same model showed that, at therapeutic doses, non-steroidal anti-inflammatory drugs (NSAIDs) had minimal effect on production of mucin by the gallbladder.[83]

NSAIDs may prevent gallstone formation by another mechanism, namely by a prokinetic effect on the gallbladder. In a human study, subjects with gallstone disease given therapeutic doses of indomethacin were found to have increased post-prandial gallbladder emptying.[84] This effect was not seen in healthy control subjects. The concentration of various eicosanoids in the gallbladder wall changes with bile cholesterol supersaturation and chronic inflammation and it may be that inhibitors of prostaglandin formation such as NSAIDs promote production of prokinetic leukotrienes or prostaglandins in diseased but not in healthy gallbladders. Further research on the use of aspirin and other NSAIDs in the prophylaxis or treatment of gallstones in intestinal failure is warranted.

Ursodeoxycholic acid

Ursodeoxycholic acid (UDCA) may also have a role to play in treatment or prophylaxis of gallstone disease in patients with intestinal failure. Use of UDCA causes bile to become richer in glycine or taurine conjugates of UDCA. A marked reduction in cholesterol crystallization was noted with use of UDCA. More recent research has shown that use of UDCA also leads to a reduction in the concentration of several crystallization-promoting factors (for example, aminopeptidase N, haptoglobin and some immunoglobulins).[85,86] Certainly, manipulation of the balance of pro-nucleating and anti-nucleating factors is a potential important avenue for future research.

Cisapride/metronidazole

Slow intestinal transit results in more primary bile acids being converted by bacteria to the more lithogenic secondary bile acids. Cisapride increases gastrointestinal transit rate (reversing any changes of octreotide treatment) and changes bile composition.[64] Thus it could be useful in preventing gallstones in patients with intestinal failure due to small bowel dysfunction.

Metronidazole, by suppressing anaerobic intestinal organisms, reduced the rise in liver enzymes associated with parenteral nutrition in Crohn's disease.[87] This may be another simple way of reducing the chance of developing gallstones.

SUMMARY

The classical triple defect theory of gallstone formation involves cholesterol supersaturation of bile, increased cholesterol crystal nucleation and reduced gallbladder contractility. These factors along with alterations in bilirubin metabolism appear to be responsible for the increased prevalence of gallstone disease in intestinal failure. Formation of biliary sludge seems to be an important intermediate in gallstone formation.

In Crohn's disease, a four- to fivefold increased prevalence of gallstone formation compared to the general population has been found. Use of TPN is also an independent risk factor in gallstone formation. Regarding Crohn's patients, earlier research suggested that cholesterol supersaturation was a dominant factor in gallstone formation, whereas more recent work has found significant increases in bilirubin levels in gallbladder bile, probably secondary to increased colonic uptake of bilirubin. Gallbladder hypocontractility and increased nucleation, possibly via mucin hypersecretion, also appear to play roles but the relative importance of each of the suggested pathogenetic mechanisms is not yet clear.

During use of TPN, impaired bile flow and prolonged gallbladder stasis have been shown. Other factors possibly play a role, but reduction in gallbladder contractility and bowel rest would appear to be dominant in gallstone formation with TPN usage.

Surgery per se leads to an increased risk of gallstone formation, as may significant weight loss, whether due to surgery or dieting. Again, gallbladder stasis has been found to be very important in these two scenarios. An increase in the cholesterol saturation index may also be important during weight loss.

In the overall picture of gallstone formation in intestinal failure (Fig. 14.2), it is difficult to determine the relative roles of the various mechanisms involved. There is a lot of overlap – for example, a patient with

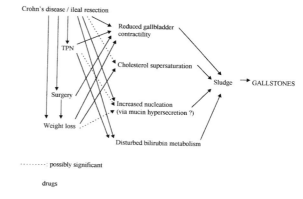

Figure 14.2 – Pathogenesis of gallstones in intestinal failure.

Crohn's disease experiences weight loss and often undergoes surgery, both of which per se increase risk of gallstone formation. However, gallbladder stasis, disturbed cholesterol, or more likely bilirubin metabolism, and changes in nucleation are all important to varying degrees.

The roles of cholecystokinin and prophylactic cholecystectomy in patients with a short bowel have yet to be agreed. Similarly, further research on the use of aspirin and UDCA in prophylaxis or treatment of gallstones is needed.

REFERENCES

1. Barbara L, Sama C, Morselli Labate AM, *et al.* A population study of the prevalence of gallstones: the Sirmione study. *Hepatology* 1987; **7**: 913–917.

2. Carey MC, Small DM. The physical chemistry of cholesterol solubility in bile: relationship to gallstone formation and dissolution in man. *J Clin Invest* 1978; **61**: 998–1026.

3. Holan KR, Holzbach RT, Herrmann RF, Cooperman AM, Claffey WJ. Nucleation time: a key factor in the pathogenesis of cholesterol gallstone disease. *Gastroenterology* 1979; **77**: 611–617.

4. Fisher R, Steltzer F, Rock E, Malmud L. Abnormal gallbladder emptying in patients with gallstones. *Dig Dis Sci* 1982; **27**: 1019–1024.

5. Portincasa P, van Erpecum KJ, vanBerge-Henegouwen G P. Cholesterol crystallisation in bile. *Gut* 1997; **41**: 138–141.

6. Crawford JM, Möckel GM, Crawford AR, Hagen SJ, Hatch VC, Barnes S, Godleski JJ, Carey MC. Imaging biliary lipid secretion in the rat: ultrastructural evidence for vesiculation of the hepatocyte canalicular membrane. *J Lipid Res* 1995; **36**: 2147–2163.

7. La Mont JT, Carey MC. Cholesterol gallstone formation. 2. Pathobiology and pathomechanics. *Prog Liver Dis* 1992; **10**: 165–191.

8. Igimi H, Carey MC. Cholesterol gallstone dissolution in bile: dissolution kinetics of crystalline cholesterol, with chenodeoxycholate, ursodeoxycholate and their glycine and taurine conjugates. *J Lipid Res* 1981; **22**: 254–263.

9. Admirand WH, Small DM. The physico-chemical basis of cholesterol gallstone formation in man. *J Clin Invest* 1968; **47**: 1043–1052.

10. Isaakson B. On the dissolving power of lecithin and bile salts for cholesterol in human gallbladder bile. *Acta Soc Med Ups* 1954; **59**: 296–304.

11. Harvey PRC, Sömjen GJ, Gilat T, Gallinger S, Strasberg SM. Vesicular cholesterol in bile. Relationship to protein concentration and nucleation time. *Biochim Biophys Acta* 1988; **958**: 10–18.

12. Kibe A, Holzbach RT. Inhibition of cholesterol crystal formation by apolipoproteins in supersaturated model bile. *Science* 1984; **255**: 514–516.

13. Lee SP, La Mont JT, Carey MC. The role of gallbladder mucus hypersecretion in the evolution of cholesterol gallstones: studies in the prairie dog. *J Clin Invest* 1981; **67**: 1712–1723.

14. Burnstein MJ, Ilson RG, Peturnka CN, Strasburg S. Evidence for a potent nucleating factor in the gallbladder of patients with gallstones. *Gastroenterology* 1983; **85**: 801–807.

15. Maki T, Matsukiro T, Susuki N, Nakamutra N. The role of sulphated glycoprotein in gallstone formation. *Surg Gyn Obs* 1974; **132**: 497–502.

16. Pemsingh RS, MacPherson BR, Scott GW. Mucus hypersecretion in the gallbladder epithelium of ground squirrels fed a lithogenic diet for the induction of cholesterol gallstones. *Hepatology* 1987; **7**: 1267–1271.

17. Shiffman ML, Shamburek RD, Schwartz CC, Sugerman HJ, Kellum JM, Moore EW. Gallbladder mucin, arachidonic acid, and bile lipids in patients who develop gallstones during weight reduction. *Gastroenterology* 1993; **105**: 1200–1208.

18. Lee SP, Nicholls JF. Nature and composition of biliary sludge. *Gastroenterology* 1986; **90**: 677–686.

19. Konikoff FM, Chung DS, Donovan JM, Small DM, Carey MC. Filamentous, helical and tubular microstructures during cholesterol crystallisation from bile. Evidence that biliary cholesterol does not nucleate classic monohydrate plates. *J Clin Invest* 1992; **90**: 1156–1161.

20. Soloway RD, Trotman BW, Ostrow JD. Pigment gallstones. *Gastroenterology* 1977; **72**: 167–182.

21. Filly B, Allen B, Minton MJ, Bernhoft B, Way LW. In vitro investigation of the origin of echoes within biliary sludge. *J Clin Ultrasound* 1980; **8**: 193–200.

22. Messing B, Bories C, Kunstlinger F, Bernier J. Does total parenteral nutrition induce gallbladder sludge formation and lithiasis? *Gastroenterology* 1983; **84**: 1012–1019.

23. Lee SP. Pathogenesis of biliary sludge. *Hepatology* 1990; **12**: 200–205.

24. Carey MC, Cahalane MJ. Whither biliary sludge? *Gastroenterology* 1988; **95**: 508–523.

25. Lee SP, Maher K, Nicholls JF. Origin and fate of biliary sludge. *Gastroenterology* 1988; **94**: 170–176.

26. Heaton KW, Read AE. Gallstones in patients with disorders of the terminal ileum and disturbed bile salt metabolism. *Br Med J* 1969; **3**: 494–496.

27. Hill GL, Mair WSJ, Goligher JC. Gallstones after ileostomy and ileal resection. *Gut* 1975; **16**: 932–936.

28. Torvik A, Hoivik B. Gallstones in an autopsy series. *Acta Chir Scand* 1960; **120**: 168–174.

29. Baker AL, Kaplan M, Norton AP, Patterson J. Gallstones in inflammatory bowel disease. *Am J Dig Dis* 1974; **19**: 109–112.

30. Kangas E, Lehmusto P, Matikainen M. Gallstones in Crohn's disease. *Hepatogastroenterology* 1990; **37**: 83–84.

31. Hutchinson R, Tyrrell PNM, Kumar D, Dunn JA, Li JKW, Allan RN. Pathogenesis of gallstones in Crohn's disease: an alternative explanation. *Gut* 1994; **35**: 94–97.

32. Cohen S, Kaplan M, Gottlieb L, Patterson J. Liver disease and gallstones in regional enteritis. *Gastroenterology* 1971; **60**: 237–245.

33. Pitt HA, Berquist WE, Mann LL, Fonkalsrud WE, Ament ME, Den Besten L. Parenteral nutrition induces calcium bilirubinate gallstones. *Gastroenterology* (abstr) 1983; **84**: 1274.

34. Bickerstaff KI, Moosa AR. Effects of resection or bypass of the distal ileum on the lithogenicity of bile. *Am J Surg* 1983; **145**: 34–40.

35. Nightingale JMD, Lennard-Jones JE, Gertner DJ, Wood SR, Bartram CI. Colonic preservation reduces the need for parenteral therapy, increases the incidence of renal stones but does not change the high prevalence of gallstones in patients with a short bowel. *Gut* 1992; **33**: 1493–1497.

36. Greig PD, Jeejeebhoy KN, Langer B, Cohen Z. A decade of home parenteral nutrition (abstr). *Gastroenterology* 1981; **80**: 1164.

37. Peterson SR, Sheldon GF. Acute acalculous cholecystitis: a complication of hyperalimentation. *Am J Surg* 1979; **138**: 814–817.

38. Barth RA, Brasch RC, Filly RA. Abdominal pseudo-tumour in childhood: distended gallbladder with parenteral hyperalimentation. *Am J Roentgenol* 1981; **136**: 341–343.

39. Roslyn JJ, Pitt HA, Mann LL, Ament ME, Den Besten L. Gallbladder disease in patients on long-term parenteral nutrition. *Gastroenterology* 1983; **84**: 148–154.

40. Roslyn JJ, Berquist WE, Pitt HA, Mann LL, Kangarloo H, DenBesten L, Ament ME. Increased risk of gall-stones in children on total parenteral nutrition. *Paediatrics* 1983; **71**: 784–789.

41. Murray FE, McNicholas M, Stack W, O'Donoghue DP. Impaired fatty-meal-stimulated gallbladder con-tractility in patients with Crohn's disease. *Clin Sci* 1992; **83**: 1–5.

42. Murray FE, Stinchcombe SJ, Hawkey CJ. Development of biliary sludge in patients on intensive care unit: results of a prospective ultrasonographic study. *Gut* 1992; **33**: 1123–1125.

43. Dowling RH, Bell GD, White J. Lithogenic bile in patients with ileal dysfunctions. *Gut* 1972; **13**: 415–420.

44. Dowling RH, Mack E, Small DM. Biliary lipid secretion and bile composition after acute and chronic interruption of the enterohepatic circulation in the rhesus monkey. *J Clin Invest* 1971; **50**: 1917–1926.

45. Kelly TR, Klein RL, Woodford JW. Alterations in gallstone solubility following distal ileal resection. *Arch Surg* 1972; **105**: 352–355.

46. Pitt HA, Lewinski MA, Muller EL, Porter-Fink V, DenBesten L. Ileal resection-induced gallstones: Altered bilirubin or cholesterol metabolism? *Surgery* 1984; **96**: 154–162.

47. Brink MA, Slors FM, Keulemans YCA, *et al.* Increased bilirubin levels in gallbladder bile in patients with ileal resection or disease. Abstract presented at seminar on 'Advances in inflammatory bowel disease', 12–13 March 1998, Amsterdam.

48. Ahonen A, Kyosola K, Penttila O. Enterochromaffin cells and macrophages in ulcerative colitis and irritable colon. *Ann Clin Res* 1976; **8**: 1–7.

49. Koch TR, Roddy DR, Carney JA, Go VLW. Peptide YY concentrations in normal ileum and colon and in idiopathic inflammatory bowel disease. *Dig Dis Sci* 1988; **33**: 1322–1328.

50. Pitt HA, King W, Mann LL, Roslyn JJ, Berquist WE, Ament ME, DenBesten L. Increased risk of chole-lithiasis with prolonged total parenteral nutrition. *Am J Surg* 1983; **145**: 106–112.

51. Lapidus A, Einarsson K. Effects of ileal resection on biliary lipids and bile acid composition in patients with Crohn's disease. *Gut* 1991; **32**: 1488-1491.

52. Lirussi F, Vaja S, Murphy GM, Dowling RH. Cholestasis of total parenteral nutrition: bile acid and bile lipid metabolism in parenterally nourished rats. *Gastroenterology* 1989; **96**: 493–502.

53. Doty JE, Pitt HA, Porter-Fink V, DenBesten L. The effects of intravenous fat and total parenteral nutrition on biliary physiology. *J Parenteral Enteral Nutr* 1984; **8**: 265–268.

54. Cano N, Cicero F, Ranieri F, Martin J, Di Costanzo T. Ultrasonographic study of gallbladder motility during total parenteral nutrition. *Gastroenterology* 1986; **91**: 313–317.

55. Doty JE, Pitt HA, Porter-Fink V, Kuchenbecker S, Den Besten L. The pathophysiology of gallbladder disease induced by total parenteral nutrition (abstr). *Gastroenterology* 1982; **82**: 1046.

56. Shuman WP, Gibbs P, Rudd PG, Mack LA. PIPIDA scintigraphy for cholecystitis: false-positives in alcoholism and total parenteral nutrition. *Am J Roentgenol* 1982; **138**: 1–5.

57. Xu QW, Shaffer EA. The potential site of impaired gallbladder contractility in an animal model of cholesterol gallstone disease. *Gastroenterology* 1996; **110**: 251–257.

58. Bolondi L, Gaiani S, Testa S, Labo G. Gallbladder sludge formation during prolonged fasting after gastro-intestinal tract surgery. *Gut* 1985; **26**: 734–738.

59. Maton PN, Selden AC, Fitzpatrick ML, Chadwick VS. Defective gallbladder emptying and cholecystokinin release in coeliac disease. Reversal by gluten-free diet. *Gastroenterology* 1985; **88**: 391–396.

60. Watts J, Dunphy JE. The role of the common bile duct in biliary dynamics. *Surg Gynecol Obstet* 1966; **122**: 1207–1218.

61. Hutton SW, Sieverd CE Jr, Vennes JA, Duane WC. The effect of sphincterotomy on gallstone formation in the prairie dog. *Gastroenterology* 1981; **81**: 663–667.

62. Bigg-Wither GW, Ho KKY, Grunstein RR, Sullivan CE, Doust BD. Effects of long-term octreotide on gall-stone formation and gallbladder function. *Br Med J* 1992; **304**: 1611–1612.

63. van Liessum PA, Hopman WPM, Pieters GFFM, *et al.* Post-prandial gallbladder motility during long-term treatment with the long-acting somatostatin analogue SMS 201-995 in acromegaly. *J Clin Endocrinol Metab* 1989; **69**: 557–562.

64. Hussaini SH, Pereira SP, Dowling RH, Wass JA. Slow intestinal transit and gallstone formation. *Lancet* 1993; **341**: 638.

65. Little JM, Avramovic J. Gallstone formation after major abdominal surgery. *Lancet* 1991; **337**: 1135–1137.

66. Harrison EC, Roschke EJ, Meyers HI, Edmiston WA, Chan LS, Tatter D, Lau FY. Cholelithiasis: a frequent complication of artificial heart valve replacement. *Am Heart J* 1978; **95**: 483–488.

67. Mabee TM, Meyer P, Den Besten L, Mason EE. The mechanism of increased gallstone formation in obese human subjects. *Surgery* 1976; **79**: 460–468.

68. Amaral JF, Thompson WR. Gallbladder disease in the morbidly obese. *Am J Surg* 1985; **149**: 551–557.

69. Liddle RA, Goldstein RB, Saxton J. Gallstone formation during weight reduction dieting. *Arch Intern Med* 1989; **149**: 1750–1753.

70. Mok HY, Von Bergmann K, Crouse JR, Grundy SM. Biliary lipid metabolism in obesity: effects of bile acid feeding before and during weight reduction. *Gastroenterology* 1979; **76**: 556–567.

71. Marzio L, Capone F, Neri M, Mezzetti A, De Angelis C, Cuccurullo F. Gallbladder kinetics in obese patients. Effect of a regular meal and low-calorie meal. *Dig Dis Sci* 1988; **33**: 4–9.

72. Greenberg GR, Mckloy RF, Adrian TE, Chadwick VS, Baron JH, Bloom SR. Inhibition of pancreas and gallbladder by pancreatic polypeptide. *Lancet* 1978; **2**: 1280–1282.

73. Johansson C, Kollberg B, Efendic S, Uvnas-Wallensten K. Effects of graded doses of somatostatin on gallbladder emptying and pancreatic enzyme output after oral glucose in man. *Digestion* 1981; **22**: 24–31.

74. Roslyn JJ, DenBesten L, Pitt HA, Kuchenbecker S, Polarek JW. Effects of cholecystokinin on gallbladder stasis and cholesterol gallstone formation. *J Surg Res* 1981; **30**: 200–204.

75. Hutton SW, Sievert CE Jr, Vennes JA, Duane WC. Inhibition of gallstone formation by sphincterotomy in the prairie dog: reversal by atropine. *Gastroenterology* 1982; **82**: 1308–1313.

76. Messing B, Aprahamian M, Rautureau M, Bories C, Bisalli A, Stock-Damle S. Gallstone formation during total parenteral nutrition: a prospective study in man (abstr). *Gastroenterology* 1984; **86**: 1183.

77. Sitzmann JV, Pitt HA, Steinborn PA, Pasha ZR, Sanders RC. Cholecystokinin prevents parenteral nutrition induced biliary sludge in humans. *Surg Gynecol Obst* 1990; **170**: 25–31.

78. Nealon WH, Upp JR, Alexander RW, Gomez G, Townsend CR, Thompson JC. Intravenous amino acids stimulate human gallbladder emptying and hormone release. *Am J Physiol* 1990; **259**: G173–G178.

79. Cohen IT, Meunier K, Hirsh MP. The effects of enteral stimulation on gallbladder bile during total parenteral nutrition in the neonatal piglet. *J Pediatr Surg* 1990; **25**: 163–167.

80. Zoli G, Ballinger A, Healy J, O'Donnell LJD, Clark M, Farthing MJG. Promotion of gallbladder emptying by intravenous aminoacids. *Lancet* 1993; **341**: 1240–1241.

81. Thompson JS. The role of prophylactic cholecystectomy in the short-bowel syndrome. *Arch Surg* 1996; **131**: 556–560.

82. Lee SP, Carey MC, LaMont JT. Aspirin prevention of cholesterol gallstone formation in prairie dogs. *Science* 1981; **211**: 1429–1431.

83. O'Leary DP, La Morte WW, Scott TE, Booker ML, Stevenson J. Inhibition of prostaglandin synthesis fails to prevent gallbladder mucin hypersecretion in the cholesterol-fed prairie dog. *Gastroenterology* 1991; **101**: 812–820.

84. O'Donnell LJD, Wilson P, Guest P, Catnach SM, McLean A, Wickham JEA, Fairclough PD. Indomethacin and post-prandial gallbladder emptying. *Lancet* 1992; **339**: 269–271.

85. Portincasa P, van Erpecum KJ, Jansen A, Renooij W, Gadellaa M, vanBerge-Henegouwen GP. Behaviour of various cholesterol crystals in bile from gallstone patients. *Hepatology* 1996; **23**: 738–748.

86. van Erpecum KJ, Stolk MFJ, van den Broek AMWC, Renooij W, van de Heijning BJM, vanBerge-Henegouwen GP. Bile concentration promotes nucleation of cholesterol monohydrate crystals by increasing the cholesterol concentration in the vesicles. *Eur J Clin Invest* 1993; **23**: 283–288.

87. Capron JP, Gineston JL, Herve MA, Braillon A. Metronidazole in prevention of cholestasis associated with total parenteral nutrition. *Lancet* 1983; **1**: 446–447.

15

Nephrocalcinosis and nephrolithiasis

Charles R. V. Tomson

*I*t has long been recognized that patients with intestinal disease are at increased risk of urinary tract stones, as a result of a high prevalence of known risk factors for stone formation including decreased urinary volume, decreased urinary pH, hyperuricosuria, hyperoxaluria and hypocitraturia. Problems associated with stone formation include repeated attacks of renal colic, obstructive uropathy (which may cause irreversible renal damage) and urinary tract infection (which in the presence of obstruction may cause pyonephrosis) (Fig. 15.1). Some patients are also at risk not only of the deposition of stones in the collecting system but also in the renal parenchyma itself (i.e. nephrocalcinosis), which may be associated with progressive impairment of renal function. Continued hyperabsorption of oxalate (enteric hyperoxaluria) may then cause systemic oxalosis, a devastating disease associated with deposition of calcium oxalate on blood vessels, cardiac-conducting tissues and muscle, bone, retina and elsewhere. For all of these reasons, and because stone formation is usually avoidable, a clear understanding of the pathogenesis of stone formation in the presence of intestinal disease is important.

This chapter is a selective review of what is known about the incidence, pathogenesis, complications and treatment of urinary tract stones in patients with intestinal disease.

PATHOGENESIS OF STONE FORMATION

Urinary stones may be formed from a number of compounds, including calcium oxalate (approximate frequency 75%), magnesium ammonium phosphate (10–20%), calcium phosphate (5%), uric acid (5%) and cystine (< 1%).[1] Patients with bowel disease are at increased risk of calcium oxalate stones and of uric acid stones. Stone formation follows three phases: nucleation, growth and aggregation. At all stages, supersaturation of urine with respect to the components of the stone are required, but stone formation also depends on other factors.

Calcium oxalate is highly insoluble, with a solubility of around 7 mg/L at 37°C in simple solution. However, urine is an extremely complex solution, containing inhibitors and promoters of crystallization. For instance, citrate and pyrophosphate form soluble complexes with calcium, thus decreasing calcium availability; magnesium forms a soluble complex with oxalate; and Tamm-Horsfall glycoprotein and other glycosaminoglycans inhibit one or several phases of calcium oxalate stone formation. Even though normal urine is supersaturated with respect to calcium oxalate, calcium oxalate crystals do not normally form in free solution, but rather by deposition on existing surfaces, such as tubular casts, sodium urate or uric acid crystals, or cell debris.[1]

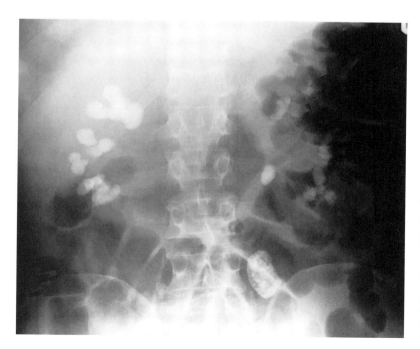

Figure 15.1 – Plain abdominal radiograph of a patient who had undergone extensive small bowel resection in 1985 as a result of spontaneous mesenteric thrombosis complicating the lupus anticoagulant syndrome. Stone formation was first reported in 1988, since when the patient had passed hundreds of calcium oxalate stones. Three months prior to this radiograph being taken he was admitted with acute renal failure, septicaemia and pyonephrosis as a result of obstruction by stones. Urinary oxalate was > 1.0 mmol/day, but fell to 0.3 mmol/day on a synthetic oxalate-free diet.

Uric acid is a weak acid, with a pK of 5.75. Undissociated uric acid is highly insoluble, with a solubility limit of 100 mg/L, whereas urate salts are very much more soluble (e.g. 1200 mg/L of urate at pH 6.5).[2] Urine pH is therefore the main determinant of uric acid solubility; the most important risk factors for uric acid stone formation are therefore high urine concentration and acid urine (Fig. 15.2). Total uric acid excretion is often normal in patients with uric acid stones, although increased production of uric acid as a result of increased purine catabolism is one cause of stone formation.[2]

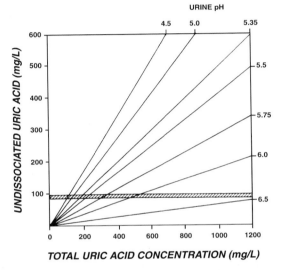

Figure 15.2 – Relationship between urine pH and solubility of uric acid. Used with permission from *Kidney International* Volume **24** page 395, 1983.[2a]

EPIDEMIOLOGY

Frequency of stone formation in patients with intestinal disease

Numerous case reports and series have documented an unexpectedly high incidence of urinary stones in patients with inflammatory bowel disease[3–14] and in patients with jejuno-ileal bypass for obesity or ileal resection for a variety of causes.[15–27] In particular, a high incidence of uric acid stones has been noted amongst patients with ileostomy.[4] Similarly, series of stone-formers have noted a history of ileostomy as a major risk factor for uric acid stones, which are frequently recurrent.[2,28] However, patients with ileostomy appear to have at least an equal incidence of calcified stones as of uric acid stones in most series (Table 15.1). Interestingly, there are no published reports of an excess incidence of stone amongst patients with chronic pancreatitis (apart from case reports of hyperparathyroidism causing both).

Parenchymal renal damage in patients with bowel disease

There are numerous reports of acute renal failure due to calcium oxalate deposition in the interstitium of the kidney, often without either a history of stone passage or even of radiological evidence of nephrocalcinosis;[29–40] in some of these there was additional evidence of immune complex damage to renal tubules, suggesting that oxalate deposition was not the

Table 15.1 – Prevalence of urinary tract stones in patients with inflammatory bowel disease

Reference	Patients	(n) with stones	% with stones	Method	Type of stone, when known
Deren *et al.*, 1962[3]	583 IBD	28	4.8	Case note	10 uric acid, 10 calcified, 2 mixed
Maratka and Nedbal, 1964[6]	74 Ileostomy	9	13	Case note	1 uric acid, 1 calcium oxalate
Bennett and Jepson, 1966[5]	72 Ileostomy	7	10	Postal	5 uric acid
Grossman and Nugent, 1967[7]	1100 IBD	35	3.2	Case note	
Gelzayd *et al.*, 1968[8]	885 IBD	64	7.2	Case note	10 uric acid, 46 calcified
Ritchie, 1971[10]	371 Ileostomy	33	10	Postal + case note verification	4 uric acid, 7 calcified
Greenstein *et al.*, 1976[12]	700 IBD	53	7.6	Case note	'Vast majority' radio-opaque
Bambach *et al.*, 1981[13]	426	40	9.4	Postal	
Kennedy *et al.*, 1982[14]	39 Ileostomy	4	10.3	Clinic review and IVU	All calcified

only mechanism.[33,37,39] Improvement of renal function after restoration of intestinal continuity was reported in some of these cases.[30,32,39]

Frequency of intestinal disease as a cause of stone formation in stone-formers

Intestinal disease is a rare cause of stone formation when compared with other causes. In one of the largest series, of 1270 adult patients evaluated according to a detailed protocol in a tertiary referral centre, abnormal urine biochemistry was found in 96%, with more than one abnormality commonly found. Enteric hyperoxaluria, in association with calcium stones, occurred in 20 (1.5%) patients, of whom seven had jejuno-ileal bypass, four ileal resection, four malabsorption, four Crohn's disease and one ulcerative colitis with ileal damage. Twenty-six (2%) patients had a chronic diarrhoeal syndrome (ten Crohn's, five jejuno-ileal bypass, four gastric resection, four small bowel resection, three ulcerative colitis), which was frequently associated with hypocitraturia, hypo-magnesuria and low urine volume.[41]

Determinants of urine volume and concentration

The concentration of lithogenic substances in urine is determined by the excretion rate of calcium, oxalate, etc and also, independently, by the excretion of water. Water excretion rate is governed by antidiuretic hormone (Vasopressin) and by renal blood flow. One of the most important correctable risk factors for stone formation in patients with intestinal disease is salt and water depletion as a result of gastrointestinal losses. In particular, patients with ileostomy or jejunostomy frequently have significantly reduced urine volume and urine sodium (reflecting avid renal sodium retention as a result of hypovolaemia).[9,42,43]

Determinants of urine pH and citrate excretion

Control of urinary citrate excretion, one of the major endogenous inhibitors of calcium oxalate crystallization in urine, is complex. Hypocitraturia (usually defined as a 24-hour urinary excretion of citrate of less than 320 mg/24 h (1.67 mmol/24 h) – although this depends on the assay method used), a known risk factor for calcium oxalate stone formation, is common in patients with malabsorption or jejuno-ileal

bypass.[18,44,45] Citrate excretion and urine pH are reduced by systemic acidosis, including that caused by gastrointestinal bicarbonate wastage, and by hypo-magnesaemia; hypocitraturia in patients with malabsorption can be corrected by oral citrate supplementation and intramuscular magnesium.[44]

SOURCES OF URINARY OXALATE

Oxalate is a metabolic end-product, and cannot be metabolized further in man. Under normal circumstances, most urinary oxalate derives from metabolism of amino acids (mainly glycine) and of ascorbic acid. Less than 10% is normally derived from dietary oxalate. Under normal circumstances, dietary oxalate is sparingly absorbed. Experiments using isotopic oxalate show that between 2 and 6% of dietary oxalate is absorbed in normal volunteers.[46,47] At first sight this would suggest that dietary oxalate is of little relevance to the formation of calcium oxalate stones. However, transient hyperoxaluria after ingestion of oxalate-rich foods[48] results in episodes of increased supersaturation of urine with respect to calcium oxalate, thereby increasing the chance of stone formation. If absorption of dietary oxalate is increased, as in enteric hyper-oxaluria, this risk is further amplified.

Metabolic production of oxalate

The major metabolic sources of oxalate are glycine catabolism and ascorbic acid catabolism. Deficiency of liver peroxisomal alanine:glyoxylate aminotransferase results in primary hyperoxaluria type 1, a rare cause of recurrent stone formation. Thiamine deficiency and pyridoxine deficiency both result in increased metabolic production of oxalate, which is accompanied by increased production and urinary excretion of glycolate, measurement of which should allow distinction between metabolic and dietary sources of increased urinary oxalate. The extent to which ascorbic acid intake contributes to oxalate excretion is complicated by the potential for conversion of ascorbate to oxalate *in vitro*, but as much as 40% of oxalate excreted may be derived from ascorbate if ascorbate intake is high.

Ileal absorption and secretion of oxalate

Normally only a small fraction of dietary oxalate is absorbed.[49] Experiments using test meals in normal subjects containing oxalate salts have shown a rise in oxalate excretion within 2 hours of ingestion, suggesting ileal absorption.[48,50,51] Experiments *in vitro* suggest that oxalate may be transported by anion exchangers on the brush border, in exchange for hydroxyl or chloride ions.[52] Transport is bi-directional. In the absence of an electrochemical gradient, the small intestine and proximal colon actively secrete oxalate into the lumen.[53] Experimental studies have suggested intestinal oxalate absorption is decreased by ascorbic acid deficiency[54] and increased by pyridoxine deficiency.[55]

Colonic absorption and secretion of oxalate

Both secretion and absorption of oxalate by the colon can be demonstrated experimentally. In normal animals and humans, the distal colon appears to be an important route of oxalate absorption.[53] Colonic oxalate absorption is increased by low dietary calcium, hyperparathyroidism and vitamin D administration, all of which reduce calcium concentrations in the colon and thus decrease the extent to which oxalate is bound to calcium in the gut lumen. As discussed below, colonic absorption of oxalate is greatly enhanced in enteric hyperoxaluria.

Dietary sources of oxalate

Determination of the oxalate content of food is complicated by methodological difficulties (including the formation of oxalate *in vitro* during the assay procedure, the presence in food of inhibitors of oxalate oxidase, used in some enzymatic oxalate assays, and the presence of highly insoluble oxalate salts), variation in oxalate content between batches of food tested (including variation in oxalate content depending on the season) and also by the fact that bio-availability is variable, depending on the method of preparation and the calcium content; sodium oxalate is much more soluble than calcium oxalate, and may therefore be lost in cooking water, but is more bio-available if ingested.[56,57] Older analytical methods utilizing colorimetric assays, though still widely quoted[58,59,60] are unreliable when compared to more modern methods.[57] For these reasons, there is no definitive information on either oxalate content of foods, or of the likely effect of ingestion of a particular foodstuff on oxalate excretion either in patients with normal gastrointestinal tracts or

those with enteric hyperoxaluria. Table 15.2 summarizes oxalate content of common foods where this is reliably known.

INFLUENCE OF CALCIUM INTAKE ON OXALATE EXCRETION AND STONE FORMATION

Epidemiological studies in men[65] and women[66] have shown that a high dietary calcium intake reduces the risk of developing renal stones. Other studies have also showed that variations in urinary calcium excretion are poorly, if at all predictive of stone recurrence, whereas the risk of recurrence appears to increase exponentially as urinary oxalate excretion increases.[67] The explanation for this paradoxical relationship between calcium intake and stone risk is twofold.

1. Studies *in vitro* and computerized iterative calculation of activity products show that the risk of calcium oxalate crystallization in urine is little affected by variations in urine total calcium concentration (as a result of the formation of soluble complexes which decreases calcium availability) but increases linearly with increasing oxalate concentration.[68] Thus, changes in urinary oxalate concentration are very much more important as a risk factor for stone formation than changes in urinary calcium concentration.

2. Oxalate is only absorbed from the gut in ionized form. Excess calcium in the gut lumen thus decreases oxalate bio-availability by the formation of insoluble calcium oxalate. Several studies have confirmed that, independent of other factors, urinary oxalate excretion decreases with increasing dietary calcium intake,[68,69] and, conversely, that dietary calcium restriction increases absorption of dietary oxalate, resulting in an increase in the probability of stone formation.[70] Similarly, administration of sodium cellulose phosphate (which decreases gut absorption of calcium) results in an increase in urinary oxalate excretion.[71] Increased intestinal absorption of calcium, as in vitamin D treatment and 'absorptive hypercalciuria' may also increase stone risk not so much because of the resulting increase in urinary calcium concentration but because of the resulting hyperabsorption of oxalate.

EFFECT OF BOWEL DISEASE ON OXALATE ABSORPTION: 'ENTERIC HYPEROXALURIA'

Numerous studies have demonstrated that absorption of oxalate from the gut is enhanced in patients with ileal disease or resection[72–87] and in those with fat mal-absorption;[88–91] absorption is normal in patients with an ileostomy[77,80,81,92] and is increased after restoration of continuity between ileum and colon,[81] indicating the colon as the major site of hyperabsorption of oxalate. This is also consistent with the observation that colonic preservation after small bowel resection is associated with a higher risk of renal stone formation.[27] The first unequivocal demonstration of increased oxalate absorption in patients with ileal disease was published in 1973: [14]C oxalate absorption was 5 times

Table 15.2 – Estimates of dietary content of some common foods, compiled from a number of sources

Food	Oxalate content (mg/100g)	Assay method	Reference
Beetroot (leaves and roots)	675	Enzymatic	Kasidas and Rose, 1980[56]
Rhubarb	600–860	Enzymatic	Kasidas and Rose, 1980[56]
	537	Gas chromatography	Hesse et al., 1979[50]
Spinach	600–750	Enzymatic	Kasidas and Rose, 1980[56]
	571	Gas chromatography	Hesse et al., 1979[50]
Okra	264	Gas chromatography	Brinkley et al., 1990[64]
Wheat bran	240	Not stated	Rao et al., 1985[62]
Peanuts	185	Enzymatic	Kasidas and Rose, 1980[56]
	116	Gas chromatography	Brinkley et al., 1990[64]
Almonds	131	Gas chromatography	Brinkley et al., 1990[64]
Bran flakes	141	Capillary electrophoresis	Hesse et al., 1979[50]
Rice bran	123	Not stated	Rao et al., 1985[62]
Chocolate	117	Enzymatic	Kasidas and Rose, 1980[56]
	140	Gas chromatography	Brinkley et al., 1981[63]
	366	Gas chromatography	Hesse et al., 1979[50]
Parsley	100	Enzymatic	Kasidas and Rose, 1980[56]
Weetabix	76.1	Capillary electrophoresis	Hesse et al., 1979[50]
Pecan nuts	12	Gas chromatography	Brinkley et al., 1981[63]
Baked beans	19	Enzymatic	Kasidas and Rose, 1980[56]
Runner beans	15	Enzymatic	Kasidas and Rose, 1980[56]
Celery	20	Enzymatic	Kasidas and Rose, 1980[56]
	61	Capillary electrophoresis	Hesse et al., 1979[50]
Carrots	10	Capillary electrophoresis	Hesse et al., 1979[50]
Strawberries	10–15	Enzymatic	Kasidas and Rose, 1980[56]
Asparagus	1.7	Gas chromatography	Hesse et al., 1979[50]
Tomato	2	Enzymatic	Kasidas and Rose, 1980[56]
	5.7	Capillary electrophoresis	Hesse et al., 1979[50]
	3.9	Gas chromatography	Hesse et al., 1979[50]
Turnip greens	6	Gas chromatography	Brinkley et al., 1990[64]
V-8 (vegetable cocktail) juice	52 mg/L	Gas chromatography	Brinkley et al., 1981[63]
	5.8	Capillary electrophoresis	Hesse et al., 1979[50]
Cranberry juice	44 mg/L	Gas chromatography	Brinkley et al., 1981[63]
Tea (2-minute infusion)	55	Enzymatic	Kasidas and Rose, 1980[56]
Tea (4-minute infusion)	72	Enzymatic	Kasidas and Rose, 1980[56]
Tea (6-minute infusion)	78	Enzymatic	Kasidas and Rose, 1980[56]
Tea (2-minute infusion)	280 mg/100 mL	Gas chromatography	Brinkley et al., 1990[64]

Results in which the method used was not stated should be treated with great caution: many of these results may have been obtained with colorimetric assays, which have been shown to be extremely unreliable compared to more modern methods. Some sources quote high levels of oxalate for a number of vegetables not listed here, including sorrel, collard greens, Swiss chard and dandelion leaves,[58–61] but data from the use of reliable assays are not available.

greater in patients with ileal resection than in control subjects, and oxalate excretion returned to normal when patients were fed a very low oxalate semisynthetic diet (Fig. 15.3).[72] On a free diet, the degree of hyperoxaluria is proportional to the amount of ileum resected (Fig. 15.4).[80] In patients with suspected malabsorption, urinary oxalate excretion after a dietary oxalate load correlates well with faecal fat excretion, leading to the suggestion of an oxalate loading test as a screening test for steatorrhoea (Fig. 15.5).[90,91]

Initially, the mechanism underlying these observations of increased oxalate absorption was unclear, but several hypotheses have emerged of which the first two are probably the most important.

Increased colonic permeability to oxalate

Observations that oxalate excretion is decreased by treatment with cholestyramine[16,72] raised the possibility that unabsorbed bile acids increased colonic permeability to oxalate. This possibility was tested directly by Fairclough et al., who perfused the surgically excluded colon in two patients with ^{14}C oxalate with and without chenodeoxycholate and showed that the bile salt increased oxalate absorption fivefold (Fig. 15.6).[78] [14]C oxalate absorption is increased in patients receiving high-dose chenodeoxycholic acid for gallstone dissolution.[79] Animal experiments confirm that long-chain fatty acids enhance colonic permeability to oxalate.[85,86]

Fat malabsorption + calcium soap formation

The finding that increasing dietary fat intake led to worsening of enteric hyperoxaluria[75] suggested that malabsorbed fat per se had an impact on oxalate absorption. Experiments in vitro showed that fatty acids increased the solubility of calcium oxalate, as a result of the formation of calcium soaps from calcium and fatty acids;[76] and in vivo, that calcium supplementation in patients with fat malabsorption decreased oxalate excretion while on a fixed oxalate intake. Urinary calcium excretion was lower in those patients with enteric hyperoxaluria compared to those with normal oxalate excretion, further supporting the hypothesis that fat malabsorption led both to calcium malabsorption as a result of the formation of calcium soaps and to enhanced colonic absorption of oxalate.

Intestinal degradation of oxalate by bacteria

Studies in animals have shown the presence of an anaerobic oxalate-degrading bacterium, Oxalobacter formigenes, within the colon, with the capacity to degrade oxalate to carbon dioxide and formate.[95] The same bacterium was cultured from 64% of normal human subjects, and contributed significantly to oxalate degradation in the colon, but was cultured less frequently from patients with Crohn's disease or steatorrhoea[96] and absent from the majority of patients with cystic fibrosis.[97] The bacteria are substrate specific, and increase in numbers in laboratory animals fed a high oxalate diet and in patients with chronic renal impairment.[98] Growth of the bacterium was inhibited by low concentrations of bile acids, leading to the suggestion that decreased bacterial degradation of oxalate in the colon contributes to enteric hyperoxaluria.[99]

Generation of oxalate from precursors in the gut

Some patients with enteric hyperoxaluria continue to show elevated urinary oxalate excretion and continue to form stones despite rigorous dietary restriction. A study in eight patients with jejuno-ileal bypass confirmed increased absorption of ^{14}C oxalate given in a test meal, with the time course of excretion suggesting colonic absorption. Urinary oxalate excretion fell, but not to normal, on a very low oxalate diet. When a protein-free low oxalate diet was substituted, urinary oxalate excretion fell further, and increased on a hydrolysed protein, low oxalate diet.[84] These observations suggested, indirectly, that oxalate was being formed in the gut, possibly as a result of bacterial degradation of dietary amino acids or creatinine to oxalate. This theory is not completely disproved by subsequent studies of the effect of non-absorbable antibiotics in patients with enteric hyperoxaluria, which have failed to show any reduction in urinary oxalate excretion.[79,85]

Renal handling of oxalate

Oxalate is freely filtered at the glomerulus, but oxalate clearance normally exceeds glomerular filtration rate by a factor of 1.3–2.0, as a consequence of secretion of oxalate in the proximal tubule. Fractional oxalate clearance is decreased by thiazide and loop diuretics and by competition with other organic anions such as urate. Enhanced tubular secretion of oxalate has been inferred

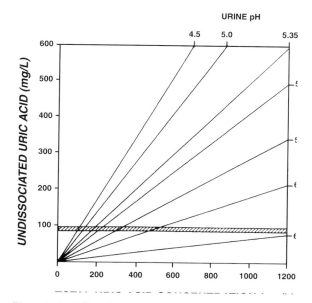

URINE pH

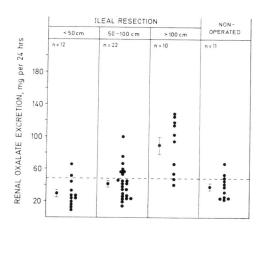

Figure 15.3 – Effect of a very low oxalate diet on urinary oxalate excretion in four patients with ileal resection and hyperoxaluria. From Chadwick *et al.*,[72] with permission. © 1973 Massachusetts Medical Society. All rights reserved.

Figure 15.5 – Relationship between faecal fat excretion and urinary oxalate excretion during oral supplementation of a fixed diet (containing 30 mg oxalate and 1000 mg calcium) with sodium oxalate, 300 mg twice daily with the lunchtime and evening meal. From Rampton *et al.*,[89] with permission.

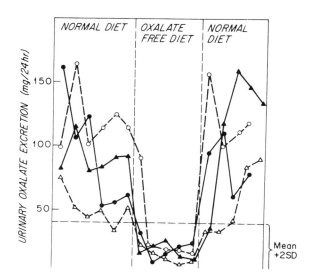

Figure 15.4 – Relationship between the length of ileum resected and urinary oxalate excretion while on a fixed diet supplying 200 mg oxalate per day. Reprinted from Hylander *et al.*,[80] by permission of Scandinavian University Press.

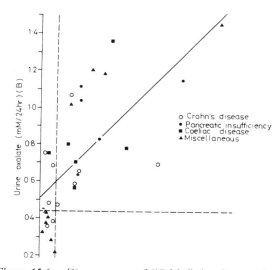

Figure 15.6 – Disappearance of ^{14}C-labelled sodium oxalate from the surgically excluded colon, perfused at 10 ml/min, with and without co-perfusion with chenodeoxycholate. Subjects were two patients who had undergone colonic exclusion for hepatic encephalopathy; one subject (filled circle) was studied twice. From Fairclough *et al.*,[78] with permission.

in one series of patients with jejuno-ileal bypass, but in this study fractional excretion of oxalate was less than 1.0 in the controls; no convincing mechanism was suggested whereby jejuno-ileal bypass should influence tubular secretion of oxalate,[100] although renal tubular acidosis as a result of renal oxalosis has been reported as a result of jejuno-ileal bypass.[30]

Vitamin deficiency

Pyridoxine deficiency could cause enhanced metabolic generation of oxalate or, possibly, enhanced ileal absorption.[24,55] Thiamine deficiency may also result in increased oxalate production.

One study has cast doubt on the relevance of enteric hyperoxaluria to stone formation. Hylander *et al.* took 87 patients with inflammatory bowel disease, classified them as having increased or normal oxalate absorption on the basis of 4-day oxalate excretion while on a standardized diet containing 200 mg oxalate, and performed intravenous pyelography in all. The prevalence of urolithiasis was 9/26 (35%) in patients with hyperoxaluria and 14/61 (23%) in patients with normal oxalate excretion, a non-significant difference. Mean oxalate excretion was no higher in patients with stones than in those without.[101] These are surprising results. The methods by which the patients were selected are not stated. The prevalence of urolithiasis is strikingly high in both groups; this is

conceivably due to the inclusion of 29 patients with ileostomy, who may be at increased risk of stone formation as a result of dehydration, acid urine and hypocitraturia, in the group with normal oxalate excretion.

In summary, there are numerous potential contributors to the increased risk of stone formation amongst patients with small bowel disease or resection (Table 15.3).

PREVENTION OF STONE FORMATION IN PATIENTS WITH INTESTINAL DISEASE

The most rational, and certainly the safest, treatment to reduce the risk of stone formation in patients who have had an ileal resection or have ileal disease is to increase water intake, and thus to make the urine more dilute, reducing supersaturation with respect to calcium, oxalate and any other potential constituents of urinary tract stones. Ideally, water intake should also be increased at night, when decreased urine flow and increased urine concentration may increase the risk of stone formation, although fluid intake should also be increased at meal-times to compensate for transient hyperoxaluria due to absorption of dietary oxalate. However, it is remarkably difficult to persuade patients

Table 15.3 – Types and causes of renal stones after ileal and colonic resection

Type of resection or area of disease	Incidence of stones (%)	Type of stone	Predisposing factors
Ileal and colonic resection (jejunostomy/ileostomy)	10–15	Calcium oxalate (50%)	Low urine volume Hypocitraturia Hypomagnesuria
		Uric acid (50%)	Low urine volume Low urine pH
Ileal resection (Jejuno-colic anastomosis)	25	Calcium oxalate	Low urine volume Enhanced oxalate absorption due to unabsorbed bile salts Decreased luminal calcium concentration due to fatty acid malabsorption Decreased bacterial degradation of oxalate Enhanced production of oxalate by gut bacteria (?) Pyridoxine deficiency Thiamine deficiency

with normal intestinal function to increase fluid intake to ensure a daily urine volume of > 3 litres.

In patients with short bowel and a retained colon, who may be even more reluctant to increase fluid intake, efforts should also be directed to minimizing gastrointestinal fluid losses, with drugs that reduce motility and/or secretions. In patients with an ileostomy or jejunostomy who have problems of renal stones, a glucose–electrolyte solution should be encouraged (Chapter 24) or slow release sodium supplements (as chloride or bicarbonate).

DIETARY MANAGEMENT

Dietary calcium restriction increases oxalate absorption and thus increases the risk of stone formation, and has no proven place in the management of stone formation. Indeed, high dietary calcium intake is likely to reduce absorption of dietary oxalate. Dietary oxalate restriction is a rational approach in patients with enteric hyper-oxaluria, although it should be admitted that the benefits of dietary oxalate restriction in reducing stone formation rate have never been demonstrated by clinical trial. At the least, patients should be advised to avoid high oxalate foods, including spinach, rhubarb, beetroot, nuts, chocolate, tea, wheat bran and strawberries. In addition, foods with lower oxalate contents, which may have no significant impact on oxalate excretion in normal volunteers or the majority of patients with calcium oxalate stones, may result in significant increases in urinary oxalate excretion in patients with greatly enhanced oxalate absorption, as in enteric hyper-oxaluria; a case can therefore be made for restriction of foods even with a moderate oxalate content – so long as this is compatible with maintenance of adequate nutritional status. Restriction of dietary oxalate and fat intake have been shown to be effective in reducing urinary oxalate excretion in metabolic ward conditions;[72,77,84] one study has confirmed that a worthwhile reduction in urinary oxalate may be obtained in out-patients with jejuno–ileal bypass as a result of advice on a low oxalate, low fat diet.[102] However, fat restriction may not be desirable for nutritional reasons. Substitution of medium-chain triglycerides may be effective in reducing oxalate absorption.[76]

DRUG THERAPY

In patients with ileostomy, sodium bicarbonate supplementation, with the aim of increasing urinary sodium excretion, urine volume and urine pH, is a rational treatment, although evidence of benefit is anecdotal only. Alternatives include citrate salts, which have the additional benefit of increasing urinary citrate excretion.

In patients with enteric hyperoxaluria, a number of treatments, designed either to decrease oxalate bio-availability in the colon or to reduce colonic permeability to oxalate, have been studied.[101–111]

Calcium salts reduce absorption of dietary oxalate in patients with ileal resection or jejuno-ileal bypass,[79,82,103–105,107–111] although one study in out-patients showed no effect.[106] This decrease may be at the expense of a rise in calcium absorption and hence urinary calcium excretion,[82] but as discussed earlier, an increment in urinary calcium concentration is of less importance to the risk of stone formation than a decrement in urinary oxalate. Calcium-containing organic marine hydrocolloid has also been shown to decrease oxalate absorption without any increase in calcium absorption, and also to ameliorate otherwise intractable diarrhoea, but has not been directly compared to equivalent molar doses of calcium given as a simple salt.[107,108] There is no evidence from long-term clinical observation that calcium treatment reduces stone recurrence rate in enteric hyperoxaluria, although, if urinary calcium excretion is carefully monitored, this is a rational treatment and should certainly be considered in patients who have formed multiple stones and have severe enteric hyperoxaluria. Neither has any comparison between the various calcium salts available been published. An analogy may be drawn with the use of calcium salts as phosphate binders in patients with renal failure. Experience in this group of patients has shown the critical importance of the timing of ingestion of calcium salts in relation to meals, and the reduction of phosphate-binding effect of calcium carbonate when co-administered with H_2 antagonists; in patients on long-term acid suppression, calcium acetate may be more effective as a phosphate binder, and this agent deserves study in enteric hyperoxaluria.

Cholestyramine has variable effects. It can be shown *in vitro* to bind oxalate.[72,73] In theory, sequestration of bile acids should ameliorate the effect of bile acids on colonic permeability to oxalate. Two reports in patients with enteric hyperoxaluria showed a significant reduction in oxalate excretion during cholestyramine treatment,[16,73] as well as dramatic improvement in diarrhoea.[73] However, other studies report no useful effect[18,79] or even an increase in urinary oxalate excretion.[106]

Aluminium salts can be shown to bind oxalate *in vitro*,[105] and by analogy with the use of aluminium hydroxide as a phosphate binder in chronic renal failure might be expected to reduce oxalate absorption if given with meals. One study, published only in abstract form, showed a halving in oxalate excretion with aluminium hydroxide in four patients with enteric hyperoxaluria,[103] but no reduction was seen in the only other published study.[106]

SUMMARY

All of the studies available on drug treatment of enteric hyperoxaluria have involved very small numbers of patients, and many were published before the methodological pitfalls of measurement of oxalate in urine were fully understood. A rational approach to the prevention of the complications of enteric hyperoxaluria requires further studies, in larger numbers of patients, using reliable oxalate assays, and ensuring proper timing of the ingestion of binding agents relative to meals. These in turn should lead to long-term studies examining the effects either of dietary restriction or of drug treatment on stone recurrence rate or progression of parenchymal renal damage. In the interim, measures designed to increase urine volume and to minimize oxalate excretion, adequately monitored by regular urine collections, should be instituted in all patients with stone formation or parenchymal renal damage attributable to enteric hyperoxaluria (Table 15.4). In patients with jejuno–ileal bypass, serious consideration should be given to restoration of intestinal continuity.[112]

Table 15.4 – Available measures to decrease risk of stone formation in patients with a short small bowel in continuity with the colon

1. Avoid salt and water depletion (consider NaCl supplements)
2. Low oxalate diet
3. Calcium supplements with meals
4. Low fat diet (if compatible with nutritional requirements)
5. Avoid systemic acidosis (consider $NaHCO_3$ supplements)
6. Magnesium supplements
7. Citrate supplements (if hypocitraturic)
8. ?Aluminium supplements with meals
9. ?Organic marine hydrocolloid supplements with meals

REFERENCES

1. Coe FL, Parks JH, Asplin JR. The pathogenesis and treatment of kidney stones. *N Engl J Med* 1992; **327**: 1141–1152.

2. Asplin JR. Uric acid stones. *Semin Nephrol* 1996; **16**: 412–424.

3. Deren JJ, Porush JG, Levitt MF, Khilnani MT. Nephrolithiasis as a complication of ulcerative colitis and regional enteritis. *Ann Intern Med* 1962; **56**: 843–853.

4. Badenoch AW. Uric acid stone formation. *Br J Urol* 1960; **32**: 374–382.

5. Bennett RC, Jepson RP. Uric acid stone formation following ileostomy. *Aust NZ J Surg* 1966; **36**: 153–158.

6. Maratka Z, Nedbal J. Urolithiasis as a complication of the surgical treatment of ulcerative colitis. *Gut* 964; **5**: 214–217.

7. Grossman MS, Nugent FW. Urolithiasis as a complication of chronic diarrheal disease. *Am J Dig Dis* 1967; **12**: 491–498.

8. Gelzayd EA, Breuer RI, Kirsner JB. Nephrolithiasis in inflammatory bowel disease. *Am J Dig Dis* 1968; **13**: 1027–1034.

9. Clarke AM, McKenzie RG. Ileostomy and the risk of urinary uric acid stones. *Lancet* 1969; **ii**: 395–397.

10. Ritchie JK. Ileostomy and excisional surgery for chronic inflammatory disease of the colon: a survey of one hospital region. *Gut* 1971; **12**: 528–540.

11. Bennett RC, Hughes ESR. Urinary calculi and ulcerative colitis. *Br Med J* 1972; **2**: 494–496.

12. Greenstein AJ, Janowitz HD, Sachar DB. The extra-intestinal complications of Crohn's disease and ulcerative colitis: a study of 700 patients. *Medicine (Baltimore)* 1976; **55**: 401–412.

13. Bambach CP, Robertson WG, Peacock M, Hill GL. Effect of intestinal surgery on the risk of urinary stone formation. *Gut* 1981; **22**: 257–263.

14. Kennedy HJ, Fletcher EWL, Truelove SC. Urinary stones in subjects with a permanent ileostomy. *Br J Surg* 1982; **69**: 661–664.

15. Dowling RH, Rose GA, Sutor DJ. Hyperoxaluria and renal calculi in ileal disease. *Lancet* 1971; **i**: 1103–1106.

16. Smith LH, Fromm H, Hofmann AF. Acquired hyperoxaluria, nephrolithiasis, and intestinal disease. Description of a syndrome. *N Engl J Med* 1972; **286**: 1371–1375.

17. Dickstein SS, Frame B. Urinary tract calculi after intestinal shunt operations for the treatment of obesity. *Surg Gynecol Obstet* 1973; **136**: 257–260.

18. O'Leary JP, Thomas WC, Woodward ER. Urinary tract stone after small bowel bypass for morbid obesity. *Am J Surg* 1974; **127**: 142–147.

19. Campbell JM, Hunt TK, Forsham PH. Jejunoileal bypass as a treatment of morbid obesity. *Arch Intern Med* 1977; **137**: 602–610.

20. Halverson JD, Wise L, Wazna M, Ballinger WF. Jejunoileal bypass for morbid obesity. A critical appraisal. *Am J Med* 1978; **64**: 461–475.

21. Joffe SN. Surgical management of morbid obesity. *Gut* 1981; **22**: 242–254.

22. Morgan SH, Watts RWE, Purkiss P, Mansell MA, Rose GA, Pilkington TRE. Jejuno-ileal bypass, hyperoxaluria, and systemic oxalosis (abstract). *Clin Sci* 1986; **71** (Suppl 15): 34p.

23. Salvatierra O, Longaker M, Crombleholme T. Bilateral renal autotransplantation with pyelovesicostomy: A surgical treatment of refractory enteric hyperoxaluria. *Surgery* 1989; **105**: 430–435.

24. Marangella M, Vitale C, Petrarulo M, Cosseddu D, Gallo L, Linari F. Pathogenesis of severe hyperoxalaemia in Crohn's disease-related renal failure on maintenance haemodialysis: successful management with pyridoxine. *Nephrol Dial Transplant* 1992; **7**: 960–964.

25. Kistler H, Peter J, Thiel G, Brunner FP. Seven-year survival of renal transplant for oxalate nephropathy due to short bowel syndrome. *Nephrol Dial Transplant* 1995; **10**: 1466–1469.

26. Backman U, Holmgren K, Vessby B, Annuk M. Longitudinal follow-up of jejunoileal bypass operated patients (abstract). *J Am Soc Nephrol* 1996; **7**: 1381.

27. Nightingale JMD, Lennard-Jones JE, Gertner DJ, Wood SR, Bartram CI. Colonic preservation reduces need for parenteral therapy, increases incidence of renal stones, but does not change high prevalence of gall stones in patients with a short bowel. *Gut* 1992; **33**: 1493–1497.

28. Melick RA, Henneman PH. Clinical and laboratory studies of 207 consecutive patients in a kidney-stone clinic. *N Engl J Med* 1958; **259**: 307–314.

29. Cryer PE, Garber AJ, Hoffsten P, Lucas B, Wise L. Renal failure after small intestinal bypass for obesity. *Arch Intern Med* 1975; **135**: 1610–1612.

30. Vainder M, Kelly J. Renal tubular dysfunction secondary to jejunoileal bypass. *J Am Med Assoc* 1976; **235**: 1257–1258.

31. Gelbart DR, Brewer LL, Fajardo LF, Weinstein AB. Oxalosis and chronic renal failure after intestinal bypass. *Arch Intern Med* 1977; **137**: 239–243.

32. Ehlers SM, Posalaky Z, Strate RG, Quattlebaum FW. Acute reversible renal failure following jejunoileal bypass for morbid obesity: a clinical and pathological (EM) study of a case. *Surgery* 1977; **82**: 629–634.

33. Drenick EJ, Stanley TM, Border WA, Zawada ET, Dornfeld LP, Upham T, Llach F. Renal damage with intestinal bypass. *Ann Intern Med* 1978; **89**: 594–599.

34. Das S, Joseph B, Dick AL. Renal failure owing to oxalate nephrosis after jejuno-ileal bypass. *J Urol* 1980; **121**: 506.

35. Mandell I, Krauss E, Millan JC. Oxalate-induced acute renal failure in Crohn's disease. *Am J Med* 1980; **69**: 628–632.

36. Canos HJ, Hogg GA, Jeffery JR. Oxalate nephropathy due to gastrointestinal disorders. *Can Med Assoc J* 1981; **124**: 729.

37. Zawada ET, Johnston WH, Bergstein J. Chronic interstitial nephritis. Its occurrence with oxalosis and antitubular basement membrane antibodies after jejunoileal bypass. *Arch Pathol Lab Med* 1981; **105**: 379–383.

38. Roberts RA, Sketris IS, MacDonald AS, Belitsky P. Renal transplantation in secondary oxalosis. *Transplantation* 1988; **45**: 985–986.

39. Verani R, Nasir M, Foley R. Granulomatous interstitial nephritis after a jejunoileal bypass: an ultrastructural and histochemical study. *Am J Nephrol* 1989; **9**: 51–55.

40. Wharton R, D'Agati V, Magun AM, Whitlock R, Kunis CL, Appel GB. Acute deterioration of renal function associated with enteric hyperoxaluria. *Clin Nephrol* 1990; **34**: 116–121.

41. Levy FL. Ambulatory evaluation of nephrolithiasis: an update of a 1980 protocol. *Am J Med* 1995; **98**: 50–59.

42. Clarke AM, Chirnside A, Hill GL, Pope G, Stewart MK. Chronic dehydration and sodium depletion in patients with established ileostomies. *Lancet* 1967; **ii**: 740–743.

43. Kennedy HJ, Al-Dukaili EAS, Edwards CRW, Truelove SC. Water and ileostomy balance in subjects with a permanent ileostomy. *Gut* 1983; **24**: 702–705.

44. Rudman D, Dedonis JL, Fountain MT, Chandler JB, Gerron GG, Fleming GA, Kutner MH. Hypocitraturia in patients with gastrointestinal malabsorption. *N Engl J Med* 1980; **303**: 657–661.

45. Nicar MJ, Skurla C, Sakhaee K, Pak CYC. Low urinary citrate excretion in nephrolithiasis. *Urology* 1983; **21**: 8–14.

46. Archer HE, Dormer AE, Scowen EF, Watts RWE. Studies on the urinary excretion of oxalate by normal subjects. *Clin Sci* 1957; **16**: 405–411.

47. Marangella M, Fruttero B, Bruno M, Linari F. Hyperoxaluria in idiopathic calcium stone disease: further evidence of intestinal hyperabsorption of oxalate. *Clin Sci* 1982; **63**: 381–385.

48. Balcke P, Zazgornik J, Sunder-Plassmann G *et al.* Transient hyperoxaluria after ingestion of food rich in oxalic acid as a high-risk factor for calcium oxalate calculi. *Proc Eur Dial Transplant Assoc* 1985; **22**: 1163–1166.

49. Finch AM, Kasidas GP, Rose GA. Urine composition in normal subjects after oral ingestion of oxalate-rich foods. *Clin Sci* 1981; **60**: 411–418.

50. Hesse A, Bach D, Strenge A, Hicking W, Vahlensieck W. The effect of dietary oxalate loads on urinary oxalate excretion. In: Rose GA, Roberston WG, Watts RWE (eds) *Oxalate in Human Biochemistry and Clinical Pathology*. Wellcome Foundation: London, 1979, pp. 100–110.

51. Prenen JAC, Boer P, Dorhout Mees EJ. Absorption kinetics of oxalate from oxalate-rich food in man. *J Clin Nutr* 1984; **40**: 1007–1010.

52. Knickelbein RG, Aronson PS, Dobbins JW. Oxalate transport by anion exchange across rabbit ileal brush border. *J Clin Invest* 1986; **77**: 170–175.

53. Hatch M, Freel R, Vaziri ND. Intestinal excretion of oxalate in chronic renal failure. *J Am Soc Nephrol* 1994; **5**: 1339–1343.

54. Farooqui S, Thind SK, Nath R, Mahmood A. Intestinal absorption of oxalate in scorbutic and ascorbic acid supplemented guinea pigs. *Acta Vitaminol Enzymol* 1983; **5**: 235–241.

55. Farooqui S, Nath R, Thind SK, Mahmood A. Effect of pyridoxine deficiency on intestinal absorption of calcium and oxalate: chemical composition of bursh border membranes in rats. *Biochem Med* 1984; **32**: 34–42.

56. Kasidas GP, Rose GA. Oxalate content of some common foods: determination by an enzymatic method. *J Hum Nutr* 1980; **34**: 255–266.

57. Holmes RP, Goodman HO, Assimos DG. Dietary oxalate and its intestinal absorption. *Scanning Microsc* 1995; **9**: 1109–1120.

58. Zarembski PM, Hodgkinson A. The oxalic acid content of English diets. *Br J Nutr* 1962; **16**: 627–634.

59. Hodgkinson A. *Oxalic Acid in Biology and Medicine*. Academic Press: London, 1977, pp. 195–209.

60. Human Nutrition Information Service. Composition of foods: vegetables and vegetable products. United States Department of Agriculture 1984: Agriculture Handbook number 8–11.

61. Pak CYC. General guidelines in medical evaluation. In: Resnick MI, Pak CYC (eds) *Urolithiasis: a Medical and Surgical Reference*. WB Saunders: London, 1990, pp. 153–172.

62. Rao PN, Jenkins IL, Robertson WG, Peacock M, Blacklock NJ. The effect of 'high fibre biscuits' on urinary risk factors for stone formation. In: Schwille PO, Smith LH, Robertson WG, Vahlensieck W (eds) *Urolithiasis and Related Clinical Research*. Plenum Press: New York, 1985, pp. 425–428.

63. Brinkley L, McGuire J, Gregory J, Pak CYC. Bioavailability of oxalate in foods. *Urology* 1981; **17**: 534–538.

64. Brinkley LJ, Gregory J, Pak CYC. A further study of oxalate bioavailability in foods. *J Urol* 1990; **144**: 94–96.

65. Curhan GC, Willett WC, Rimm EB, Stampfer MJ. A prospective study of dietary calcium and other nutrients and the risk of symptomatic kidney stones. *N Engl J Med* 1993; **328**: 833–838.

66. Curhan GC, Willett WC, Speizer FE, Spiegleman D, Stampfer MJ. Comparison of dietary calcium with supplemental calcium and other nutrients as factors affecting the risk for kidney stones in women. *Ann Intern Med* 1997; **126**: 497–504.

67. Robertson WG, Peacock M. The cause of idiopathic calcium stone disease: hypercalciuria or hyperoxaluria? *Nephron* 1980; **26**: 105–110.

68. Smith LH, Diet and hyperoxaluria in the syndrome of idiopathic calcium oxalate lithiasis. *Am J Kidney Dis* 1991; **17**: 370–375.

69. Lemann J, Pleuss JA, Worcester EM, Hornick L, Schrab D, Hoffmann RG. Urinary oxalate excretion increases with body size and decreases with increasing dietary calcium intake among healthy adults. *Kidney Int* 1996; **49**: 200–208.

70. Messa P, Marangella M, Paganini L, Codardini M, Cruciatti A, Turrin D, Filiberto Z, Mioni G. Different dietary calcium intake and relative supersaturation of calcium oxalate in the urine of patients forming renal stones. *Clin Sci* 1997; **93**: 257–263.

71. Hayashi Y, Kaplan RA, Pak CYC. Effect of sodium cellulose phosphate therapy on crystallization of calcium oxalate in urine. *Metabolism* 1975; **24**: 1273–1278.

72. Chadwick VS, Modha K, Dowling RH. Mechanism for hyperoxaluria in patients with ileal dysfunction. *N Engl J Med* 1973; **289**: 172–176.

73. Stauffer JQ, Humphreys MH, Weir GJ. Acquired hyper-oxaluria with regional enteritis after ileal resection. Role of dietary oxalate. *Ann Intern Med* 1973; **79**: 383–391.

74. Hofmann AF, Tacker MM, Fromm H, Thomas PJ. Smith LH. Acquired hyperoxaluria and intestinal disease. Evidence that bile acid glycine is not a precursor of oxalate. *Mayo Clin Proc* 1973; **48**: 35–42.

75. Earnest DL, Johnson G, Williams HE, Admirand WH. Hyperoxaluria in patients with ileal resection: an abnormality in dietary oxalate absorption. *Gastroenterology* 1974; **66**: 1114–1122.

76. Earnest DL, Williams HE, Admirand WH. A physico-chemical basis for treatment of enteric hyperoxaluria. *Trans Assoc Am Physicians* 1975; **88**: 224–234.

77. Dobbins JW, Binder HJ. Importance of the colon in enteric hyperoxaluria. *N Engl J Med* 1977; **296**: 298–301.

78. Fairclough PD, Feest TG, Chadwick VS, Clark ML. Effect of sodium chenodeoxycholate on oxalate absorption from the excluded colon – a mechanism for 'enteric' hyperoxaluria. *Gut* 1977; **18**: 240–244.

79. Caspary WF, Tonissen J, Lankisch PG. Enteral hyperoxaluria. Effect of cholestyramine, calcium, neomycin, and bile acids on intestinal oxalate absorption in man. *Acta Hepato-Gastroenterol* 1977; **24**: 193–200.

80. Hylander E, Jarnum S, Juel Jensen H, Thale M. Enteric hyperoxaluria: dependence on small intestinal resection, colectomy, and steatorrhoea in chronic inflammatory bowel disease. *Scand J Gastroenterol* 1978; **13**: 577–588.

81. Modigliani R, Labayle D, Aymes C, Denvil R. Evidence for excessive absorption of oxalate by the colon in enteric hyperoxaluria. *Scand J Gastroenterol* 1978; **13**: 187–192.

82. Barilla DE, Notz C, Kennedy D, Pak CYC. Renal oxalate excretion following oral oxalate loads in patients with ileal disease and with renal and absorptive hypercalciurias. Effect of calcium and magnesium. *Am J Med* 1978; **64**: 579–585.

83. Tiselius H-G, Ahlstrand C, Lundstrom B, Nilsson M-A. ^{14}C-oxalate absorption by normal persons, calcium oxalate stone formers, and patients with surgically disturbed intestinal function. *Clin Chem* 1981; **27**: 1682–1685.

84. Hofmann AF, Laker MF, Dharmsathaphorn K, Sherr HP, Lorenzo D. Complex pathogenesis of hyperoxaluria after jejunoileal bypass surgery. Oxalogenic substances in diet contribute to urinary oxalate. *Gastroenterology* 1983; **84**: 293–300.

85. Nordenvall B, Hallberg D, Larsson L, Nord CE. Intestinal flora and oxalate excretion in patients with enteric hyperoxaluria. In: Schwille PO, Smith LH, Robertson WG, Vahlensieck W (eds) *Urolithiasis and Related Clinical Research*. Plenum Press: New York, 1985, pp. 139–142.

86. Lindsjo M, Danielson BG, Fellstrom B, Lithell H, Ljunghall S. Intestinal absorption of oxalate and calcium in patients with jejunoileal bypass. *Scand J Urol Nephrol* 1989; **23**: 283–289.

87. Obialo CI, Clayman RV, Matts JP, Fitch LL, Buchwald H, Gillis M, Hruska KA and the POSCH Group. Pathogenesis of nephrolithiasis post-partial ileal bypass surgery: Case–control study. *Kidney Int* 1991; **39**: 1249–1254.

88. McDonald GB, Earnest DL, Admirand WH. Hyperoxaluria correlates with fat malabsorption in patients with sprue. *Gut* 1977; **18**: 561–566.

89. Andersson H, Gillberg R. Urinary oxalate on a high-oxalate diet as a clinical test of malabsorption. *Lancet* 1977; **ii**: 677–678.

90. Rampton DS, Kasidas GP, Rose GA, Sarner M. Oxalate loading test: a screening test for steatorrhoea. *Gut* 1979; **20**: 1089–1094.

91. Rampton DS, McCullough DA, Sabbat JS, Salisbury JR, Flynn JV, Sarner M. Screening for steatorrhoea with an oxalate loading test. *Br Med J* 1984; **299**: 1419 (published erratum: *Br Med J* 1984; **288**: 1728).

92. Duce AM, Jerez E, Rapado A, Cajigal R. Intestinal absorption of oxalic acid in ileostomized patients. *Acta Chir Scand* 1988; **154**: 297–299.

93. Saunders DR, Sillery J, McDonald GB. Regional differences in oxalate absorption by rat intestine: evidence for excessive absorption by the colon in steatorrhoea. *Gut* 1975; **16**: 543–554.

94. Dobbins JW, Binder HJ. Effect of bile salts and fatty acids on the colonic absorption of oxalate. *Gastroenterology* 1976; **70**: 1096–1100.

95. Argenzio RA, Liacoz JA, Allison MJ. Role of intestinal oxalate degrading bacteria in the pathogenesis of enteric hyperoxaluria (abstract). *Gastroenterology* 1985; **88**: 1309.

96. Allison MJ, Cook HM, Milne DB, Gallagher S, Clayman RV. Oxalate degradation by gastrointestinal bacteria from humans. *J Nutr* 1986; **116**: 455–460.

97. Sidhu H, Hoppe B, Hesse A, Tenbrock K, Bromme S, Rietschel E, Peck AB. Absence of Oxalobacter formigenes in cystic fibrosis patients: a risk factor for hyperoxaluria. *Lancet* 1998; **352**: 1026–1029.

98. Camici M, Balestri PL, Lupetti S, Colizzi V, Falcone G. Urinary excretion of oxalate in renal failure. *Nephron* 1982; **30**: 269–270.

99. Argenzio RA, Liacox JA, Allison MJ. Intestinal oxalate-degrading bacteria reduce oxalate absorption and toxicity in guinea pigs. *J Nutr* 1988; **118**: 787–792.

100. Lindsjo M, Fellstrom B, Danielson BG, Kasidas GP, Rose GA, Ljunghall S. Hyperoxaluria or hypercalciuria in nephrolithiasis: the importance of renal tubular functions. *Eur J Clin Invest* 1990; **20**: 546–554.

101. Hylander E, Jarnum S, Frandsen I. Urolithiasis and hyperoxaluria in chronic inflammatory bowel disease. *Scand J Gastroenterol* 1979; **14**: 475–479.

102. Nordenvall B, Backman L, Burman P, Larsson L, Tiselius H-G. Low-oxalate, low-fat diet in hyperoxaluria patients following jejunoileal bypass. *Acta Chir Scand* 1983; **149**: 89–91.

103. Earnest DL, Gancher S, Admirand WH. Treatment of enteric hyperoxaluria with calcium and aluminium (abstract). *Gastroenterology* 1976; **70**: A23–881.

104. Hylander E, Jarnum S, Nielsen K. Calcium treatment of enteric hyperoxaluria after jejunoileal bypass for morbid obesity. *Scand J Gastroenterol* 1980; **15**: 349–352.

105. Laker MF, Hoffmann AF. Effective therapy of enteric hyperoxaluria: in vitro binding of oxalate by anion-exchange resins and aluminum hydroxide. *J Pharm Sci* 1981; **70**: 1065–1067.

106. Nordenvall B, Backman L, Larsson L, Tiselius H-G. Effects of calcium, aluminium, magnesium, and cholestyramine on hyperoxaluria in patients with jejunoileal bypass. *Acta Chir Scand* 1983; **149**: 93–98.

107. Lindsjo M, Fellstrom B, Ljunghall S, Wikstrom B, Danielson BG. Treatment of enteric hyperoxaluria with calcium-containing organic marine hydrocolloid. *Lancet* 1989; **ii**: 701–704.

108. Lindsjo M, Backman U, Ejerblad S, Fellstrom B, Wikstrom B, Danielson BG. Therapy with an organic marine hydrocolloid in patients with Crohn's disease with intractable diarrhoeas and enteric hyperoxaluria. *J Am Soc Nephrol* 1990; **1**: 336 (abstract).

109. D'Cruz DH, Gertner DJ, Kasidas GP, Rampton DS, Rose GA, Samuell CT. Failure of Allopurinol to modify urinary composition in enteric hyperoxaluria. *Br J Urol* 1989; **64**: 231–234.

110. Harper J, Mansell MA. Treatment of enteric hyperoxaluria. *Postgrad Med J* 1991; **67**: 219–222.

111. McLeod RS, Churchill DN. Urolithiasis complicating inflammatory bowel disease. *J Urol* 1992; **148**: 974–978.

112. Dean P, Joshi S, Kaminski DL. Long-term outcome of reversal of small intestinal bypass operations. *Am J Surg* 1990; **159**: 118–124.

16

Intestinal adaptation

R. Goodlad, J. Nightingale and R. Playford

INTRODUCTION

*I*ntestinal adaptation is the process that attempts to restore the total gut absorption of macronutrients, macrominerals and water, to that pertaining before an 'insult' (usually an intestinal resection). This process may involve an increased appetite and food consumption (hyperphagia), and structural and functional changes within the remaining gut. The gut has high rates of cell division, second only to the haemopoietic system, which allow it to adapt rapidly to altered circumstances and demands.

CHANGES OF ADAPTATION

The factors likely to maximize survival after an intestinal resection include weight loss (to reduce the nutritional requirements), an increased food intake (to compensate for malabsorption), slowing of intestinal transit and increasing intestinal absorptive area (to promote absorption). The stomach and colon could take on some of the absorptive functions of the small intestine.[1]

Hyperphagia

Weight loss occurs in all patients after a major intestinal resection, and with time a compensatory increase in food intake occurs to overcome macronutrient malabsorption. As much as 50% of macronutrients may not be absorbed in patients who ultimately manage without the need for parenteral nutrition.[2,3]

Structural adaptation

Stassoff is credited with being the first person to note small bowel 'hypertrophy' and increased absorption in the remaining small intestine of dogs after a large resection of small intestine.[4] After a resection of mainly jejunum in animals (leaving some ileum and an intact colon), there is structural adaptation with dilatation and elongation of the remaining intestine (compensatory hypertrophy), and the villi become longer, crypts deepen and the cell number over a given length of villus increases (epithelial hyperplasia),[5–8] but the size of the cell does not change. These changes are much more marked in an ileal than a jejunal remnant.[6,7]

In man, various case reports have described dilatation of the stomach, duodenum, jejunum, ileum and colon after a massive small bowel resection.[9–15] There is a risk that the findings in some reports reflect not structural adaptation but bowel dilatation proximal to an anastomosic stricture. One report suggests that an increase in bowel length occurred,[9] however a very carefully documented set of observations in one unique patient does not support this.[16] The patient had a mesenteric infarction and was left with 105 cm of small intestine (95 cm jejunum and 10 cm terminal ileum) and a functioning colon. She subsequently had four caesarean sections over 5 years; on each occasion bowel length and diameter was measured and showed no change from the measurements taken at the time of the original resection.[16]

Jejunum–colon

There is little evidence for structural jejunal adaptation in patients with jejunum anastomosed to a functioning colon. Two reports of jejunal biopsies from 4 patients with jejunum anastomosed to colon showed epithelial hyperplasia,[17,18] and a larger study of 10 patients showed, not hyperplasia, but atrophy in most such patients.[19]

Jejunostomy

No structural changes have been observed in biopsies from the distal duodenal mucosa in patients with an established jejunostomy.[20]

Functional adaptation

Functional adaptation is demonstrated by measuring increases (with time or compared with normal subjects) in the absorption of macro- and/or micronutrients over a given length of bowel. Functional adaptation may be the result of structural changes, a slowing of transit rate or intracellular molecular events (e.g. increased transport and/or enzyme activity). No changes in the activity of mucosal enzymes have been demonstrated.[21] There is no evidence that remaining jejunum acquires any of the specialized transport functions of the ileum (e.g. vitamin B_{12} or bile salt absorption), or develops tight intracellular junctions.

Jejunum–colon

In patients with jejunum in continuity with a functioning colon there is a small reduction in faecal weight in the 3 months following a small bowel resection.[22] There is also increased jejunal absorption of macronutrients, water, sodium, glucose and calcium with time,[18,23–25] and an increased chance of the patient being able to stop parenteral nutrition.[26]

Jejunostomy

Patients who have an ileostomy following a colectomy (usually for ulcerative colitis) have a reduction in intestinal output over the first 4 months.[27–29] This is not the case, however, when there has also been an ileal resection. Hill et al. showed, in a study of patients who had an 'ileostomy' after an ileal resection, that there was no decrease in ileostomy water, sodium and potassium losses from 11 days after the resection to 6 months.[29] Nightingale et al. demonstrated no change in the nutritional/fluid requirements of patients with a jejunostomy from 6 to 24 months after their last resection.[30]

There is no good evidence for structural adaptation in either group, however there is evidence for functional adaptation in patients with jejunum anastomosed to a functioning colon and in patients with an ileostomy. Patients with a jejunostomy show no structural or functional adaptive changes.

TIME COURSE OF ADAPTIVE CHANGES

Initial changes are very rapid. In the rat, there is an increase in mucosal DNA synthesis within 24–36 hours after a bowel resection. Villus epithelial hyperplasia, probably occurring as a result of increased crypt cell production rather than villus tip cell loss, is evident at 1–2 weeks and maximal at 1 month.[7]

In 1959, Pullan described three clinical phases (Ch. 12) after intestinal resection in man that left the colon remaining. In phase 2 (which follows the large fluid losses of phase 1), the emphasis shifts from fluid balance to nutritional support, and over the next 12–24 months the diarrhoea improves and the amount of nutritional support is reduced or stopped. It is during this phase that most adaptation is occurring. In phase 3 there is no further improvement and no major adaptive changes occur.[31]

While major adaptive changes are evident within a few weeks in those with a retained colon, the full benefits may take years to be complete. For example, intestinal calcium absorption may continue to increase for more than 2 years after the resection.[25] The need for continuing parenteral nutrition is apparent earlier: if parenteral nutrition is needed for 2 years after a bowel resection, the chances of subsequently being able to stop it are 6%.[26]

FACTORS INVOLVED IN INTESTINAL ADAPTATION

The study of the mechanism of growth control and adaptation in the intestine has focused on four main areas, namely luminal nutrition, pancreatico-biliary secretions, trophic hormones and specific growth factors (Fig. 16.1).

Luminal nutrients

The control of cell renewal in the gastrointestinal tract is complex and multifactorial. The bowel shows a remarkable ability to adapt to changes in dietary modification. Major reductions in the weight of the small intestine and colon take place during fasting or when a patient receives total parenteral nutrition (TPN) and these rapidly reverse on the re-introduction of a normal diet. Studies in the late 1970s and 1980s examined the effects of chemically defined diets (elemental diets) on small intestinal and colonic growth. They showed that elemental diets maintained intestinal mass well into the proximal small intestine, but the colon became atrophic to a similar extent to that seen with parenteral feeding.[32,33] Hyperplasia is seen if food intake is increased after an intestinal resection; a similar situation occurs in animals exposed to the cold which have hyperphagia followed by epithelial cell hyperplasia.

The presence of food within the intestinal lumen ('luminal nutrition') is the most potent stimulus for intestinal epithelial cell proliferation,[34] thus there is an increasing consensus that patients who are receiving parenteral nutrition in an intensive care environment should continue to receive some nutrition via the enteral route to prevent mucosal atrophy. Some studies suggest that this results in a lower infection rate, possibly because of reduced bacterial translocation.[35] The action of the luminal nutrients may be direct, as has been suggested for glutamine and the short-chain fatty acids, or may be indirect via hormones or specific growth factors. Supplementation of an elemental diet with glutamine, the preferred substrate for the enterocyte, in an attempt to maintain intestinal mass has produced conflicting reports.[36]

The presence of nutrients in the colon may be important in causing small intestinal adaptation. A colonic infusion of glucose (compared with mannitol) in rats caused jejunal adaptation (measured by an increase in the crypt cell production rate, mucosal wet weight, DNA and protein content per unit length of

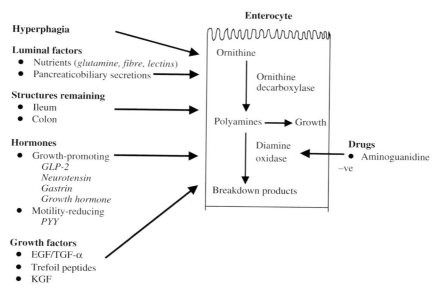

Figure 16.1 – Factors affecting intestinal adaptation.

small intestine).[37] The authors found raised levels of plasma enteroglucagon and suggested that this was the colonic growth factor that stimulated small bowel growth.[37] Short-chain fatty acids play a part in small bowel adaptation, as reduction of colonic carbohydrate fermentation in rats (by giving metronidazole) reduced small intestinal adaptation.[38]

Colonic adaptation

Most of the literature on intestinal adaptation has concentrated on the small intestine, and few accounts of colonic adaptation following surgical interventions are available. This may reflect both the interests of the investigators and the fact that adaptation of the colon is more difficult to quantify as the proliferation rates are slower than in the small bowel. Papers on colonic adaptation also tend to reflect a different perspective, focusing predominantly on the effects of diet, especially dietary 'fibre'. Different regions of the colon vary in their sensitivity to dietary manipulation, hormones and growth factors.[39,40]

Dietary manipulation of colonic growth is relatively easy to achieve as most absorption of simple components occurs in the proximal small bowel. Fibre-free elemental diets will therefore effectively starve the colon, leading to distal atrophy.[41,42] This atrophy can be reversed by the addition of dietary fibre, and it was at first thought that these effects were caused by mechanical distension (bulk). However, inert bulk does not

reverse the atrophy.[43] The effects of fibre on colonic proliferation are marked, but are not seen in germ-free rats,[44] indicating that it is the products of fibre fermentation (short-chain fatty acids; SCFAs) that are trophic. SCFAs, which include acetic, propionic and butyric acid, stimulate cell division *in vivo*. However, *in vitro* their main action is to increase cell differentiation. SCFAs can also stimulate cell migration.[45] When the colon is considered as a fermentation chamber, it follows that any material that cannot be digested by endogenous enzymes acts as a substrate for the colonic microflora. Plant fibre, starches resistant to amylase, intestinal mucins and sloughed cells can all be fermented in the colon to give SCFAs that can be absorbed and metabolized by the host.[46,47] The effects of fibre are predominantly indirect, but some trophic effects, especially on the small bowel, can be direct[48] and may be linked to viscosity.[49] In addition to its effects on the colon, fibre can also directly stimulate proliferation in the gastric glands[50] and the intestinal muscle layers.[42,51,52]

Further evidence that SCFAs are trophic to the colon has been provided by infusion studies.[53] There is debate about the mechanisms underlying this adaptation: many believe it to be caused by 'luminal nutrition' as colonocytes preferentially metabolize SCFAs, especially butyrate. The fact that colonocytes metabolize SCFAs does not necessarily imply however that they use it as a preferred fuel – it could be that it is their task to 'detoxify' the SCFAs.

Plant lectins – a group of agents that can influence cell division in the intestine – are a large group of non-immune proteins that recognize and reversibly bind to specific carbohydrate groups. They are omnipresent constituents of plants and are abundant in the diet. Cell-surface molecules, including receptors, are often glycosylated, and lectins presumably act by binding to these.[54] Certain lectins, such as those from peanuts and kidney beans, increase the proliferation of intestinal cells of animals and in human colonic explants.[55] Other lectins are internalized and bind to the nuclear membrane; in the case of those present in mushrooms they are internalized and inhibit growth.

Pancreatico-biliary secretions

Pancreatico-biliary secretions are important luminal growth factors.[56–58] Gastric and duodenal juices both increase the size of ileal villi, however the effect of pancreatico-biliary secretions is even greater.[1] Diversion of pancreatico-biliary secretions causes distal hyperplasia. The effect is not solely due to the enzymatic digestion of macronutrients giving luminal nutrition: infusions of pancreatic extracts into isolated intestinal segments caused greater villous hyperplasia than an amino acid mixture,[56] and in rats the effect of a pancreatico-biliary diversion is still seen when they are fed an elemental diet.[57] Rats given total parenteral nutrition develop marked pancreatic atrophy[59] which can further impair the adaptive response.

Hormones

Some of the most convincing evidence that circulating factors (hormones) are involved in gut adaptation comes from cross-circulation and non-continuity experiments. Intestinal segments surgically out of continuity with the main flow of digesta can still respond to intestinal resection, implying the action of a systemic factor.[60] Similar conclusions were obtained in early parabiosis (cross-circulation) studies.[61] The identity of the circulating trophic factors is, however, still not definitively established.

Gastrin

The physiological role of gastrin in human gut adaptation is still unclear but must be considered as hypergastrinaemia has been described after a major intestinal resection (Ch. 12). Infusions of gastrin into animal models have major effects on stomach growth and especially on gastric endocrine cell growth.[62] The gastric hyperplasia, which is associated with acid-induced inhibition in rats, is mediated via gastrin.[63] In rats, life-long gastrin enterochromaffin-like (ECL) cell hyperplasia[64,65] can lead to non-metastasizing carcinoid tumours of low malignancy.[66] This led to concern over long-term use of acid suppressants in humans. However, present evidence suggests that rats may be particularly prone to these types of tumours[67] and, more importantly, it must be remembered that gastric carcinoids are relatively rare in man. This is true even in patients who have massive hypergastrinaemia (several times greater than that found in patients taking high-dose acid suppressants) associated with the Zollinger–Ellison syndrome or pernicious anaemia.[68] The original suggestion[69] that gastrin has a general trophic role throughout the gastrointestinal tract was not supported by infusion studies.[70] Studies using gastrin-deficient mice generated through targeted gene disruption found a marked change in gastric architecture but no difference in the cell proliferation rate in the stomach; however, cell proliferation was reduced in the colon.[71]

It has been suggested that it may not be gastrin itself but its intermediates, such as glycine-extended gastrin, that are trophic. Mice that overexpress glycine-extended gastrin show a large increase in colonic mucosal thickness and colonic proliferation.[72]

Enteroglucagon

Enteroglucagon was for many years considered a front-runner as the active agent in causing intestinal adaptation. Enteroglucagon-producing tumours were associated with villus enlargement.[73,74] Many studies have shown excellent correlation between crypt cell production rate and plasma enteroglucagon[75,76] and have demonstrated enhanced intestinal transport.[77] All of these studies provided only circumstantial evidence, as pure enteroglucagon was difficult to synthesize until the late 1990s. When synthetic enteroglucagon was infused into parenterally fed rats, it had little effect on gastrointestinal cell proliferation.[78]

Glucagon-like peptide-2 (GLP-2)

Enteroglucagon is only one member of a family of related peptides derived from the pre-pro glucagon family of peptides, and the active member is now thought to be glucagon-like peptide-2. GLP-2 is an enterocyte-specific growth hormone that in mice causes small and large bowel villus/crypt growth and increases small and large bowel length and weight, and in pigs reduces gastric antral motility.[79–82] It seems likely that it is the most important mucosal growth-stimulating hormone.[83]

It is not surprising to find that GLP-2 levels are low in patients with a jejunostomy as the L cells that produce it in the ileum and colon have been removed;[84] however, it may explain why patients with a jejunostomy show no evidence of structural or functional adaptation after a resection.[85] In contrast, patients with a short bowel and preserved colon have high plasma levels of GLP-2,[86] and this may explain why they undergo a degree of adaptation after a resection. It will be interesting to see if GLP-2 levels gradually increase after a resection (correlating with the degree of intestinal adaptation) and whether GLP-2 levels can be used to measure the amount of intestinal adaptation that has occurred.

Peptide YY

Peptide YY, like GLP-2, is produced by the L cells of the ileum and colon; it slows gastric emptying and small bowel transit and may be responsible for the 'ileal' and 'colonic' brakes.[87] At physiological doses in man, peptide YY increases small bowel transit time and reduces stimulated intestinal secretion.[88] Peptide YY serum levels are high in patients with a retained colon and low in patients with a jejunostomy,[89] thus it may be responsible for part of the functional adaptation that occurs in patients with a retained colon. It is unlikely to be responsible for any structural changes as it does not induce gut growth in rats fed only with parenteral nutrition.[90,91]

Neurotensin

Neurotensin is produced in the ileum. Neurotensin levels are low in patients with a jejunum in continuity with a functioning colon and also in patients with a jejunostomy.[89] Infusion experiments in rats suggest a potential trophic effect on the small intestine but not the colon.[92]

Growth hormone

Growth hormone stimulates the development of most tissues during development and stimulates mitosis in the duodenal crypts of hypophysectomized rats.[93] It increases small and large bowel mass and increases sodium, water and amino acid absorption from the small bowel. Growth hormone influences plasma levels of other circulating hormones (e.g. gastrin and insulin-like growth factor-1) and these gastrointestinal effects

might be mediated through intermediary trophic hormones. Preliminary studies suggest that growth hormone may be of value in preserving gut function in septic patients on intensive care units.[94] Prolactin, which is closely related to growth hormone, may have similar effects, especially during lactation.

Insulin

Manipulation of endogenous levels of insulin had no effect on the crypt cell production rate.[95]

Growth factors/cytokines

Growth factors and cytokines are extracellular signalling proteins or peptides, the cytokines being generally considered as local mediators in cell-to-cell communication[96] while the growth factors were originally defined on the basis of their stimulation of growth or cell division. Some of these factors have relatively broad sites of action: for example, epidermal growth factor (EGF) acts on multiple organs by several different actions, including influencing gastric acid secretion, gut growth and repair.

Many growth factors were named soon after their isolation and were classed on the basis of nanogram concentrations stimulating DNA synthesis in serum-deprived cell cultures. Consequently, the physiological role of many 'growth factors' is still not known despite the abundance of information regarding their genes, structure and receptor signalling pathways. It is likely that the main biological roles of many of these factors are different to that which might be deduced from their name. Many have more than one action, thus they may have proliferative or anti-proliferative effects on different tissues as well as effects unrelated to proliferation.[97,98] The action of growth factors may also differ according to the state of development of the target cell type; therefore the importance of individual growth factors may vary during fetal, neonatal and adult development.

Although many papers have examined the effect of an individual peptide on mucosal function or repair, it has been difficult to understand their overall role in mucosal homeostasis as the site of production, mechanism of action and change in concentration at sites of injury vary according to the peptide being examined. We have therefore found it useful to devise a functional classification of these peptides based on their overall role in maintaining gut growth or in stimulating repair.[99] They can be considered as belonging to one of three broad groups: mucosal integrity peptides, luminal surveillance peptides, and rapid-response peptides. This classification requires a distinction between protective actions and repair mechanisms. Some protective actions can be very rapid – 'cytoprotection', for example, can occur within minutes – while other mechanisms may take days. These actions can be mediated via several different routes including maintainance of blood flow or alteration of other mucosal regulatory proteins. Whatever the cause of mucosal injury, the healing process tends to occur in two main phases: the initial restitutive response in which epithelial migration attempts to cover the defect (this process starts within one hour of the injury), and a later increase in proliferation that begins about 24 hours after injury. It is necessary to distinguish between factors influencing the processes of restitution and those influencing proliferation (the two not being mutually exclusive). It is now becoming apparent that growth factors can be subclassified along these lines.[100]

Mucosal integrity peptides

The mucosal integrity peptides include transforming growth factor alpha and pancreatic secretory trypsin inhibitor which are constitutively expressed in the mucosa throughout the gastrointestinal tract and function to maintain normal mucosal integrity.

Transforming growth factor alpha (TGF-α) is a 50 amino acid peptide, with 35% sequence homology to EGF, that is present in the gastrointestinal mucosa throughout the gastrointestinal tract (though not in secretions) and binds to the 'EGF' receptor. It is important to note, however, that its major distribution is in the superficial (non-proliferative) zones. It may therefore be that its major role is to maintain cell migration and differentiation as opposed to proliferation. TGF-α 'knock-out' mice have a relatively normal phenotype;[101] studies suggest that they have an increased susceptibility to injurious agents to the colon[102] but they do not have an increased susceptibility to indomethacin-induced small intestinal injury.[103]

Luminal surveillance peptides

Epidermal growth factor (EGF) is the most studied example of the luminal surveillance peptides. It is continuously secreted into the lumen but may only be of major importance in the stimulation of mucosal repair following a breach in the mucosa. There is now a wealth of detailed structural and genetic information about the EGF molecule and its receptor (EGFR; c-erbb1).[104] Epidermal growth factor (EGF) was first isolated from the submandibular salivary glands of mice and found to stimulate precocial eyelid

Table 16.1 – Gastrointestinal functions of EGF[98]

Action	Effect	Possible secondary message
Proliferation		
Cell division	↑	
Protection		
Acid secretion	↓	Protein kinase C, cAMP
Bicarbonate secretion	↑	Prostaglandins
Mucus secretion	↑	Prostaglandins
GI blood flow	↑	β-Adrenergic, NO, prostaglandins
Restitution	↑	Cell migration, prostaglandins
Mucosal protection	↑	Proliferation, polyamines, mucus, trefoil peptides
Digestion/absorption		
Amylase secretion-pancreas	↑(↓)	cAMP phospholipase C
NaCl and glucose uptake	↑	Brush border area, Na+-glucose co-transporter, lipids
Chloride secretion	↓(↑)	Phosphatidylinositol 3-kinase
Permeability	↑	
Motility		
Longitudinal smooth muscle contraction	↑	Prostaglandins
Circular smooth muscle contraction	↑	(desensitizes) not prostaglandins
Gastric emptying/small bowel transit	↓	

( ): = Some studies suggest the opposite effect.

opening and tooth eruption. Human EGF, originally known as urogastrone, was independently identified in the urine of pregnant women. It is formed as a pre-pro molecule of 1217 amino acids which is processed by the salivary glands to the mature EGF_{1-53} peptide. EGF is predominantly produced in the salivary glands and the Brunner's glands of the duodenum. It is also present in lower concentrations in many biological fluids, such as plasma and milk. When administered systemically, EGF, like many growth factors, has a wide range of actions on the gut (Table 16.1, Fig. 16.2). EGF is partially digested to a less active form in the stomach by gastric juice and completely digested by fasting small intestinal juice, but not if food is present. It probably only binds to damaged areas of bowel.

The physiological role of EGF, however, continues to be a matter of some controversy.[105] One of the major problems in understanding its role is that in the majority of the previous studies EGF was administered systemically whereas, in a physiological context, EGF is present within the gut lumen. Attempts to understand its physiology have focused on four main areas: intraluminal administration, distribution of the EGF receptor, removal of the salivary glands and the production of knock-out mice.

Intraluminal administration. At first thought, this approach seems the most logical as it attempts to reproduce the physiological site of delivery. EGF administered via this route stimulates growth of the bowel in the neonatal rat and also in damaged bowel (where the permeability is increased). However, there is continuing controversy about the potential influence of intraluminal EGF in the adult non-damaged gut. Discrepancies between reports are likely to be the result of different methodological approaches (e.g. species studied, dosages or bolus versus continuous infusions of EGF). One of the earliest studies reported that intraluminal administration of EGF into totally parenterally fed rats was not trophic to the bowel.[106] Subsequently, however, it was shown that EGF is digested into less active forms in gastric juice and was completely digested into inactive forms in the fasted (or TPN-fed) bowel because residual luminal proteases were present within the small intestine.[107,108] The original TPN-fed rat experiment was therefore reproduced, but also examining the effect of adding co-infusions of soya bean trypsin inhibitor to prevent the digestion of intraluminal EGF. Under these circumstances, a trophic response to luminal EGF was found, particularly when the trypsin inhibitor was co-infused.[109] The bowel under these circumstances may

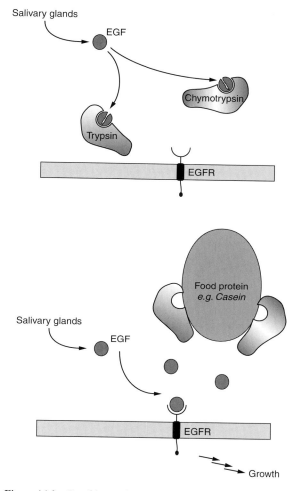

Figure 16.2 – Possible mechanism behind the trophic effect of food. EGF is digested in the small intestine in the fasted state by unopposed proteases (a). The presence of food proteins may block the active sites of the proteases, allowing the luminal EGF to interact with its receptor (b).

not, however, be normal, as TPN-fed animals have increased gut permeability. Studies examining the effect of luminal EGF on animal models involving resection and adaptation suffer from the same problem: surgical manipulation and anastomosis may well expose any (basolaterally placed) EGF receptors to the luminal surface.

Distribution of the EGF receptor. If the EGF is to stimulate a trophic response, it must interact with its receptor. The earlier literature provides apparently conflicting reports, although most of the more recent studies in the rat suggest that the EGF receptor is restricted to the basolateral membranes only.[110] Our recent studies in humans suggest that, in the normal adult gastrointestinal tract, the EGF receptor is localized only on basolateral membranes.[111] In the non-damaged bowel, luminal EGF is therefore unlikely to be able to reach its receptor. Preliminary immunolocalization studies, however, suggest that the distribution might be different in damaged human bowel.

Removal of the salivary glands. Removal of the salivary glands from rats markedly reduces the concentration of EGF present in gastric juice; however, gastric ulceration does not occur spontaneously and gastric acid secretion does not change.[112] Several studies suggest that mucosal growth within the stomach of the animals is reduced by this procedure, although the small intestine and colon are probably not affected.[113] Caution has to be shown, however, in extrapolating these results from rats to man.

Production of knock-out mice. Recent advances in molecular biology allow us to 'knock out' the gene of interest in mice strains. Disruption of the EGF receptor in such 'knock-out' mice had major effects in many organs of the body including the gut, where severe intestinal ulceration was seen.[114] The phenotype from different strains varied markedly, other groups finding no evidence of colitis.[115,116] These findings emphasize the need to show caution in extrapolating the results from mice to humans. In addition, it is important to note that when the EGF receptor is knocked out, all ligands for this receptor, which include TGF-α and amphiregulin, are also inactivated.

Taken together, the studies to date suggest that the major role of EGF is to stimulate repair at sites of injury and that it plays a relatively minor role in the maintenance of the normal gut growth in the human adult.

Rapid-response peptides

The rapid-response peptides are the trefoil peptide family (e.g. spasmolytic polypeptide); their production is rapidly unregulated at sites of damage and is likely to be of particular importance in the early stages of mucosal repair. The trefoil peptide family obtain their name from the original description of their structure, when it was likened to a three-leaf structure. They were first found in pancreatic juice. They are very stable and are not absorbed in the small bowel but reach the colon where they are broken down by colonic bacteria. Their action is extremely rapid and they are the first peptides produced after the gut is damaged (even before TGF-α). Although they are present in the normal gut, their expression is markedly unregulated at sites of injury in conditions such as inflammatory bowel disease and peptic ulceration.[117]

Administration of trefoil peptides systemically[118] and, at much higher doses, into the gut lumen,[119] has been shown to reduce injury and stimulate repair in models of gastric injury. In addition, transgenic mice that overexpress a trefoil peptide have been shown to have an increased resistance to small intestinal injury,[120] suggesting that the trefoil peptides may play an important role in the repair process. This idea is supported by recent studies showing that 'knock-out' of the trefoil peptide intestinal trefoil factor (ITF; TFF3) resulted in a relatively normal phenotype in mice but that these mice had a markedly increased sensitivity to injurious agents.[121] This family of peptides therefore occupies an unusual position in the role of peptides in mucosal integrity and repair in that they stimulate the repair process, probably by initiating restitution,[118,122] without stimulating proliferation.[118,123]

Other peptides

The list of peptides involved in mucosal integrity and repair continues to grow. Table 16.2 lists some of the more common peptides researched in the area of intestinal growth and adaptation. Three further peptides worthy of mention are transforming growth factor beta (TGF-β), basic fibroblast growth factor (β-FGF) and keratinocyte growth factor (KGF). TGF-β may function to turn off proliferation of the enterocytes once they have left the crypt; in addition, it may also act as an intermediary signalling peptide for pro-migratory effects of EGF and TGF-α on epithelial cells.[124] β-FGF is present in the normal gastric mucosa and is a potent stimulant of proliferation. Preliminary studies suggest that TGF-β tissue levels are reduced in patients with gastric ulcers and that recombinant β-FGF can stimulate ulcer healing in humans.[32] KGF, originally known as FGF-7, has been demonstrated to markedly stimulate proliferation of hepatocytes and epithelial cells throughout the rat gastrointestinal tract,[125] and can alter crypt branching.[126] Moreover, KGF, like EGF, also stimulates mucus production, but unlike EGF does not stimulate cell migration and is not cytoprotective.[127]

Table 16.2 – Overview of action of some gastrointestinal agents that may affect small intestinal adaptation

Agent	Action						
	Proliferation	Acid secretion	Cell migration	Cytoprotection	Mucus secretion	Chloride production	Muscle contraction
Dietary factors							
Lectins	↑/↓			?			
SCFAs	↑		↑				
Hormones							
Enteroglucagon	↑	↓					
Gastrin	(↑)	↑					
Neurotensin	↑						
Somatostatin	↓						
Insulin	–						
PYY	–						
GH	↑						
Bombesin							
Mucosal integrity peptides							
TGF-α	↑	↓		↑	↑		
(20×> in gut)							
Luminal surveillance peptides							
EGF	↑	↓	↑	↑	↑	↑/↓	↑
Rapid response (trefoil) peptides							
TFF1 (pS2)	–	–	↑	↑		–	
TFF2 (SP)	(↑/↓)		↑	↑			(↓)
TFF3 (ITF)	–		↑	↑		↑	
TGF-β	↓(↑)		↑				
β-FGF	↑						
KGF (FGF7)	↑	↓	–	–	↑		
Others							
Prostaglandins	↑		(↑)				
IGF-I	↑						
IGF-II	↑						
FGF							
PDGF							
VEGF							

TFF = trefoil factor: TFF1 was pS2, TFF2 was SP (spasmolytic peptide), TFF3 was ITF (intestinal trefoil peptide); FGF = fibroblast growth factor; IGF = insulin-like growth factor; PDGF = platelet-derived growth factor; VEGF = vascular endothelial growth factor.

THERAPIES TO PROMOTE ADAPTATION

Many treatments have been tried in order to enhance intestinal growth (e.g. fibre, growth hormone, glutamine, EGF, GLP-2, aminoguanidine). Studies using peptides to slow intestinal transit (e.g. peptide YY or an analogue[128]) have not yet been performed.

Fibre, growth hormone and glutamine

The value of fibre supplementation is of great interest, but caution must be shown in assuming that the available 'fibre supplements', including drinks and yoghurts, have the same clinical outcome as a natural high-fibre diet which will be rich in many more nutrients.[129] It is also possible that some supplements, if they stimulate proliferation, may also increase the risk of carcinogenesis.[130] Some intervention studies appear either to show no effect[131] or to substantiate this view.[132,133]

An uncontrolled study, in which subcutaneous growth hormone (mean 0.11 mg/kg/d, range 0.03–0.14), oral glutamine (30 g) and a high-carbohydrate low-fat diet were given for 4 weeks, found that 57% of 47 patients (all but 4 had a colon remaining and all but 7 had received parenteral nutrition for 2 or more years) were able to stop parenteral nutrition.[134] The beneficial effect on stool weight reduction and protein absorption was greatest with the three treatments together; diet or glutamine alone was not effective.[134,135] Two subsequent randomized double-blind placebo-controlled cross-over trials have shown no clinical benefit from this treatment.[136,137] In the first study of 8 patients (6 had a jejunostomy and 2 a retained colon, all had received parenteral nutrition for more than 2 years, and all were taking no anti-diarrhoeal or antisecretory drugs), subcutaneous growth hormone (0.14 mg/kg/d), oral glutamine (0.63 g/kg/d) and a high-carbohydrate, low-fat diet was given for 21 days. While it showed significantly greater sodium and potassium absorption and a slowing of gastric emptying and 2-hour stomal output; there was no change in stool output, fat or nitrogen absorption or small bowel morphology.[136] In the second study, 8 patients who had received parenteral nutrition for more than 3 years and had a short bowel (4 had a retained colon) received the same dose of growth hormone and glutamine for 28 days; 5 days after treatment was stopped there was no significant improvement in the absorption of energy, carbohydrate, nitrogen, water, sodium or magnesium.[137] There are concerns that patients with acromegaly are more prone to colonic polyps and colon cancer, thus long-term therapy with growth hormone may entail risks.[138]

Epidermal growth factor

Systemic administration of recombinant EGF may prove to be of value in treating ulcerative conditions of the gastrointestinal tract. An infusion of recombinant epidermal growth factor 100 ng/kg/h for two 6-day periods with 5 days between the courses was given to one infant with microvillous atrophy. It stimulated crypt cell proliferation and increased villus height but did not improve absorption of xylose.[139] Another report, using the same treatment regimen in an infant with necrotizing enterocolitis, showed benefit.[140]

Luminal, as opposed to systemic, administration of EGF may be of clinical value but will probably need to be delivered in a site-specific release formulation or co-administered with protease inhibitors to preserve biological activity.

GLP-2

GLP-2 400 μg, a dose that exceeds physiological levels, was given twice a day by subcutaneous injection to 8 patients with a jejunostomy for 35 days. Energy absorption improved by a mean of 3.5%, stool weight reduced by 11%, body weight increased by 1.2 kg and the gastric emptying of solids slowed.[141] This may represent an important new treatment for patients with a jejunostomy in whom GLP-2 levels are very low. A new preparation of GLP-2, with alanine substituted by glycine at position 2, is resistant to the enzyme dipeptidyl peptidase IV which degrades GLP-2.

Aminoguanidine

Within an epithelial cell, ornithine is converted by ornithine decarboxylase to polyamines (putrescine, spermidine and spermine) which are responsible for inducing epithelial hyperplasia.[142] Their concentration in jejunostomy fluid rises on refeeding;[143] this may be due to the nutrients, mucosal blood flow, a neural or a humoral mechanism. Any mechanism that increases the synthesis or slows the removal of polyamines could lead to cellular hyperplasia and improved absorption. Aminoguanidine, which inhibits diamine oxidase and thus reduces polyamine breakdown, has been used successfully in animals to induce epithelial hyperplasia and increased nutrient absorption.[144]

Colostrum

A novel nutritional adjuvant, which appears to give hope for the prevention and treatment of gastrointestinal injury, is bovine colostrum. Colostrum is rich in growth factors (including EGF) and antibacterial peptides. Clinical trials are presently under way in which it is being used to prevent chemotherapy-induced and indomethacin-induced gut injury.[145]

Recombinant peptides

The advent of molecular biology now allows a variety of recombinant growth factors to be produced relatively cheaply. Recombinant peptides may well prove useful for conditions such as necrotizing enterocolitis, chemotherapy-induced mucositis and inflammatory bowel disease. Caution must be shown in administering potent growth factors via the systemic circulation, as there is some clinical concern over uncontrolled proliferation in potentially pre-malignant cells throughout the body. Luminal administration of growth factors could reduce these risks but problems of proteolytic digestion will require specific formulations.

Grow small intestinal mucosa

A novel, still experimental, way of improving absorption in those with a retained colon is to replace colonic mucosa with small intestinal mucosa and thus to try to change colonic function to that of the small intestine.[146]

SUMMARY

The control of gut growth and adaptation is complex. Following a large resection of small intestine, food intake increases (hyperphagia) to cope with malabsorption. Structural and functional adaptation occurs in the ileum after a predominantly jejunal resection. Functional, but not structural, jejunal adaptation occurs after an ileal resection that leaves the colon in situ. There is no evidence for structural or functional jejunal adaptation in patients with a jejunostomy. Specific dietary modification (e.g. high polysaccharide) continues to offer the potential for improved clinical outcome. Treatments to induce adaptation are directed mainly at increasing mucosal growth (e.g. EGF, GLP-2 and possibly KGF). Drugs that reduce transit (e.g. peptide YY or an analogue) show potential as future treatments.

REFERENCES

1. Williamson RCN, Chir M. Intestinal adaptation. *N Engl J Med* 1978; **298:** 1393–1402, 1444–1450.

2. Messing B, Pigot F, Rongier M, Morin MC, Ndeindoum U, Rambaud JC. Intestinal absorption of free oral alimentation in very bowel syndrome. *Gastroenterology* 1991; **100:** 1502–1508.

3. Crenn P, Beloucif L, Morin MC, Thuillier F, Messing B. Adaptive hyperphagia and net digestive absorption in short bowel patients. *Gastroenterology* 1997; **112:** A356.

4. Stassoff B. Experimentelle Untersuchungen uber die Kompensatorischen Vorgange bei Darmresektionen. *Beitr Klin Chir* 1914; **89:** 527–586.

5. Flint J M. The effect of extensive resections of the small intestine. *Bull Johns Hopkins Hosp* 1912; **23:** 127–144.

6. Nygaard K. Resection of the small intestine in rats. III. Morphological changes in the intestinal tract. *Acta Chir Scand* 1967; **133:** 233–348.

7. Dowling R H, Booth C C. Structural and functional changes following small intestinal resection in the rat. *Clin Sci* 1967; **32:** 139–149.

8. Weser E, Hernandez M H. Studies of small bowel adaptation after intestinal resection in the rat. *Gastroenterology* 1971; **60:** 69–75.

9. McClenahan JE, Fisher B. Physiologic effect of massive small intestinal resection and colectomy. *Am J Surg* 1950; **79:** 684–688.

10. Martin J R, Patee C J, Gardener C, Marien B. Massive resection of the small intestine. *Can Med Assoc J* 1953; **69:** 429–433.

11. Trafford HS. The outlook after massive resection of small intestine, with a report of two cases. *Br J Surg* 1956; **44:** 10–13.

12. Clayton BE, Cotton DA. A study of malabsorption after resection of the entire jejunum and proximal half of the ileum. *Gut* 1961; **2:** 18–22.

13. Meyer HW. Sixteen-year survival following extensive resection of small and large intestine for thrombosis of the superior mesenteric artery. *Surgery* 1961; **51:** 755–759.

14. Kinney JM, Goldwyn RM, Barr JS Jr, Moore FD. Loss of the entire jejunum and ileum, and the ascending colon: Management of a patient. *JAMA* 1962; **179:** 529–532.

15. Anderson C M. Long-term survival with six inches of small intestine. *Br Med J* 1965; **1:** 419–422.

16. Butler DB. Compensatory mechanisms following massive small bowel resection for intestinal volvulus. *Surg Gynecol Obstet* 1959; **109:** 479–481.

17. Porus RL. Epithelial hyperplasia following massive small bowel resection in man. *Gastroenterology* 1965; **48:** 753–759.

18. Weinstein LD, Shoemaker CP, Hersh T, Wright HK. Enhanced intestinal absorption after small bowel resection in man. *Arch Surg* 1969; **99:** 560–562.

19. De Francesco A, Malfi G, Delsedime L *et al.* Histological findings regarding jejunal mucosa in short bowel syndrome. *Transplant Proc* 1994; **26:** 1455–1456.

20. O'Keefe SJD, Haymond MW, Bennet WM, Oswald B, Nelson DK, Shorter RG. Long-acting somatostatin analogue therapy and protein metabolism in patients with jejunostomies. *Gastroenterology* 1994; **107:** 379–388.

21. Bury KD. Carbohydrate digestion and absorption after massive resection of the small intestine. *Surg Gynecol Obstet* 1972; **135**: 177–187.

22. Cosnes J, Carbonnel F, Beaugerie L, Ollivier J-M, Parc R, Gendre J-P, Le Quintrec Y. Functional adaptation after extensive small bowel resection in humans. *Eur J Gastroenterol Hepatol* 1994; **6**: 197–202.

23. Althausen TL, Doig RK, Uyeyama K, Weiden S. Digestion and absorption after massive resection of the small intestine. II. Recovery of the absorptive function as shown by intestinal absorption tests in two patients and a consideration of compensatory mechanisms. *Gastroenterology* 1950; **16**: 126–134.

24. Dowling RH, Booth CC. Functional compensation after small bowel resection in man: Demonstration by direct measurement. *Lancet* 1966; **ii**: 146–147.

25. Gouttebel MC, Saint Aubert B, Colette C, Astre C, Monnier L H, Joyeux H. Intestinal adaptation in patients with short bowel syndrome. Measurement by calcium absorption. *Dig Dis Sci* 1989; **34**: 709–715.

26. Messing B, Crenn P, Beau P, Boutron-Ruault MC, Rambaud J-C, Matuchansky C. Long-term survival and parenteral nutrition dependence in adult patients with the short bowel syndrome. *Gastroenterology* 1999; **117**: 1043–1050.

27. LeVeen HH, Lyons A, Becker E. Physiologic adaptation to ileostomy. *Am J Surg* 1962; **103**: 35–41.

28. Wright HK, Cleveland JC, Tilson MD, Herskovic T. Morphology and absorptive capacity of the ileum after ileostomy in man. *Am J Surg* 1969; **117**: 242–245.

29. Hill GL, Mair WSJ, Goligher JC. Impairment of 'ileostomy adaptation' in patients after ileal resection. *Gut* 1974; **15**: 982–987.

30. Nightingale JMD, Lennard-Jones JE, Gertner DJ, Wood SR, Bartram CI. Colonic preservation reduces the need for parenteral therapy, increases the incidence of renal stones but does not change the high prevalence of gallstones in patients with a short bowel. *Gut* 1992; **33**: 1493–1497.

31. Pullan JM. Massive intestinal resection. *Proc R Soc Med* 1959; **52**: 31–37.

32. Hull MA, Knifton A, Filipowicz B, Brough JL, Vautier G, Hawkey CJ. Healing with basic fibroblast growth factor is associated with reduced indomethacin induced relapse in a human model of gastric ulceration. *Gut* 1997; **40**: 204–210.

33. Morin CL, Ling V, Bourassa D. Small intestinal and colonic changes induced by a chemically defined diet. *Dig Dis Sci* 1980; **25**: 123–128.

34. Levine GM, Deren JD, Yezdimir E. Small bowel resection: Oral intake is the stimulus for hyperplasia. *Dig Dis* 1976; **21**: 542–546.

35. Rennie MJ. EPIC: Infection in intensive care in Europe. *Br J Intens Care* 1993; **3**: 27–36.

36. Souba WW, Herskowitz K, Austgen TR, Chen MK, Salloum RM. Glutamine nutrition: theoretical considerations and therapeutic impact. *J Parent Enteral Nutr* 1990; **14**: 237S–243S.

37. Miazza B M. Hyperenteroglucagonaemia and small intestinal mucosal growth after colonic perfusion of glucose in rats. *Gut* 1985; **26**: 518–524.

38. Aghdassi E, Plapler H, Kurian R et al. Colonic fermentation and nutritional recovery in rats with massive small bowel resection. *Gastroenterology* 1994; **107**: 637–642.

39. Park HS, Goodlad RA, Ahnen D J, Winnett A, Sasieni P, Lee CY, Wright NA. Effects of epidermal growth-factor and dimethylhydrazine on crypt size, cell-proliferation, and crypt fission in the rat colon – cell-proliferation and crypt fission are controlled independently. *Am J Pathol* 1997; **151**: 843–852.

40. Maleckapanas E, Fligiel SEG, Jaszewski R, Majumdar APN. Differential responsiveness of proximal and distal colonic mucosa to gastrin. *Peptides* 1997; **18**: 559–565.

41. Janne P, Carpentier Y, Willems G. Colonic mucosal atrophy induced by a liquid elemental diet in rats. *Am J Dig Dis* 1977; **22**: 808–812.

42. Goodlad RA, Wright NA. The effects of addition of cellulose or kaolin to an elemental diet on intestinal cell proliferation in the mouse. *Br J Nutr* 1983; **50**: 91–98.

43. Goodlad RA, Lenton W, Ghatei MA, Adrian TE, Bloom SR, Wright NA. Effects of an elemental diet, inert bulk and different types of dietary fibre on the response of the intestinal epithelium to refeeding in the rat and relationship to plasma gastrin, enteroglucagon, and PYY concentrations. *Gut* 1987; **28**: 171–180.

44. Goodlad RA, Ratcliffe B, Fordham JP, Wright NA. Does dietary fibre stimulate intestinal epithelial cell proliferation in germ free rats? *Gut* 1989; **30**: 820–825.

45. Wilson AJ, Gibson PR. Short-chain fatty acids promote the migration of colonic epithelial-cells in-vitro. *Gastroenterology* 1997; **113**: 487–496.

46. Cummings JH, Englyst HN. Gastrointestinal effects of food carbohydrate. *Am J Clin Nutr* 1995; **61**: 938s–945s.

47. Englyst HN, Quigley NW, Hudson GJ. Definition and measurement of dietary fibre. *Eur J Clin Nutr* 1995; **49(suppl 3)**: S48–62.

48. Wyatt GM, Horn N, Gee JM, Johnson IT. Intestinal microflora and gastrointestinal adaptation in the rat in response to non-digestible dietary polysaccharides. *Br J Nutr* 1988; **60**: 197–207.

49. Pell JD, Johnson IT, Goodlad RA. The effects of, and interactions between fermentable dietary fibre and lipid in germ free and conventional mice. *Gastroenterology* 1995; **108**: 1745–1752.

50. Goodlad RA, Ratcliffe B, Lee CY, Wright NA. Dietary fibre and the gastrointestinal tract: differing trophic effects on muscle and mucosa of the stomach, small intestine and colon. *Eur J Clin Nutr* 1995; **49(suppl 3):** S178–S181.

51. Jacobs LR. Differential effects of dietary fibers on rat intestinal circular muscle cell size. *Dig Dis Sci* 1985; **30:** 247–252.

52. Stark A, Nyska A, Zuckerman A, Madar Z. Changes in intestinal tunica muscularis following dietary fiber feeding in rats. A morphometric study using image analysis. *Dig Dis Sci* 1995; **40:** 960–966.

53. Kripke SA, Fox AD, Berman JA, Settle RG, Rombeau JL. Stimulation of intestinal mucosal growth with intra-colonic infusion of short chain fatty acids. *J Parent Enteral Nutr* 1989; **13:** 109–116.

54. Pusztai A. Dietary lectins are metabolic signals for the gut and modulate immune and hormone functions. [Review] [47 refs]. *Eur J Clin Nutr* 1993; **47:** 691–699.

55. Ryder SD, Parker N, Ecclestone D, Haqqani MT, Rhodes JM. Peanut lectin stimulates proliferation in colonic explants from patients with inflammatory bowel disease and colon polyps. *Gastroenterology* 1994; **106:** 117–124.

56. Altmann GG. Influence of bile and pancreatic secretions on the size of the intestinal villi in the rat. *Am J Anat* 1971; **132:** 167–178.

57. Weser E, Heller R, Tawil T. Stimulation of mucosal growth by bile and pancreatic secretions in the ileum after jejunal resection. *Gastroenterology* 1977; **73:** 524–529.

58. Williamson RCN, Bauer FLR, Ross JS, Malt RA. Contributions of bile and pancreatic juice to cell proliferation in ileal mucosa. *Surgery* 1978; **5:** 570–576.

59. Johnson LR, Copeland EM, Dudrick SJ, Lichtenberger LM, Castro GA. Structural and hormonal alterations in the gastrointestinal tract of parenterally fed rats. *Gastroenterology* 1975; **68:** 1177–1183.

60. Williamson RC, Buchholtz TW, Malt RA. Humoral stimulation of cell proliferation in small bowel after transaction and resection in rats. *Gastroenterology* 1978; **75:** 249–254.

61. Laplace JP. Compensatory hypertrophy of the residual small intestine after partial enterectomy. A neuro-humoral feedback? *Annales de Recherches Veterinaires* 1980; **11:** 165–177.

62. Walsh JH. Role of gastrin as a trophic hormone. *Digestion* 1990; **47:** 11–16.

63. Carlsson E, Havu N, Mattsson H, Ekman L. Gastrin and gastric enterochromaffin-like cell carcinoids in the rat. *Digestion* 1990; **47:** 17–23.

64. Tielemans Y, Hakanson R, Sundler F, Willems G. Proliferation of enterochromaffin like cells in omeprazole-treated hypergastrinernic rats. *Gastroenterology* 1989; **96:** 723–729.

65. Eissele R, Roskopf B, Koop H, Adler G, Arnold R. Proliferation of endocrine cells in the rat stomach caused by drug-induced achlorhydria. *Gastroenterology* 1991; **101:** 70–76.

66. Havu N. Enterochromaffin-like cell carcinoids of gastric mucosa in rats after life-long inhibition of gastric secretion. *Digestion* 1986; **35:** 42–55.

67. Holt S, Powers RE, Howden CW. Antisecretory therapy and genotoxicity. *Dig Dis Sci* 1991; **36:** 545–547.

68. Berlin RG. Omeprazole-gastrin and gastric endocrine cell data from clinical studies. *Dig Dis Sci* 1991; **36:** 129–136.

69. Johnson LR. Regulation of gastrointestinal growth. In: Johnson LR (ed) *Physiology of the digestive tract*. Raven Press, New York, 1981, pp 169–196.

70. Ekundayo A, Lee CY, Goodlad RA. Gastrin and the growth of the gastrointestinal tract. *Gut* 1995; **36:** 203–208.

71. Koh TJ, Goldenring JR, Ito S et al. Gastrin deficiency results in altered gastric differentiation and decreased colonic proliferation in mice. *Gastroenterology* 1997; **113:** 1015–1025.

72. Koh TJ, Dockray GJ, Varro A, Cahill RJ, Dangler CA, Fox JG, Wang TC. Overexpression of glycine-extended gastrin in transgenic mice results in increased colonic proliferation. *J Clin Invest* 1999; **103:** 1119–1126.

73. Gleeson MH, Bloom SR, Polak JM, Henry K, Dowling RH. Endocrine tumour in kidney affecting small bowel structure, motility, and absorptive function. *Gut* 1971; **12:** 773–782.

74. Stevens FM, Flanagan RW, O'Gorman D, Buchanan KD. Glucagonoma syndrome demonstrating giant duodenal villi. *Gut* 1984; **25:** 784–791

75. Al-Mukhtar MYT, Polak JM, Bloom SR, Wright NA. The role of pancreatico-biliary secretions in intestinal adaptation after resection, and its relationship to plasma enteroglucagon. *Br J Surg* 1983; **70:** 398–400.

76. Goodlad RA, Ghatei MA, Domin J, Bloom SR, Gregory H, Wright NA. Plasma enteroglucagon, peptide YY and gastrin in rats deprived of luminal nutrition, and after urogastrone-EGF administration. A proliferative role for PYY in the intestinal epithelium? *Experientia* 1989; **45:** 168–169.

77. Rudo ND, Rosenberg IH. Chronic glucagon administration enhances intestinal transport in the rat. *Proc Soc Exp Biol Med* 1973; **142**: 521–525.

78. Bloom SR. Gut hormones in adaptation. *Gut* 1987; **28**: 31–35.

79. Drucker DJ, Erlich P, Asa SL, Brubaker PL. Induction of intestinal epithelial proliferation by glucagon-like peptide 2. *Proc Natl Acad Sci USA* 1996; **93**: 7911–7916.

80. Goodlad RA, Ghatei MA, Brynes AE, Wright NA, Bloom SR. Enteroglucagon has little effect on gastrointestinal epithelial cell proliferation in rats, whilst glucagon-like peptide 11 (GLP-11) is a major mitogen. *Regul Pept* 1997; **71**: 53.

81. Drucker DJ. Epithelial-cell growth and differentiation. I. Intestinal growth-factors. *Am J Physiol* 1997; **273**: G3–G6.

82. Druker DJ. Glucagon-like peptide 2. *Trends Endocrinol Metab* 1999; **10**: 153–156.

83. Dunphy JL, Fuller PJ. Enteroglucagon, bowel growth and GLP-2. *Mol Cell Endocrinol* 1997; **132**: 7–11.

84. Jeppesen PB, Hartmann B, Hansen BS, Thulesen J, Holst JJ, Mortensen PB. Impaired stimulated glucagon-like peptide 2 response in ileal resected short bowel patients with intestinal failure. *Gut* 1999; **45**: 559–563.

85. Nightingale JMD. Short gut, short answer? *Gut* 1999; **45**: 478–479.

86. Jeppesen PB, Hartmann B, Thulesen J, Hansen BS, Holst JJ, Poulsen SS, Mortensen PB. Elevated plasma glucagon-like peptide 1 and 2 concentrations in ileum-resected short bowel patients with a preserved colon. *Gut* 2000; **47**: 370–376.

87. Nightingale JMD, Kamm MA, van der Sijp JRM *et al.* Disturbed gastric emptying in the short bowel syndrome. Evidence for a 'colonic brake'. *Gut* 1993; **34**: 1171–1176.

88. Playford RJ, Domin J, Beacham J, Parmar KB, Tatemoto K, Bloom SR, Calam J. Preliminary report: role of peptide YY in defence against diarrhoea. *Lancet* 1990; **335**: 1555–1557.

89. Nightingale JMD, Kamm MA, van der Sijp JRM, Walker ER, Ghatei MA, Bloom SR, Lennard-Jones JE. Gastrointestinal hormones in the short bowel syndrome. PYY may be the 'colonic brake' to gastric emptying. *Gut* 1996; **39**: 267–272.

90. Savage AP, Gornacz GE, Adrian TE, Ghatei MA, Goodlad RA, Wright NA, Bloom SR. Is raised plasma peptide YY after intestinal resection in the rat responsible for the trophic response? *Gut* 1985; **26**: 1353–1358.

91. Goodlad RA, Ghatei MA, Dornin J, Bloom SR, Wright NA. Is peptide YY trophic to the intestinal epithelium of parenterally fed rats? *Digestion* 1990; **46**: 177–181.

92. Wood JG, Hoang HD, Bussjaeger LJ, Solomon TE. Neurotensin stimulates growth of small intestine in rats. *Am J Physiol* 1988; **255**: G813–G817.

93. Leblond CP, Carriere RM. The effect of growth hormone and thyroxine on the mitotic rate of the intestinal mucosa in rats. *Endocrinology* 1955; **56**: 261–271.

94. Shimoda N, Tashiro T, Yamamori H, Takagi K, Nakajima N, Ito I. Effects of growth hormone and insulin-like growth-factor-1 on protein-metabolism, gut morphology, and cell mediated-immunity in burned rats. *Nutrition* 1997; **13**: 540–546.

95. Goodlad RA, Lee CY, Gilbey S, Ghatei MA, Bloom SR. Insulin and intestinal epithelial cell proliferation. *Exp Physiol* 1993; **78**: 697–705.

96. Alberts B, Bray D, Lewis J, Raff M, Roberts K, Watson JD. *Molecular biology of the cell.* Garland Publishing, New York, 1994.

97. Sporn MB, Roberts AB. Peptide growth factors are multifunctional. *Nature* 1988; **332**: 217–219.

98. Uribe JM, Barrett KE. Nonmitogenic actions of growth factors: an integrated view of their role in intestinal physiology and pathophysiology. *Gastroenterology* 1997; **112**: 255–268.

99. Playford RJ. Peptides and gastrointestinal mucosal integrity. *Gut* 1995; **37**: 595–597.

100. May FEB, Westley BR. Trefoil proteins: their role in normal and malignant cells. *J Pathology* 1997; **183**: 4–7.

101. Mann GB, Fowler KJ, Gabriel A, Nice EC, Williams RL, Dunn AR. Mice with a null mutation of the TGF alpha gene have abnormal skin architecture, wavy hair, and curly whiskers and often develop corneal inflammation. *Cell* 1993; **73**: 249–261.

102. Egger B, Procaccino F, Lakshmanan J *et al.* Mice lacking transforming growth factor α have an increased susceptibility to dextran sulfate-induced colitis. *Gastroenterology* 1997; **113**: 825–832.

103. Macdonald CE, Playford RJ, Khatri M, Goodlad RA. Transforming growth factor α knockout mice have smaller small intestines, larger large intestines, but no increased sensitivity to NSAID induced small intestinal injury. *Gut* 1998; **42(suppl 1)**: A3.

104. Barnard JA, Beauchamp RD, Russell WE, DuBois RN, Coffey RJ. Epidermal growth factor-related peptides and their relevance to gastrointestinal pathophysiology. *Gastroenterology* 1995; **108**: 564–580.

105. Playford RJ, Wright NA. Why is epidermal growth factor present in the gut lumen? *Gut* 1996; **38**: 303–305.

106. Goodlad RA, Wilson TJ, Lenton W, Gregory H, McCullagh KG, Wright NA. Intravenous but not intra-gastric urogastrone-EGF is trophic to the intestine of parenterally fed rats. *Gut* 1987; **28:** 573–582.

107. Playford RJ, Marchbank T, Calnan DP, Calam J, Royston P, Batten JJ, Hansen HF. Epidermal growth factor is digested to smaller, less active forms in acidic gastric juice. *Gastroenterology* 1995; **108:** 92–101.

108. Playford RJ, Woodman AC, Clark P *et al*. Effect of luminal growth factor preservation on intestinal growth. *Lancet* 1993; **341:** 843–848.

109. Marchbank T, Goodlad RA, Lee CY, Playford RJ. Luminal epidermal growth-factor is trophic to the small-intestine of parenterally fed rats. *Clin Sci* 1995; **89:** 117–120.

110. Thompson JS, Van-Den Berg M, Stokkers PCF. Developmental regulation of epidermal growth factor receptor kinase in rat intestine. *Gastroenterology* 1994; **107:** 1278–1287.

111. Playford RJ, Hanby AM, Gschmeissner S, Peiffer LP, Wright NA, McGarrity T. The epidermal growth-factor receptor (EGF-r) is present on the basolateral, but not the apical, surface of enterocytes in the human gastrointestinal-tract. *Gut* 1996; **39:** 262–266.

112. Skov-Olsen P. Role of epidermal growth factor in gastroduodenal mucosal protection. *J Clin Gastroenterol* 1988; **10:** S146–S151.

113. Skinner KA, Soper BD, Tepperman BL. Effect of sialoadenectomy and salivary gland extracts on gastro-intestinal mucosal growth and gastrin levels in the rat. *J Physiol Lond* 1984; **351:** 1–12.

114. Miettinen PJ, Berger JE, Meneses J, Phung Y, Pedersen RA, Werb Z, Derynck R. Epithelial immaturity and multiorgan failure in mice lacking epidermal growth factor receptor. *Nature* 1995; **376:** 337–341.

115. Sibilia M, Wagner EF. Strain-dependent epithelial defects in mice lacking the EGF receptor. *Science* 1995; **269:** 234–238.

116. Threadgill DW, Dlugosz AA, Hansen LA *et al*. Targeted disruption of mouse EGF receptor: effect of genetic background on mutant phenotype. *Science* 1995; **269:** 230–234.

117. Wright NA, Poulsom R, Stamp G *et al*. Trefoil peptide gene expression in gastrointestinal epithelial cells in inflammatory bowel disease. *Gastroenterology* 1993; **104:** 12–20.

118. Playford RJ, Marchbank T, Chinery R *et al*. Human spasmolytic polypeptide is a cytoprotective agent that stimulates cell migration. *Gastroenterology* 1995; **108:** 108–116.

119. Babyatsky MW, deBeaumont M, Thim L, Podolsky DK. Oral trefoil peptides protect against ethanol- and indomethacin-induced gastric injury in rats. *Gastroenterology* 1996; **110:** 489–497.

120. Playford RJ, Marchbank T, Goodlad RA, Lee CY, Chinery RA, Poulsom R, Hanby AM. Transgenic mice which overexpress the human trefoil peptide, pS2, have an increased resistance to intestinal damage. *Proc Natl Acad Sci USA* 1996; **93:** 2137–2142.

121. Mashimo H, Wu DC, Podolsky DK, Fishman MC. Impaired defence of intestinal mucosa in mice lacking intestinal trefoil factor. *Science* 1996; **274:** 262–265.

122. Dignass A, Lynch-Devaney K, Kindon H, Thim L, Podolsky DK. Trefoil peptides promote epithelial migration through a transforming growth factor beta-independent pathway. *J Clin Invest* 1994; **94:** 376–383.

123. Marchbank T, Wesley BR, May FEB, Calnan DP, Playford RJ. Dimerization of human pS2 (TFF1) plays a key role in its protective/healing effects. *J Pathol* 1998; **185:** 153–158.

124. Dignass AU, Podolsky DK. Cytokine modulation of intestinal epithelial cell restitution: central role of trans-forming growth factor beta. *Gastroenterology* 1993; **105:** 1323–1332.

125. Housley RM, Morris CF, Boyle W *et al*. Keratinocyte growth factor induces proliferation of hepatocytes and epithelial cells throughout the rat gastrointestinal tract. *J Clin Invest* 1994; **94:** 1764–1777.

126. Goodlad RA, Mandir N, Meeran K, Ghatei MA, Bloom SR, Playford RJ. Does the response of the intestinal epithelium to keratinocyte growth factor vary according to the method of administration? *Regul Pept* 2000; **87:** 83–90.

127. Playford RJ, Marchbank T, Mandir N *et al*. Effects of keratinocyte growth factor (KGF) on gut growth and repair. *J Pathol* 1998; **184:** 316–322.

128. Litvak DA, Iseki H, Evers M *et al*. Characterization of two novel proabsorptive peptide YY analogs, BIM-43073D and BIM-43004C. *Dig Dis Sci* 1999; **44:** 643–648.

129. Wasan H, Goodlad RA. 'Fibre' supplemented foods may damage your health. *Lancet* 1996; **348:** 319–320.

130. Alberts DS, Martinez ME, Roe DJ *et al*. Lack of effect of a high-fiber cereal supplement on the recurrence of colorectal adenomas. Phoenix Colon Cancer Prevention Physicians' Network. *N Engl J Med* 2000; **342:** 1156–1162.

131. Faivre J, BonithonKopp C, Kronborg O, Rath U, Giacosa A. A randomized trial of calcium and fiber supplementation in the prevention of recurrence of colorectal adenomas. A European intervention study. *Gastroenterology* 1999; **116:** G0238.

132. Schatzkin A, Lanza E, Corle D et al. Lack of effect of a low-fat, high-fiber diet on the recurrence of colorectal adenomas. Polyp Prevention Trial Study Group. *N Engl J Med* 2000; **342**: 1149–1155.

133. Wasan H, Goodlad RA. 'Fibre' supplemented foods may damage your health. *Lancet* 1996; **348**: 319–320.

134. Byrne TA, Persinger RL, Young LS, Ziegler TR, Wilmore DW. A new treatment for patients with short-bowel syndrome: Growth hormone, glutamine, and a modified diet. *Ann Surg* 1995; **222**: 243–255.

135. Byrne TA, Morrissey TB, Nattakom TV, Ziegler TR, Wilmore DW. Growth hormone, glutamine, and a modified diet enhance nutrient absorption in patients with severe short bowel syndrome. *J Parenter Enteral Nutr* 1995; **19**: 296–302.

136. Scolapio JS, Camilleri M, Fleming CR et al. Effect of growth hormone, glutamine, and diet on adaptation in short-bowel syndrome: a randomized, controlled study. *Gastroenterology* 1997; **113**: 1074–1081.

137. Szkudlarek J, Jeppesen PB, Mortensen PB. Effect of high dose growth hormone with glutamine and no change in diet on intestinal absorption in short bowel patients: a randomised, double blind, crossover, placebo controlled study. *Gut* 2000; **47**: 199–205.

138. Delhougne B, Deneux C, Abs R et al. The prevalence of colonic polyps in acromegaly: a colonoscopic and pathological study in 103 patients. *J Clin Endocrinol Metab* 1995; **80**: 3223–3226.

139. Walker-Smith JA, Phillips AD, Walford N, Gregory H, Fitzgerald JD, MacCullagh K, Wright NA. Intravenous epidermal growth factor/urogastrone increases small-intestinal cell proliferation in congenital microvillous atrophy. *Lancet* 1985; **ii**: 1239–1240.

140. Sullivan PB, Brueton MJ, Tabara ZB, Goodlad RA, Lee CY, Wright NA. Epidermal growth factor in necrotising enteritis. *Lancet* 1991; **338**: 53–54.

141. Jeppesen PB, Hartmann B, Thulesen J et al. Treatment of short bowel patients with Glucagon-like peptide-2 (GLP-2), a newly discovered intestinotrophic, anti-secretory, and transit modulating peptide. *Gastroenterology* 2000; **118**: A178–A179.

142. Luk GD, Baylin SB. Polyamines and intestinal growth – increased polyamine biosynthesis after jejunectomy. *Am J Physiol* 1983; **245**: G656–G660.

143. Thompson JS, Laughlin K. Relationship of jejunostomy and urine polyamine content to refeeding and intestinal structure and function. *J Parenter Enteral Nutr* 1989; **13**: 13–17.

144. Rokkas T, Vaja S, Murphy GM, Dowling RH. Aminoguanidine blocks intestinal diamine oxidase (DAO) activity and enhances the intestinal adaptive response to resection in the rat. *Digestion* 1990; **46(suppl 2)**: 447–457.

145. Playford RJ, Adenekan RO, Marchbank T, Boulton R, Johnson W, Goodlad RA. Bovine colostrum is prophylactic against indomethacin-induced intestinal injury. *Gastroenterology* 1997; **112**: A394.

146. Campbell FC, Tait IS, Flint N, Evans GS. Transplantation of cultured small bowel enterocytes. *Gut* 1993; **34**: 1153–1155.

Section 4

Treatment of intestinal failure

17

Assessment of nutritional and fluid status

Khursheed N. Jeejeebhoy

Nutritional health is maintained by a state of equilibrium in which nutrient intake and requirements balance. Protein-energy malnutrition occurs when net nutrient intake (nutrient intake corrected for abnormally large faecal or urinary losses) is less than requirements. Protein-energy malnutrition leads to a succession of metabolic abnormalities, physiological changes, reduced organ and tissue function, and loss of body mass. Concurrent stresses such as trauma, sepsis, inflammation and burns accelerate loss of tissue mass and function. Ultimately, critical loss of body mass and function occur resulting in death (Fig. 17.1).

The evaluation of the nutritional status is a broad topic, and to be of clinical importance the ideal method should be able to predict whether the individual would have increased morbidity and mortality in the absence of nutritional support. In short, can it predict the occurrence of nutrition-associated complications (NAC) and thus predict outcome? Unfortunately, disease and nutrition interact so that disease in turn may cause secondary protein-energy malnutrition, or protein-energy malnutrition may adversely influence the underlying disease. Thus patient outcomes are multi-factorial and attempting to formulate the influence of protein-energy malnutrition on outcome based on single parameters or simple models fails to consider the many interacting factors. This complexity has been recognized in the recent recommendations of the American Dietetic Association.[1]

Traditional nutritional science was first developed in the field of agriculture where the effect of nutrition was entirely judged by the amount of meat on the carcass of animals and the production of proteins by the liver. This approach was embodied in the initial attempts to assess nutritional status in humans as given below under 'Traditional nutritional assessment indices'. These techniques lacked the ability to predict outcome and to detect early changes in function, which occur with nutritional support. In this document some of the traditional nutritional assessment indices are discussed, then more recent assessment methods are evaluated with a view to:

1. To specifically assess the risk of morbidity and mortality resulting from protein-energy malnutrition.

2. To identify and separate the causes and consequences of protein-energy malnutrition and disease in the individual patient.

3. To assess if the patient will clinically benefit from nutritional support.

TRADITIONAL NUTRITIONAL ASSESSMENT INDICES

Nutritional status has been traditionally defined by body composition, plasma protein concentrations, immune competence and multivariate analysis.[2,3]

Body composition

Assessment of nutritional status based on body composition involves detecting the loss (or gain) of body components relative to previous measurements and relating the values in a given patient to normal standards. The former is affected by the reproducibility and error in the measurements themselves, while the latter is dependent upon the normal range of values. A person who starts off at the upper end of the normal range may be classified as 'normal' despite considerable changes in the measured value. Therefore, it is possible for a person to be in a negative nutritional state for a long time before anthropometric measurements fall below normal.

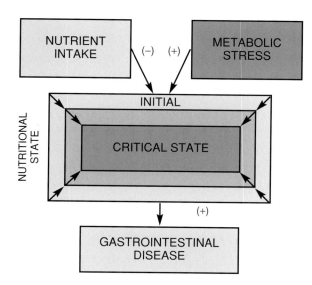

Figure 17.1 – Factors influencing nutritional status.

Body weight and weight loss

Body weight is a simple measure of total body components and is compared to an 'ideal' or desirable weight. This comparison can be made by using formulas such as the Hamwi formula or to tables.[4] However, a simple approach which gives as much information as tables is the calculation of the body mass or Quetelet index (BMI). BMI is calculated as weight in kilograms divided by height in meters squared (Appendix 1). A BMI of 14–15 kg/m^2 is associated with significant mortality. However, measurements of body weight in patients in hospital, intensive care units (ICUs), those with liver disease, cancer and renal failure are confounded by changes in body water due to underhydration, oedema, ascites and dialysate in the abdomen.

Unintentional weight loss greater than 10% is a good prognosticator of clinical outcome.[5,6] (See Appendix 2 for percent weight loss chart.) However, it may be difficult to determine true weight loss. Morgan et al.[7] have shown that the accuracy of determining weight loss by history was only 0.67 and the predictive power was 0.75. Hence 33% of patients with weight loss would be missed and 25% of those who have been weight-stable would be diagnosed as having lost weight. Furthermore, the nutritional significance of changes in body weight can again be confounded by changes in hydration status.

Anthropometry

Triceps and subscapular skinfold thicknesses provide an index of body fat, and mid-arm muscle circumference provides a measure of muscle mass. Although these measurements seem to be useful in population studies their reliability in individual patients is less clear. The most commonly used standards for triceps skinfold thickness and mid-arm muscle circumference are those reported by Jelliffe,[8] which are based on measurements of European male military personnel and low-income American women, and those reported by Frisancho,[9] which are based on measurements of White males and females participating in the 1971–1974 United States Health and Nutrition Survey. The use of these standards to identify protein-energy malnutrition in many patients is problematic because of the restricted database and the absence of correction factors for age, hydration status and physical activity on anthropometric parameters. Several studies have demonstrated that 20–30% of healthy control subjects would be considered undernourished based on these standards[10,11] and that there is poor correlation between the Jellife and Frisancho standards in classifying patients.[11] Although attempts have been made to create standards for diseases such as dialysis patients[12] the validity of standards have been questioned and interpretation of the data may be limited by inter-rater variability.[13] Hall et al.[14] found considerable inconsistencies when anthropometric measurements were performed by three different observers. The coefficient of variation was 4.7% for arm circumference and 22.6% for triceps skinfold thickness. Therefore, a change in arm muscle circumference (arm circumference minus triceps skinfold thickness) of at least 2.68 cm was needed to demonstrate a true change in a given patient (See Appendix 3 for Mid-Arm Muscle Circumference chart). These considerations in particular apply to patients in ICUs, and those with liver and renal disease where oedema is a major problem in assessing skinfolds and arm circumference.

Creatinine–height index

The excretion of creatinine in the urine is related to muscle mass (creatinine–height index (CHI)). Normalized for height the 24-hour creatinine excretion is an index of muscle mass. In theory it is a good and simple way of assessing the lean body mass. However, it is dependent upon complete 24-hour urine collections and urinary losses or oliguria may result in an inappropriate diagnosis of protein-energy malnutrition. Patients on diuretics, such as those with cardiac and liver failure and those with renal disease, are especially likely to have low excretions of creatinine.

Serum proteins

Albumin

This protein is one of the most extensively studied and over the past 30 years there are about 19 000 citations to it in the Index Medicus! Several studies have demonstrated that a low serum albumin concentration correlates with an increased incidence of medical complications.[15–17] In addition a low serum albumin is associated with increased mortality in general, examples are elderly nursing home patients[18] and dialysis patients.[19] An understanding of albumin physiology clarifies why serum albumin concentration correlates with disease severity in hospitalized patients but may be inappropriate as a measure of nutritional status per se.[20]

The concentration of serum albumin represents the net summation of many events – albumin synthesis, albumin degradation, albumin losses from the body, exchange between intra- and extravascular albumin compartments, and the volume in which albumin is distributed. Albumin is highly water-soluble and resides in the extracellular space. The total body pool of albumin in a normal 70 kg man is about 300 g (3.5–5.3 g/kg). Approximately one-third of the total pool constitutes the intravascular compartment and two-thirds the extravascular compartment.[21] The concentration of albumin in blood is greater than that in lymph or other extracellular fluids, and the ratio of intravascular to extravascular albumin concentration varies from tissue to tissue. Within 30 minutes of initiating albumin synthesis, the hepatocyte secretes albumin into the bloodstream.[22] Once albumin is released into plasma, its half-life is 20 days. During steady state conditions ~14 g of albumin (200 mg/kg) are produced and degraded daily. Thus, each day about 5% of the total albumin pool is degraded and replaced by newly synthesized albumin. Equilibration of albumin in the intravascular compartment is rapid and occurs within minutes after albumin enters the bloodstream. Equilibration between intra- and extravascular albumin occurs more slowly. Every hour about 5% of the plasma albumin pool exchanges with extravascular albumin so that the total plasma albumin mass exchanges with extravascular albumin each day. Because the rate of equilibration varies among tissues complete equilibration may take 7–10 days.

Protein-calorie malnutrition causes a decrease in the rate of albumin synthesis because adequate nutrient intake is important for polysomal aggregation and maintenance of cellular RNA levels needed for protein synthesis. Within 24 hours of fasting, the rate of albumin synthesis decreases markedly.[23] However, a short-term reduction in albumin synthesis has little impact on albumin levels because of albumin's low turnover rate and large pool size. Indeed, plasma albumin concentration may actually increase during short-term fasting because of contraction of intravascular water.[24] Even during chronic protein-energy malnutrition plasma albumin concentration is often maintained because of a compensatory decrease in albumin degradation and a transfer of extravascular albumin to the intravascular compartment. Prolonged protein-calorie restriction induced experimentally in human volunteers[25] or observed clinically in patients with anorexia nervosa[26] causes marked reductions in body weight but little change in plasma albumin concentration. A protein-deficient diet with adequate calories in elderly persons causes a decrease in lean body mass and muscle function without a change in plasma albumin concentration.[27]

Hospitalized patients may have low levels of plasma albumin for several reasons. Inflammatory disorders cause a decrease in albumin synthesis,[28] an increase in albumin degradation,[29] and an increase in albumin transcapillary losses.[30] Gastrointestinal and some cardiac diseases increase albumin losses through the gut, while renal diseases may cause considerable albuminuria. Wounds, burns and peritonitis cause major losses from the injured surface and in certain circumstances an increase in albumin losses through the gut, kidneys, or damaged tissues. Because the exchange between intra- and extravascular albumin is so large, even small changes in the percentage of exchange can cause significant changes in plasma albumin levels. The normal rate of albumin exchange between intra- and extravascular compartments is more than 10 times the rate of albumin synthesis or degradation. During serious illness vascular permeability increases dramatically. Albumin losses from plasma to the extravascular space were increased twofold in patients with cancer cachexia and threefold in patients with septic shock. Plasma albumin levels will not increase in stressed patients until the inflammatory stress remits and is not affected by nutritional intake. For example, albumin levels fail to increase in patients with cancer after 21 days of intensive nutritional therapy[31] and in nursing home patients after enteral feeding through a gastrostomy.[18]

Prealbumin

Prealbumin is a transport protein for thyroid hormones and exists in the circulation as a retinol-binding–prealbumin complex.[32] The turnover rate of this protein is rapid with a half-life of 2–3 days. It is synthesized by the liver and is catabolized partly in the kidneys. Protein-energy malnutrition reduces the levels of prealbumin and refeeding restores levels.[33] However, prealbumin levels fall without protein-energy malnutrition in infections[34,35] and in response to cytokine[36] and hormone infusion.[37] Renal failure increases[38] while liver failure may cause decreased levels. Although, prealbumin is responsive to nutritional changes it is influenced by several disease-related factors making it unreliable as an index of nutritional status in patients.

Immune competence

Immune competence, as measured by delayed cutaneous hypersensitivity (DCH), is affected by severe protein-energy malnutrition. While it is true that immune competence as measured by DCH is reduced in protein-energy malnutrition, several diseases[39] and drugs influence this measurement making it a poor predictor of protein-energy malnutrition in sick patients. The following factors non-specifically alter DCH in the absence of protein-energy malnutrition:

1. Infections (viral, bacterial and granulomatous)

2. Uraemia, cirrhosis, hepatitis, trauma, burns and haemorrhage

3. Steroids, immunosupressants, cimetidine, warfarin and perhaps aspirin

4. General anaesthesia and surgery.

Hence in the critically sick patient many factors can alter DCH and render it valueless in assessing the state of nutrition. Meakins et al.[40] have shown that simply draining an abscess can reverse anergy. Immunity is therefore neither a specific indicator of protein-energy malnutrition nor is it easily studied.[41]

Serum cholesterol

Low levels are seen in undernourished patients. However, very low levels are seen in patients with liver disease, renal disease and malabsorption. In addition, low levels correlate with mortality.[19,42]

Discriminant analysis

Buzby et al.[43] developed a prognostic nutritional index (PNI), calculated retrospectively from multiple parameters, to predict the occurrence of complications. It depends largely on the levels of plasma albumin and transferrin. In a prospective study, the PNI, measured in patients before gastrointestinal surgery, was found to provide a quantitative estimate of postoperative complications.

CLINICAL ASSESSMENT OF NUTRITIONAL STATUS

The clinical assessment of nutritional status attempts to identify the initial nutritional state and the interplay of the factors influencing the progression or regression of nutritional abnormalities. Therefore, a clinical nutritional assessment is a dynamic process which is not limited to a single 'snapshot' at the moment of measurement but provides a picture of current nutritional status and insight into the patient's future status. The clinical assessment of nutritional status involves a focused history and physical examination in conjunction with selected laboratory tests aimed at detecting specific nutrient deficiencies and patients who are at high risk for future nutritional abnormalities.

History

The nutritional history should evaluate the following questions:

1. Has there been a recent change in body weight and was the change intentional or unintentional?

2. Is dietary intake adequate? The patient should be questioned about their habitual diet and any change in diet pattern. Has the number, size, and contents of meals changed? Are nutrient supplements being taken? A diary documenting food intake may be useful when the history is inconclusive.

3. What is the reason(s) for the change in dietary intake? Has appetite changed? Is there a disturbance in taste, smell, or the ability to chew or swallow food? Has there been a change in mental status or increased depression? Has there been a change in the ability to prepare meals? Are there gastrointestinal symptoms, such as early satiety, postprandial pain, nausea, or vomiting? Is the patient taking medications that affect food intake?

4. Is there evidence of malabsorption? Does the patient have gastrointestinal disease? Has there been a change in bowel habits?

5. Are there symptoms of specific nutrient deficiencies including macrominerals (e.g. sodium, potassium, calcium or magnesium), micronutrients, and water?

Physical examination

The physical examination corroborates and adds to the findings obtained by history:

Anthropometric assessment

Current body weight should be compared with previously recorded weights, if available (Appendix 1). Weight for height should be compared with standard normal values (Appendix 2). A search for evidence demonstrating depletion of body fat and muscle masses should be made. A general loss of adipose tissue can be judged by clearly defined bony, muscular and venous outlines, and loose skinfolds. A fold of skin, pinched between the forefinger and thumb, can detect the adequacy of subcutaneous fat. The presence of hollow cheeks, buttocks and perianal area suggests body fat loss. An examination of the temporalis, deltoids, and quadriceps muscles should be made to search for muscle wasting.

Assessment of muscle function

Strength testing of individual muscle groups should be made to evaluate for generalized and localized muscle weakness. In addition, a general evaluation of respiratory and cardiac muscle function should be made.

Fluid status

An evaluation for dehydration (hypotension, tachycardia, postural changes, mucosal xerosis, dry skin, and swollen tongue) and excess body fluid (oedema, ascites) should be made.

Evaluation for specific nutrient deficiencies (Tables 17.6–17.9)

Rapidly proliferating tissues, such as oral mucosa, hair, skin, and bone marrow are often more sensitive to nutrient deficiencies than are tissues that turn over more slowly.

Laboratory tests

The results of the history and physical examination may lead to a suspicion of specific nutrient deficiencies, which can be further corroborated by appropriate diagnostic laboratory tests.

SUBJECTIVE GLOBAL ASSESSMENT

A clinical method for evaluating nutritional status, termed subjective global assessment (SGA), encompasses historical, symptomatic and physical parameters.[44,45] This approach defines undernourished patients as those who are at increased risk for medical complications and who will presumably benefit from nutritional therapy. The basis of this assessment is to determine whether nutrient assimilation has been restricted because of decreased food intake, maldigestion or malabsorption, whether any effects of protein-energy malnutrition on organ function and body composition have occurred, and whether the patient's disease process influences nutrient requirements. The specific features of the history and physical examination used in the SGA are listed in Table 17.1.

Table 17.1 – Features of subjective global assessment

History
1. Weight change and height
   Current: Height   _____ cm
                 Weight   _____ kg
   Overall loss in past 6 months: _____ kg
                                     _____ %
   Change in past 2 weeks (use + or −): _____ kg
                                         _____ %

2. Dietary intake change (relative to usual intake)
   No change
   Change: Duration _____ days
   Type: Suboptimal solid diet
                Hypocaloric liquids
                Starvation
   Supplement: (circle)
                Nil
                Vitamin
                Minerals

3. Gastrointestinal symptoms that persisted for > 2 weeks
   None
   Nausea
   Vomiting
   Diarrhoea
   Pain: At rest
                On eating

4. Functional capacity
   No dysfunction
   Dysfunction: Duration _____ days
                 Type: Working suboptimally
                          Ambulatory but not
                             working
                          Bedridden

5. Disease and its relation to nutritional requirements
   Primary diagnosis: _____
   Metabolic demand (stress):
                No stress
                Moderate stress
                High stress (burns, sepsis, severe
                   trauma)

Physical status (for each trait specify: 0 = normal, 1 = mild deficit, 2 = established deficit)
   Loss of subcutaneous fat
   Muscle wasting
   Oedema
   Ascites
   Mucosal lesions
   Cutaneous and hair changes

SGA Grade _____

A: well nourished; B: moderate or suspected protein-energy malnutrition; C: severe protein-energy malnutrition

The history used in the SGA focuses on five areas. The percentage of body weight lost in the previous 6 months is characterized as mild (< 5%), moderate (5–10%), and severe (> 10%). The pattern of loss is also important and it is possible for a patient to have significant weight loss but still be considered well-nourished if body weight (without oedema or ascites) recently increased. For example, a patient who has had a 10% body weight loss but regained 3% of that weight over the past month, would be considered well-nourished. Dietary intake is classified as normal or abnormal as judged by a change in intake and whether the current diet is nutritionally adequate. The presence of persistent gastrointestinal symptoms, such as anorexia, nausea, vomiting, diarrhoea and abdominal pain, which have occurred almost daily for at least 2 weeks, is recorded. The patient's functional capacity is defined as bedridden, suboptimally active, or full capacity. The last feature of the history concerns the metabolic demands of the patient's underlying disease state. Examples of high-stress illnesses are burns, major trauma and severe inflammation, such as acute colitis. Moderate-stress diseases might be a mild infection or limited malignant tumour.

The features of the physical examination are noted as normal, mild, moderate, or severe alterations. The loss of subcutaneous fat measured in the triceps region and the mid-axillary line at the level of the lower ribs. These measurements are not precise, but are merely a subjective impression of the degree of subcutaneous tissue loss. The second feature is muscle wasting in the temporal areas and in the deltoids and quadriceps, as determined by loss of bulk and tone detectable by palpation. A neurological deficit will interfere with this assessment. The presence of oedema in the ankle and sacral regions and the presence of ascites are noted. Co-existing disease such as renal or congestive failure will modify the weight placed on the finding of oedema. Mucosal and cutaneous lesions are recorded, as are colour and appearance of the patient's hair.

The findings of the history and physical examination are used to categorize patients as being well-nourished (category A), having moderate or suspected protein-energy malnutrition (category B), or having severe protein-energy malnutrition (category C). The rank is assigned on the basis of subjective weighting. Equivocal information is given less weight than definitive data. Fluid shifts related to onset or treatment of oedema or ascites must be considered when interpreting changes in body weight. In general, a patient who has experienced weight loss and muscle wasting but is currently eating well and is gaining weight is classified as well nourished. A patient who has experienced moderate weight loss, continued compromised food intake, continued weight loss, progressive functional impairment, and has a 'moderate-stress' illness is classified as moderately undernourished. A patient who has experienced severe weight loss, continues to have poor nutrient intake, progressive functional impairment and muscle wasting is classified as severely undernourished independent of disease stress. Baker et al.[44] and Detsky el al.[45] found that the use of SGA in evaluating hospitalized patients gives reproducible results and there was more than 80% agreement when two blinded observers assessed the same patient.

Illustrative cases

Case 1

A 60-year-old woman was admitted to the hospital for elective resection of a colon carcinoma. She had lost 10% of her initial weight over 8 months before admission. However, she recently gained weight after therapy with nutritional supplements was initiated. She continued to work and was active. On physical examination, there was no loss of muscle or fat. She is SGA A.

Case 2

A 40-year-old man with an acute exacerbation of Crohn's disease had lost 10% of his body weight within the previous 2 weeks and was ingesting mostly liquids to avoid gastrointestinal discomfort. He was ambulatory but was not going to work. On physical examination, he had slight loss of subcutaneous tissue manifested by a reduced buccal fat pad and loose skinfolds over the arms. He is SGA B.

Case 3

A 67-year-old man with oesophageal cancer had minimal food intake for almost 3 months. He lost 15% of his body weight during the previous 4 months and is continuing to lose weight. He was able to move around the house but had marked muscle weakness and fatigue and did not walk outdoors. On physical examination, he lacked subcutaneous tissue, had hollow temples, deltoid wasting and mild pitting oedema. He is SGA C.

Comparison of SGA with traditional methods?

To make a meaningful comparison, Detsky *et al.*[45] compared the predictive accuracy of the different techniques done on the same individuals in a prospective analysis of 59 surgical patients. In that study preoperative SGA was a better predictor of postoperative infectious complications than serum albumin, serum transferrin, delayed cutaneous, hypersensitivity, anthropometry, creatinine–height index and the prognostic nutritional index. Combining SGA with some of the 'traditional' markers of nutritional status increased the ability to identify patients who developed complications (from 82% to 90%) but also increased the percentage of patients identified as 'undernourished' but who did not develop a postoperative complication (from 25% to 30%). Therefore, increasing assessment sensitivity also increases the number of patients who might receive unnecessary nutrition support. How does SGA perform in predicting complications in conditions other than preoperative patients? In studies done by others it has been used and shown to predict complications in general surgical patients,[46] patients on dialysis,[47–49] and liver transplant patients.[50,51]

At present there is no 'gold standard' for evaluating nutritional status, and the reliability of any nutritional assessment technique as a true measure of nutritional status has never been validated. No prospective controlled clinical trials have demonstrated that providing nutrition support to patients judged to be undernourished influences clinical outcome. However, a retrospective subgroup analysis of a large multicentre trial found that parenteral nutrition given preoperatively to patients diagnosed as severely undernourished by SGA or a nutritional risk index (based on serum albumin and body weight change) decreased postoperative infectious complications.[52] We recommend that nutritional assessment involve a careful clinical evaluation with additional laboratory studies as needed to help determine specific nutrient deficiencies or severity of illness. This information should be used in a prognostic fashion to decide which patients might benefit from nutritional therapy.

FUNCTIONAL TESTS OF PROTEIN-ENERGY MALNUTRITION

SGA identifies patients at risk of complications by clinically assessing changes in intake of food, body composition and function. Functional impairment in protein–energy malnutrition has been previously studied by examining changes in immune function,[41] ability to perform work in an ergometer[53] and in changes of heart rate during maximal exercise.[54] The use of exercise tolerance by ergometers and measurement of heart rate are useful for population studies but difficult for sick patients with cardio-respiratory impairment and for patients under intensive care. They also are dependent upon the previous exercise status of the individual. An early study showing the role of impaired function in predicting postoperative complications showed that the strength of the handgrip was predictive of the development of postoperative complications.[55] However, the direct relationship of dietary intake to function as a measure of the effect of nutritional manipulation was shown by Russell *et al.*[56]

In order to study critically ill patients it was necessary to develop a method that did not require the co-operation of the patient and was not affected by sepsis, drugs, trauma, surgical intervention and anaesthesia. In order to do this we selected a method developed by Edwards[57] to study muscle fatigue. It consisted of measuring the contraction of the adductor pollicis muscle in response to an electrical stimulus of the ulna nerve at the wrist. When the nerve is stimulated at the above site with unidirectional square wave pulses lasting only 50–70 microseconds at a range of frequencies from 10 to 50 Hz there is a progressive increase in force with a maximal attained at 50 Hz. The plotted results constitute a force-frequency curve. In addition when the nerve is stimulated at 20 Hz for 2 seconds and then the stimulus is switched off, the muscle relaxes after the initial contraction and the rate of this relaxation can be measured. Finally if the stimulus at 20 Hz is continued any loss of power represents fatigue of an objective nature (not due to voluntary relaxation). By studying two pure models of human starvation and refeeding, namely the starving obese subject and the anorexic patient being refed, we showed that starvation causes the ratio of the force at 10 Hz/50–100 Hz to double and the relaxation rate to slow from a mean of about 10% of maximal force lost/10 milliseconds to 5–6%. In addition we showed the development of fatigue. Refeeding corrected these changes prior to gain in body nitrogen.[25,56,58] In other studies, Lenmarken *et al.*[59] consider the relaxation rate to be a good index of the nutritional status. More importantly Zeiderman and McMahon[60] have shown that, in a group of preoperative surgical patients, the combination of an abnormal force-frequency curve and slow relaxation rate was the most specific and sensitive predictor of NACs when compared with other parameters of nutritional status such as hand-grip strength, arm muscle circumference, albumin and transferrin levels. Windsor and Hill[61] have shown that muscle function including handgrip, respiratory muscle strength and relaxation rate of the adductor pollicis were the main indicators of surgical complications rather than weight loss. In patients with inflammatory bowel disease, Christie and Hill[62] have confirmed our earlier observation that muscle function is restored before body composition.[26,56] They showed early restoration of muscle function prior to significant increase in body protein. Furthermore, Chan et al.[63] demonstrated that intravenous feeding rapidly restores muscle function in preoperative undernourished patients.

It is clear from the above findings that there is good evidence that muscle function is an index of nutritional changes and of the risks of complications in the sick individual. Preliminary studies suggest that the function changes rapidly on feeding; however, it is not clear whether the restoration of function is associated with an improvement in outcome. Studies by Hill and colleagues[61,62] suggest that grip strength, respiratory muscle strength and function by electrical stimulation all demonstrate changes with nutrition. The question is which one(s) should be used for assessment? The study by Ziederman and McMahon[60] suggests that electrical stimulation has greater predictive power over grip strength. Also respiratory muscle strength needs elaborate instrumentation in a pulmonary function laboratory, good cardio–respiratory status and cooperation. We therefore feel that the relaxation rate of single twitches may be a simple, non-invasive and reproducible way of studying function in sick patients.

MEASUREMENT OF BODY COMPOSITION

The body consists of compartments or components. There are over 35 well-recognized components and these are organized into five levels of increasing complexity: atomic, molecular, cellular, tissue-system and whole body. In healthy weight stable subjects there are relatively constant relationships between these components which are correlated with each other. For example, the atomic level component nitrogen is 16% of the molecular level component protein.

Isotope dilution

Total body water, measured by isotope dilution, is usually the largest molecular level component. Water maintains a relatively stable relationship to fat-free body mass and thus measured water isotope dilution volumes allow prediction of fat-free body mass and fat (i.e. body weight minus fat-free body mass). The relationship between total body water and other body composition components may change with disease and this should be considered when interpreting data from hospitalized or chronically ill patients. The usual approach is to measure a dilution volume using one of three isotopes, tritium, deuterium, or ^{18}O-labelled water. This first step allows estimation of a dilution volume of one of the three isotopes. In the second step it is assumed that the proportion of fat-free body mass as water is constant at 0.732. This allows calculation of fat-free body mass and fat. Relationship to outcome has not been studied.

Bioimpedance analysis

Bioimpedance analysis (BIA) is a method of estimating body fluid volumes by measuring the resistance to a high frequency, low amplitude alternating electric current (50 kHz at 500–800 mA). The amount of resistance measured (R) is inversely proportional to the volume of electrolytic fluid in the body, and to a lesser extent on the proportions of this volume. A regression equation is then developed based between a reference measurement of fat-free body mass (i.e. isotope dilution) and the measured R, height and other variables. Recent research in this area has focused on separate measurements of extra- and intracellular water. In healthy adults it is possible to predict total body water within 2–3 litres. Much more variable results are observed in diseased patients, owing in part to the population-specific nature of BIA. Relationship to outcome has not been studied in hospitalized patients and the method is not yet fully validated for use in all disease states.

Dual-energy X-ray absorptiometry

Dual-energy X-ray absorptiometry (DEXA) is a method developed originally for the measurement of bone density and mass. Systems today also quantify soft tissue composition, and it possible to measure total and regional fat, bone mineral and bone mineral-free lean components with DEXA. The method is based on the attenuation characteristics of tissues exposed to X-rays at two peak energies. Mathematical algorithms allow calculation of the separate components using various physical and biological models. Software can be used to measure regions separately if desired. A typical whole body scan takes approximately 30 minutes and exposes the subject to ~ 1 mrem radiation. The method provides the first accurate and practical means of measuring bone mineral mass and offers a new opportunity to study appendicular muscle mass. Again there is no data indicating whether DEXA can predict outcome in hospital patients.

Whole-body counting/neutron activation

The elements potassium (K), nitrogen (N), phosphorus (P), hydrogen (H), oxygen (O), carbon (C), sodium (Na), chloride (Cl) and calcium (Ca) can be measured with a group of techniques referred to as whole-body counting/*in vivo* neutron activation analysis. Shielded whole body counters can count the gamma-ray decay of naturally occurring ^{40}K. The method is safe and can be used in children and pregnant women. The ^{40}K counts can be used to estimate total body potassium, which in turn can be used to calculate body cell mass and fat-free body mass. Prompt gamma neutron activation analysis can be used to measure total body N and H. Nitrogen can be used to calculate total body protein. Delayed gamma neutron activation measures total body Ca, Na, Cl and P. These elements can be used to calculate bone mineral mass and extracellular fluid volume. Lastly, inelastic neutron scattering methods measure total body oxygen and carbon. Carbon is useful in models designed to quantify total body fat. Whole body counting-neutron activation methods are important because they provide a means of estimating all major chemical components *in vivo*. These methods are considered the standard for evaluating the body composition components of nutritional interest, including body cell mass, fat, fat-free body mass, skeletal muscle mass and various fluid volumes. Refeeding the undernourished subject by mouth or by parenteral nutrition results in a rapid increase in total body K but not N. In animal studies it has been shown that this increase in total body K is the result of improved membrane voltage and an increase in the intracellular ionic potassium. The findings are consistent with improved cell energetics demonstrated by nuclear magnetic resonance spectroscopy and the improved muscle function shown concurrently. Loss of total body K is a good predictor of poor outcome in a variety of conditions associated with protein-energy malnutrition.[64–67]

Computerized axial tomography and magnetic resonance imaging

These methods measure components at the tissue-system level of body composition, including skeletal muscle, adipose tissue, visceral organs and brain. Computerized axial tomography (CT) systems measure X-ray attenuation as the source and detector rotate in a perpendicular plane around the subject. Magnetic resonance imaging (MRI) systems measure nuclear relaxation times from nuclei of atoms with a magnetic moment that are aligned within a powerful magnetic field. Clinical systems are based on hydrogen, although it is possible to create images and spectrographs from phosphorus, sodium and carbon. The collected data are transformed into high-resolution images, and this allows quantifying whole-body or regional body composition. A large number of studies in phantoms, cadavers and *in vivo* validate these methods. There are no studies of imaging methods in relation to outcome.

CONCLUSIONS ABOUT NUTRITIONAL ASSESSMENT

Thus protein-energy malnutrition (protein-energy malnutrition) result in a continuum which starts when the patient fails to eat enough to meet needs and progresses through a series of functional changes which precede any changes in body composition which are related to the duration of reduced intake and its severity. To base the definition of protein-energy malnutrition on any one of these changes is inappropriate. Only by recognizing the different facets of protein-energy malnutrition can we define its various manifestations in relation to our clinical objectives. At present, SGA combined with selected objective parameters provides the best clinical way of meeting these objectives. In future, muscle function may be useful in determining optimal nutrient intake early in the course of feeding. Techniques such a BIA, DEXA and MRI combined with spectroscopy may provide powerful tools in the future.

ASSESSMENT OF FLUID STATUS

Water and salt are critically important constituents of the body, and disturbances of salt and water have quicker and more profound effects on health than nutrients. Body water comprises 73% of the lean body mass but 54% of body weight because fat does not contain water. Consequently, obese persons have less water in relation to body weight. Of total body water, 40% is the volume in which chloride is distributed and is extracellular; 60% resides in cells and is called the intracellular water in which body potassium and magnesium is distributed. The assessment of fluid status depends upon recognizing that body fluids are composed of isotonic saline and free water. The changes in the normal saline content alters the volume of the extracellular fluid and leaves the electrolyte concentration unchanged, while changes in free water alter the osmolarity and change plasma sodium concentration.

Clinically the status is assessed by:

1. History of conditions which can cause deficits or overload.
2. History of symptoms suggestive of abnormal fluid status.
3. Physical examination.
4. Biochemical tests.

Reduced saline compartment: reduced in extracellular fluid volume

There is a history of losses such as diarrhoea, large stomal and intestinal fistula output and/or vomiting. When the changes are mild with less than 10% reduction of extracellular fluid volume (ECF), the patients may have very few complaints except for rapid weight loss. When there is a greater reduction of ECF then there are symptoms of marked weight loss, dizziness and palpitations on changing from a recumbent to an erect posture, weakness, thirst and fainting. On examination there is postural tachycardia and fall in systolic blood pressure on changing posture. In normal individuals or those with < 7% volume depletion the pulse will rise by 10 beats/minute, the systolic pressure will fall by 5–10 mm and the diastolic will rise by 5–10 mm when the posture is changed from a recumbent to an erect state. With greater loss of the ECF the pulse rises by 20 beats/minute and the postural change in systolic pressure will be 20 mm or more without a similar compensatory rise in the diastolic pressure. Weight loss always occurs, with severe depletion (> 15%) the jugular venous wave is not seen even when the patient is lying flat. The changes in blood pressure may be missed unless the blood pressure is taken only after waiting for 10 minutes after change of position. The clinical features of ECF volume depletion are summarized in Table 17.2.

On biochemical testing the plasma sodium concentration is normal unless the patient has been drinking water to quench thirst, in which case the plasma sodium may fall below the normal range (hyponatraemia). When patients have a short bowel, losses of fluid from a jejunostomy, which is isotonic will cause serious volume contraction but leave the plasma sodium, potassium, chloride and bicarbonate concentrations normal. Losses from other sites can change the plasma electrolyte picture as indicated in Table 17.3. In addition renal urine electrolytes will show a marked reduction in sodium concentration < 10 mmol/L.

Increased saline compartment: increased in ECF

This condition occurs after vigorous resuscitation with sodium-containing fluids, in protein-energy malnutrition, heart failure, renal and hepatic diseases. The symptoms of saline overload are rapid weight gain, swelling of the extremities and abdomen, and breathlessness. On examination there may be one or more of

Table 17.2 – History and clinical features of ECF depletion

History	Symptoms	Physical signs
Losses of fluid: vomiting and diarrhoea Renal disease with diuresis Diuretic therapy	Weakness, thirst, dizziness, postural symptoms	Weight loss Dry mucous membranes Reduced skin turgor Reduced central venous pressure Postural changes in pulse > 10 beats/min and a fall in systolic pressure > 15 mm

Table 17.3 – Changes in plasma electrolytes with conditions resulting in loss of ECF

Clinical condition	Sodium	Potassium	Chloride	Bicarbonate
Vomiting	Normal	Low	Low	High
Jejunostomy losses	Normal	Normal	Normal	Normal
Pancreatic fistula	Normal	Normal	High	Low
Ileostomy	Normal	Normal or low	Normal or high	Normal or low
Diarrhoea	Normal	Low	High	Low

the following: acute weight gain, pitting oedema, ascites, raised jugular venous pressure and pleural effusion. In this condition the plasma electrolytes will be normal unless the patient has received diuretics and continues to drink water or receive fluids without sodium (e.g. isotonic glucose).

Increased free water: hyponatraemia

A very common cause of hyponatraemia is drinking excessive amounts of water due to thirst when there is loss of saline through vomiting, diarrhoea or diuretics. Another equally common cause if the infusion of isotonic glucose instead of saline in patients with losses of saline or overhydration with isotonic glucose in the postoperative state. A summary of the causes of hyponatraemia is given in Table 17.4.

Table 17.4 – Causes of hyponatraemia

Salt depletion with excessive water intake
   Diarrhoea and water drinking

Sequestration
   Burns, pancreatitis, peritonitis, ascites

Severe cardiac failure

Endocrine disturbances
   Adrenal insufficiency
   Hypothyroidism

Pathological water drinkers
   Inappropriate infusion of isotonic glucose

Drugs
   Morphine, clofibrate, barbiturates, tricyclics and
      antineoplastic agents

Syndrome of inappropriate ADH secretion (SIADH)
   Cerebral disease
   Pulmonary disease
   Neoplasia
   Porphyria

Clinically the plasma sodium has to fall below 125 mmol/L for the patient to become symptomatic. The patient complains of lethargy and nausea, then as the sodium level falls between 120 and 110 mmol/L, there is progressive mental confusion and when it falls below 110 mmol/L coma and seizures may occur. Care must be taken not to correct hyponatraemia too rapidly as central pontine myelinolysis can rapidly result.

Laboratory changes in hyponatraemia consist of a reduced plasma sodium concentration and a reduced plasma osmolarity. Pseudo-hyponatraemia occurs because all increased concentration of lipid or glucose in the plasma. Under the circumstances possible osmolarity is normal. The next question is whether hyponatraemia is associated with inappropriate anti-diuretic hormone (ADH) secretion alone or with ECF volume contraction. In the presence of normal renal function the presence of ECF volume contraction results in reduced urinary sodium and increased serum uric acid. When the inappropriate ADH secretion occurs without ECF volume contraction the urine sodium is increased and the plasma uric acid is low.

Reduced free water: hypernatraemia

Loss of water in excess of salt can occur as a result of losses from the gastrointestinal tract, kidneys, skin and due to inappropriate infusion of sodium-containing fluids. Diarrhoea associated with the ingestion of osmotic laxatives such as lactulose, diabetes insipidus, excessive sweating and the infusion of hypertonic saline into children or unconscious patients are factors which could result in hypernatraemia. A summary of the factors that cause hypernatraemia is given in Table 17.5.

Clinically hypernatraemia causes symptoms by dehydration of the brain and these are identical to those of hyponatraemia. However, given time the

Table 17.5 – Causes of hypernatraemia

Gastrointestinal losses
  Diarrhoea, fistula and vomiting

Renal losses
  Osmotic diuresis
  Diabetes insipidus

Skin losses
  Sweating
  Burns

Iatrogenic causes
  Infusion of hypertonic saline or bicarbonate to infants or
    comatose patients

brain restores brain volume by generating intracellular idiogenic osmoles[68] and therefore clinical effects depend not only upon the degree of hypernatraemia but also the rate of its development. Clinically it is important to differentiate between hypernatraemia with associated ECF contraction, which has the characteristics of ECF contraction, and pure water loss without postural hypotension. This condition is due to diabetes insipidus.

Abnormalities of acid-base balance

A complete analysis of acid-base disturbances is beyond the scope of this chapter. However, a summary of causes and key diagnostic features relevant to gastrointestinal diseases is given in Table 17.6. Mixed disorders are recognized by a difference between expected changes in pCO_2 or HCO_3 and those observed. The fall in pCO_2 in metabolic acidosis should be $1.5 \times [HCO_3] + 8 \pm 2$, if it is below this value the patient has both metabolic acidosis and respiratory alkalosis.

Potassium

Potassium is an intracellular ion and small shifts between the ECF and the intracellular fluid (ICF) can have profound effects on the circulating potassium levels. Since the circulating potassium concentration influences cell membrane polarization, changes in plasma potassium concentration has profound effects on cardiac and skeletal muscle contractility.

Hypokalaemia

The causes of hypokalaemia are given in Table 17.7. The clinical features are those of malaise, muscle weakness, restless leg syndrome, and even tetany can occur when the plasma potassium falls below 3 mmol/L; paralysis and rhabdomyolysis can occur if the plasma potassium falls below 2.5 mmol/L. At these levels cardiac ventricular ectopic rhythms and tachycardia can occur. Patients can develop digitalis toxicity. Renal water conservation is reduced and polyuria and loss of free water can occur causing hypernatraemia and thirst. When the plasma potassium falls below 3.0 mmol/L there is flattening of

Table 17.6 – Disturbances of acid-base equilibrium

Metabolic state	pH	HCO_3	pCO_2	Anion gap	Common causes
Metabolic acidosis	< 7.35	Reduced	Reduced	Reduced	Diarrhoea, pancreatic and biliary fistula, ureterosigmoidostomy
				Increased	Lactic or ketoacidosis
Respiratory acidosis	< 7.35	Increased	Increased	Normal	Respiratory depression due to narcotics, CNS disturbances
					Paralysis of the ventilatory apparatus
Metabolic alkalosis	> 7.44	Increased	Normal	Normal or low	Vomiting
					Chloride diarrhoea
					Hyperaldosteronism
					Excessive bicarbonate loads
Respiratory alkalosis	> 7.44	Normal or low	Low	Normal	Hepatic encephalopathy
					Hyperventilation
					Salicylate poisoning
					Hypoxaemia

Anion gap: Plasma (Na + K)–(Cl +HCO_3). Normal range 12–18 mmol/L.

Table 17.7 – Causes of hypokalaemia

Gastrointestinal losses
    Vomiting
    Diarrhoea, laxative abuse, fistula losses

Renal losses
    Diuretics
    Hyperaldosteronism
    Renal tubular acidosis

Poor diet
    Tea and toast diet
    Alcoholism

the T wave in the ECG and the development of a large U wave. ST depression can also occur.

Hyperkalaemia

The causes of hyperkalaemia are summarized in Table 17.8. Hyperkalaemia alters cardiac contractility and changes in the ECG occur early with a peaking of the T wave, prolonged P-R interval and widening of the QRS complex. There is tingling in peripheral muscles and progressive paralysis, which may mimic a Guillian–Barré syndrome.

Table 17.8 – Causes of hyperkalaemia

Pseudohyperkalaemia
    Haemolysis
    Increased WBC or platelets
Renal failure
Drugs
    Potassium sparing diuretics
    Angiotensin converting enzyme inhibitors

Adrenal insufficiency

Tissue necrosis and rhabdomyolysis

Magnesium

Magnesium is mainly an intracellular ion but the plasma levels are quite reliable as an index of deficiency. However, with mild deficiency the plasma levels may be normal but the urinary excretion is reduced. The causes of magnesium deficiency are summarized in Table 17.9. Clinically patients present with apathy, weakness, anorexia and nausea. On examination there may be neuromuscular hyper-irritability with tremors, stridor and positive Trousseau's and Chvostek's signs.

Table 17.9 – Causes of magnesium deficiency

Gastrointestinal losses
    Malabsorption syndromes but not pancreatic deficiency
    Short bowel
    Prolonged diarrhoea
    Parenteral nutrition

Endocrine disease
    Hyperparathyroidism

Alcoholism

Dietary deficiency

Diuretic therapy

The plasma magnesium levels are usually below 0.7 mmol/L. The 24-hour urine magnesium falls to below 3.0 mmol even when the plasma levels are normal. When the plasma magnesium fall below 0.4 mmol/L, hypocalcaemia may develop as bone becomes resistant to the action of parathormone. It is the associated hypocalcaemia that causes carpo-pedal spasm. Magnesium deficiency causes increased renal losses of potassium and can result in hypokalaemia. This hypokalaemia can only be corrected after magnesium has been given.

REFERENCES

1. ADA's definition for nutrition screening and assessment. *J Am Diet Assoc* 1994; **94**: 838–839.

2. Blackburn GL, Bistrian BR, Maini BS, Schlamm HT, Smith MF. Nutritional and metabolic assessment of the hospitalized patient. *J Parenter Enteral Nutr* 1977; **1**: 11–22.

3. Detsky AS, Baker JP, Mendelson RA, Wolman SL, Wesson DA, Jeejeebhoy KN. Evaluating the accuracy of nutritional assessment techniques applied to hospitalized patients: methodology and comparisons. *J Parenter Enteral Nutr* 1984; **8**: 153–159.

4. Robinson JD, Lupkiewicz SM, Palenik L, Lopez LM, Ariet M. Determination of ideal body weight for drug dosage calculations. *Am J Hosp Pharm* 1983; **40**: 1016–1019.

5. Stanley KE. Prognostic factors for survival in patients with inoperable lung cancer. *J Natl Cancer Inst* 1980; **65**: 25–32.

6. Dewys WD, Begg C, Lavin PT, *et al.* Prognostic effect of weight loss prior to chemotherapy in cancer patients. Eastern Cooperative Oncology Group. *Am J Med* 1980; **69**: 491–497.

7. Morgan DB, Hill GL, Burkinshaw L. The assessment of weight loss from a single measurement of body weight: the problems and limitations. *Am J Clin Nutr* 1980; **33**: 2101–2105.

8. Jelliffe DB. The assessment of the nutritional status of the community: with special reference to field surveys in developing regions of the world. WHO monograph. WHO, Geneva, 1966.

9. Frisancho AR. New norms of upper limb fat and muscle areas for assessment of nutritional status. *Am J Clin Nutr* 1981; **34**: 2540–2545.

10. Harries AD, Jones LA, Heatley RV, Rhodes J. Malnutrition in inflammatory bowel disease: An anthropometric study. *Hum Nutr Clin Nutr* 1982; **36**: 307–313.

11. Thuluvath PJ, Triger DR. How valid are our reference standards of nutrition? *Nutrition* 1995; **11**: 731–733.

12. Nelson EE, Hong CD, Pesce AL, Peterson DW, Singh S, Pollak VE. Antropometric norms for the dialysis population. *Am J Kidney Dis* 1990; **16**: 32–37.

13. Gray GE, Gray LK. Antropometric measurements and their interpretation: principles, practices and problems. *J Am Diet Assoc* 1980; **77**: 534–539.

14. Hall JC, O'Quigley J, Giles GR, Appleton N, Stocks H. Upper limb anthropometry: the value of measurement variance studies. *Am J Clin Nutr* 1980; **33**: 1846–1851.

15. Anderson CF, Wochos DN. The utility of serum albumin values in the nutritional assessment of hospitalized patients. *Mayo Clin Proc* 1982; **57**: 181–184.

16. Reinhardt GF, Myscofski JW, Wilkens DB, Dobrin PB, Mangan JE Jr, Stannard RT. Incidence and mortality of hypoalbuminemic patients in hospitalized veterans. *J Parenter Enter Nutr* 1980; **4**: 357–359.

17. Apelgren KN, Rombeau JL, Twomey PL, Miller RA. Comparison of nutritional indices and outcome in critically ill patients. *Crit Care Med* 1982; **10**: 305–307.

18. Kaw M, Seka G. Long-term follow up of consequences of percutaneous endoscopic gastrostomy (PEG) in nursing home patients. *Dig Dis Sci* 1994; **39**: 738–743.

19. Lowrie EG, Lew N. Death risk in hemodialysis patients: The predictive value of commonly measured variables and the evaluation of death rate differences between facilities. *Am J Kidney Dis* 1990; **15**: 458–482.

20. Klein S. The myth of serum albumin as a measure of nutritional status. *Gastroenterology* 1990; **99**: 1845–1846.

21. Jeejeebhoy KN. Cause of hypoalbuminaemia in patients with gastrointestinal and cardiac disease. *Lancet* 1962; **i**: 343.

22. Rothschild MA, Oratz M, Schreiber SS. Albumin synthesis. *N Engl J Med* 1972; **286**: 748–757.

23. James WPT, Hay AM. Albumin metabolism: Effect of the nutritional state and the dietary protein intake. *J Clin Invest* 1968; **47**: 1958–1972.

24. Broom J, Fraser MH, McKenzie K, *et al*. The protein metabolic response to short-term starvation in man. *Clin Nutr* 1986; **5**: 63.

25. Keys A, Brozek J, Henschel A, Mickelsen O, Taylor HL. *The Biology of Human Starvation*. University of Minnesota Press: Minneapolis, 1950.

26. Russell DMcR, Prendergast PJ, Darby PL, Garfinkel PE, Whitwell J, Jeejeebhoy KN. A comparison between muscle function and body composition in anorexia nervosa: the effect of refeeding. *Am J Clin Nutr* 1983; **38**: 229–237.

27. Castaneda C, Charnley JM, Evans WJ, Crim MC. Elderly women accommodate to a low-protein diet with losses of body cell mass, muscle function, and immune response. *Am J Clin Nutr* 1995; **62**: 30–39.

28. Moshage HJ, Janssen JAM, Franssen JH, Hafkenscheid JCM, Yap SH. Study of the molecular mechanism of decreased liver synthesis of albumin in inflammation. *J Clin Invest* 1987; **79**: 1635–1641.

29. Cohen S, Hansen JDL. Metabolism of albumin and gamma-globulin in Kwashiorkor. *Clin Sci* 1962; **23**: 411.

30. Fleck A, Hawker F, Wallace PI, Raines G, Trotters J, Ledingham I, Calman KC. Increase vascular permeability: a major cause of hypoalbuminemia in disease and injury. *Lancet* 1985; **1**: 781–784.

31. Gray GE, Meguid MM. Can total parenteral nutrition reverse hypoalbuminemia in oncology patients? *Nutrition* 1990; **6**: 225–228.

32. Waits RP, Yamada T, Uemichi T, Benson MD. Low plasma concentrations of retinol-binding protein in individuals with mutations affecting position 84 of the transthyretin molecule. *Clin Chem* 1995; **41**: 1288–1291.

33. Prealbumin in Nutritional Care Consensus Group. Measurement of visceral protein status in assessing protein and energy malnutrition: standard of care. *Nutrition* 1995; **11**: 169–171.

34. Hedlund JU, Hansson LO, Ortqvist AB. Hypoalbuminemia in hospitalized patients with community-acquired pneumonia. *Arch Intern Med* 1995; **155**: 1438–1442.

35. Winkler MF, Gerrior SA, Pomp A, Albina JE. Use of retinol-binding protein and prealbumin as indicators of response to nutrition therapy. *J Am Diet Assoc* 1989; **89**: 684–687.

36. Nieken J, Mulder NH, Buter J, Vellenga E, Limburg PC, Piers DA, de Vries EG. Recombinant human interleukin-6 induces a rapid and reversible anemia in cancer patients. *Blood* 1995; **86**: 900–905.

37. O'Riordain MG, Ross JA, Fearon KC, Maingay J, Farouk M, Garden OJ, Carter DC. Insulin and counterregulatory hormones influence acute-phase protein production in human hepatocytes. *Am J Physiol* 1995; **269**: E323–E330.

38. Cano N, Di Costanzo-Dufetel J, Calaf R, *et al.* Prealbumin retinol binding protein-retinol complex in hemodialysis patients. *Am J Clin Nutr* 1988; **47**: 664–667.

39. Dowd PS, Heatley RV. The influence of under-nutrition on immunity. *Clin Sci Mol Med* 1984; **66**: 241–248.

40. Meakins JL, Christou NV, Shizgal HM, MacLean LD. Therapeutic approaches to anergy in surgical patients. Surgery and levamisole. *Ann Surg* 1979; **190**: 286–296.

41. Dominioni L, Diogini R. Immunological function and nutritional assessment. *J Parenter Enteral Nutr* 1987; **11** (Suppl 5): 70S–72S.

42. Degoulet P, Legrain M, Reach I, *et al.* Mortality risk factors in patients treated by hemodialysis. *Nephron* 1983; **31**: 103–110.

43. Buzby GP, Mullen JP, Matthews DC. Prognostic nutritional index in gastrointestinal surgery. *Am J Surg* 1980; **139**: 160–167.

44. Baker JP, Detsky AS, Wesson DE, *et al.* Nutritional assessment: a comparison of clinical judgment and objective measurements. *N Engl J Med* 1982; **306**: 969–972.

45. Detsky AS, McLaughlin JR, Baker JP, Johnston N, Whittaker S, Mendelson RA, Jeejeebhoy KN. What is subjective global assessment of nutritional status? *J Parenter Enteral Nutr* 1987; **11**: 8–13.

46. Hirsch S, de Obaldia N, Petermann M, Rojo P, Barrientos C, Iturriaga H, Bunout D. Subjective global assessment of nutritional status: further validation. *Nutrition* 1991; **7**: 35–37.

47. Fenton SSA, Johnston N, Delmore T, *et al.* Nutritional assessment of continuous ambulatory peritoneal dialysis patients. *Trans Am Soc Artif Organs* 1987; **23**: 650–653.

48. Young GA, Kopple JD, Lindholm B, *et al.* Nutritional assessment of continuous ambulatory peritoneal dialysis patients: An international study. *Am J Kidney Dis* 1990; **17**: 462–471.

49. Enia G, Sicuso C, Alati G, Zoccali C. Subjective global assessment of nutrition in dialysis patients. *Nephrol Dial Transplant* 1993; **8**: 1094–1098.

50. Hasse J, Strong S, Gorman MA, Liepa G. Subjective global assessment: alternative nutrition-assessment technique for liver-transplant candidates. *Nutrition* 1993; **9**: 339–343.

51. Pikul J, Sharpe MD, Lowndes R, Ghent CN. Degree of preoperative malnutrition is predictive of post-operative morbidity and mortality in liver transplant recipients. *Transplantation* 1994; **57**: 469–472.

52. The Veterans Affairs total parenteral nutrition co-operative study group. Perioperative total parenteral nutrition in surgical patients. *New Engl J Med* 1991; 325–532.

53. Desai ID, Garcia Tavares ML, Dutra de Oliveira BS, *et al.* Anthropometric and cycloergometric assessment of the nutritional status of the children of agricultural migrant workers in Southern Brazil. *Am J Clin Nutr* 1981; **34**: 1925–1934.

54. Spurr GB, Barac-Nieto M, Maksud MG. Functional assessment of nutritional status: heart rate response to submaximal work. *Am J Clin Nutr* 1979; **32**: 767–778.

55. Klidjian AM, Foster KJ, Kammerling RM, Cooper A, Karran SJ. Relation of anthropometric and dynamo-metric variables to serious post-operative complications. *Br Med J* 1980; **2**: 899–901.

56. Russell DMcR, Leiter LA, Whitwell J, Marliss EB, Jeejeebhoy KN. Skeletal muscle function during hypocaloric diets and fasting: a comparison with standard nutritional assessment parameters. *Am J Clin Nutr* 1983; **38**: 229–237.

57. Edwards RHT. Physiological analysis of skeletal muscle weakness and fatigue. *Clin Sci Mol Med* 1978; **54**: 463–470.

58. Brough W, Horne G, Blount A. Irving MH, Jeejeebhoy KN. Effect of nutrient intake, surgery, sepsis and long term administration of steroids on muscle function. *Br Med J* 1986; **293**: 983–988.

59. Lenmarken C, Sandstedt S, Schenck HV, Larsson J. The effect of starvation on skeletal muscle function in man. *Clin Nutr* 1986; **5**: 99–103.

60. Zeiderman MR, McMahon MJ. The role of objective measurement of skeletal muscle function in the pre-operative patient. *Clin Nutr* 1989; **8**: 161–166.

61. Windsor JA, Hill GL. Weight loss with physiologic impairment: a basic indicator of surgical risk. *Ann Surg* 1988; **207**: 290–296.

62. Christie PM, Hill GL. Effect of intravenous nutrition on nutrition and function in acute attacks of inflammatory bowel disease. *Gastroenterology* 1990; **99**: 730–736.

63. Chan STF, McLaughlin SJ, Ponting GA, Biglin J, Dudley HA. Muscle power after glucose-potassium loading in undernourished patients. *Br Med J* 1986; **293**: 1055–1056.

64. Kotler DP, Tierney AR, Wang J, Pierson RN Jr. Magnitude of body-cell-mass depletion and the timing of death from wasting in AIDS. *Am J Clin Nutr* 1989; **50**: 444–447.

65. Halliday AW, Benjamin IS, Blumgart LH. Nutritional risk factors in major hepatobiliary surgery. *J Parenter Enteral Nutr* 1988; **12**: 43–48.

66. Lehr K, Schober O, Hundeshagen H, Pichlmayr R. Total body potassium depletion and the need for pre-operative nutritional support in Crohn's disease. *Ann Surg* 1982; **196**: 709–714.

67. Mann MD, Bowie MD, Hansen JD. Total body potassium and serum electrolyte concentrations in protein energy malnutrition. *S Afr Med J* 1975; **49**: 76–78.

68. Pollock AS, Arieff AI. Abnormalities of cell volume regulation and their functional consequences. *Am J Physiol* 1980; **239**: F195–205.

18

Insertion and care of enteral feeding tubes

A. Mensforth and J. Nightingale

INTRODUCTION

Most patients, except those with severe intestinal failure, have enough gut to absorb adequate macronutrients and fluid. Oral energy intake can be increased and dietary modifications made in order to maximize absorption (Ch. 25). If the addition of sip feeds fails to improve a patient's nutritional status, enteral feeding may be given to utilize the gut for longer periods (e.g. with an overnight enteral feed[1,2]).

Enteral feeding is usually preferred to parenteral nutrition as it is more physiological, less expensive and prevents biliary sludge formation. It may also maintain the gut barrier function to prevent endotoxin and bacterial translocation[3-5] which could lead to sepsis and multi-organ failure.

This chapter outlines the methods of inserting enteral feeding tubes and advises upon their subsequent care.

ACCESS ROUTES TO THE GUT

There are many ways to access the gut (Box 18.1, Fig. 18.1). Direct feeding into the colon/rectum has been successful in the past but is not currently used.[6] If there is a mucus fistula to defunctioned ileum or colon, however, saline or the effluent from a high stoma may be instilled into it to help with fluid/nutrient balance; this can be unpleasant and technically difficult.

Box 18.1 – Ways of providing enteral nutritional support

Nasal tube
Nasogastric
Nasoduodenal/jejunal

Pharyngostomy/oesophagostomy

Gastrostomy
Surgical
Percutaneous endoscopic (PEG)
Percutaneous fluoroscopic (PFG)

Duodenostomy/jejunostomy
Surgical (open surgical, needle catheter or laparoscopic)
Percutaneous endoscopic via gastrostomy (PEGJ)
Percutaneous fluoroscopic via gastrostomy (PFGJ)
Percutaneous endoscopic (PEJ)

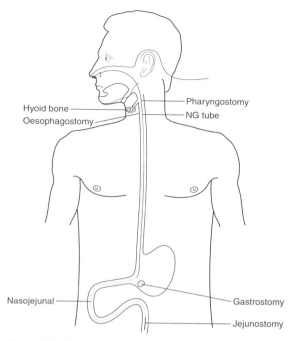

Figure 18.1 – Enteral routes for feeding.

NASOENTERIC FEEDING

An enteral feed may be given by a tube passed through the nose into the stomach, duodenum or jejunum (nasogastric, nasoduodenal and nasojejunal feeding). It has become traditional to insert enteral feeding tubes through the nose rather than the mouth as it is thought to be more comfortable for the patient and eliminates the possibility of the tube being bitten. Fine bore naso- or oro-enteral tubes are chosen for short-term feeding (up to 4–6 weeks) and a gastrostomy or jejunostomy tube for long-term enteral feeding.

Feed may be delivered into the stomach if there are no problems with aspiration or inadequate/delayed gastric emptying (e.g. if opiate drugs have been given). The stomach tolerates hypertonic feeds, higher feeding rates and bolus feeding better than the small intestine. After abdominal surgery, owing to increased sympathetic activity, the stomach may take 1–2 days to regain its motor function and the colon may take 3–5 days, but the motor and absorptive functions of the small bowel usually remain normal.[7-9] Thus post-pyloric feeding may be started safely within 12 hours of surgery/trauma, especially if the patient is already undernourished. Many units wait for at least 24 hours to allow for the 'ebb phase' of hypometabolism and some surgeons delay for 5 days, often to 'protect a distal anastomosis'.[10,11] Bowel sounds are an un-reliable indicator of bowel function as they are generated mainly by the stomach and colon. It is helpful if access for feeding, via the gut, is achieved at the time of surgery (e.g. by nasojejunal tube or needle jejunostomy).

Nasogastric tubes

Nasogastric tubes are generally marketed for single use; however, the manufacturers of some tubes advocate cleaning and re-passing of the same tube on the same patient if it is accidentally dislodged. The maximum rate of flow through an enteral feeding system depends mainly upon the tube diameter and length, and less upon the viscosity and temperature of the feed.[12]

Material

Fine-bore nasogastric tubes are made of polyvinyl chloride (PVC), latex, polyurethane or silicone, and are available in a variety of sizes and lengths. Polyurethane is preferred to polyvinyl chloride (PVC) and latex as it is more resistant to kinking. Polyurethane allows the tube wall to be thinner than with silicone, so that while its outer diameter is the same its internal diameter is larger, so allowing high flow rates. Naso-gastric tubes made from PVC tend to lose plasticizers after a few days; they become brittle and rarely can cause pressure necrosis of soft tissues. PVC tubes are damaged by radiotherapy. PVC tubes require changing after 7–10 days, whereas polyurethane or silicone tubes can remain in situ for a month. Many tubes are impregnated with a water-activated lubricant to help insertion, and many are radio-opaque.

Diameter

Large-bore Ryles tubes, used for gastric drainage, are uncomfortable and may be associated with rhinitis, oesophageal reflux, and oesophageal strictures. Fine-bore tubes (1.4–4.0 mm diameter, 4–12 Fr★) are more comfortable and cause less trauma to the nasopharynx and oesophagus. Fine-bore tubes are more easily

★ Fr stands for French Gauge, which is the same as CH (from Charrière, a Frenchman who described the measurement) and is the external circumference of a tube in millimetres. To derive Fr from the tube diameter, multiply by π.

displaced by coughing or vomiting than large-bore tubes, and there is a greater chance of them being accidentally inserted into a bronchus, especially in an unconscious patient. The presence of an endotracheal tube does not preclude the tube being passed down the trachea into a lung.

Quoted tube size is based on external diameter; the internal diameter is usually about one millimetre less. The diameter of a tube is the single most important limitation to flow, and an increase in internal diameter from 1 mm to 2 mm results in a 10-fold increase in flow. The limitation to flow is rarely clinically relevant; for example an 8 FG 100 cm long tube connected to a giving set and a feed container will discharge 100 ml of 24°C solution (viscosity 4.25 cps which is similar to/higher than most feeds) at a pressure of 75 cm water (about the height of a drip stand) within 5 minutes.[12] The fine-bore tubes used in clinical practice vary from 1.4 mm (4 FG) for small infants, to 2.7–4.0 mm (8–12 FG) for older children and adults. All com-mercially available feeds can be administered with good flow through an 8 FG tube though even smaller tubes may suffice (e.g. infants may be fed boluses via a 4 FG tube with no problems). Only if there is a need to give drugs through the tube, or if gastric juice needs to be aspirated regularly in adults, is a larger tube required.

Length

The total length of a nasogastric tube varies between 40 and 90 cm and is selected to ensure a manageable amount of external tubing. The longer the tube, the greater is the resistance to flow.[12] A weighted tip on a nasogastric tube does not make the tube easier to pass or less likely to become displaced.[13]

Insertion of nasogastric tubes

The method of insertion is outlined in Box 18.2. The tube must not be forced, and special care must be taken if a tube is considered necessary in a patient with mucositis or oesophageal varices. The tube may be passed through the mouth if there is a severe rhinitis. Soft, pliable nasogastric tubes made of polyurethane or silicone generally have a guidewire to aid insertion, while those made of PVC do not. There is still a small risk of misplacement (1.3%),[17] oesophageal or pulmonary perforation. There is a high rate of naso-gastric tubes 'falling out'. This 'non-elective removal' has been reported to be as high as 25% within the first 24 hours.[13]

Box 18.2 – Passing a nasogastric tube

Equipment

Tray, nasogastric tube, sterile/boiled water, hypo-allergenic tape or other fixative, glass of water, lubricating jelly, 10 and 50 ml syringe, blue litmus/pH paper, measuring tape.

Method

1. Explain the procedure and arrange a signal for patient to give if he/she wants the procedure to stop.
2. Sit the patient upright and do not tilt the head backwards (if insertion is difficult it can be helpful to put the head forwards and/or turn it to one side).
3. Measure the distance from the xiphisternum to an earlobe and from there to the nose (50–60 cm in adults).
4. Check that the nostrils are patent by getting patient to sniff with each nostril occluded in turn.
5. Wash and dry your hands.
6. Put out the equipment. Mark the tube with the measured distance. If there is a guidewire in the tube, remove it and flush the tube with 10 ml water, then reinsert the guidewire; this allows the wire to be withdrawn freely. Check that the guidewire does not protrude through the end of the tube and that it is freely mobile within the tube.
7. The clearest nostril may be sprayed with lignocaine. Lubricate the tube with a small amount of lubricating jelly (or water).
8. Gently slide the tube backwards along the floor of the clearest nostril. At a distance of 10–15 cm the tube can usually be seen at the back of the pharynx. If possible, at this point ask the patient to take a mouthful of water and hold it. Ask the patient to swallow and at that moment advance the tube 5–10 cm, stop when the swallowing stops and repeat 3–6 times. If the patient becomes distressed, continually coughs or becomes blue, remove the tube. If there is difficulty passing the tube, the patient can turn his/her head either way by 90°[8] and flex the head.
9. When the mark (at 50–60 cm in adults) is reached, stop advancing the tube and gently remove the guidewire. Do not attempt to replace the guidewire when the tube is in situ as it may exit from the side of the tube and cause a perforation.

10. Check the tube position by aspirating 2–5 ml gastric juice and check that the pH is less than 4 using the litmus/pH paper. If so, the tube is in the correct position and can be secured at the nose and feeding begun. If not, the tube may not be in the stomach or the stomach may not be producing acid (e.g. if the patient is taking a proton inhibitor drug); an abdominal radiograph is then needed to confirm the position of the tube tip. Auscultating for bubbles is unreliable as bubbles can be heard even if the tube is in the lung.

Additional comments

- The end of the tube can be left in a glass of water as the tube is inserted. If the tube then enters the lung, there should be bubbles in the water.
- If the patient is heavily sedated or has had a general anaesthetic, the head can be flexed to 30° and the larynx lifted anteriorly.[14]

Methods for passing a nasojejunal tube

When the tube is in the stomach (60 cm), the guidewire inside the tube can be removed and a 30° bend made 3 cm from the tip. The wire is then carefully replaced. This allows the tube to be rotated to assist its passage through the pylorus.[15] In addition, when the tube is at 60 cm, the patient is turned onto his/her right side and the tube advanced to about 70 cm. This usually results in passage of the tube; if not, the stomach can be rapidly inflated with 500–1000 ml of air before the tube is advanced further.[16] Rotating the tube clockwise[8] and giving 10 mg intravenous metoclopramide may also help the tube pass the pylorus.[16] The tube position should be checked radiologically and ideally screened so that the tube tip is positioned at or beyond the duodeno-jejunal flexure.

Checking position of nasogastric tubes

The intragastric position of a nasogastric tube should be confirmed before using the tube for feeding or administering medication. This should be carried out every time the tube is used; failure to do so may result in feed or medication being delivered to the lungs. There are four methods for checking position of the tube.

Aspiration

Two to five millilitres of gastric juice is aspirated through the nasogastric tube using a 50 ml syringe. A 50 ml syringe exerts less negative pressure and so is less likely than a smaller syringe to create a vacuum and cause damage. The aspirate is checked, using either blue litmus paper (which turns pink when exposed to acid) or pH paper, and should show an acidic fluid with a pH of less than 4.[18,19] Care in interpreting the pH is advised if little fluid is aspirated and much lubricating jelly has been used, as lubricating jelly has an acidic pH. Fluids aspirated from the respiratory and intestinal tract or from a patient receiving a proton pump inhibitor all have an alkaline pH. In future, a means of both measuring pH and detecting a gastric (e.g. pepsin) or intestinal enzyme (e.g. trypsin) may become available.

Problems

No aspirate in syringe. If this occurs, check that the correct/usual length of tubing is visible externally and that the tube is firmly secured to the face. If a longer length of tube than expected is visible, the tube may have slipped back and thus needs to be removed or re-sited. If the tube appears to be of correct length, it may be that the tip is not in contact with gastric contents; in this case, the position of the patient can be changed (i.e. to lie on the left or right side, sit up, etc.) and aspiration again attempted. Alternatively, if some oral intake is possible, the patient can be given a drink to increase the volume of the gastric contents before another attempt is made to aspirate the stomach. If these methods fail, the tube may be advanced a short distance (2–5 cm) and aspiration again tried. This may not be possible with some polyurethane tubes.

Aspirate is not acidic. This may occur if the patient is taking antacids, H_2 antagonists or proton pump inhibitors. A confirmatory abdominal radio-graph may be needed.

Auscultation

Air is injected into the stomach via the nasogastric tube and at the same time the observer listens with a stethoscope over the upper abdomen; bubbling should be heard. This method can be falsely reassuring and bubbles may be heard when the tube is in the lung base. This technique should not be relied upon.

A feeding tube can be attached to a specially adapted stethoscope; if the tube is in the trachea or bronchi, loud breath sounds are heard.[20]

Abdominal radiography

Abdominal radiography is the definitive way to confirm the correct position of a radio-opaque naso-gastric tube. Most tubes have radio-opaque markings, or contain a radio-opaque compound (e.g. bismuth trioxide). Although it is a reliable method, it is only indicative of the position of the tube at the time of x-ray, and is therefore not necessarily correct at the time the patient starts feeding, when aspiration should again be done. It may be used as a check on initial placement of the tube if acidic gastric juice cannot be aspirated. Many community hospitals, and patients at home, do not have access to x-ray facilities and so do not have this ultimate checking system. When tubes are dislodged frequently (e.g. in patients with neuro-logical problems), repeated x-rays are not practical and the radiation exposure becomes unacceptable. An additional problem is that feeding is delayed while a patient is waiting for a radiograph and its interpre-tation.

Laryngoscopy

If the patient is unconscious, the tube can be visualized passing into the upper oesophagus using a laryngo-scope or endoscope.

Nasoduodenal and nasojejunal tubes

Post-pyloric feeding may be indicated when there is delayed gastric emptying (gastroparesis or atony) or an increased risk of aspiration (large hiatus hernia). Nasoduodenal/jejunal tubes may be single lumen (as for a nasogastric tube but of a longer length) or double lumen, allowing feeding into the small intestine while aspirating gastric secretions. A nasojejunal tube which develops a spiral coil when the guidewire is removed (Bengmark) can be inserted into the stomach and in most patients will pass spontaneously into the small bowel, probably being carried there by the fasting migrating myoelectrical complex (Ch. 2). This type of tube may stay in position more reliably than a straight tube.[21]

Insertion of a nasoduodenal/jejunal tube

Post-pyloric tube placement may be difficult, and various techniques have been adopted (Box 18.2). A randomized prospective trial in 1993 showed that tubes with weighted tips were less likely than unweighted tubes to pass through the pylorus.[22] This may be because a weighted tip naturally falls into the antrum to a level below that of the pylorus. Fluoroscopic techniques are generally successful[23,24] and almost as often successful as endoscopic placement.[24] Endoscopic placement may be difficult.[25] If the nasoenteral tube is grasped with forceps and taken to the distal duodenum/proximal jejunum using a paediatric colonoscope, it easily becomes displaced during withdrawal of the endoscope, even when the guidewire has been left within the tube. It is technically easier to position a long guidewire through an endoscope into the jejunum, and then withdraw the endoscope completely to leave the guidewire in situ. The wire can be re-routed through the nose (using a short tube passed through the nose and out of the mouth). The lubricated nasoenteric tube is passed over the guidewire into the jejunum while being careful to maintain the same length of guidewire outside the patient.

It may be advantageous to give metoclopramide,[22] erythromycin or cisapride just prior to any insertion procedure to increase gastric emptying and help the tube pass the pylorus. Neostigmine may also be used, but careful cardiac monitoring is needed as it may cause a severe bradycardia. A plain abdominal radiograph should be taken 8–12 hours after insertion to confirm position, except in pregnant women.

A polyurethane tube of 105–145 cm can be expected to last about 10 days; the longer-length tubes can be positioned further into the intestine and allow more free tube outside the nose; they do not block more frequently than shorter ones.[26]

Confirmation of position of nasoduodenal/nasojejunal tubes

In hospital, an abdominal radiograph is usually taken to confirm the position of a post-pyloric feeding tube; however this is not possible if the patient is at home or is pregnant. The following auscultation and aspiration techniques may then be used to attempt confirmation that the tube is situated beyond the pylorus, but they are not conclusive.[8] If air is injected down the tube during insertion, the loudest place that bubbling is heard (with a stethoscope) is initially on the left side of the abdomen (in the stomach) then, when the tube is past the pylorus, on the right side of the abdomen. In addition, the volume of air that can be aspirated from a post-pyloric tube, after 60 ml air has been instilled, is usually about 10 ml as compared to 40 ml if the tube

is in the stomach. A more reliable method is to aspirate fluid which should show a pH change from less than or equal to 4 in the stomach, to greater than or equal to 6 in the duodenum/small bowel. Other techniques for placing a transpyloric tube include the use of ultrasound, gastrointestinal magnetic imaging[27] or an electromyogram.[8]

Securing of nasoenteric tubes

A nasoenteric tube can be secured with a non-allergenic fixative on the maxilla, and the tube can be hooked over the ear. A technique of making a nasal bridle for confused patients has been described. A catheter is passed through one nostril and brought out of the mouth (as done initially for re-routing a tube from the mouth to the nose). Surgical ribbon is taped to the catheter coming out of the mouth. The catheter is pulled gently back out of the nose and a 15 cm length of ribbon is left emerging from one nostril. The procedure is repeated through the other nostril, and the ribbon is cut 15 cm from the nose. Thus ribbon passes into one nostril, goes round the nasal septum, and exits through the other nostril. The ends of the tape are tied through tape fastened round the nasoenteric tube.[28,29] This sounds unpleasant but the technique is very effective and causes only minor discomfort to the patient.

CERVICAL PHARYNGOSTOMY AND OESOPHAGOSTOMY

A tube with its insertion in the neck above the cricoid cartilage is termed a pharyngostomy; one below the cricoid is an oesophagostomy. Either may be performed after maxillofacial surgery, often performed for head/neck cancer. These are basically blind procedures that carry not only the risks of any operation but also the risk of pharyngeal or oesophageal leaks or salivary fistulas. The tubes are just as visible as nasoenteric tubes and are extremely uncomfortable for the patient, as whenever the neck is moved it pulls on the tube. Now that percutaneous endoscopic or radiologically guided enterostomies can be made, usually prior to surgery, pharyngostomy and oesophagostomy are rarely performed except in the very rare circumstance that, for anatomic reasons, a nasoenteric tube, gastrostomy or jejunostomy cannot be placed.

Cervical pharyngostomy was first described by Shumrick in 1967.[30] It can be performed using open dissection, a percutaneous approach,[31] or a combination of both. The pyriform sinus is located with an index finger passed down the lateral pharyngeal wall until below the hyoid bone; a right-angle forceps is inserted through the mouth and pushed out in this position. A small stab incision is made through the skin, then mainly blunt dissection is used to reach the forceps, which are pushed out of the side of the neck. Tape is grasped and pulled back into the pharynx, Kelly forceps hold onto the tape, so are pulled from outside the neck into the pharynx, the proximal end of an already in situ orogastric tube is grasped by the Kelly's forceps and pulled out through the skin incision.[32] If a long-term pharyngostomy is required, a more definitive incision is made along the anterior border of the sternocleidomastoid muscle, and it and the carotid sheath are retracted laterally. The exit site is made as before but the pharyngeal mucosa is sutured to the cervical skin.

Cervical oesophagostomy was described by Klopp in 1951.[33] The approach is usually on the left side of the neck as the oesophagus lies to the left of the midline in this area. A formal dissection requires a 4–6 cm oblique supraclavicular incision. The sterno-cleidomastoid muscle is retracted laterally after careful open dissection that does not damage the thyroid or its vessels, trachea, recurrent laryngeal nerve, carotid sheath and contents or thoracic duct. A tube is then inserted through a 5 mm incision in the lateral wall of the oesophagus. The tube feeds into the stomach and either exits through the lower end of the incision or from a separate stab incision.[34]

For both procedures the position of the feeding tube tip can be checked as for other nasoenteric tubes.

GASTROSTOMY FEEDING

A gastrostomy may be inserted surgically, endoscopically or under radiological/ultrasound guidance. It means that the patient can be fed without having to swallow and is likely to receive a greater amount of the prescribed feed than from a nasoenteric tube.[35,36] Gastrostomy feeding devices are currently made from polyurethane or silicone, and may vary in diameter from 9 Fr to 20 Fr. As with nasogastric tubes, the smallest diameter that is adequate for feeding is chosen. Thin tubes are cosmetically most acceptable to patients. Gastrostomy tubes differ in appearance, but share most of the same features. An inner radio-opaque

fixation device (a soft flange or a balloon) sits against the anterior stomach wall. It prevents the tube from being accidentally pulled out and, as long as it is held securely against the gastric mucosa, it prevents leakage of gastric contents. An external fixation device is positioned comfortably against the skin and is adjusted to accommodate weight changes. It prevents migration of the tube through the pylorus, and also prevents leakage and soreness due to excessive inward/outward movement of the tube.

Endoscopically placed gastrostomy

An endoscopic gastrostomy can be inserted, under light sedation and using local anaesthetic, in over 95% of adult patients. A gastrostomy placed at endoscopy is a less expensive procedure than one placed at open operation. It may not be possible to insert an endoscopic gastrostomy safely if a patient has had a gastrectomy, has ascites, hepatomegaly, a neoplastic/infiltrative disease of the gastric wall, an obstructing oesophageal lesion, a coagulation problem or is in the later stages of pregnancy. It may be difficult if the patient is obese and if it is not possible to bring the anterior gastric wall into contact with the anterior abdominal wall.

All techniques involve gastric insufflation to bring the stomach wall into apposition with the abdominal wall, percutaneous placement of a tapered cannula into the stomach, passage of guidewire/thread into the stomach, placement of the gastrostomy and verification of its position. There are three ways in which an endoscope can be used to help position a gastrostomy tube: by a pull (traction), push, or observational technique. The tubes inserted by the first two methods are commonly referred to as PEGs (percutaneous endoscopic gastrostomies). The pull technique was introduced in 1980[37] and takes only 15–20 minutes to perform (Box 18.3).[38,39] The push technique is similar to the pull technique except that a 300 cm flexible-tipped guidewire is inserted into the stomach instead of a thread, the wire is snared and brought out through the mouth, and the gastrostomy tube is pushed over it down through the mouth and into the stomach.[40] No significant differences have been found between the push and pull techniques in terms of procedure time or complications.[41,42]

Some studies show benefit from giving antibiotics (e.g. a single dose of 2.2 g co-amoxiclav 30 minutes before the procedure) to avoid peristomal wound

Box 18.3 – Pull method for placing a percutaneous endoscopic gastrostomy

1. The procedure is explained to the patient/relative/carer and written informed consent obtained. The platelets and INR may need to be corrected if there is a risk of bleeding. The patient is fasted for 6 hours before the procedure. Prophylactic antibiotics may be given half an hour before the procedure. Some units may stop H$_2$ antagonists/PPI for 1–3 days before the procedure, and some carefully clean the mouth with an antiseptic mouthwash immediately before the procedure.

2. The PEG inserter (A1) sets up a trolley near to the endoscopy table and examines the patient's abdomen for scars and enlarged organs. The size and position of the aorta is noted. The patient is sedated with an intravenous injection of a short-acting benzodiazepine. The gastric smooth muscle is relaxed by an intravenous injection of 20 mg hyoscine butylbromide.

3. The endoscopist (A2) performs a full upper gastrointestinal endoscopy, noting in particular any evidence of a hiatus hernia or oesophagitis (a duodenal biopsy and test for *Helicobacter pylori* may be done). The patient is turned onto the back. The stomach is distended with air. A1 pushes a finger gently into the epigastric region about halfway between xiphisternum and umbilicus, A2 sees if this is visible in the gastric antrum. The site of maximum indentation is chosen. If no indentation is seen, the endoscope light power is turned to full brightness and A1 observes if the light can be seen through the abdominal wall. Sometimes, on transillumination a shadow from the transverse colon can be seen and this area must be avoided. These two techniques locate the route that the PEG's sheathed trochar (with air valve) will take to enter the stomach. Originally, the site chosen for a gastrostomy was one-third of the distance from umbilicus to left costal margin in the mid-clavicular line. Although the PEG can be inserted anywhere in the abdomen, the rectus abdominis muscles and abdominal creases are best avoided.

4. A1 washes and dries hands, opens the dressing pack, and puts on sterile gloves. Antiseptic solution is poured into a small container. 5 ml of 1% lignocaine solution is drawn up.

5. A1 cleans a 15 cm area of abdominal skin and puts a small dressing towel below the intended insertion site. Using a small, then a long injection needle, the skin and route to the stomach (including peritoneum) are anaesthetized with about 2–3 ml of 1% lignocaine solution. The longer needle can often be seen by A2 to enter the stomach. If this can be done there is rarely any problem in subsequently inserting the sheathed trochar. The PEG set is opened and tipped onto the open dressing pack.

6. A1 makes a 1–3 mm vertical skin incision about 5 mm deep with a pointed scalpel. The sheathed trochar is carefully inserted along the line by which the long needle entered the stomach; it is advanced with short jabs. Sometimes the needle can only be made to fully enter the stomach with the help of biopsy forceps used by A2. When 1–2 cm are free inside the stomach, the trochar is removed to leave the sheath in place; the latter may need a cap over it to prevent air escaping.

7. A narrow long thread is inserted down the sheath. A2 catches this in the stomach with biopsy forceps or a snare and withdraws the thread up into the endoscope. A1 must take care that not all the thread is pulled up into the endoscope. The endoscope is withdrawn and the thread is left coming out of the mouth.

8. The PEG is held by A1 and tied to the thread. A1 then pulls the PEG down through the mouth into the stomach and, using gentle traction, pulls the dilating end of the PEG out onto the abdominal wall.

9. The dilating end of the PEG is cut off and attachments made according to the manufacturer's instructions. The patient returns to the ward with clear written instructions about subsequent care for the next 2 weeks.

infection[43–45] though others have been less encouraging.[46,47] An antiseptic mouthwash before the procedure may also be beneficial.

The observer technique involves first distending the stomach with air via a nasogastric tube; the abdominal assistant then introduces a needle and guidewire into the stomach. Under endoscopic observation (the endoscope can be used to push the stomach towards the anterior abdominal wall), the tract is dilated and a peel-away introducer sheath is passed into the stomach. A balloon catheter is then passed into the stomach, inflated, and the sheath removed.[48,49] This technique may be less prone to entry site infections as the tube has not passed through the mouth.

The external fixation device (disc/plate) is made of non-irritant material and provides a secure external grip on the catheter, keeping it in contact with the skin; it also prevents the tube from kinking/looping. It may alter the tube angle by 90 degrees.

Problems

Complications requiring surgery occur in fewer than 5% of patients; the procedure-related mortality rate is 0.3–2%.[44,50–52] Most deaths are caused by the underlying illness. The main problems are infection of the insertion site and peristomal leakage.[53,54] Other rare early problems include peritonitis, septicaemia, tube dislodgement, pulmonary aspiration, bowel perforation, gastro-colic fistula and necrotizing fasciitis.[55] Bleeding problems should be avoided if coagulation abnormalities are corrected before the procedure.

Complications are more common in under-nourished patients (e.g. those with cancer/HIV infection)[54,55] and mortality is higher during the first month in patients with previous aspiration or urinary tract infections or those who are older than 75 years.[56]

A benign pneumoperitoneum is common and can be seen on abdominal or chest x-rays in as many as 38% of patients.[57,58] It is important to recognize this as a normal finding – it does not mean that the patient has a significant bowel perforation.

In the long term, aspiration pneumonia may occur in 23% of patients.[59]

Button gastrostomy

When a gastrostomy tract has become established, the catheter may be replaced with a button-type gastrostomy, especially in children.[60] The button-type gastrostomy (14–28 FG) consists of a small catheter with an internal water or saline balloon containing 5–20 ml. It is anchored externally with a flange, and the button opening is flush with the skin. The button has a duckbill anti-reflux valve, which prevents leakage of gastric contents. A feeding extension clicks into it when in use, and a cap fits into it when not in use. It has the advantage of being level with the skin and so more convenient and cosmetically acceptable.

When inserting a button for the first time, the length of the abdominal wall tract is measured by inserting a balloon catheter with measurements along its side. The balloon is inflated with 5 ml air and pulled back, the length of the tract is measured and a suitable size button is selected. If the shaft length is too long, the balloon does not sit close to the gastric mucosa. This may cause leakage of the stomach contents around the button shaft. If the shaft is too short, skincare may be difficult and soreness can result. If the tube is tight or painful, a lateral abdominal x-ray is performed to check that the balloon is in the stomach, not the peritoneal cavity. The balloon volume should be checked every 7 days, as there is always a small loss of volume.

Surgical gastrostomy

A surgical gastrostomy may be fashioned at the time of other abdominal surgery using the Stamm technique;[61] a laparoscopic technique has also been described.[62] The Stamm technique uses concentric submucosal purse-string sutures (two rows) that invaginate the serosa about a mushroom-tipped tube passed into the anterior stomach wall at the junction of the body and antrum. An exit separate from the laparotomy incision is made for the tube. The gastric serosa is sutured to the peritoneum and transversalis fascia.[63]

Surgical gastrostomy is rarely performed as percutaneously inserted gastrostomies are quicker to accomplish, avoid a general anaesthetic, and usually have a lower incidence of stomal leakage and wound infection.[64–66] Ho and Ngo showed no difference in the complications following a PEG, laparoscopic or open gastrostomy.[67] A PEG or, rarely, a balloon catheter can be inserted at the time of surgery, though the latter may be difficult to connect to a giving set and may not last as long.

Percutaneous fluoroscopic gastrostomy (PFG)

The technique for insertion of a PFG is outlined in Box 18.4.[68] Often a PFG or PFGJ (percutaneous fluoroscopically placed gastrojejunostomy) succeeds when a PEG has not been possible,[69,70] though it does not allow the upper gastrointestinal tract to be carefully inspected. A study of 133 patients who underwent percutaneous non-endoscopic gastrostomy placement found a 1.5% incidence of major complications requiring operative intervention and a 3% incidence of minor complications;[65] this may be less than with a PEG.[70]

Box 18.4 – Radiological method of placing a percutaneous gastrostomy

A gastrostomy tube can be placed using ultrasound or x-ray guidance (fluoroscopically) or both.

1. Ultrasound may be used to determine the position of the liver and transverse colon relative to the stomach. Occasional injections of air into the colon via a rectal tube can be used to delineate the transverse colon, but too much gas makes ultrasound difficult.
2. A nasogastric tube is passed into the stomach, and the stomach is distended with air.
3. Upon selection of a site in the mid-body of the stomach, an aseptic technique is used, gloves are worn, the skin is cleaned and the area draped with towels. The skin, subcutaneous tissues and peritoneum are injected with local anaesthetic.
4. The abdominal wall is punctured with a needle through which a T fastener is passed to anchor the anterior gastric wall to the abdominal wall. One to four of these may be inserted.
5. The abdominal wall between the anchoring clasps is punctured with a needle inside a sheath. Using fluoroscopic guidance, the needle is inserted into the stomach and then withdrawn, leaving the sheath in place.
6. A water-soluble contrast agent may be injected to confirm the position of the sheath within the stomach.
7. A wire is passed into the stomach and the sheath removed. The opening may be dilated using progressively larger dilators. A catheter (pigtail or balloon type) is passed into the stomach over the wire. The wire is removed and the threads to a pigtail catheter released or a balloon inflated.
8. Contrast may again be injected through the catheter to try to ensure that there is no leakage into the peritoneal cavity. If a jejunal tube is needed a catheter can be inserted through the pylorus into the duodenum or jejunum.
9. An external fixing device is attached and sutured to the skin.

POST-PYLORIC FEEDING

Percutaneous gastro–jejunostomy

If a percutaneous endoscopic gastro-jejunostomy (PEGJ) is to be done, a large (e.g. 15 FG) gastrostomy tube is inserted and through this the jejunostomy tube is passed with a stiffening wire in its centre. The patient is re-intubated with a long endoscope (e.g. a paediatric colonoscope), the end of the jejunostomy tube is grasped by biopsy forceps, and the tube is taken slowly (using the push-pull techniques of colonoscopy) about 30–50 cm distal to the pylorus (at or beyond the duodeno-jejunal flexure). The endoscope is withdrawn to the gastric body while the forceps are advanced to keep the jejunal tube in position. The biopsy forceps let go of the tube and are gently shaken as they are withdrawn to try to prevent the jejunostomy tube from returning into the stomach. When the forceps have been fully withdrawn, the stiffening wire is removed from the jejunostomy tube. The view from the endoscope will show the tube passing through the pylorus. An abdominal radiograph is done to confirm the post-pyloric position of the jejunostomy tube tip. Only when the tip is considered to be in a satisfactory position is the tube cut and connected to the inner gastrostomy tube. Some tubes allow the stomach to be drained at the same time as the jejunal feed is given. If the tube cannot be placed endoscopically, it may be done radiologically (PFGJ), which may be easier if the PEG has been inserted through the greater curve of the stomach.

There have, in the past, been many difficulties with PEGJ tubes.[71–73] In particular, PEGJ tubes often become displaced back into the stomach[73] or become disconnected and the whole tube passes through the PEG and into the gut. A PEGJ does not necessarily prevent aspiration,[71] though a patient with a PFGJ is less likely to develop pneumonia than one with a PEG.[74] Tube blockage, leakage, migration or fracture occurred in 53% of PEGJs compared to 24% of PEGs in a mean follow-up of 275 days.[72] Newer designs of jejunostomy tube with a distal flexible, non-weighted tip that can easily be grasped with biopsy forceps may be better; though the connection of the jejunostomy tube to the gastrostomy tube can still become detached and result in the tube being lost into the gut.

Percutaneous endoscopic jejunostomy

A technique similar to PEG insertion can be used to insert a percutaneous endoscopic jejunostomy (PEJ) in patients who have had a gastrectomy. Sometimes a paediatric colonoscope can be positioned in the distal duodenum, the duodeno-jejunal flexure or beyond, and under radiological guidance a needle inserted into the bowel just distal to the scope. If thread can be introduced through a medium-sized needle (the large introducers supplied with a PEG set are usually too big and do not penetrate the bowel) then a PEG-type tube can be inserted in the usual way (to prevent the thread being cut, the needle must be completely withdrawn as the thread is pulled into the endoscope). Radiological screening also helps to prevent other structures (especially the transverse colon) being entered with the needle.

Surgical needle jejunostomy

It is difficult at surgery to manipulate a nasoenteric tube round the duodenum and into the jejunum. It can be difficult to both aspirate the stomach and feed into the small bowel at the same time, though tubes are available to do this. For these reasons a needle jejunostomy is often inserted at the time of operation (Box 18.5).[75–79] A laparoscopic method of inserting a needle jejunostomy has been described.[80] Complications are common, especially tube dislodgement or

---

Box 18.5 – Surgical placement of a needle jejunostomy

At the end of the laparotomy a needle jejunostomy may be inserted. This takes about 20 minutes.

1. A loop of jejunum about 10–30 cm distal to the duodeno-jejunal flexure or gastro-intestinal anastomosis is selected and orientated. The distance should be sufficiently great to allow tension-free apposition to the abdominal wall.
2. A 1 cm diameter purse-string absorbable suture is placed on the antimesenteric border of the jejunum at the site selected for jejunal catheter insertion. The ends are left untied.
3. A submucosal tunnel is created on the antimesenteric border using a 12–14 gauge hollow needle with a retractable obturator.

With the obturator withdrawn, the needle is pushed into the seromuscular layer within the purse-string suture. The obturator is advanced and the blunt end used to create an intramural tract for 2.5–5.0 cm before the obturator is withdrawn and the sharp needle is advanced into the lumen. If the needle tip position is uncertain, 10 ml of air can be injected into the bowel and distension observed; if there is resistance the needle is withdrawn and another attempt is made to enter the bowel lumen.

4. If present, the flexible J end of the guidewire is identified and put into the catheter (but not so that it protrudes from the catheter). The catheter (with guidewire) is then advanced through the needle into the bowel lumen.
5. The needle is removed while grasping the catheter within the bowel; the catheter is advanced for 20–45 cm. If necessary, the J end of the guidewire may be advanced to just beyond the distal end of the catheter to help passage. Care is taken to prevent the catheter from kinking or curling within the bowel. The guidewire is removed and the purse-string is tied.
6. In addition to the submucosal tunnel, a short (2–3 cm) Witzel tunnel is often made by suturing two parts of the seromuscular layer (from the same circumference) together around the catheter, so covering the catheter. The sutures must not be tight enough to cause occlusion of the catheter or to cause tissue necrosis.
7. A second sheathed hollow needle that can be split (or that has a sheath that can be split) is inserted through the left abdominal wall at a position where there will be no tension on the bowel. The catheter is fed through this (or if necessary the needle is removed) and the needle (or introducer) is split and removed.
8. The jejunum is stitched to the anterior abdominal wall using 2–3 sutures around the catheter.
9. The catheter is placed in an external fixative device (retainer) which is sutured with non-reactive monofilament sutures to the skin.
10. The site may be covered with a clear dressing and any attachments are connected to the catheter. Catheter patency is confirmed using 20 ml air, saline or contrast.

obstruction,[79,81] and the outcome is no better than for a well-placed and cared-for surgical tube jejunostomy.[82] The bowel can kink at the catheter entry point, so causing obstruction, or leakage can occur. The incidence of aspiration pneumonia is still high at about 16%.[80] The tube is always left in for 3–5 weeks, even if feeding has stopped, so that a tract can become established and the purse-string suture holding the tube will have dissolved. This may take longer if the patient is taking steroids.

CARE OF A PATIENT RECEIVING ENTERAL FEEDING

Skin care

Each day, after the insertion of a percutaneous gastrostomy or jejunostomy, the site should be cleaned gently with unperfumed soap and water and the tube gently rotated by 90°, but not pushed inwards. A loose absorbent dressing may be needed. Full healing occurs 10–14 days after placement. After that no dressing is needed and the patient can move, bathe and shower as normal with the tube capped. If a 9 FG PEG is used, the skin incision is so small that early PEG problems are very rare;[83] however, peritonitis, fasciitis and pericatheter leaks are reported.[84]

After 2–4 weeks the anterior gastric or jejunal wall becomes adherent to the abdominal wall so that an intraperitoneal leak is improbable. Thus, after the first two weeks and then every week, the external fixing plate should be undone, the tube pushed in and rotated, and the skin cleaned and dried. The tube is pulled with light traction and the external fixing device is reattached. If the external fixing device is positioned while the patient lies supine, it may be tight when sitting/standing and have to be loosened. The external fixation device may also need loosening as the patient puts on weight. If the tube is kept too tight and not rotated, epithelial overgrowth can occur.[85,86]

The skin around a gastrostomy or jejunostomy tube is kept clean and dry to prevent soreness/infection; the use of gauze and talcum powder is discouraged. Creams are kept off the tube as these can cause the external fixing device to slip. If the external fixing device slips when dry, it should be replaced. Patients are advised to cover the tube with a waterproof dressing when swimming.

Leakage of gastric contents onto the skin should not occur if the stoma is healthy and the external fixation device correctly positioned. When it does happen, however, it can result in extreme soreness because of the low pH of the gastric juice. It requires a review of the tube and skin care to prevent recurrence. A barrier cream is useful to protect the skin in the interim. The advice of a stoma care nurse may help to deal with these problems. The formation of granulation tissue may be prevented by regular rotation of the tube. Silver nitrate can be gently applied to areas of excessive granulation tissue but can burn the surrounding skin, so an antibacterial/steroid cream is often preferred.

Mouth care

Patients, especially those who have no oral intake, are advised to clean their mouth with a mouthwash and to brush teeth and gums twice daily. They may need artificial saliva if their mouth is too dry. Some patients like to have something to taste (sweet) in their mouths when they feed. For patients on an intensive care unit, the normal or induced production of saliva can be useful because of saliva's bactericidal activity. Lemon and glycerine swabs are avoided as they lower the pH in the mouth to 2.3–3.9, which can cause decalcification of teeth.

Care of the feeding tube

Enteral feeding tubes are used for the administration of feeds, water and, if necessary, medications (Box 18.6); they may become blocked by feed or medication solidifying within the tube. Feed may block the tube if there is a failure to flush the tube, interrupted feeding (e.g. due to a pump malfunction) or if the feed is of a high viscosity and contains whole protein. Acidic fluids with a pH of less than 5 (e.g. gastric acid or fruit juices) and the warmth of the body may cause casein–derived feeds to coagulate and thus block the tube. However, feeds containing free amino acids, small peptides (elemental or peptide feeds), egg albumin or whey proteins do not coagulate at a pH of less than 5[12,87] and thus can be used if recurrent blockage occurs. Crushed tablets and potassium and iron preparations are especially likely to block tubes. Many drugs are in a hyperosmolar solution which, in addition to making line blockage more likely, may cause nausea and diarrhoea.[88]

To prevent blockage, the tube should be kept clean by flushing with water (usually 30–50 ml of fresh tap water, cooled boiled water or sterile water in accordance with

Box 18.6 – How to set up an enteral feed

1. Check the expiratory date on the feed, which should be at room temperature. Record the time/date the feed was set up. Invert the feed container 2–3 times.
2. Wash and dry your hands. (Some units recommend putting on gloves.)
3. Remove the cover from the feeding container and clean the inferior surface with spirit.
4. Close the giving set clamp/roller, then spike the feeding container and attach the giving set.
5. Invert the container and hang it on the drip stand. For gravity feeding, the feeding container should be one metre above the proximal end of the feeding tube.
6. Remove the distal cap from the tubing and slowly open the roller/clamp to prime the giving set.
7. Flush the feeding tube with the prescribed quantity (usually 50 ml) of cooled boiled or sterile water.
8. Connect the giving set to the feeding tube.
9. Insert the drip chamber or length of tubing into the pump.
10. Set the pump rate, unclamp the giving set and run.

Approximate drip rates★

ml/h	drips/min
125	35
100	28
75	21
50	14
25	7

$$\text{drips/min} = \frac{\text{ml/h} \times 17}{60}$$

★ The drip rate is affected by viscosity of feed, temperature of feed and giving set material.

local policy) before and after administering feed or medication. A 50 ml syringe is used for flushing, fitting either directly onto the feeding tube or onto the side port of a giving set. The quantity of water used to flush the tube should be sufficient to clear the tube and meet the patient's fluid requirements. Some units recommend that the tube be flushed weekly with a carbonated drink (e.g. Coca Cola®, 7 Up®, or a sodium bicarbonate solution) or pineapple juice, followed by cooled boiled or sterile water, to prevent blockage. Drugs should not

be given through an enteral feeding tube, if possible; if such administration is necessary, they should be obtained in liquid form after establishing compatibility. When more than one medication is required, the tube should be flushed after each medication to prevent the two from mixing within the tube.

It may be possible to clear a blocked tube by flushing with warm water, a carbonated drink, pineapple juice or sodium bicarbonate solution. Cranberry juice is less effective than Coca Cola® or water in preventing blockage.[89] An alkalinized solution of pancreatic enzymes (Viokase® at pH 7.9 with sodium bicarbonate) is effective in unblocking most lines,[90] and the same mixture has been advocated for giving after a feed and a water flush to prevent tube blockage.[91] This solution can be made by adding 5 ml of water to one crushed tablet of Viokase® and one of sodium bicarbonate.

Before the enteral feeding tube is connected to a giving set, air is allowed to come out. Some 'backflow' of gastric contents into tube is normal and is a reassuring sign of the correct position of the tube within the stomach, though it may be perceived by a carer to be a problem.

Some types of gastrostomy or jejunostomy tube have a clip/clamp on the tube to prevent leakage when the feeding ports are open. If left closed when the tube is not in use, these clamps can cause damage to the tube, which may eventually break at the point where the clamp was located.

It may be possible to replace certain parts of an enteral feeding tube (e.g. the Luer lock end) if damaged.

Gastric aspirates

It is uncommon for a nasogastric tube to be inserted routinely after abdominal surgery to 'decompress the stomach' as patients with a tube in place have more infective complications and it is longer before they can take food orally.[92] Sedative drugs and high circulating catecholamine levels delay gastric emptying. If a gastrostomy or nasogastric tube has been inserted post-operatively or in an intensive therapy unit, the residual volume should not prevent feeding from starting, but care must be taken when aspirating more than 200 ml from a nasogastric tube or 100 ml from a gastrostomy tube.[93] If, more than 2 hours after starting to feed, there is an aspirate of more than 200 ml or more than 2 times the hourly feeding rate, gastric emptying is likely to be delayed and extra care is needed, however the feed does not necessarily need to be stopped. Some intensive therapy units aspirate all the gastric contents every 4 hours and replace 200 ml. Metoclopramide 10–20 mg three times a day (0.1–0.2 mg/kg in children) orally or intravenously, domperidone 10 mg four times a day, cisapride 10 mg four times a day, erythromycin 125–250 mg four times a day (3 mg/kg in children over one hour) or, rarely, neostigmine 1 mg may all be used to increase the gastric emptying rate. If a high gastric aspirate is preventing feeding, jejunal feeding should be considered.

A fine-bore feeding tube used to aspirate gastric fluid is much more likely to become blocked as the acid coagulates casein-derived protein.[94]

Feeding regimen

Starter regimens/feeding rates

Traditionally, a gastrostomy or jejunostomy is not used for 6 hours after insertion (and possibly longer after surgery/trauma), then water 25 ml/h increasing over 6 hours to 75–85 ml/h is commenced. Feeding starts at 12 hours at a reduced rate of 20–45 ml/h for the next 12 hours, before being increased (sometimes over 2–4 days) to the amount needed to meet the patient's requirements.[95] Our unit starts the feed at 25 ml/h and increases it every 4 hours in 25 ml/h increments until the calculated rate is reached. With an overnight feed the rate rarely exceeds 150 ml/h.

With continuous infusions in patients who have had some oral intake in the last week, starter regimens that either dilute[96] or reduce the feed volume[97] are not necessary and may prolong the period of negative nitrogen balance. However, if vomiting/bloating or diarrhoea (not related to antibiotic therapy) occurs, the feed rate may be reduced for a trial period.

Energy/composition

If high-energy feed is given, hepatic steatosis, osmotic diarrhoea, refeeding syndrome, uraemia or hypercapnia may occur. Care must be taken not to overfeed a patient who is being ventilated as energy requirements are likely to be 1000 kcal/24 h less than calculated; a feed with less carbohydrate is usually given. Ten to thirty per cent of tube-fed patients will have hyperglycaemia[98] and may need to be given an oral hypoglycaemic agent or subcutaneous insulin before starting the feed. It is important not to underfeed patients. Keeping a patient 'nil by mouth' while wait-

ing for investigations, stopping feeding because of a high nasogastric aspirate, cardiac problems or the tube 'falling out' can all worsen the problems of under-nutrition.

If a patient has a non-functioning gut and full nutrient requirements are being met by parenteral nutrition, minimal enteral feeding (10 ml/h) with or without added glutamine is often given on the basis that it may preserve the gut's barrier function and prevent villous atrophy,[4] however there is no good evidence in man that it reduces bacterial trans-location.[99]

Most commercial feeds contain 1.0–1.5 kcal/ml and are nutritionally complete. In the long term, a feed containing fibre (fructo-oligosaccharide) is often given as it may result in a normal formed stool. If a patient is being fed into the jejunum and a polymeric diet has caused symptoms of dumping syndrome, then an iso-osmolar peptide feed may be given.

Feeding method

Gravity, a pump or a syringe can be used to deliver a feed, which may be given continuously, intermittently or by boluses.

Continuous feeding keeps the intragastric pH high/neutral;[100] this used to be thought to protect against haemorrhage from 'stress ulceration' in critically ill patients. If the gastric contents are not acidic, however, they will not be bactericidal and the stomach can become colonized by enteral bacteria.[101,102] The gastric contents can reflux up the oesophagus and spill over into the lungs where micro-organisms can cause pneumonia and an increased mortality.[103] Administration of cimetidine increases the risk of patients on a ventilator developing pneumonia.[104] Bile reflux into the duodenum raises gastric pH and predisposes to colonization of the lower respiratory tract by gastric bacteria.[105] Four Gram-negative bacteria (*Escherichia coli*, *Enterobacter cloacae*, *Klebsiella pneumoniae* and *Serratia marcescens*) are mainly responsible for stomach-to-airway colonization. At a pH of less than 2.7, all four bacterial species are killed within 90 minutes,[106] thus a period free from a feed that allows a normal low gastric fasting pH to be reached should be beneficial. An additional problem in ventilated critically ill patients is that their gastric motility is disrupted, making them more likely to have viable bacteria in their stomach.[107]

The time a patient should be rested from a feed has not been determined; Bonten *et al.* showed that colonization of the stomach, oropharynx and trachea was the same with 4 hours fasting every 24 h as with continuous feeding.[108] With 8 hours fasting every 24 h, the incidence of pneumonia on an intensive therapy unit fell from 54% to 12%.[109] A break in feeding (probably of 4–8 hours) allows both the stomach pH to return to normal and catch-up time to ensure that all of a feed is given.

Continuous and intermittent feeding is usually done via a pump, which provides a resistance to flow, so preventing excessive amounts of feed abruptly being delivered into the stomach/small bowel. Whole protein feeds may be of high viscosity but the pump is not needed to generate a high pressure.[12] It would be cheaper and simpler for most patients to use gravity feeding with a variable or fixed resistance to control the feeding rate.

In bolus feeding, boluses of 200–400 ml feed are generally given into the stomach over 20 minutes (range 15–60).[110] Bolus feeding may cause bloating and diarrhoea and, if given into the jejunum, may cause a dumping type syndrome. Bolus feeding can be done by pouring the feed into an inverted 50 ml syringe which has had the plunger removed. The syringe is then either connected directly to the feeding tube or via an extension tube and the feed is run in slowly. If the rate is too slow the plunger can be replaced and the feed gently injected. The syringes can be washed between uses, depending upon local policies. They need to be replaced weekly as they become hard to use.

Drugs

Drugs should be given in liquid form and the tube flushed before and after use. Care should be exercised if digoxin and fibre, or warfarin and vitamin K/E are given together as they may make digoxin and warfarin, respectively, less effective. Sucralfate that is allowed to mix with enteral feed in the stomach or in an enteral tube can form a solid mass. Phenytoin can interact with protein, so it is given 2 hours before or 2 hours after enteral feeding.

Contamination of feeds

An enteral feed is an ideal culture medium and can easily become contaminated. The feeding tube itself is also an important reservoir for bacteria, including those that are multi-resistant.[111] The factors that determine whether contamination will cause a problem are the dose of infecting organism, the route

of administration (stomach or jejunum) and host resistance, which is reduced in elderly, undernourished or immunosuppressed patients.

Unacceptable contamination of a feed is said to occur when there are more than 10^4 colony-forming units per ml of feed, and levels greater than this have been associated with diarrhoea.[112] In ventilated patients the organisms that contaminate a feed have often come from the gut.[105] Contamination is common if a feed is hung for more than 24 hours.[113] It is important that asepsis is maintained in the preparation and delivery of a feed, especially for those patients on the intensive therapy unit, immunocompromised patients, patients taking proton pump inhibitors or H_2 antagonists, and neonates. Hand washing is the single most important measure to prevent contamination. A mask should be worn if the carer has a cold, sore throat or respiratory tract infection. No part of the system that comes into contact with the feed should touch the hands, clothes, skin or any non-disinfected surface.[114,115] The number of manipulations to a feed should be kept to a minimum. A recessed spike on the giving set helps to reduce the chance of contact and thus contamination of the feed. Bottles with a ring pull that need decanting should be avoided as the feed is usually poured over the area the thumb has touched to remove the ring. If a feed has to be decanted it should be hung for a short time.

Acidifying an enteral feed preserves gastric acidity and reduces gastric colonization in critically ill patients and thus may reduce the incidence of pneumonia.[116]

Patient position

Patients should always be fed in the semi-supine position (propped up) for nasogastric or gastrostomy feeding and for 30 minutes after finishing, as there is a high and often unrecognized risk of aspirating the feed. While this position does not prevent aspiration, it reduces its frequency and severity.[19]

Equipment

Pumps

Most pumps in Europe give a flow rate that varies from 1 to 300 ml/h and they comply with European Device Standards. It is suggested that no more than 500 ml be given over 4–6 hours without a pump. An enteral feeding pump should not be able to generate a pressure of more than 15 psi, and syringes smaller than 50 ml should not be used as they can exceed this pressure. A parenteral nutrition pump should never be used as this generates high pressures. Pumps may have alarms for occlusion, air in the line or low battery.

Several small portable pumps with carrying packs are available and allow feeding to occur while the patient is mobile.

Drip stands

A large hospital drip stand is often provided, but small bedside stands are available. The LITRE (Looking Into The Requirements for Equipment) group in United Kingdom has designed a small portable drip stand that can be used for carrying a feeding bag for enteral or parenteral nutrition.

Dry goods

The feeding catheter connects to a flexible giving set, which in turn connects to the nutrient-feeding bag (Fig. 18.2).

Feeding tube. The position of the feeding tube should be regularly checked by looking at the markers

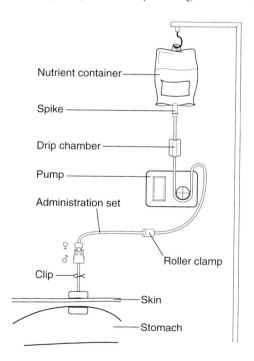

- Nutrient container
- Spike
- Drip chamber
- Pump
- Administration set
- Roller clamp
- Clip
- Skin
- Stomach

Figure 18.2 – Diagram of an enteral feed being given through a gastrostomy.

on its side to ensure that it has not slipped out. Some jejunal feeding systems allow the stomach to be drained while feeding continues into the jejunum. Tubes with a balloon may not last as long as those with a flange. A PEG tube may last for 2 years, a jejunostomy tube for a shorter time of about 6 months. There is no difference in blockage between an 8, 10 or 12 FG feeding tube, though it is harder to aspirate fluid from the smaller tube,[117] and leakage and peristomal infections were not significantly more common with a 20 FG compared to a 12 FG tube.[118] A radiologically placed gastrostomy will last about 6–12 months.

Connectors. European Standards state that the connector on the end of an enteral giving set shall not connect with a female Luer lock fitting. This prevents an enteral feed from being connected by mistake to an intravenous catheter. All the same, care should be taken to label the delivery system to prevent its contents from being accidentally administered intravenously, especially as adapters that change male Luer lock or push–in connections to female ones are available. 'All parts, joints and connectors of an enteral giving set and catheter shall withstand a linear tensile strength of 15 N without disconnection, rupture or cracking' and there should be no leakage when the system is pressurized to a minimum of 150 kPa with water for 2 minutes.[119]

Giving set/nutrient containers/syringes. There may be local policies concerning the feed administration sets and handling procedures. The feed administration set and nutrient containers are discarded after a single use while syringes may be washed and reused.

Disconnecting an enteral feed

An enteral feed is disconnected after hands have been washed; the tube is flushed with cooled boiled or sterile water, then capped off. All feeding equipment except syringes is discarded. An open nutrient container can be refrigerated and reused for 24 hours only.

Discharge planning

Before discharge from hospital, the patient/carer must be trained in the setting up/taking down of a feed, flushing the tube, giving medication through the tube, care of the exit site, prevention and treatment of tube blockage, and repair of the hub. They must understand some basic anatomy and physiology as well as how to set up and operate the pump (if used). They must have made arrangements for delivery so that there is an uninterrupted supply of the feed/dry goods. They should have contact numbers in case of illness or if they have problems with the equipment. They should have follow-up appointments arranged. All patients, those receiving enteral nutrition, are reviewed at least annually by a specialist nutrition team (see also Ch. 23).

Monitoring

When an enteral feed is first started, especially if the patient is very undernourished, haemoglobin, clotting, sodium, potassium, urea, creatinine, liver and bone chemistry and magnesium are measured, as is a random urinary sodium concentration. Within the first 24 hours of starting the feed the serum phosphate and potassium are measured. These tests, along with serum magnesium, are done at least weekly for 2 weeks, then every 2–12 months depending upon the clinical condition of the patient.

The patient is ideally weighed daily in hospital, but often this is not possible; mid-arm muscle circumference may be determined and measured every week until discharge, then every few months.

Psychosocial implications

It is difficult for a patient to feel that he/she is part of the family if he/she cannot eat; fortunately, patients with intestinal failure are usually able to eat normally and use the feeding as a way of getting extra energy, usually at night. They can lead a moderately normal life and can bathe/shower/swim 2 weeks after a gastrostomy or jejunostomy has been inserted.

Problems of enteral tubes

The long-term problems include tube blockage, aspiration, leakage around entry site or at the connection and discharge at exit site (Ch. 31).

Tube removal/replacement

A percutaneously inserted tube should not be removed until at least 14 days after insertion, as a fibrous tract needs to have become established to prevent intraperitoneal leakage. A gastrostomy tube with an internal fixation device that deflates can be removed by withdrawing air/water from it and gently pulling. If it does not come out easily, however, it may need to be removed in the same way as a tube with a non-deflating internal fixation device. If a gastrostomy tube is pushed inwards to check that it is free, then pulled upon and transected as near to the skin as possible, it will usually pass through the gut with no problems;[120] however, in a few cases (2%) the tube does not pass.[121] This method may be appropriate if the patient has a normal gut (no Crohn's disease or distal strictures). If a gastrostomy tube with a rigid internal fixation device is removed endoscopically, the tube is pushed 1–2 cm inwards and a polypectomy snare is put over the internal fixation device and tightened round the tube. The tube is cut about 5 cm from its skin entry point and the endoscopist withdraws the scope and tube. The patient is usually kept nil by mouth for 12 hours following tube removal. Abdominal fistulae rarely develop, even in patients with Crohn's disease.[122] If there is significant epithelial overgrowth and the tube is painful or infected, a needle knife can be used to cut the tube out.[123]

If a tube comes out accidentally it should ideally be replaced within 12 hours, or the tract may completely close over. A flexible guidewire is often the easiest way of finding the tract. Its soft end can be inserted into the tract. An endoscopist can see the wire emerge in the stomach and can catch it with a polypectomy snare or grasping forceps. The wire is pulled up into the endoscope, which is withdrawn to leave the wire coming out of the mouth. A new PEG is tied to this and pulled into position in the usual way by the assistant at the abdominal wall. Another option is to dilate the tract with dilators of gradually increasing diameter and to insert a button or balloon-type gastrostomy.

When a PEG/PEJ tube needs replacement because of breakage/leakage that cannot be corrected with repair kits/replacement parts, it can usually be done endoscopically. The PEG can be transected about 10 cm from the exit site and a 1 mm hole cut 5–10 mm from the end; the introducing thread from the new PEG set is put through the newly cut side hole and out of the end of the PEG, where it is tied. The old PEG can then be removed, using a polypectomy snare, through an endoscope as already described. The thread will emerge from the mouth and the new PEG is attached to this and pulled into position in the usual way. An alternative method, after transecting the PEG, is to push the double-looped introducing thread of the new PEG out through the lumen of the old PEG and into the stomach. The closed polypectomy snare from the endoscope is pushed through this loop, and then opened; this traps the thread round the snare. The snare is then put round the internal fixation device and closed; the thread is caught in this and, when the PEG is removed, the thread will again come out of the mouth ready to be attached to a new PEG.

When a PEG is removed it is sometimes replaced with a button, especially in children.

REFERENCES

1. McIntyre PB, Wood SR, Powell-Tuck J, Lennard-Jones JE. Nocturnal nasogastric tube feeding at home. *Postgrad Med J* 1983; **59:** 767–769.

2. Aiges H, Markowitz J, Rosa J, Daum F. Home nocturnal supplemental nasogastric feedings in growth-retarded adolescents with Crohn's disease. *Gastroenterology* 1989; **97:** 905–910.

3. Moore FA, Moore EE, Poggetti R, McAnena OJ, Peterson VM, Abernathy CM, Parsons PE. Gut bacterial translocation via the portal vein: a clinical perspective with major torso trauma. *J Trauma* 1991; **31:** 629–638.

4. Buchman AL, Moukarzel AA, Bhuta S *et al.* Parenteral nutrition is associated with intestinal morphologic and functional changes in humans. *J Parenter Enteral Nutr* 1995; **19:** 453–460.

5. Kudsk KA, Croce MA, Fabian TC *et al.* Enteral versus parenteral nutrition. Effect on septic morbidity after blunt and penetrating abdominal trauma. *Ann Surg* 1992; **215:** 503–513.

6. Randall HT. Enteral nutrition: Tube feeding in acute and chronic illness. *J Parenter Enteral Nutr* 1984; **8:** 113–136.

7. Woods JH, Erickson LW, Condon RE, Schulte WJ, Sillin LF. Postoperative ileus: a colonic problem? *Surgery* 1978; **84:** 527–532.

8. Levy H. Nasogastric and nasoenteral feeding tubes. *Gastrointest Endoscop Clin North Am* 1988; **8:** 529–549.

9. Gluckman DL, Halser MH, Warren WD. Small intestinal absorption in the immediate post-operative period. *Surgery* 1966; **60:** 1020–1025.

10. Moore EE, Moore FA. Immediate enteral nutrition following multisystem trauma: a decade perspective. *J Am Coll Nutr* 1991; **10:** 633–648.

11. Carr CS, Ling KDE, Boulos P, Singer M. Randomised trial of safety and efficacy of immediate postoperative enteral feeding in patients undergoing gastrointestinal resection. *Br Med J* 1996; **312:** 869–871.

12. Elia M, Crozier C, Martin S, Neale G. Flow and aspiration of artificial feeds through nasogastric tubes. *Clin Nutr* 1984; **2:** 159–166.

13. Keohane PP, Attrill H, Silk DBA. Clinical effectiveness of weighted and unweighted 'fine bore' nasogastric feeding tubes in enteral nutrition: a controlled clinical trial. *J Clin Nutr Gastroenterol* 1986; **1:** 189–193.

14. Moore DM, Calcaterra TC. Inserting and securing the nasogastric tube. *Laryngoscope* 1987; **97:** 1460.

15. Zaloga GP. Bedside method for placing small bowel feeding tubes in critically ill patients. *Chest* 1991; **100:** 1643–1646.

16. Schulz MA, Santanello SA, Monk J, Falcone RE. An improved method for transpyloric placement of nasoenteric feeding tubes. *Int Surg* 1993; **78:** 79–82.

17. McWey RE, Curry NS, Schabel SI, Reines D. Complications of nasoenteric feeding tubes. *Am J Surg* 1988; **155:** 253–257.

18. Metheny NA, Clouse RE, Clark JM, Reed L, Wehrle MA, Wiersema L. pH testing of feeding-tube aspirates to determine placement. *Nutr Clin Pract* 1994; **9:** 185–190.

19. Metheny N. Minimizing respiratory complications of nasoenteric tube feedings: State of the science. *Heart Lung* 1993; **22:** 213–223.

20. Kirby DF, Delegge MH, Fleming CR. American Gastroenterological Association technical review on tube feeding for enteral nutrition. *Gastroenterology* 1995; **108:** 1282–1301.

21. Bengmark S. Progress in peri-operative enteral tube feeding. *Clin Nutr* 1998; **17:** 145–152.

22. Lord LM, Weiser-Maimone A, Pulhamus M, Sax HC. Comparison of weighted vs unweighted enteral feeding tubes for efficacy of transpyloric intubation. *Parenter Enteral Nutr* 1993; **17:** 271–273.

23. Gutierrez ED, Balfe DM. Fluoroscopically guided nasoenteric feeding tube placement: Results of a 1-year study. *Radiology* 1991; **178:** 759–762.

24. Ott DJ, Mattox HE, Gelfand DW, Chen NW, Wu WC. Enteral feeding tubes: placement by using fluoroscopy and endoscopy. *Am J Roentgenol* 1991; **157:** 769–771.

25. Van Stiegmann GV, Pearlman NW. Simplified endoscopic placement of nasoenteral feeding tubes. *Gastointest Endosc* 1986; **32:** 349–350.

26. Mathus-Vliegen EMH, Tytgat GNJ, Merkus MP. Feeding tubes in endoscopic and clinical practice: the longer the better? *Gastrointest Endosc* 1993; **39:** 537–542.

27. Gabriel SA, Ackermann RJ, Castresana MR. A new technique for placement of nasoenteral feeding tubes using external magnetic guidance. *Crit Care Med* 1997; **25:** 641–645.

28. Zweng TN, Hill BB, Strodel WE. An improved technique for securing nasoenteral feeding tubes. *J Am Coll Surg* 1996; **183:** 268–270.

29. Popovich MJ, Lockrem JD, Zivot JB. Nasal bridle revisited: an improvement in the technique to prevent unintentional removal of small-bore nasoenteric feeding tubes. *Crit Care Med* 1996; **24:** 429–431.

30. Shumrick DA. Pyriform sinusostomy; a useful technique for temporary or permanent tube feeding. *Arch Surg* 1967; **94:** 277–279.

31. Gaggiotti G, Orlandoni G, Boccoli G, Caporelli SG, Patrizi I, Masera N. A device to perform percutaneous cervical pharyngostomy (PCP) for enteral nutrition. *Clin Nutr* 1989; **8:** 273–275.

32. Lyons JH. Cervical pharyngostomy. A safe alternative for gastrointestinal decompression. *Am J Surg* 1974; **127:** 387–391.

33. Klopp CT. Cervical esophagostomy. *J Thorac Cardiovasc Surg* 1951; **21:** 490–491.

34. Ketcham AS. Elective esophagostomy. *Am J Surg* 1962; **104:** 682–685.

35. Park RHR, Allison MC, Lang J et al. Randomised comparison of percutaneous endoscopic gastrostomy and nasogastric tube feeding in patients with persisting neurological dysphagia. *Br Med J* 1992; **304:** 1406–1409.

36. Norton B, Homer-Ward M, Donnelly MT, Long RG, Holmes GKT. A randomised prospective comparison of percutaneous endoscopic gastrostomy and nasogastric tube feeding after acute dysphagic stroke. *Br Med J* 1996; **312:** 13–16.

37. Gauderer ML, Ponsky JL, Izans RJ. Gastrostomy without laparotomy: a percutaneous endoscopic technique. *J Pediatr Surg* 1980; **15:** 872–875.

38. Ponsky JL, Gauderer MWL. Percutaneous endoscopic gastrostomy: a nonoperative technique for feeding gastrostomy. *Gastrointest Endosc* 1981; **27:** 9–11.

39. Beasley SW, Catto-Smith AG, Davidson PM. How to avoid complications during percutaneous endoscopic gastrostomy. *J Pediatr Surg* 1995; **30:** 671–673.

40. Sachs BA, Vine HS, Palestrant AM, Ellison HP, Shropshire D, Lowe R. A nonoperative technique for establishment of a gastrostomy in the dog. *Invest Radiol* 1983; **18:** 485–487.

41. Hogan RB, DeMarco DC, Hamilton JK, Walker CO, Polter DE. Percutaneous endoscopic gastrostomy – to push or pull. A prospective randomized trial. *Gastrointest Endosc* 1986; **32:** 253–258.

42. Mamel JJ. Percutaneous endoscopic gastrostomy. *Am J Gastroenterol* 1989; **84:** 703–710.

43. Akkersdijk WL, van Bergeijk JD, van Egmond T, Mulder CJJ, van Berge Henegouwen GP, van der Werken C, van Erpecum KJ. Percutaneous endoscopic gastrostomy (PEG): Comparison of push and pull methods and evaluation of antibiotic prophylaxis. *Endoscopy* 1995; **27:** 313–316.

44. Jain NK, Larson DE, Schroeder KW, Burton DD, Cannon KP, Thompson RL, DiMagmo EP. Antibiotic prophylaxis for percutaneous endoscopic gastrostomy. A prospective, randomized, double-blind clinical trial. *Ann Intern Med* 1987; **107:** 824–828.

45. Preclik G, Grune S, Leser HG et al. Prospective, randomised, double blind trial of prophylaxis with single dose of co-amoxiclav before percutaneous endoscopic gastrostomy. *Br Med J* 1999; **319:** 881–884.

46. Sturgis TM, Yancy W, Cole JC, Proctor DD, Minhas BS, Marcuard SP. Antibiotic prophylaxis in percutaneous endoscopic gastrostomy. *Am J Gastroenterol* 1996; **91:** 2301–2304.

47. Jona SK, Neimark S, Panwalker AP. Effect of antibiotic prophylaxis in percutaneous endoscopic gastrostomy. *Am J Gastroenterol* 1985; **80:** 438–441.

48. Russell T, Brotman M, Norris F. Percutaneous gastrostomy: a new simplified and cost effective technique. *Am J Surg* 1984; **184:** 130–137.

49. Miller RE, Kummer BA, Kotler DP, Tiszenkel HI. Percutaneous endoscopic gastrostomy. Procedure of choice. *Ann Surg* 1986; **204:** 543–545.

50. Ponsky JL, Gauderer MWL, Stellato TA, Aszodi A. Percutaneous approaches to enteral alimentation. *Am J Surg* 1985; **149:** 102–105.

51. Larson DE, Burton DD, Schroeder KW, DiMagno EP. Percutaneous endoscopic gastrostomy. Indications, success, complications, and mortality in 314 consecutive patients. *Gastroenterology* 1987; **93:** 48–52.

52. Hull MA, Rawlings J, Murray FE et al. Audit of outcome of long–term enteral nutrition by percutaneous endoscopic gastrostomy. *Lancet* 1993; **341:** 869–872.

53. Chowdhury MA, Batey R. Complications and outcome of percutaneous endoscopic gastrostomy in different patient groups. *J Gastroenterol Hepatol* 1996; **11:** 835–839.

54. Amann W, Mischinger HJ, Berger A et al. Percutaneous endoscopic gastrostomy (PEG). 8 years of clinical experience in 232 patients. *Surg Endosc* 1997; **11:** 741–744.

55. Fox VL, Abel SD, Malas S, Duggan C, Leichtner AM. Complications following percutaneous endoscopic gastrostomy and subsequent catheter replacement in children and young adults. *Gastrointest Endosc* 1997; **45:** 64–71.

56. Light VL, Slezak FA, Porter JA, Gerson LW, McCord G. Predictive factors for early mortality after percutaneous endoscopic gastrostomy. *Gastrointest Endosc* 1995; **42:** 330–335.

57. Gottfried EB, Plumser AB, Clair MR. Pneumo-peritoneum following percutaneous endoscopic gastrostomy. *Gastrointest Endosc* 1986; **32:** 397–399.

58. Pidala MJ, Slezak FA, Porter JA. Pneumoperitoneum following percutaneous endoscopic gastrostomy. Does timing matter? *Surg Endosc* 1992; **6:** 128–129.

59. Cogen R, Weinryb J. Aspiration pneumonia in nursing home patients fed via gastrostomy tubes. *Am J Gastroenterol* 1989; **84:** 1509–1512.

60. Gauderer MWL, Picha GJ, Izant RJ. The gastrostomy "button" – a simple, skin-level, nonrefluxing device for long-term enteral feedings. *J Pediatr Surg* 1984; **19:** 803–805.

61. Stamm M. Gastrostomy by a new method. *Med News* 1894; **65:** 324–326.

62. Murphy C, Rosemurgy AS, Albrink MH, Carey LC. A simple technique for laparoscopic gastrostomy. *Surg Gynecol Obstet* 1992; **174:** 424–425.

63. Gallagher MW, Tyson KRT, Ashcraft KW. Gastrostomy in pediatric patients: an analysis of complications and techniques. *Surgery* 1973; **74:** 536–539.

64. Grant JP. Comparison of percutaneous endoscopic gastrostomy with Stamm gastrostomy. *Ann Surg* 1988; **207:** 598–603.

65. Ho C-S, Yee CAN, McPherson R. Complications of surgical and percutaneous non-endoscopic gastrostomy: Review of 233 patients. *Gastroenterology* 1988; **95:** 1206–1210.

66. Ruge J, Vazquez RM. An analysis of the advantages of Stamm and percutaneous endoscopic gastrostomy. *Surg Gynecol Obstet* 1986; **162:** 13–16.

67. Ho HS, Ngo H. Gastrostomy for enteral access. A comparison among placement by laparotomy, laparoscopy, and endoscopy. *Surg Endosc* 1999; **13:** 991–994.

68. Preshaw RM. A percutaneous method for inserting a feeding gastrostomy tube. *Surg Gynecol Obstet* 1981; **152:** 658–660.

69. Hicks ME, Surratt RS, Picus D, Marx MV, Lang EV. Fluoroscopically guided percutaneous gastrostomy and gastroenterostomy: Analysis of 158 consecutive cases. *Am J Roentgenol* 1990; **154:** 725–728.

70. Wollman B, D'Agostino HB, Walusi Wigle JR, Easter DW, Beale A. Radiologic, endoscopic, and surgical gastrostomy: An institutional evaluation and meta-analysis of the literature. *Radiology* 1995; **197:** 699–704.

71. DiSario JA, Foutch PG, Sanowski RA. Poor results with percutaneous endoscopic jejunostomy. *Gastrointest Endosc* 1990; **36:** 257–260.

72. Wolfsen HC, Kozarek RA, Ball TJ, Patterson DJ, Botoman VA. Tube dysfunction following percutaneous endoscopic gastrostomy and jejunostomy. *Gastrointest Endosc* 1990; **36:** 261–263.

73. Henderson JM, Strodel WE, Gilinsky NH. Limitations of percutaneous endoscopic jejunostomy. *Parenter Enteral Nutr* 1993; **17:** 546–550.

74. Hoffer EK, Cosgrove JM, Levin DQ, Herskowitz MM, Sclafani SJ. Radiological gastrojejunostomy and percutaneous endoscopic gastrostomy: a prospective, randomized comparison. *J Vasc Interv Radiol* 1999; **10:** 413–420.

75. Delany HM, Carnevale NJ, Garvey JW. Jejunostomy by a needle catheter technique. *Surgery* 1973; **73:** 786–790.

76. Delaney HM, Carnevale N, Garvey JW, Moss CM. Postoperative nutritional support using needle catheter feeding jejunostomy. *Ann Surg* 1977; **186:** 165–170.

77. Gerndt SJ, Orringer MB. Tube jejunostomy as an adjuvant to esophagectomy. *Surgery* 1994; **115:** 164–169.

78. Sarr MG. Needle catheter jejunostomy: an unappreciated and misunderstood advance in the care of patients after major abdominal operations. *Mayo Clin Proc* 1988; **63:** 565–572.

79. Eddy VA, Snell JE, Morris JA. Analysis of complications and long term outcome of trauma patients with needle catheter jejunostomy. *Am Surg* 1996; **62:** 40–44.

80. Duh Q-Y, Way LW. Laparoscopic jejunostomy using T-fasteners as retractors and anchors. *Arch Surg* 1993; **128:** 105–108.

81. Gogen R, Weinryb J, Pomerantz C, Fenstemacher P. Complications of jejunostomy tube feeding in nursing facility patients. *Am J Gastroenterol* 1991; **86:** 1610–1613.

82. Haun JL, Thompson JS. Comparison of needle catheter versus standard tube jejunostomy. *Am Surg* 1985; **51:** 466–469.

83. Litchfield BL, Nightingale JMD. Outcomes of percutaneous endoscopic gastrostomy tube insertion 1991–7. *Proc Nutr Soc* 1999; **58:** 138A.

84. Chung RS, Schertzer M. Pathogenesis of complications of percutaneous endoscopic gastrostomy. A lesson in surgical principles. *Am Surg* 1990; **56:** 134–137.

85. Klein S, Heare BR, Soloway RD. The 'buried bumper syndrome': a complication of percutaneous endoscopic gastrostomy. *Am J Gastroenterol* 1990; **85:** 448–451.

86. Lipscomb GR, Brown CM, Wardle T, Rees WDW. Blocked gastrostomy tubes. *Lancet* 1994; **343:** 801–802.

87. Marcuard SP, Perkins AM. Clogging of feeding tubes. *J Parenter Enteral Nutr* 1988; **12:** 403–405.

88. Niemiec PW, Vanderveen TW, Morrison JI, Hohenwarter MW. Gastrointestinal disorders caused by medication and electrolyte solution osmolality during enteral nutrition. *J Parenter Enteral Nutr* 1983; **7:** 387–389.

89. Metheny N, Eisenberg P, McSweeney M. Effect of feeding tube properties and three irrigants on clogging rates. *Nurs Res* 1998; **37:** 165–169.

90. Marcuard SP, Stegall KL, Trogdon S. Clearing obstructed feeding tubes. *J Parenter Enteral Nutr* 1989; **13:** 81–83.

91. Sriram K, Jayanthi V, Lakshmi RG, George VS. Prophylactic locking of enteral feeding tubes with pancreatic enzymes. *J Parenter Enteral Nutr* 1997; **21:** 353–356.

92. Cheatham ML, Chapman WC, Key SP, Sawyers JL. A meta-analysis of selective versus routine nasogastric decompression after elective laparotomy. *Ann Surg* 1995; **221:** 469–478.

93. McClave SA, Snider HL, Lowen CC *et al.* Use of residual volume as a marker for enteral feeding intolerance: prospective blinded comparison with physical examination and radiographic findings. *J Parenter Enteral Nutr* 1992; **16:** 99–105.

94. Powell KS, Marcuard SP, Farrior ES, Gallagher ML. Aspirating gastric residuals causes occlusion of small-bore feeding tubes. *J Parenter Enteral Nutr* 1993; **17:** 243–246.

95. Wicks C, Gimson A, Vlavianos P *et al.* Assessment of the percutaneous endoscopic gastrostomy feeding tube as part of an integrated approach to enteral feeding. *Gut* 1992; **33:** 613–616.

96. Keohane PP, Attrill H, Love M, Silk DBA. Relationship between osmolality of diet and gastrointestinal side effects in enteral nutrition. *Br Med J* 1984; **288:** 678–680.

97. Rees RGP, Keohane PP, Grimble GK, Frost PG, Attrill H, Silk DBA. Elemental diet administered nasogastrically without starter regimens to patients with inflammatory bowel disease. *J Parenter Enteral Nutr* 1986; **10:** 258–262.

98. Vanlandingham S, Simpson S, Daniel P, Newmark SR. Metabolic abnormalities in patients supported with enteral tube feeding. *J Parenter Enteral Nutr* 1981; **5:** 322–324.

99. MacFie J, Bradford I, O'Boyle C, Mitchell CJ. Bacterial translocation and nutritional support. *Br J Intens Care* 1996; 195–201.

100. Valentine RJ, Turner WW, Borman KR, Weigelt JA. Does nasoenteral feeding afford adequate gastroduodenal stress prophylaxis? *Crit Care Med* 1986; **14:** 599–601.

101. du Moulin GC, Hedley-Whyte J, Paterson DG, Lisbob A. Aspiration of gastric bacteria in antacid-treated patients: a frequent cause of post-operative colonisation of the airway. *Lancet* 1982; **i:** 342–345.

102. Garvey BM, McCambley JA, Tuxen DV. Effects of gastric alkalinization on bacterial colonization in critically ill patients. *Crit Care Med* 1989; **17:** 211–216.

103. Jacobs S, Chang RWS, Lee B, Bartlett FW. Continuous enteral feeding: a major cause of pneumonia among ventilated intensive care unit patients. *J Parenter Enteral Nutr* 1990; **14:** 353–356.

104. Craven DE, Kunches LM, Kilinsky V, Lichtenberg DA, Make BJ, McCabe WR. Risk factors for pneumonia and fatality in patients receiving continuous mechanical ventilation. *Am Rev Respir Dis* 1986; **133:** 792–796.

105. Inglis TJJ, Sherratt MJ, Sproat LJ, Gibson JS, Hawkey PM. Gastroduodenal dysfunction and bacterial colonisation of the ventilated lung. *Lancet* 1993; **341:** 911–913.

106. Mehta S, Archer JF, Mills J. pH-dependent bactericidal barrier to gram-negative aerobes: its relevance to airway colonisation and prophylaxis of acid aspiration and stress ulcer syndromes – study in vitro. *Intensive Care Med* 1986; **12:** 134–136.

107. Dive A, Moulart M, Jonard P, Jamart J, Mahieu P. Gastroduodenal motility in mechanically ventilated critically ill patients: A manometric study. *Crit Care Med* 1994; **22:** 441–447.

108. Bonten MJM, Gaillard CA, van der Hulst R, de Leeuw PW, van der Geest S, Stobberingh EE, Soeters PB. Intermittent enteral feeding: The influence on respiratory and digestive tract colonization in mechanically ventilated intensive-care-unit patients. *Am J Respir Crit Care Med* 1996; **154:** 394–399.

109. Lee B, Chang RWS, Jacobs S. Intermittent nasogastric feeding: a simple and effective method to reduce pneumonia among ventilated ICU patients. *Clin Intensive Care* 1990; **1:** 100–102.

110. McAtear CA (ed) Current perspectives on enteral nutrition in adults. A report by the British Association for Parenteral and Enteral Nutrition, 1999.

111. Bussy V, Marechal F, Nasca S. Microbial contamination of enteral feeding tubes occurring during nutritional treatment. *J Parenter Enteral Nutr* 1992; **16:** 552–557.

112. Anderson KR, Norris DJ, Godfrey LB, Avent CK, Butterworth CE Jr. Bacterial contamination of tube-feeding formulas. *J Parenter Enteral Nutr* 1984; **8:** 673–678.

113. Kohn CL. The relationship between enteral formula contamination and length of enteral delivery set usage. *J Parenter Enteral Nutr* 1991; **15:** 567–571.

114. Anderton A, Aidoo KE. The effect of handling procedures on microbial contamination of enteral feeds. *J Hosp Infect* 1988; **11:** 364–372.

115. Anderton A. Reducing bacterial contamination in enteral tube feeds. *Br J Nursing* 1995; **4:** 368–376.

116. Heyland DK, Cook DJ, Schoenfeld PS, Frietag A, Varon J, Wood G. The effect of acidified enteral feeds on gastric colonization in critically ill patients: Results of a multicenter randomized trial. *Crit Care Med* 1999; **27:** 2399–2406.

117. Methy N, Eisenberg P, McSweeney M. Effect of feeding tube properties and three irrigants on clogging rates. *Nurs Res* 1988; **37:** 165–169.

118. Duncan HD, Bray MJ, Kapadia SA *et al.* Prospective randomized comparison of two different sized per- cutaneous endoscopically placed gastrostomy tubes. *Clin Nutr* 1996; **15:** 317–320.

119. Sterile enteral feeding catheters and giving sets for single use. BS EN 1615: 1997

120. Korula J, Harma C. A simple and inexpensive method of removal or replacement of gastrostomy tubes. *JAMA* 1991; **265:** 1426–1428.

121. Mollitt DL, Dokler ML, Evans JS, Jeiven SD, George DE. Complications of retained internal bolster after pediatric percutaneous endoscopic gastrostomy. *J Pediatr Surg* 1998; **33:** 271–273.

122. Nightingale JMD. Gastrostomy placement in patients with Crohn's disease. *Eur J Gastroenterol Hepatol* 2000; **12:** 1073–1075.

123. Nightingale JMD. PEG removal with needle knife (in preparation).

19

Insertion and care of parenteral feeding catheters

Sally Magnay and Jeremy Nightingale

Parenteral nutrition is used when the gut is not functioning, is functioning insufficiently, is being left to 'rest' or if enteral nutrition is unsuccessful. Traditionally medical staff have placed parenteral feeding lines, but in some progressive units dedicated nutrition nurses successfully insert both central and peripheral feeding lines.[1] More commonly nursing staff care for, and teach about, the continuing care of feeding lines following insertion. This chapter provides a practical guide about central and peripheral feeding line insertion and the subsequent care of the lines.

CENTRAL AND PERIPHERAL FEEDING

The routes for parenteral nutrition can be described according to the position of the catheter tip as either large, medium or small vein feeding (Table 19.1). Previous descriptions have addressed the site of catheter insertion as either central or peripheral. This may lead to confusion as peripheral nutrition may be given through a short cannula with its insertion site and tip in a small vein (e.g. on the back of the hand or on the forearm), or via a catheter inserted into the basilic vein with its tip in the axillary vein.

Table 19.1 – Parenteral nutrition routes

Catheter tip	Venous insertion site	Type of nutrition
Large vein	Subclavian/jugular/cephalic vein	Central
	Cubital fossa (PICC)	Central
Medium vein	Brachial vein in cubital fossa	Peripheral
Small vein	Vein on back of hand	Peripheral

Nomenclature is most clear when both insertion site and catheter tip position are named (e.g. with peripherally inserted central catheters (PICCs)). PICCs are long small diameter catheters inserted into the basilic vein in the cubital fossa with their tip at the superior vena caval (SVC)/ right atrial (RA) junction.

CATHETER MATERIALS

The ideal catheter material is flexible, strong, chemically inert, non-thrombogenic, radio-opaque and does not kink. It should have a measurement scale on its side. The wall of the vein may be damaged by pressure, if the catheter material is relatively inflexible, and this can lead to thrombosis.[2] Small diameter flexible catheters that effectively float in the bloodstream are less likely to cause injury.

The chemical composition of a catheter is probably the most important factor in causing thrombophlebitis of peripheral veins. Most plastics contain additives that may produce a chemical phlebitis. Rubber, polyethylene, polyvinylchloride, Teflon® and uncoated polyurethane are all thrombogenic.[2–6] For parenteral nutrition either a polyurethane-hydromer or silicone elastomer (also called silicone rubber or silastic) catheter is used because they are biologically relatively inert. When compared, thrombophlebitis occurred less frequently with the polyurethane-hydromer-coated catheter.[7,8]

The coating of a polyurethane-hydromer catheter contains a hydrophobic polymer made from polyvinylpyrrolidone and anisocyanate prepolymer. When a hydromer-coated catheter is wetted, water is absorbed onto the coating and the resulting gel acts as a barrier between the blood and the catheter material so that platelets do not adhere to it. This gives the practical advantage that when wetted by body fluids (e.g. blood) the catheter becomes slippery, which makes the passage of the catheter up a peripheral vein relatively easy and so less likely to cause trauma to the vein. It also has the advantage of being physically stronger than a silicone elastomer catheter, allowing its external diameter to be reduced; in addition, it does not easily kink. Thus polyurethane-hydromer catheters are used when the insertion site is a medium or small vein. Silicone elastomer catheters, which are soft and flexible, are commonly used for long-term central vein feeding where they can last for 10 years without problems.

Some catheters have an antimicrobial (e.g. minocycline) incorporated into the material.[9] Other catheters have an extra cuff (VitaCuff®) containing collagen impregnated with silver ions; the collagen cuff swells to 2–3 times its original size and the silver acts as an antimicrobial.[10]

CATHETER INSERTION

Guidelines relating to the standards for parenteral nutrition catheter insertion are shown in Table 19.2. Some types of large vein catheter are shown in Figure 19.1.

Table 19.2 – Standards for parenteral nutrition catheter insertion (modified from BAPEN)[11]

1. There is a training programme for medical and nursing staff in the techniques of central line insertion and management.

2. Written guidelines are available for staff and patient/carers about the insertion and subsequent management of feeding catheters.

3. The insertion of a feeding catheter is a planned procedure.

4. Informed consent is obtained.

5. Adequate sedation/analgesia is given for the duration of the procedure.

6. The insertion and subsequent care of the line are performed using a strict aseptic technique.

7. If the catheter tip should be in a large vein, its position is confirmed by radiology and documented before feeding commences.

8. The catheter is fixed securely in place. Its connections are appropriate in diameter, length and material to prevent accidental damage, removal or contamination.

9. The feeding catheter (or one lumen of a multilumen catheter) is dedicated for parenteral feeding.

LARGE-VEIN NUTRITION

A catheter placed in a central vein has a lower risk of causing mechanical phlebitis due the relatively small size of the catheter compared to the large diameter of the vein and a lower risk of chemical phlebitis due to the rapid dilution of a high osmolality acidic feed. A catheter that has its tip positioned in a large central vein is ideally inserted in an aseptic environment with imaging facilities and by or under the supervision of fully trained and experienced clinicians. The catheter tip should lie at the junction of the SVC/RA. A more proximal location within the SVC increases the risk of venous thrombosis, whereas a more distal location risks cardiac perforation and cardiac tamponade. A chest radiograph is taken and used to check the catheter tip position before parenteral nutrition is commenced. The subclavian vein is commonly cannulated by physicians and radiologists using the infraclavicular approach and by surgeons 'cutting down' onto the cephalic vein.

Subclavian catheter placement

The blind percutaneous infraclavicular approach to the subclavian vein has been traditionally performed in the aseptic condition of the operating theatre, but now is in many centres satisfactorily performed in a clean quiet area of a ward[1,12] or in a radiology department. Cannulation of the subclavian vein can be done accurately using ultrasound guidance[13,14] though it may not necessarily result in fewer complications.[15] Introduction of a catheter can be over a needle or guidewire, or through a cannula.

Prior to insertion of a long-term catheter, the patient should be sensitively consulted about the optimum position of the exit site. Some women will prefer that the exit is as low as possible so that they can continue to wear low cut dresses. A patient's occupation and hobbies should be taken into account as these can affect the safety of the catheter (e.g. shooting). The site is marked. If the patient is agitated or confused the catheter may be tunnelled over the shoulder to exit on the back medial to the scapula. Some units check the patient's platelet count and INR prior to insertion.

It is important to have good lighting, access to emergency equipment, sufficient space for the operator and their assistant to undertake the aseptic procedure and the patient should be positioned above the height of the operator's waist. Informed consent is obtained and sedation administered via a peripheral vein on the opposite side to that on which the line will be inserted. A pulse oximeter is attached to the patient to warn of hypoxia. Oxygen and suction equipment are positioned nearby. Prophylactic antibiotics are not usually given unless the patient has a prosthetic heart valve.

Subclavicular approach

Insertion of long-term cuffed feeding line The equipment needed is variable but includes a gown, gloves, sterile drapes, needles, syringes, dissecting scissors, scalpel, suturing equipment, cleaning solution, local anaesthetic, a feeding line (Hickman or the smaller Broviac type of line), tunneller, split introducer, Seldinger wire and needle.

1. Patient lies supine, ideally with the head and shoulders positioned lower than the body (some put a small sandbag or rolled pillow between the shoulders). The operator selects the right or left subclavian vein. There is a tendency to choose the right as there is less risk of damaging the thoracic duct and thus of causing a chylothorax. The side furthest away from any abdominal stomas or fistulae is chosen. If the right subclavian vein is selected, the following anatomical

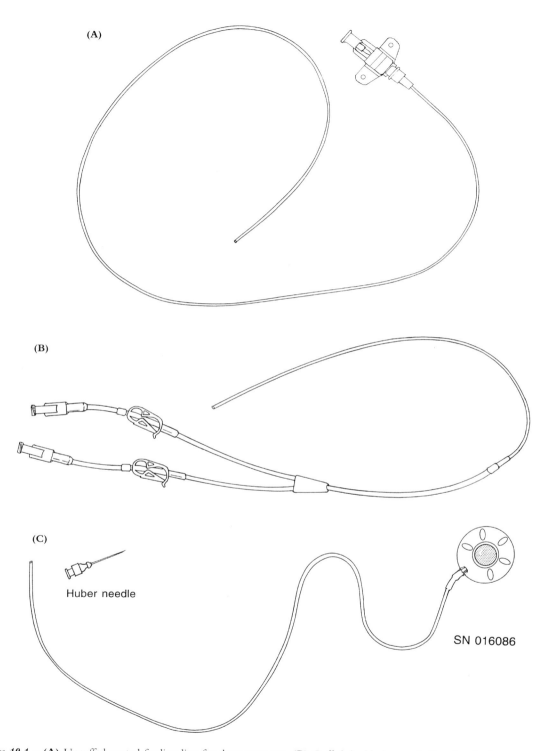

(A)

(B)

(C)

Huber needle

SN 016086

Figure 19.1 – **(A)** Uncuffed central feeding line for short-term use. **(B)** Cuffed double lumen feeding line for long-term use in haematology patients (single lumen is preferred). **(C)** Portacath for long-term feeding.

landmarks are noted: the tip of the left shoulder, supra sternal notch, the junction of the lateral one-third and middle two-thirds of the right clavicle, the site of the right internal jugular vein and carotid artery.

2. The operator 'scrubs up', puts on a sterile gown and gloves, then checks the equipment on the operating trolley.

3. The operator cleans the chosen site with a chlorhexidine in spirit solution. Sterile drapes are put over the patient's hair and round approximate 30 cm² of skin, which leaves all anatomical landmarks visible except the left shoulder tip, which can be felt.

4. Once the skin is dry, a local anaesthetic (lignocaine 1%) is injected intradermally about 1–2 cm below the junction of the lateral one-third and medial two-thirds of the clavicle. An assistant then holds the patient's right hand and pulls gently down towards the patient's feet. The patient turns their head away from the operator and the head of the operating table is lowered. The needle is changed to a longer one, re-introduced and passed under the clavicle, then it is redirected aiming to pass both under the sternal notch and at the left shoulder tip for a distance of about 5 cm. The syringe aspirates every few millimetres before injecting local anaesthetic, usually the subclavian vein will be encountered.

5. The operator may change their gloves, then make a small 1 cm transverse skin incision over the site of the intradermal local anaesthetic injection. Blunt dissection may be done (closed scissors are inserted and opened) to make it easier for the introduction of a splittable introducer. Then the 18 gauge needle from the catheterization pack is connected to a 10–20 ml syringe (some fill this with saline) and advanced in the same way as for the local anaesthetic, with gentle suction being applied from the syringe until there is a good flashback of venous blood into the syringe indicating that the vein has been entered. Holding the needle still, the syringe is removed and the soft end of the guidewire is pushed gently down the needle for a distance of about 30 cm. Hardly any pressure is put on the guidewire. Keeping the guidewire in position, the needle is withdrawn.

6. While the guidewire is left in position and covered lightly with a piece of sterile gauze, the subcutaneous tunnel is made. The tunnel is usually about 15 cm long, the exit site is chosen to be approximately midway between the mid point of the sternum and the nipple position of a man. The exit site should be on a flat area of chest, well away from the moist warm potentially bacteria prone axilla. Skin creases should be avoided. This aids security and comfort by making the catheter easier to anchor, and it reduces the chance of bacterial infection. Local anaesthetic is inserted at the exit site and along the line of the tunnel with 3–4 injections. A small 1 cm vertical incision is made at the exit site. Blunt dissection is performed by opening and closing surgical scissors in the line of the tunnel for a distance of about 7 cm from the exit site. The tunnel is created by pushing, with a rotating action, either a hollow plastic tube into the exit site and up towards the entry site or attaching the feeding catheter to a sharp-ended metal tunnelling rod and pushing this up. Some blunt dissection is usually needed to get the tunnelling instrument out of the entry site. Care should also be taken to maintain a superficial approach so that the Dacron® cuff will easily be felt below the skin. A single pass may reduce the chances of the patient developing a haematoma, infection or pain.

7. The catheter may be primed with either saline or heparinized saline, reducing the risk of air entering the venous circulation. The catheter is positioned in the tunnel either by putting it into the hollow plastic tunneller or it is pulled behind a metal rod. The dacron cuff is positioned halfway up the tunnel. It must not be at the exit site as cuffs situated adjacent to the exit site readily become infected, which can lead to the loss of the catheter.

8. The tunnelling rod is removed from the catheter, and the length of catheter needed estimated by lying the catheter on the chest wall in the shape of the sub-clavian vein and SVC (usually about 15–20 cm of catheter will be needed). The catheter is then cut. Care needs to be taken not to contaminate the catheter.

9. The rigid dilator surrounded by the splittable intro-ducer are advanced over the guidewire, checking that the guidewire remains free all the time until the wings of the splittable introducer are close to the patient's skin. The guidewire and rigid introducer are removed leaving the splittable introducer in position. The catheter is then quickly fed through the splittable introducer (forceps may be needed). If the catheter cannot immediately be fed into the splittable intro-ducer the operator may temporarily place their thumb over the splittable introducer to reduce bleeding and prevent air from entering the venous circulation.

10. The working field may be covered and the catheter tip position checked radiologically. However, with experience the operator can achieve a good position. The ideal position for the tip is the SVC/RA junction.

11. If the position is good, the splittable introducer is slowly peeled apart as the catheter is advanced into the vein (non-toothed forceps may be needed to prevent the catheter coming out), until the entire catheter is in place and the sheath has been completely split and removed.

12. Five millilitres of 50 units/ml heparin is instilled into the lumen of the catheter and the line is either capped or connected to a saline infusion.

13. One stitch is put over the insertion and exit site. The long threads from the exit site are tied round the catheter to help prevent it from being pulled out. The entry and exit sites may be sprayed with povidone-iodine. Adhesive sterile gauze dressings are placed over the cannulation and exit sites (Fig. 19.2). The catheter is curled round or over the dressing and taped to prevent traction.

14. The patient is advised to stay in bed for 2–3 hours for the effect of sedation to wear off. A postero-anterior chest radiograph is taken about 3 hours after the procedure to check the catheter tip position and to warn of a pneumothorax. If the catheter tip position is satisfactory then parenteral nutrition may be started.

Providing the catheter is mechanically stable and not infected, connective tissue will grow into the interstices of the cuff over the following 6 weeks. Sutures are removed after 2–3 weeks, but if the patient is receiving corticosteroids they are left in for at least 5 weeks.

Insertion of non-cuffed short-term feeding line If a non-cuffed line is used, the tunnel may be much shorter (5–10 cm). After the subclavian vein has been cannulated, the central needle is withdrawn leaving a plastic sheath in situ, the catheter is fed quickly through this for a measured distance (marks on the catheter usually make this easy). The plastic sheath is removed then the tunnel is made. Local anaesthetic is applied, but no incision made at the exit site. In order to reduce the risk of piercing the catheter with the tunnelling needle, the tunnelling needle without its plastic sheath is pushed from the entry site down the tunnel and out of the exit site. The exit site may need to be enlarged to about 2 mm. About 5 mm of plastic sheath is then pushed gently onto the needle at the exit site. The tunneller needle is gently pulled while the plastic sheath is pushed until the plastic sheath exits from the entry site. The tunneller needle is removed, the catheter is fed down this and the plastic cannula withdrawn. The attachments are put on the end of the feeding line, which is then flushed. A plastic clip, sutured to the skin may be used to hold the line in position.

Cephalic vein approach

The cephalic vein lies in the deltopectoral groove and is well placed for surgical insertion of a long-term venous feeding catheter. A 1–3 cm incision is made approximately 1–2 cm below the lateral end of the clavicle. The cephalic vein in the clavipectoral fascia is identified and is controlled by proximal and distal ligatures. A subcutaneous tunnel is created in the same way as described in the percutaneous approach, with the tunnelling rod and catheter exiting at the subclavicular incision. The required length of the catheter is decided and advanced into the cephalic vein via a venotomy made between the proximal and distal ligatures. The tip of the catheter is located at the SVC/RA junction. The ligatures supporting the catheter are tied. The lumen is checked by venous aspiration and flushed with heparinized saline. The clavicular incision is sutured with a subcutaneous catgut suture first, then finally with 2–3 silk skin sutures, which are left in for approximately a week. The exit site of the catheter is secured using the same method as the percutaneous approach.

Other large vein access sites

The internal jugular vein, which is relatively quick and easy to cannulate, may be used with the catheter being tunnelled down onto the anterior chest wall. However, this site is usually avoided, as such a catheter is often uncomfortable for the patient.

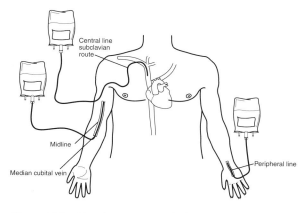

Central line subclavian route

Midline

Median cubital vein

Peripheral line

Figure 19.2 – Dressing over a single lumen cuffed large-vein feeding line.

The femoral vein can be used with the tunnel being on the anterior abdominal wall, but the risks of catheter-related sepsis and venous thrombosis are high, though better than first reported.[16] The tip is positioned at IVC/RA junction. The IVC can be cannulated percutaneously via a translumbar route entering the vein at L2–3 level below the renal veins.[10] Thoracotomy with placement in the azygous vein has been used.[10] The use of an arterio-venous fistula is associated with a high risk of early closure of the fistula.

The implantable venous access device

The first fully implantable venous access device (port) appeared in 1982.[17] Since that time they have gained in popularity and are now used widely and may have fewer complications than cuffed lines.[18] They consist of a vascular catheter and a subcutaneous port. The port segment is a cone-shaped chamber made of either stainless steel, titanium or plastic covered with a self-sealing compressed silicone septum that can be punctured up to 2000 times by a non-coring needle. Ports are available in single or dual lumen configurations with a pre-attached or attachable silicone rubber or polyurethane catheter. The port is inserted into a subcutaneous pocket created over the upper chest wall. The catheter is placed either after percutaneous subclavian vein cannulation or after a cutdown onto the cephalic vein.

Immediately after a port has been placed, an access needle is placed in the port and heparin is locked into it. This is done because swelling and inflammation will make access to the port very difficult for the next week. It is especially important to do this if the port is not going to be used within the next 4 days. When the non-coring needle is in place it must be secured safely and comfortably in place with a sterile gauze dressing. A plastic sterile dressing may then be placed on top to allow the patient to bathe or shower, but should be removed immediately the activity has finished.

Some patients needing home parenteral nutrition choose to have a port in preference to an external segment catheter. A port has a better cosmetic appearance and is less restrictive to social, sporting (especially swimming) and hygiene activities. However, not all patients given the choice of a venous access device will choose a port. The requirement to puncture the skin with a needle to access the port will be an unacceptable feature of this system for some people, particularly patients requiring nightly feeds.[19] It is possible for the needle to stay in situ for several days, but the reason for having a port is then negated.

Complications associated with large vein catheter insertion

Insertion-related complications are reported in 3–12% patients[20] (Table 19.3) and are less if they are inserted by a nutrition team.[21]

Table 19.3 – Insertion-related complications of central vein catheterization

- Malposition (cardiac arrhythmia's or perforation)
- Subclavian artery puncture (haemothorax or haemomediastinum)
- Pneumothorax
- Air or catheter embolism
- Nerve injuries (brachial plexus, phrenic or recurrent laryngeal nerve)
- Thoracic duct damage

Malposition

When using a subclavian approach, the catheter can pass up into the jugular vein, a clue to this is that the patient may complain of a pain in their ear when the guidewire is inserted. The catheter can advance into the ventricle or pass into the opposite subclavian vein. The catheter can be redirected using radiological guidance or it may (especially if cuffed) need to be replaced. Rarely the guidewire can induce cardiac arrhythmias, if so it is withdrawn or cardiac perforation and tamponade have been described. Rarely a catheter can be malpositioned in the pleural cavity or mediastinum and this will cause a pleural or pericardial effusion respectively when the feeding is started.

Subclavian artery puncture

It is not uncommon during insertion to puncture the subclavian artery. If so the needle is removed and firm pressure applied for 5 minutes. If the patient's coagulation status is normal, another attempt can be made on the same side. Blood can collect in the pleural space (haemothorax) or mediastinum (haemomediastinum) following arterial puncture.

The catheter entry site is observed for signs of bleeding after catheter insertion and blood pressure is monitored. If bleeding occurs, a pressure dressing is applied over the exit site and coagulation studies may be performed.

Pneumothorax

If air is aspirated during cannulation of the subclavian vein, a pneumothorax is likely to develop. This is often not apparent until several hours after the procedure when the patient complains of pleuritic chest pain and breathlessness; a physical examination reveals tachypnoea, tachycardia, a hyperresonant lung with reduced breath sounds. An immediate post-insertion chest radiograph may have been normal; hence one is usually done about 3 hours after insertion. A small pneumothorax may be asymptomatic and can be left alone, larger ones can be aspirated and only rarely is a chest drain needed. Subcutaneous emphysema can occur but is most common when a chest drain is inserted for too short a distance and one of the drainage holes is in the subcutaneous tissue.

Air/catheter embolism

Care is taken to ensure a closed system is maintained at all times during the procedure. If an air embolism is ever suspected (e.g. if the catheter suddenly becomes detached) the catheter is clamped as near to the skin as possible and the patient is positioned on their left side with their head tilted downwards. Rarely part of the catheter can break away and pass as an embolus to the lungs. It can be left alone but if an abscess develops may have to be surgically removed.

Nerve injuries

If the introduction needle hits the brachial plexus, numbness and tingling can develop in the arm and/or specific muscles can become weak. The exact pattern of weakness depends upon which part of the brachial plexus has been damaged. A neuropraxia can follow and may take several months to resolve. Rarely the phrenic nerve is damaged resulting in diaphragmatic paralysis; the recurrent laryngeal or vagus nerves can also be damaged causing hoarseness.

Thoracic duct damage

This can occur from left subclavian vein cannulation and rarely causes a chylothorax.

Peripherally inserted central catheter

As nutrient infusions into small or medium-sized veins are associated with a high risk of thrombophlebitis, there is a tendency for units to site the tip of feeding lines in a large vein. This was first reported in 1975[22] and can be done using a long catheter inserted into a medium-sized vein. A PICC is made of radio-opaque silicone rubber or polyurethane-hydromer and comes with a single or dual lumen. PICCs are inserted into the basilic, median cubital or cephalic veins in the ante-cubital fossa and the tip of the PICC terminates at the SVC/RA junction. Their insertion can be done at the patient's bedside by a trained nurse.[23] As PICCs are placed by cannulating a peripheral vein, they are easier to insert, associated with fewer insertion complications than centrally placed lines[24] and are less expensive than Hickman-type catheters. PICCs are available in a variety of sizes from 2 to 5 CH, in common with large-vein catheters they are either open-ended or have a Groshung valve incorporated into their tip.

PICCs are suitable for short to intermediate venous access for parenteral nutrition and they compare favourably with centrally placed venous access devices. They may be used in preference to the subclavian vein if a patient has abnormal clotting or cannot lie flat. They are not suitable for patients who use crutches or a wheelchair. However, they are dependent upon good peripheral venous access. They require an experienced team approach and a consistent standardized procedure for insertion and maintenance. In the USA, PICCs are widely used for patients in the community requiring long-term parenteral therapy and they are gaining in popularity in the UK especially for intravenous drug administration. However, they remain less ideal for long-term parenteral feeding due to the risk of dislodgement of the catheter. The exit site position on the arm restricts normal arm movement making daily living activities difficult. There is a theoretical worry about excessive arm movement causing much catheter tip movement, which in turn may traumatize the vein.

Insertion procedure for a PICC

The equipment needed includes a gown, gloves, sterile drapes, cleaning solution, local anaesthetic cream, PICC line, securing mechanism (Steri-strips® and Stat-lock®) and a plastic dressing (e.g. Opsite IV 3000®).

1. A local anaesthetic cream is usually applied over the skin near a vein in the elbow region and slightly above approximately 1 hour prior to insertion.

2. The insertion area is cleansed thoroughly with chlorhexidine in spirit.

3. The area is surrounded with sterile drapes.

4. The operator 'scrubs up' and puts on sterile gown and gloves. The required length of PICC line is measured pre-insertion in anticipation of the final tip location.

5. The needle is inserted into the basilic vein. Catheter insertion is performed above the bend of the elbow, or 0.5–1 inch below, to prevent kinking of the line when the arm is bent. Lubricating the line with sterile normal saline may help insertion. The PICC line is then gradually advanced through the needle. The patient is asked to turn their head towards the operator and to flex it so preventing the catheter from entering the external jugular vein.

6. The catheter is secured (e.g. with Steri-strips® and a Stat-lock® dressing). A small gauze square or release dressing is placed over the entry site, then a plastic dressing (e.g. Opsite IV 3000®) is applied over the exit site for security, a light bandage (or Tubigrip®) is applied again for security and comfort (Fig. 19.3).

7. A chest X-ray is taken to ascertain the position of the catheter tip.

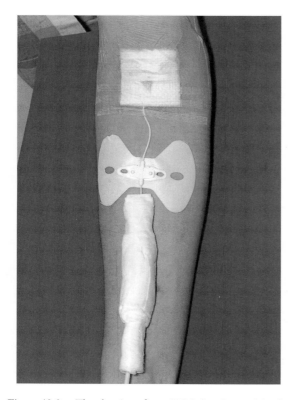

Figure 19.3 – The dressings for a PICC line inserted in the cubital fossa.

MEDIUM-VEIN NUTRITION

Peripheral parenteral nutrition with the entry site in a medium-sized vein and the catheter tip in the axillary vein is popular. It may be considered when it is anticipated that the patient's requirement for nutritional support is likely to be for less than 2–4 weeks, or if large vein access is likely to be difficult (e.g. if there is large vein thrombosis, anatomical anomalies or coagulation defects). This type of feeding may be preferable to central feeding as the catheter is easier to insert and manage, less likely to have complications and is less expensive.[25] It has been more successful than parenteral nutrition through a small vein as thrombophlebitis does not always occur.

The peripheral route is not suitable if the peripheral veins have been damaged by venepuncture or intravenous treatments, if the patient has renal impairment and may need the veins for creation of an arteriovenous fistula for dialysis, if the patient's nutritional requirements are very high or if it is anticipated that parenteral nutrition will be needed for longer than 2–4 weeks.

Choosing a suitable vein

The larger the peripheral vein used the better as this allows good blood flow around the cannula, thereby dispersing the infused fluids and having a lower risk of causing thrombophlebitis. The basilic or occasionally the cephalic veins are used for medium vein feeding. Whenever possible the cannula is inserted above the ante-cubital fossa to avoid occluding the line when the arm is bent. This can prove difficult in practice, as the upper arm veins lie increasingly deeper as they ascend. A venous bifurcation avoids the problem of the veins rolling to one side when the needle is inserted. A palpable vein, though often not visible, is often very firmly embedded in the tissues and relatively easy to cannulate. It is best to avoid a vein over or in the immediate vicinity of an artery because of the potential risk of creating an arterio-venous fistula and it is best to avoid one over a joint as the cannula may bend and become dislodged. Veins in the feet immobilize the patient and so increase the risk of thrombosis.

Choice of catheter

A small 18–23 French gauge polyurethane-hydromer-coated, radio-opaque catheter of 15–20 cm long is used and allows blood to flow around it thereby helping dilute vaso-irritative solutions. This type of catheter is often referred to as a midline catheter. The catheter tip should be 15 cm from an insertion site near the cubital fossa. This is much closer to the insertion site than previously reported as 40 cm for 'half-way' venous catheters.[26] These catheters should last for more than 5 days[27] and most are likely to be functional for up to 2 weeks. A short extension set is used to reduce catheter movement at the exit site. The insertion procedure is much the same as for a PICC.

SMALL-VEIN NUTRITION

After the introduction of Intralipid® allowed feeding solutions to become less hyperosmolar, it again became possible to consider parenteral nutrition through a small vein.[28] Small-vein parenteral nutrition is administered through a short plastic cannula inserted into the small veins on the forearm, on the back of the hand, or on the scalp of babies. The limiting feature of this type of parenteral feeding is the high incidence of thrombophlebitis which means that a cannula does not often remain patent for more than 3 days.[29–32] It is recommended that a cannula used for feeding in a small vein is re-sited every 1–2 days.

CARE OF FEEDING LINES

Within a multi-disciplinary nutrition team, the clinical nurse specialist usually plays the leading role in drawing up and implementing protocols for catheter management. These include monitoring, reporting and managing any complications following catheter insertion, caring for the catheter entry and exit sites, changing the infusion, capping off the line, detecting problems of hypo- or hyperglycaemia, venous thrombosis, line occlusion or infection. The role involves a large educational commitment for training patients, carers and staff.

The main principles of care are to minimize the risk of complications such as infection, trauma to the catheter and air from entering the system. Catheter care protocols, which will differ between units, help achieve this. The procedures outlined (Tables 19.4–19.6) should act only as a starting point from which to base practice.

Skin cleaning

Chlorhexidine (either 2% aqueous solution or 0.5% solution in 70% ethyl alcohol) results in fewer

Table 19.4 – Guidelines for dressing/re-dressing the catheter entry site

Equipment
  Trolley
  Chlorhexidine in spirit spray
  Chlorhexidine in spirit solution
  Dressing pack (gallipot, forceps and gauze squares)
  Sterile gloves
  Wound swab
  Sterile porous non-adhesive dressing
  Tape

Procedure
1. Wipe working surface with warm water and detergent. Then spray with chlorhexidine in spirit.
2. Wash hands.
3. Make patient comfortable. Loosen old dressing, being careful not to pull catheter or touch skin at entry site.
4. Open sterile dressing pack on sterile field. Pour chlorhexidine solution into gallipot, put dressing and gloves onto sterile field. Remove and discard old dressing.
5. Observe:
   - The entry site for redness or discharge. Obtain a swab for culture if necessary. Record the site appearance and state if pyrexial and on the microbiology form. Redress daily if redness or discharge is present.
   - That the dacron cuff on Broviac or Hickman catheters is not visible. Note the integrity of any sutures. Look for any kinks in the catheter as these will weaken the material and may lead to catheter blockage.
6. Put on sterile gloves, clean around the entry site using gauze soaked in chlorhexidine in spirit. Wipe from the entry site outwards. Allow to dry.
7. Apply new dressing. Neatly coil the catheter on top of dressing and tape securely in place.
8. In hospital the dressing should be checked daily and changed weekly. Between dressing changes it should not be disturbed if it is clean and dry.
9. Ideally the cuff should be felt under the skin at least 2–3 cm from the exit site.

catheter-related infections than povidone-iodine.[33,34] A chlorhexidine in spirit spray is commonly used.

Dressing and line security

Sterile mechanical phlebitis can be caused by the powder on gloves used at the time of insertion or when the dressing has been changed. It is recommended that non-powdered gloves be used. If they are not available, gloved hands should be washed in sterile water before use.

Table 19.5 – Guidelines for changing parenteral nutrition bag

The parenteral nutrition bag must be stored in the refrigerator and removed at least one hour prior to use, to bring the temperature of the feed to room temperature. In some units the bag comes with a giving set and if used a click-lock attached.

Equipment
    Trolley
    Parenteral nutrition feeding bag
    Volumetric infusion pump
    Chlorhexidine in spirit spray
    Sterile gloves
    Dressing pack (gallipot, gauze squares and dressing towel)

Procedure
1. Check patient details and the expiry date of the bag. Leave the light protective cover on the parenteral nutrition-feeding bag. Hang on drip stand touching only the handle.
2. If feed is in progress, switch off pump and clip or clamp feeding line. Remove the old line from the pump.
3. Wash hands with detergent under warm running water for at least 1 minute. Ensure hands are thoroughly dried.
4. Clean working surface (usually a trolley) with chlorhexidine in spirit spray.
5. Open a dressing towel onto the working surface, touching only the corners. Put opened administration set and sterile gloves onto dressing towel.
6. Put a second sterile towel under feeding-line connection. Lift up feeding-line and spray line connection. Drop line onto sterile towel. Spray bottom of feeding bag.
7. Wash hands or clean with a hand rub, put on sterile gloves (now only sterile or sprayed equipment may be touched).
8. Unravel administration set and spike feeding bag, keep other end on sterile towel. Prime the line using gravity into sterile gallipot.
9. Disconnect old line and securely reconnect new line.
10. Gloves can be taken off. Insert administration set into pump and set the rate and volume to be infused. Remove clamp/undo clip and start infusion.
11. Check the infusion after 15 minutes for possible leakage and then at regular intervals.

Table 19.6 – Guidelines for capping off a line

Equipment
    Chlorhexidine in spirit spray
    2 dressing towels
    10 ml of 50 units heparin
    Sterile gloves
    10 ml syringe
    Filter straw
    Injectable cap (or Interlink cap and straw)

Procedure
1. Switch off pump and clamp feeding line.
2. Wash hands with detergent under warm running water. Ensure hands are thoroughly dried.
3. Clean working surface. Put heparin ampoule down in one corner of working surface and spray. Open one dressing towel onto working surface and drop onto it gloves, 10 ml syringe, filter straw, injectable cap (or interlink cap and straw).
4. Put other dressing towel down near to the hub connection. Spray feeding-line and hub connection with chlorhexidine in spirit spray. Place line onto sterile towel.
5. Wash hands with detergent under warm running water for at least 1 minute. Ensure hands are thoroughly dried. Put on sterile gloves. Break cap off heparin solution and draw up 10 ml through the filter straw.
6. Disconnect feeding-line. Attach syringe to line, unclamp line, inject 10 ml heparin, reclamp line and put on injectable cap (if Interlink system is used, put Interlink cap on line, then inject heparin through the Interlink straw).
7. Remove gloves.
8. A line that is not used will need to be flushed with heparin twice weekly. The cap should be changed every week.

their transparency. However, fluids, either from seepage back down the catheter, sweat or blood, may collect under them and become infected.[35] Transparent dressings that are porous to water vapour (e.g. Opsite IV 3000®) may be better.[36]

Medium- and small-vein catheters are not sutured to the skin, therefore extra care is taken to ensure security of the site. The insertion site is covered with a sterile adhesive dressing which is also more comfortable for the patient. All care is aseptically carried out and the veins inspected daily for thrombophlebitis.

If a line has withdrawn no attempt should ever be made to push it back. Referring to the original measurements will indicate how much has come out. A chest radiograph will show the catheter tip position. Prior to delivery of intravenous drugs or fluids, it is

A sterile porous dressing with an incorporated sterile pad is the dressing of choice for large-vein catheters exiting on the chest wall (e.g. Mepore® or Primapore® dressings). Transparent film dressings, while providing secure catheter retention and acting as a bacterial barrier, allow for ease of inspection through important to ensure that the lumen is patent by flushing with saline.

Infusion rate

The rate of a feed should not be increased in order to 'catch up' if a feed is running behind time, as this can increase the risk of hyperglycaemia and phlebitis. The rate of feeding should gradually be reduced over the last hour to prevent rebound hypoglycaemia.

Catheter-related sepsis

The greatest problem of parenteral feeding is to reduce/eliminate the chance of developing catheter-related sepsis (CRS). CRS can be reduced to almost zero by employing a nutrition nurse specialist who implements meticulous care of the catheter using aseptic techniques with sterile equipment and antiseptic solutions.[37]

Some important general principles about caring for a line to reduce the chance of CRS are as follows:

- Only experienced staff should touch a feeding line. A catheter handled by many people is more likely to become infected than one handled by a few.

- Single lumen catheters, with an integrated hub, are less likely to become infected than double or triple lumen ones.[38,39]

- There should only be one connection to a feeding catheter (3-way taps should not be used).[39]

- A catheter should be used only for parenteral nutrition. Ideally no other drugs/solutions should be put through the catheter. However, if they are to be administered they are drawn up through a filter straw, especially if a glass ampoule has had to be broken.

- Blood should not be taken from the line except for blood cultures if CRS is suspected.

- Additions to the feed are done in a compounding unit and rarely on the ward.

In the short-term, micro-organisms may gain access from the exit site, but after 2 weeks the hub connection is the most common site of contamination and the site from which most cases of CRS arise.[40,41] CRS may less commonly arise from the exit site or from a septicaemia from a distant site (e.g. urine or teeth). *Staphlococcus epidermidis*, *Enterobacter*, *Streptococcus faecalis*, *Staph. aureus* and various *Candida* species are the most commonly implicated organisms. CRS remains one of the most common and serious complications of parenteral nutrition. It can be fatal.

Diagnosis can be difficult, as patients frequently have other sources of sepsis which could explain the symptoms of pyrexia and malaise. The diagnosis becomes relatively certain when the patient suffers a rigor shortly after the commencement of a feed; this is most obvious if the patient is not feeding continuously. The issue of whether the infusion should be continued when there is a suspected CRS is controversial and many would advocate the immediate cessation of the infusion, with the taking of central and peripheral blood. When taking blood cultures under aseptic conditions from the feeding line, up to 10 ml of blood is taken which includes the residue in the line. The line may then be locked with heparinized saline or, if the patient has no other access source and needs fluid, the feeding bag may be changed to saline. While awaiting the results of the cultures, systemic antibiotics (e.g. vancomycin or gentamicin) are given. Catheter salvage is possible using urokinase and an antibiotic lock for *Staph. epidermidis*, but success is unlikely if the organism is *Staph. aureus* or *Candida* (Chapter 32). A quarter of patients with *candidal* feeding-line infections will have involvement of their eyes.[42] Salvage is doubtful when the patient has a port, and there is the potential risk of recrudescence and metastatic infection that could result in endocarditis or osteomyelitis.

Central vein thombosis

Central vein thombosis may be suspected if the patient complains of a headache, pain in the chest or neck, swollen face or arm. There may be pyrexia in the absence of an infection or an unexplained tachycardia (Chapter 32). The precipitating factors are as for peripheral vein thrombophlebitis (PVT) with catheter sepsis, dehydration and a distal catheter tip position (e.g. in brachocephalic or subclavian vein) being especially important. The volume and osmolality of current parenteral nutrition, solutions is considerably lower than those used in the early days of central parenteral nutrition and most adult patients require less than 2000 kcal/day or 30 kcal/kg/day.[43]

Peripheral vein thrombophlebitis

Peripheral venous cannulation aims to minimize the risk of damage to small veins, which have a relatively poor blood supply and are thus vulnerable. PVT results from inflammation of the vein intima and the inflammation leads on to thrombosis and subsequent occlusion of the vein. It is a major factor that limits the use of both small- and medium-vein feeding. PVT occurs when two or more of the following are noted at the insertion site or proximal to it: pain, erythema, swelling, excessive warmth or a palpaple venous cord.[44] PVT is the major problem of medium- and small-vein catheterization and needs to be detected early. All peripheral lines should be inspected daily and if there is any evidence of PVT the line is removed and re-sited.

Trauma at the venepuncture site may cause a temporary reduction in blood flow sufficient to initiate an inflammatory reaction and subsequent thrombosis. If venous thrombosis becomes a recurring problem, coagulation studies may be necessary (antithrombin III, lupus anticoagulant, protein C, S and activated protein C resistance).

Risk factors for peripheral venous thrombophlebitis

The nutrient solution, the catheter and the properties of the vein influence the chance of thrombophlebitis occurring (Table 19.7). The two most

Table 19.7 – Factors increasing risk of thrombophlebitis

---

1. Composition of nutrient solution
   - high osmolality
   - acidic pH
   - high potassium
   - low lipid
   - particulate matter
   - drug additives

2. Catheter
   - material (rubber, polyethylene, polyvinyl chloride and teflon)
   - large diameter
   - long length
   - poor flexibility
   - bacterial colonization
   - intermittent infusion

3. Properties of vein
   - insertion trauma
   - small diameter
   - low flow (e.g. if patient dehydrated)
   - movement of catheter
   - catheter in situ a long time

4. Absence of a nutrition support team

---

common causes of thrombophlebitis are chemical due to the high osmolality and low pH of the infused fluids, and mechanical due to vein trauma during insertion.

A major factor in facilitating the widespread use of peripheral feeding, particularly for short-term nutritional support, has been the reduction in osmolality achieved by using lipid emulsions in addition to carbohydrate as an energy source. Infusion-related thrombophlebitis is significantly less frequent in patients who receive 'all-in-one' compounded bags, rather than receiving the lipid solution separately.[31] A high osmolality feed (low in lipid) is more likely to result in thrombosis than one of low osmolality (high lipid content). Glucose solutions are acidic, a 10% unbuffered glucose has a pH of 3.5–4.5 and caused thrombophlebitis in 18% compared with 5% when a buffered glucose solution at pH 6.8 was given.[45] The risk is reduced if 2000 kcal or 11 gm N are given daily. A high amino acid or potassium content increase the risk of thrombosis.[46] An infusion rate of less than 2 L/24 hours makes catheter occlusion likely, however a rate of greater than 3.5 l/24 hours is difficult to get through the fine-bore cannula.[47] A line that is not used (e.g. in cyclical parenteral nutrition) is more prone to causing thrombophlebitis.

The catheter-related factors that relate to thrombophlebitis are length, diameter, flexibility and biocompatibility of the material (hydrophilic surface). Longer catheters have a higher chance of causing thrombophlebitis than shorter ones.[32] If a catheter becomes infected it is likely to cause a secondary thrombophlebitis, thus strict aseptic techniques in caring for the catheter are vital. Securing the catheter with sutures or sterile wound closure material and an adhesive dressing (e.g. Stat-lock®) may reduce catheter movement inside the vein. If the vein was small and the catheter only just fitted into the vein at insertion, heat can be applied to the insertion site for up to 20 minutes 4 times daily.

A strict aseptic insertion technique is one of the most important factors in preventing thrombophlebitis.[48] Glyceryl trinitrate patches over the vein distal to the insertion site cause veno-dilation and increase blood flow; thereby reducing the risk of thrombophlebitis.[30,49] A similar application of a nonsteroidal anti-inflammatory drug gel over the site of a peripheral infusion may prove beneficial. Heparin (1 IU/ml) alone[50] or with hydrocortisone (5 mg/ml)[51] in the nutrient feeding bag reduce the chance of thrombophlebitis but they are not added to the bags by many units as both drugs may cause osteoporosis in the long-term.

Catheter occlusion

Persistent withdrawal occlusion (PWO) has been described as sluggish or absent blood withdrawal, even though some fluids may be infused.[52] PWO can occur if there is an anatomical obstruction, if the catheter tip is wrongly positioned or if the catheter is kinked (especially with PICC). Changing the patient's position (e.g. raising their arms above their heads or asking them to cough) can sometimes rectify the problem and allow blood to be aspirated. While thrombus, lipid and precipitate can all cause PWO, the commonest cause is a fibrin sheath formed around the catheter.[53,54]

A fibrin sheath is a collection of fibrin and platelets that can be demonstrated in 40% of all catheters with radiological screening after radio-opaque dye has been injected down the catheter.[55] It starts from where the catheter enters the vein and spreads towards the tip. It does not generally cause a problem until it surrounds the catheter tip when it may classically act as a one-way valve such that a solution can be infused down the catheter but not withdrawn.

Treatment of catheter occlusion

When trying to flush a line (or administer drugs) a 2 ml or 5 ml syringe should not be used as they generate a very high pressure which can cause the catheter to herniate and rupture. If there is difficulty with either flushing the line or withdrawing blood, the patient is asked to raise their arms and cough. If these measures restore the catheters patency, the exact position of the catheter tip is rechecked with a chest X-ray. If they do not work, a urokinase lock is usually tried on the assumption that the occlusion is due to a fibrin sheath. Initially, 5000 units of urokinase in 2–5 ml solution are inserted into the catheter and left for 10–60 minutes before being aspirated. If there is any difficulty in injecting the urokinase, a three-way tap can be attached to the end of the catheter. Two syringes, one empty and one containing the urokinase, are then attached to the three-way tap. A gentle rocking action between the two syringes will ensure that the urokinase is well distributed within the lumen. After giving a treatment, an attempt is made to aspirate blood with a 50 ml syringe.

If the bolus of urokinase does not work, radio-opaque contrast may be put down the line to define

the problem. If definitely due to a fibrin sheath a urokinase infusion (40 000 units/hour of 5000 units/ml) may be given for 6 hours (this has had an immediate success rate of 58%,[56] or t-PA (10 000 units) left in the line for 4 hours has been successful in 83%.[57] Lipid occlusion may occur in up to 30% patients when lipid is incorporated into all feeding bags,[58] it may be treated with 3 ml of 70% alcohol[59,60] or prevented by giving 10 ml of 20% ethanol after the feed.[61] Precipitate causing line occlusion is a formulation issue that may cause problems in children when the amount of calcium and phosphate in the feed is high; it can be cleared with 0.2–0.5 ml of 0.1 N hydrochloric acid being put in the line for 20 minutes.[62]

Goodwin and Carlson stressed the importance of the flushing technique in preventing vascular access device occlusion.[63] They recommend a rapid pushing–pausing or pulsating action. This creates turbulence in the lumen, thus decreasing the risk of fibrin or platelets being deposited. Occlusion of a vascular access port can be treated with 10 ml of 0.1 N sodium hydroxide solution.[64]

Catheter damage

Catheter repair kits should be available and staff familiar with their application. A skillful repair to a damaged/split line prevents the trauma and risk of a fresh insertion and can maintain the integrity of a line for several years. However, the line often becomes infected before the repair is done.

Air/bubbles in line

If air has entered the line, the line is immediately clamped as close to the exit site as possible. Using an aseptic procedure the hub connection is undone and the air is flushed out of the system before reconnecting or capping off the line.

ISSUES ABOUT EQUIPMENT

There is an increasing choice of equipment available, especially connections and catheter types.

Closed connection devices

Closed intravenous connection devices also called needleless systems (e.g. Bionector®, Interlink®, Clicklock® or Safesite®) are now commonly favoured in the UK. Although to date little conclusive data are available, manufacturers of these devices claim that they help to reduce the incidence of CRS by maintaining a closed system at all times and that they reduce the risk of needle stick injury.

The National Nurses Nutrition Group (NNNG) undertook a survey in 1996, which concluded that closed connection devices were beneficial in terms of cost-effectiveness, savings in nursing time and decreasing the risk of air embolism. However, sometimes there were problems with the catheter leaking, cracking and being difficult to flush. They did not show any evidence of reduced CRS or needlestick injuries.[65]

These devices are no substitute for careful catheter management and should be changed weekly, whenever damaged or if blood flashback occurs.

Valved catheters

The Bard Groshong valve is a three-way valve incorporated into the tip of a large-vein catheter which, in the absence of a negative or positive pressure, remains in the closed position. It opens inward when negative pressure is applied for aspiration and outward with positive pressure used for infusion. It should prevent blood from the venous circulation entering the lumen, so making catheter occlusion less common, and should reduce the risk of air entering the line; thus heparin should not need to be flushed into the line. While generally performing well,[66] they were no better than Hickman-type lines in terms of CRS or thrombosis formation, and they malfunctioned more frequently.[67]

Filters

Although intravenous solutions may appear clear to the naked eye, they contain particles of 1–25 microns, which can induce sterile inflammation and cause granulomas elsewhere such as lungs and brain.[68] The particles consist of glass, cotton fibres, precipitated proteins, microcrystalline drug particles, degenerative products of interactions between fluids and glass, plastic and even rubber stoppers. Some arise from glass ampoules[69] and some from syringes themselves.[70]

A 0.2-micron filter reduces the incidence of thrombophlebitis[71] especially when intravenous antibiotics are given.[72] However, a larger filter is needed if lipid is infused and Intralipid (particles < 1.4 μm) will pass through a 5-micron filter without disruption of the emulsion.[73] It would seem sensible to draw up all drugs and solutions that are to be given intravenously through a filter straw, and it may be advisable to have a filter in the infusion line but it can reduce flow and cause blockage.

Feeding pumps

The pump of choice is a volumetric pump to ensure a constant, accurate low-pressure infusion. Drip counters are not recommended, as they are inaccurate in the measurement of parenteral nutrition fluid. For patient comfort one that makes little noise, has few false alarms and has lights that can be dimmed is best.[74]

REMOVAL OF A FEEDING LINE

The patient is placed in the head down position or flat, to prevent air embolism. The skin is cleaned with chlorhexidine in spirit, the operator wears gloves and drapes towels around the area. Any remaining stitches, including those securing the line, are removed. A non-cuffed feeding line is removed by gently withdrawing the catheter at a slow, constant rate. The tip is not allowed to touch anything, its tip (about 3 cm) is cut off using sterile scissors; it is then sent for culture. The catheter is inspected to ensure that it is complete.

A long-term catheter with dacron cuff is removed by injecting local anaesthetic around the dacron cuff, then making a 1 cm incision beside the upper end of the cuff. Using blunt dissection the catheter just above the cuff is located (a surgical hook may be put round it), the fibrin sheath round the line is cut and pealed away clearly exposing the line. The cuff is dissected out, and once free, the line can be gently removed using gentle traction. Once the tip has come out and its tip cut off for microbiology, the catheter needs to be cut near the exit site so the distal end can be removed. One or two sutures will be needed to close the incision. A small pressure dressing is applied to the incision site.

The removal of a port is a longer procedure than removing a cuffed line and many patients will choose to have this done under a general anaesthetic. Some will choose a local anaesthetic after sedation and analgesics have been given.

REFERENCES

1. Hamilton H, O'Byrne M, Nickolai L. Central lines inserted by clinical nurse specialists. *Nursing Times* 1995; **91**: 38–39.

2. Handfield-Jones RPC, Lewis HBM. Rubber tubing as a cause of infusion thrombophlebitis. *Lancet* 1952; **1**: 585–588.

3. Indar R. The danger of indwelling polyethylene cannulae in deep veins. *Lancet* 1959; **i**: 284–286.

4. Madan M, Alexander DJ, McMahon MJ. Influence of catheter type on occurrence of thrombophlebitis during peripheral intravenous nutrition. *Lancet* 1992; **339**: 101–103.

5. Nachnan GH, Lessin LS, Motomiya T, Jensen WN. Scanning electron microscopy of thrombogenesis on vascular catheter surfaces. *N Engl J Med* 1972; **286**: 139–140.

6. Borow M, Crowley JG. Evaluation of central venous catheter thrombogenicity. *Acta Anaesthesiol Scand* 1985; **Suppl 81**: 59–64.

7. Everitt NJ, Madan M, Alexander DJ, McMahon MJ. Fine bore silicone rubber and polyurethane catheters for delivery of complete intravenous nutrition via a peripheral vein. *Clin Nutr* 1993; **12**: 261–265.

8. Linder L-E, Curelaru I, Gustavsson B, Hansson H-A, Stenqvist O, Wojciechowski J. Material thrombogenicity in central venous catheterization; a comparison between soft, antebrachial catheters of silicone elastomer and polyurethane. *J Parenter Enteral Nutr* 1984; **8**: 399–406.

9. Darouiche RO, Raad II, Heard SO, *et al*. A comparison of two antimicrobial-impregnated central venous catheters. *N Engl J Med* 1999; **340**: 1–8.

10. Denny DF Jr. Placement and management of long-term central venous access catheters and ports. *Am J Roentgenol* 1993; **161**: 385–393.

11. Sizer T (ed). *Standards and Guidelines for Nutritional Support of Patients in Hospital*. A report by a working party of the British Association for Parenteral and Enteral Nutrition, 1996.

12. Payne-James JJ, de Gara CJ, Doherty J, Cribb R, Rana S, Silk DBA. Nutritional Support in Hospitals in the UK: National Survey. *Health Trends* 1990; **22**: 8–12.

13. Lameris JS, Post PJM, Zonderland HM, Gerritsen PG, Kappers-Klunne MC, Schutte HE. Percutaneous placement of Hickman catheters: comparison of sonographically guided and blind techniques. *Am J Roentgenol* 1990; **155**: 1097–1099.

14. Ubhi SS, Rees Y, Veitch PS. Ultrasound guided subclavian vein catheterisation. *Ann R Coll Surg Engl* 1991; **73**: 227–228.

15. Mansfield PF, Hohn DC, Fornage BD, Gregurich MA, Ota DM. Complications and failures of subclavian-vein catheterization. *N Engl J Med* 1994; **331**: 1735–1738.

16. Moncrief JA. Femoral catheters. *Ann Surg* 1958; **147**: 166–172.

17. Niederhuber JE, Ensminger W, Gyves JW, Liepman M, Doan K, Cazzi E. Totally implanted venous and arterial access system to replace external catheters in cancer treatment . *Surgery* 1982; **92**: 706–712.

18. Howard L, Claunch C, McDowell R, Timchalk M. Five years' experience in patients receiving home nutritional support with the implanted reservoir: a comparison with the external catheter. *J Parenter Enteral Nutr* 1989; **13**: 478–483.

19. Magnay S, Wheatley C, Wood S, Forbes A. Comparison of implanted ports with Broviac/Hickman-style tunnelled catheters for long-term home parenteral nutrition: the patient's view. *Proc Nutr Soc* 1995; **54**: 103A.

20. Mughal MM. Complications of intravenous feeding catheters. *Br J Surg* 1989; **76**: 15–21.

21. DeJong PCM, von Meyenfeldt MR, Rouflart M, Wesdorp RIC, Soeters PB. Complications of central venous catheterization of the subclavian vein: The influence of a parenteral nutrition team. *Acta Anaesthiol Scand* 1985; **Suppl 81**: 48–52.

22. Hoshal VL. Total intravenous nutrition with peripherally inserted silicone elastomer central venous catheters. *Arch Surg* 1975; **110**: 644–646.

23. Merrell SW, Peatross BG, Grossman MD, Sullivan JJ, Harker WG. Peripherally inserted central venous catheters. Low-risk alternatives for ongoing venous access. *West J Med* 1994; **160**: 25–30.

24. Brown J. Peripherally inserted central catheters: use in home care. *J Intravenous Nurs* 1989; **12**: 144–147.

25. May J, Sedman P, Mitchell C, MacFie J. Peripheral and central parenteral nutrition: a cost-comparison analysis. *Health Trends* 1993; **25**: 129–132.

26. Linder LE, Wojciechowski J, Zachrisson BF, Curelaru I, Gustavsson B, Hultman E, Bylock A. 'Half-way' venous catheters. IV. Clinical experience and thrombogenicity. *Acta Anaesthiol Scand* 1985: **Suppl 81**: 40–46.

27. Kohlhardt SR, Smith RC. Fine-bore silicon catheters for peripheral intravenous nutrition in adults. *Br Med J* 1989; **299**: 1380–1381.

28. Deitel M, Kaminsky V. Total nutrition by peripheral vein: the lipid system. *Can Med Assoc J* 1974; **111**: 152–154.

29. Isaacs JW, Millikan WJ, Stackhouse J, Hersh T, Rudman D. Parenteral nutrition of adults with a 900 milliosmolar solution via peripheral veins. *Am J Clin Nutr* 1977; **30**: 552–559.

30. Khawaja HT, Campbell MJ, Weaver PC. Effect of transdermal glceryp trinitrate on the survival of peripheral intravenous infusions: a double-blind prospective clinical study. *Br J Surg* 1988; **75**: 1212–1215.

31. Nordenstrom J, Jeppsson B, Loven L, Larsson J. Peripheral parenteral nutrition: effect of a standardised compounded mixture on infusion phlebitis. *Br J Surg* 1991; **78**: 1391–1394.

32. May J, Murchan P, MacFie J, Sedman P, Donat R, Palmer D, Mitchell CJ. Prospective study of the aetiology of infusion phlebitis and line failure during peripheral parenteral nutrition. *Br J Surg* 1996; **83**: 1091–1094.

33. Rannem T, Ladefoged K, Hegnhoj J, Hylander E, Moller E, Bruun B, Jernum S. Catheter-related sepsis in long-term parenteral nutrition with Broviac catheters. An evaluation of different disinfectants. *Clin Nutr* 1990; **9**: 131–136.

34. Maki DG, Ringer M, Alvarado CJ. Prospective randomised trial of povidone-iodine, alcohol, and chlorhexidine for prevention of infection associated with central venous and arterial catheters. *Lancet* 1991; **338**: 339–343.

35. Conly JM, Grieves K, Peters B. A prospective, randomized study comparing transparent and dry gauze dressings for central venous catheters. *J Infect Dis* 1989; **159**: 310–319.

36. Fincham Gee C, Noble W. Transparent film dressings. *Nursing* 1990; **4**: 39–41.

37. Keohane PP, Jones BM, Astrill H, Cribb A, Northover J, Frost P, Silk DBA. Effects of catheter tunnelling and nutrition nurse on catheter sepsis during parenteral nutrition. *Lancet* 1983; **ii**: 1388–1390.

38. McCarthy MC, Shivers JK, Robison RJ, Broadie TA. Prospective evaluation of single and triple-lumen catheters in parenteral nutrition. *J Parenter Enteral Nutr* 1987; **11**: 259–262.

39. Stotter AT, Ward H, Waterfield AH, Hilton J, Sim AJW. Junctional care the key to preventing catheter sepsis in intravenous feeding. *J Parenter Enteral Nutr* 1987; **11**: 159–162.

40. Sitges-Serra A, Puig P, Linares J, Perez JL, Ferrero N, Jaurrieta E, Garau J. Hub colonisation as the initial step in an outbreak of catheter-related sepsis due to coagulase negative staphylococci during parenteral nutrition. *J Parenter Enteral Nutr* 1984; **8**: 668–672.

41. Weightman NC, Simpson EM, Speller DCE, Mott MG, Oakhill A. Bacteraemia related to indwelling central venous catheters; prevention, diagnosis and treatment. *Eur J Clin Microbiol Infect Dis* 1988; **7**: 125–129.

42. Nightingale JMD, Simpson AJ, Wood SR, Lennard-Jones JE. Fungal feeding-line infections: beware the eyes and teeth. *J R Soc Med* 1995; **88**: 258–263.

43. Payne-James JJ, Khawaja HT. First choice for total parenteral nutrition: the peripheral route. *J Parenter Enteral Nutr* 1993; **17**: 468–478.

44. Elia M. Changing concepts of nutrient requirements in disease: implications for artificial nutritional support. *Lancet* 1995; **345**: 1279–1284.

45. Elfving G, Saikku K. The effect of pH on the incidence of infusion thrombophlebitis. *Lancet* 1966; **1**: 953.

46. Gazitua R, Wilson K, Bistrian BR, Blackburn GL. Factors determining peripheral vein tolerance to amino acid infusions. *Arch Surg* 1979; **114**: 897–900.

47. Everitt NJ, McMahon MJ. Peripheral intravenous nutrition. *Nutrition* 1994; **10**: 49–57.

48. Lodge JPA, Chisholm EM, Brennan TG, MacFie J. Insertion technique, the key to avoiding infusion phlebitis: a prospective clinical trial. *Br J Clin Pract* 1987; **41**: 816–819.

49. Khawaja HT, Williams JD, Weaver PC. Transdermal glyceryl trinitrate to allow peripheral total parenteral nutrition: a double-blind placebo controlled feasibility study. *J R Soc Med* 1991; **84**: 69–72.

50. Tanner WA, Delaney PV, Hennessy TP. The influence of heparin on intravenous infusions: a prospective study. *Br J Surg* 1980; **67**: 311–312.

51. Makarewicz PA, Freeman JB, Fairfull-Smith R. Prevention of superficial phlebitis during peripheral parenteral nutrition. *Am J Surg* 1988; **151**: 126–129.

52. Mayo D, Pearson D. Chemotherapy extravasation: a consequence of fibrin sheath formation around venous access devices. *Oncol Nurs Forum* 1995; **22**: 675–680.

53. Hoshal VL Jr, Ause RG, Hoskins PA. Fibrin sleeve formation on indwelling subclavian central venous catheters. *Arch Surg* 1971; **102**: 353–358.

54. Stephens LC, Haire WD, Kotulak GD. Are clinical signs accurate indicators of the cause of central venous catheter occlusion? *J Parenter Enteral Nutr* 1995; **19**: 75–79.

55. Schneider TC, Krzywda E, Andris D, Quebbeman EJ. The malfunctioning silastic catheter – Radiological assessment and treatment. *J Parenter Enteral Nutr* 1986; **10**: 70–73.

56. Haire WD, Lieberman RP. Thrombosed central venous catheters: restoring function with 6-hour urokinase infusion after failure of bolus urokinase. *J Parenter Enteral Nutr* 1992; **16**: 129–132.

57. Atkinson JB, Bagnall HA, Gomperts E. Investigational use of tissue plasminogen activator (t-PA) for occluded central venous catheters. *J Parenter Enteral Nutr* 1990; **14**: 310–311.

58. Messing B, Beliah M, Girard-Pipau F, Leleve D, Bernier JJ. Technical hazards of using nutritive mixtures in bags for cyclical intravenous nutrition: comparison with standard intravenous nutrition in 48 gastroenterological patients. *Gut* 1982; **23**: 297–303.

59. Pennington CR, Pithie AD. Ethanol lock in the management of catheter occlusion. *J Parenter Enteral Nutr* 1987; **11**: 507–508.

60. Werlin SL, Lausten T, Jessen S, *et al*. Treatment of central venous catheter occlusions with ethanol and hydrochloric acid. *J Parenter Enteral Nutr* 1995; **19**: 416–418.

61. Johnston DA, Walker K, Richards J, Pennington CR. Ethanol flush for the prevention of catheter occlusion. *Clin Nutr* 1992; **11**: 97–100.

62. Duffy LF, Kerzner B, Gebus V, Dice J. Treatment of central venous catheter occlusions with hydrochloric acid. *J Pediatr* 1989; **114**: 1002–1004.

63. Goodwin M, Carlson I. The peripherally inserted central catheter: A retrospective look at three years of insertions. *J Intraven Nurs* 1993; **16**: 92–103.

64. Ter Borg F, Timmer J, De Kam SS, Sauerwein HP. Use of sodium hydroxide solution to clear partially occluded vascular access ports. *J Parenter Enteral Nutr* 1993; **17**: 289–291.

65. Colagiovanni L. Closed IV connection devices: Their use in parenteral nutrition – results of the survey. *National Nurses Nutrition Group Newsletter* 1996; Sept: 3–4.

66. Delmore JE, Horbelt DV, Jack BL, Roberts DK. Experience with the Groshong long-term central venous catheter. *Gynecol Oncol* 1989; **34**: 216–218.

67. Pasquale MD, Campbell JM, Magnant CM. Groshong versus Hickman catheters. *Surg Gynecol Obstet* 1992; **174**: 408–410.

68. Garvan JM, Gunner BW. The harmful effects of particles in intravenous fluids. *Med J Aust* 1964; **II**: 1-6.

69. Shaw NJ, Lyall EGH. Hazards of glass ampoules. *Br Med J* 1985; **291**: 1390.

70. Taylor SA. Particulate contamination of sterile syringes and needles. *J Pharm Pharmacol* 1982; **34**: 493–495.

71. Falchuk KH, Peterson L, McNeil BJ. Microparticulate-induced phlebitis. Its prevention by in-line filtration. *N Engl Med* 1985; **312**: 78–82.

72. Allcutt DA, Lort D, McCollum CN. Final inline filtration for intravenous infusions: a prospective hospital study. *Br J Surg* 1983; **70**: 111–113.

73. Rubin M, Bilik R, Gruenewald Z, *et al*. Use of 5-micron filter in administering 'all-in-one' mixtures for total parenteral nutrition. *Clin Nutr* 1986; **4**: 163–168.

74. Carter D, Wheatley C, Martin R, *et al*. Nights of bright lights and noisy pumps – home parenteral feeding. *Proc Nutr Soc* 1996; **55**: 149A.

20

Designing parenteral and enteral regimens

Edgar Pullicino and Marinos Elia

*W*ide ranges of enteral (EN) and parenteral nutritional (PN) regimens are required for different types of patients with intestinal failure. The patients range from the premature newborn infants with necrotizing enterocolitis to adults with a short bowel, and from those requiring short-term nutritional support in hospital to long-term support at home. The regimens must be of proven efficacy and based on an understanding of nutrient requirements in the different groups of patients.

This chapter considers how requirements vary with clinical state in both adults and children, including neonates. The nutrient requirements of growing infants and children vary with age, but recommendations at any specified age are based on extrapolations from other age groups. Enteral feeds come from the manufacturers already compounded, while parenteral feeding bags are usually compounded within a hospital and most of the components need to be specified. Thus this chapter details mainly the design of a parenteral regimen.

ENERGY REQUIREMENTS

In sick patients a period of negative energy balance, particularly over a prolonged period of time, depletes the body of glycogen, protein and fat. This negative energy balance can be corrected by administering more energy than total energy expenditure (TEE). In general about 0.2 grams of tissue are accreted for every kcal deposited under anabolic conditions. Whilst total energy intake (EI) can be readily calculated from the intake of individual macronutrients with known energy densities, TEE over a prolonged period of time can only be calculated directly by continuous 24-hour calorimetry or tracer techniques. More often, TEE is calculated by adding together the perceived components of TEE (Table 20.1). The calculations are the same for parenteral and enteral regimens.

Basal metabolic rate (BMR)

BMR is classically measured in relaxed, motionless subjects after an overnight fast in thermoneutral ambient conditions. Its most important determinant is the size of the lean body mass. Equations that estimate BMR from body weight and height are popular and have been established from measurements of BMR in large numbers of healthy volunteers. These equations include the Roberston-Reid,[1] Fleish[2] and Harris-Benedict[3] equations, which have been found to overestimate BMR of healthy volunteers by a mean of 0%, +2.5% and +4.1% respectively.[4] However, these equations do not necessarily apply to patients with disease (e.g. sepsis which frequently accompanies intestinal failure (IF)), undernutrition, or disturbances in hydration (e.g. oedema).

Table 20.1 – To work out a parenteral regimen

1) Calculate total energy needed.
    Basal Metabolic Rate (BMR) – Harris-Benedict equation (kcal/day)
    Men   66 + (13.7 × weight (kg)) + (5.0 × height (cm)) − (6.8 × age (yr))
    Female 655 + (9.6 × weight (kg)) + (1.8 × height (cm)) − (4.7 × age (yr))
    <u>Additional factors to add</u>: Stress factor for disease (+13% for every degree C rise in body temperature)
                                       Physical activity (+10% for inactive subjects)
                                       Growth/Repletion
                                       Dietary induced thermogenesis (10%)
2) Calculate amino acid requirement:
    0.15–0.30 gN/kg/day
    Add repletion (0.1 gN per kg weight lost)
3) Calculate amino acid energy:
    gN × 27
4) Calculate maximum amount of fat allowed (2g fat/kg)★
5) Calculate CHO energy as:
    Total energy − (fat energy + amino acid energy)
6) Calculate fat: CHO calorie ratio and ensure it is about 40:60
7) Check safety of derived glucose, amino acid and lipid infusion rates
8) Calculate/estimate volumes of water, sodium, potassium, magnesium, calcium and phosphate

★ Many nutrition units divide the non-amino acid energy by 2 to give a fat:CHO energy ratio of 50:50. The exact ratio then is varied so that all the contents of a commercial lipid container are used in the feeding bag.

Stress factor

Sepsis increases BMR by 5–40%.[5,6] Fever raises BMR by approximately 13% per °C rise in body temperature (7.2% for every °Fahrenheit).[7] Intestinal irradiation, chemotherapy, bowel infarction and major surgery also raise BMR (0–30%).

Physical activity

IF patients, who are bed-bound or mechanically ventilated and minimally active have an estimated physical activity component of about 10% of BMR. In contrast, ambulant adult IF patients receiving cyclic nocturnal PN at home have been reported to have a physical activity component of about 30% of BMR.[8] Similar, if not higher, values occur in children.

Growth/repletion

Additional energy is required for tissue repletion or for normal growth in children (about 5 kcal/g of tissue deposited[9]). A positive energy balance (EI > TEE) of about 500 kcal/day in adults can achieve slow weight gain, but faster repletion can be achieved with higher intakes.

Diet-induced thermogenesis

Enteral or parenteral feeding induces a rise in energy expenditure that is proportional to the EI ((diet-induced thermogenesis) DIT approximates to 10% of the metabolizable EI).[8–10]

Malabsorption

In patients with intestinal failure enteral tube feeding may be poorly tolerated and the absorption is poor (50% or more of the energy may not be absorbed), so that nutrients may have to be given in increased amounts and often continuously.

Total energy requirements

After the BMR has been calculated, the effect of disease ('stress') on BMR is taken into account, either through measurements or predictions (Tables 20.1 and 20.2). The final or desirable energy intake also takes into account, physical activity, and any desirable changes in energy stores and DIT. The requirements may vary during the course of disease or during growth. For example, premature infants require approximately 120 kcal/kg/day. Energy requirements decrease with age.

Table 20.2 – Sequential design for macronutrients of a PN regimen for 40-year-old man of 50 kg (1.7 m)

		Metabolic stress/weight loss		
		Nil/15 kg	Mild/20 kg	Moderate/20 kg
1:	Target Energy Intakes:			
	BMR (Harris Benedict) (kcal)	1334	1334	1334
+	allowance for sepsis (kcal)	0	10% of BMR = 133	20% of BMR = 267
+	allowance for activity (kcal)★	133	146	160
+	allowance for repletion (kcal)	500	500	500
+	allowance for dietary induced thermogenesis (kcal)	218	235	251
=	Total energy needed (kcal)	2185	2348	2512★★
2:	Nitrogen needed (gN)†	9.0	12.0	14.5
3:	Amino acid energy (Kcal)	243	324	391
4:	Maximum fat allowance (Kcal)‡	1000	1000	1000
5:	CHO energy (Kcal)	942	1024	1121
6:	Fat : CHO energy ratio	51:49	49:51	47:53
7a:	CHO in g/kg body weight	5.0	5.5	6.0
7b:	N in g/kg body weight	0.18	0.24	0.29
7c:	fat in g/kg body weight	2.0	2.0	2.0

★: 10% of (BMR + stress factor).

†: Give 0.15, 0.20, 0.25, 0.30 g N/kg body weight for absent, mild, moderate, severe metabolic stress respectively. Give extra 0.1 g N per kg of body weight lost.

‡: Maximum fat allowance (2g fat/kg/d) has been used; assume that the energy content of 500 ml of a 20% fat emulsion (~1000 kcal) (~100 gm) is used.

★★ Please note this patient is malnourished and therefore excess energy can be given to replete his stores.

PARENTERAL NUTRITION

The recommended intakes for intravenous nutrients (RIV) vary with the nutrient. RIV for total amino acids (AA) have been largely based on nitrogen (N) balances, and RIV for specific amino acids on additional measurements of circulating and tissue concentrations. The RIV for vitamins have been largely based on studies of oral intake with additional increments for disease and repletion of stores. The recommendations are also based on measurements of vitamin status and on losses during preparation, storage and administration of PN admixtures (e.g. photo-degradation of vitamin A, oxidation of vitamin C). Parenteral doses of trace elements have been largely based on those for oral intake, multiplied by a factor for absorption, which varies from < 0.1 to 1.0, depending on the trace element. Further adjustments are made to take into account losses in gastrointestinal effluents and measurements of trace element status.

The step-wise reasoning behind the design of a tailored PN regimen attempts to provide enough nitrogen to optimize tissue nitrogen deposition. It then deals with constraints such as volume restriction or maximum safe doses of macronutrients by compro-mising on the less critical fat: CHO ratio (Table 20.1). If, with time, there is a significant change in body composition the regimen must be recalculated.

Energy

Energy is administered in parenteral admixtures containing macronutrients with different energy densities: fats (9.4 kcal/g), carbohydrates (CHO) (~3.75 kcal/g glucose) and amino acids (~27 kcal/g nitrogen). The carbon skeletons of these macro-nutrients may be variably oxidized, deposited in tissues, or inter-converted.

Carbohydrate

Fructose, xylitol, sorbitol and glycerol all have their potential merits as carbohydrates in PN but glucose (e.g. dextrose monohydrate at 3.4 kcal/g) is both popular and most widely available. Calorimetric studies by King *et al.*[11] have shown that infusing dextrose (as the sole non-protein energy source) at approximately 7 g/kg/day will produce a non-protein respiratory quotient (npRQ) of approximately 1.0 in patients with mild metabolic stress. At this point, fat oxidation gives way completely to oxidation of glucose. With more rapid glucose infusions, up to about 30% of the extra glucose infused will be diverted into synthesis of new fat, a process that dissipates a large amount of the extra energy infused. In severely stressed patients with intestinal failure (e.g. peritonitis, post-radiotherapy enteritis) net fat oxidation (npRQ < 1) is likely to persist despite glucose infusions.[12] Such high rates of glucose infusion should normally be avoided. Non-protein calories are often supplied to such patients using approximate fat:CHO calorie ratio of 40:60. This ratio is not critical and varies from centre to centre. However, glucose-only feeds are to be discouraged because they are often associated with higher volumes and osmolalities. They result in higher rates of CO_2 production (a possible clinical disadvan-tage in pulmonary disease), and they are more likely to produce hyperosmolar complications and essential fatty acid deficiency, than those that contain fat.

Pre-term infants are often started on 6–10 mg dextrose/kg/min, whilst monitoring glucose tolerance, which usually improves with post-natal age.

Lipid

Adult fat infusions are increased cautiously to a dose that does not usually exceed 2 g fat/kg/day or 0.15 g fat/kg/h. During cyclic PN, gross lipaemia at 6 hours after ending the infusion indicates the need to reduce the dose of lipid administered since continuation may lead to impaired reticuloendothelial and immune function and impaired gas diffusion across the lung. During continuous lipid infusions, plasma triglycerides are typically kept below 400 mg/dl. Twenty per cent lipid emulsions may be preferable to 10% lipid emul-sions because of their lower phospholipid:triglyceride ratio, which is associated with less inhibition by phospholipid lysosomes of the clearance of infused triglycerides from plasma.

In newborn infants an initial, continuous, separate, infusion of less than 1 g fat/kg/day is slowly increased to a maximum of 3 g fat/kg/day. Higher infusion rates are more likely to have adverse consequences includ-ing impaired pulmonary gas exchange, and possibly reduced host defence against bacteraemia (a common accompaniment of necrotizing enterocolitis).[13]

The infusion of a minimum of 0.5 g fat/kg/day will prevent essential fatty acid (EFA) deficiency, which can develop rapidly on continuous glucose-amino acid infusions in the absence of lipid. Conversion of infused fatty acids to longer polyunsaturated fatty acids (PUFA), which are necessary for brain development, is slow in infants. Since PUFA are not available for intra-venous use they are given enterally if tolerated.

During the preparation of fat emulsions for intravenous use, soya-bean oil or coconut oil are fractionated yielding long-chain triglycerides (LCT) (14–24 carbon atoms) or medium-chain triglycerides (MCT) (6–12 carbon atoms),[14] emulsified by addition of phosphatidyl-choline and rendered isosmolar to plasma by the addition of glycerol. While there are many advantages of giving lipid, it is not considered appropriate to give it with no glucose, partly because some tissues have a particular preference or need for glucose (leucocytes, repairing tissues, brain), and partly because lean tissue is more rapidly accreted in the presence of glucose. In addition, large doses of parenteral lipids can have detrimental effects (see above).

Medium-chain triglycerides Compared to LCT, MCT are more soluble in phospholipid, and are present in higher concentrations on the surface of fat droplets, which makes them more accessible to tissue lipases. Their greater tissue availability is complemented by their ability to cross the hepatocyte mitochondrial membrane independently of carnitine.[15] Therefore, MCT are cleared more rapidly from plasma, and are oxidized more rapidly than LCT. They are also alleged to cause less depression of immune function[16] and to be more effective in sparing protein in the catabolic patient. Their energy density (8.3 kcal/g) is only slightly lower than that of LCT (9.4 kcal/g). Since MCT do not contain essential n3- and n6- fatty acids (EFAs), commercial preparations are only available as a 50:50 MCT/LCT admixtures. Their use might be considered in the following situations:

Neonates Newborn infants are at risk of developing tissue carnitine deficiency, and infants of low gestational age are at an even greater risk.[17] MCT may be used in such patients because they enter the mitochondrion in a carnitine-independent fashion, where they are oxidized to ketone bodies. Hyperketonaemia, which may have detrimental effects, is prevented by concomitant administration of LCT and/or glucose. MCT have a lower affinity for plasma albumin. This property, together with their faster clearance from plasma, makes them less prone to displace bilirubin from its binding sites on albumin. This minimizes the danger of brain damage by free bilirubin, which crosses the blood–brain barrier.

Patients with PN-associated liver dysfunction Balderman et al.[18] found that PN-associated rises in transaminases, liver size and liver density occurred less frequently with MCT/LCT infusions than with LCT infusions alone.

Patients at risk of infusional hyperlipidaemia The half-life of infused MCT is only about half that of LCT. The faster clearance of MCT droplets may be due to their smaller size and less inhibition of lipoprotein lipase (LPL) by fatty acids released during their hydrolysis, and their metabolism by different biochemical pathways (see above).

Nitrogen

The doses of amino acids, which yield approximately 27 kcal/g N, required to meet patient requirements can be calculated using Table 20.3.[19] Many patients with intestinal failure will be nutritionally depleted through malabsorption or protein-losing enteropathy, and they may require extra N (up to 0.1 g N/kg/day) to replete the protein losses. The nitrogen is more likely to be retained in depleted patients than non-depleted patients in energy balance. Furthermore, approximately 1–2 mg N is retained per kcal of energy administered in excess of energy expenditure in non-stressed patients, and possibly more in depleted patients. In metabolically stressed patients, nitrogen losses may exceed 20 g/day, and positive balances are difficult to achieve, even with increased energy and N intake.[20]

Table 20.3 – Approximate recommended intakes of intravenous amino acids[19]

Metabolic stress	Example	Nitrogen (g/kg/day)
Nil	Healed extensive intestinal resection	0.15
Mild	Mild Crohn's disease in small intestinal remnant	0.20
Moderate	Crohn's fistula with abscess	0.25
Severe	Intestinal failure associated with acute pancreatitis or severe infection	0.25–0.30

One gram of nitrogen is equivalent to approximately 7.33 g of intravenous amino acids or 6.25 g of oral protein. Give extra 0.1 g N per kg of body weight lost. One mole of amino acid (typically ~ 110 g) contains one mole of water (18 g) derived from the hydrolysis of protein.

Specific amino acids

Most commercial parenteral nutrition solutions lack glutamine because of concerns about its instability (spontaneous degradation to ammonia and pyro-glutamic acid). However, free glutamine can be added to PN solutions shortly before use. The alternative is to use a stable dipeptide (e.g. alanyl-L-glutamine). Glutamine is a non-essential amino acid that acts as a carbon and nitrogen carrier, e.g. between skeletal muscle, which produces glutamine, and the small intestine, which utilizes it. Glutamine is an important oxidative fuel for the enterocyte, an essential precursor for nucleotide synthesis,[21] which is necessary during rapid cell division (especially epithelial and immune cells) and a regulator of acid base balance. In rats, glutamine-enriched PN has been reported to reduce intestinal villus damage after 5-fluorouracil (5-FU) administration,[22] minimize intestinal disuse-atrophy[23] and restore mucosal integrity associated with experimental endotoxaemia.[24] In man, although intravenous glutamine supplementation may improve post-operative nitrogen balance,[25] beneficial effects on mucosal growth and absorption are not proven[26,27] or are limited to case studies.[28] However, PN regimens enriched with glutamine have been reported to improve N balance and reduce hospital stay in patients undergoing bone marrow transplantation and major colonic surgery.[29,30]

Other amino acids, which have putative benefits, but which have not always been present in PN solutions include arginine, which may be an important immunonutrient, and taurine, which may act as an oxidant scavenger during persistent inflammation.

Neonates

An infant tolerating 7 mg/kg/min of intravenous dextrose can be started cautiously on a paediatric amino acid solution (PAA) increasing to a maximum of 0.34 g N (approximately 2.5 g AA/kg/day) while monitoring serum ammonia and urea levels. Modern PAA contain an amino acid mixture that aims to establish a circulating amino acid profile that is similar to that of healthy breast-fed term infants (or to that of umbilical cord-blood in pre-term infants).[31] However, this cannot always be achieved because some amino acids are unstable, too acidic, or potentially toxic. Furthermore, several solutions contain a variety of 'non-essential' amino acids that may become conditionally essential during the metabolic demands of refeeding. The following are examples: arginine, because its synthesis may not meet the demands of the urea cycle, and because of possible immune-enhancing properties; cysteine, because of absence of cystathionase in fetal liver; and taurine,[32] because low circulating

concentrations are observed in infants receiving long-term PN. The low taurine concentrations may result from the loss of taurine-conjugated bile salts in patients without a functioning terminal ileum or due to an inadequate supply of its precursor (cysteine) in PN admixtures. Therefore, it is recommended that these amino acids are included in neonatal PN solutions.

Water, sodium and potassium

Typical daily parenteral intakes of water, sodium and potassium in patients without abnormal gastro-intestinal fluid losses are about 2.5–3.0 litres, 90 mmol and 80 mmol respectively. However, changes in the underlying condition of the patient, particularly large variations in the loss of gastrointestinal effluents, will effect the requirements.

Patients with intestinal failure may have variable losses of fluids and electrolytes from stool, stoma or fistulae. A clinical guide to the additional quantities of electrolytes that need to be replaced can be established from the composition of different intestinal effluents (Chapter 2). Patients with an end-jejunostomy have the highest losses of water, sodium and divalent cations. It is important to replace these losses, especially when there are large fluid outputs. For example, each litre of most effluents contains about 100 mmol of sodium (Chapter 24). However, it is also important to remember that acute disease may reduce the capacity of the kidneys to excrete a sodium and water load, predisposing to dilutional hyponatraemia and refeeding oedema. Potassium and magnesium depletion will aggravate renal water handling, while protein-losing enteropathy will produce further sodium retention through hyperaldosteronism.

PN regimens should also take into account potassium losses from gastrointestinal effluents, renal losses due to diuretics or amphotericin,[33] glucose-induced entry of the ion into cells, and deposition into lean tissue such as muscle (approximately 3 mEq of K+ per gram nitrogen deposited).[34] The circulating potassium concentration can act as crude but practical guide to the dose administered.

Micronutrients

Trace elements and vitamins (Tables 20.4 and 20.5)

For many trace elements RIV is often much lower than the recommended nutrient intake for enteral

Table 20.4a – Recommended mineral and trace element intakes in enteral and parenteral regimens★

	ENTERAL Adult (a) dose/day	PARENTERAL Adult (b) dose/day	Comments
Sodium (Na) mmol	70	50–100	Healthy gut absorbs > 95%, IF patients may require more than 200 mmol/day. Intestinal losses increase during high enteral intake and decrease during ORS administration
Chloride (Cl) mmol	70	50–100	Healthy gut absorbs > 90%, IF patients may need more than 200 mmol/day
Potassium (K) mmol	90	50–100	Suspend K administration if oliguria develops
Calcium (Ca) mmol	17.5	6–10	Healthy gut absorbs up to 40%, IF patients may need up to 120 mmol/day[62] patients with a functioning colon have lower Ca requirements[68]
Phosphorus (P) mmol	17.5	20–40	Healthy gut absorbs 50 to 60%, IF patients need up to 40 mmol/day
Magnesium (Mg) mmol	12.3	6–12	Healthy gut absorbs up to 75%, for clinical hypomagnesaemia give 17 mmol Mg iv over 30 minutes before starting TPN: steatorrhoea, nephrotoxic drugs, alcohol increase requirements[69]
Zinc (Zn) µmol	142	38–62	Oral phytate, Ca, Zn reduce absorption, IF patients require 1200 µg (18 µmol) per litre of intestinal effluent, renal losses of Zn increased during amino acid infusions
Copper (Cu) µmol	19	4.7–7.8	Oral phytates, Vitamin C, Cd, Zn reduce absorption, diarrhoeal losses not proportional to effluent volume, increase Cu intake in diarrhoea, reduce intake in liver dysfunction
Chromium (Cr)★ ★µmol	0.48	0.19–0.29	Glucose loading increases urinary clearance
Selenium (Se) µmol	0.95	0.51–1.01	High losses in pus + fistula fluids
Manganese (Mn)★ ★µmol	25	1.1–1.8	Absorption: adults < 4%, neonates up to 50%, > 90% excreted in bile
Molybdenum (Mo)★ ★µmol	0.52–4.17		Excreted mostly in urine, significant increased losses in short bowel syndrome; 300 µg (3 µmol)/day iv recommended in SBS patients[70]
Iodine (I) µmol	1		PN addition of 1 µg (0.008 µmol)/kg/day recommended only in depleted patients

★ Amounts not adjusted for absorption or excess loss of nutrient. a: amounts based on oral Reference Nutrient intakes (★★ or safe intake)[60] b: refers to patients without excess gi loss[61,62,63]

Table 20.4b – Recommended mineral and trace element intakes in enteral and parenteral regimens★

	ENTERAL Preterm (b, c) dose/kg/day	ENTERAL Term (a) dose/day	PARENTERAL Preterm (d, e) dose/kg/day	PARENTERAL Term (e, f) dose/kg/day	Comments
Sodium (Na) mmol	1.3–3	9	3–5	2–4	Beware of hyponatraemia due to high insensible water loss, hypotonic diarrhoea, immature renal tubular Na reabsorption
Chloride (Cl) mmol	1.4–3.2	9	3–5	2–3	Doses of Cl above 6 mmol/kg/day may cause hyperchloraemic acidosis
Potassium (K) mmol	2–5	20	1–2	2–3	Beware of non-oliguric hyperkalaemia due to immature distal tubular secretion of K
Calcium (Ca) mmol	1.9–5.7	13.1	1.5–2.2	0.2–1.2	During low fluid intakes Ca and PO4 in PN should be in a 1:1 molar ratio and should not exceed 15 mmol/l[66]
Phosphorus (P) mmol	1.8–4.8	12.9	1.5–2.2	1–2	
Magnesium (Mg) mmol	0.3–0.8	2.3	0.3–0.4	0.12–0.5	Danger of hypermagnesaemia in renal insufficiency
Zinc (Zn) µmol	9.3–27.9	61	6.1	3.8	PN intakes refer to stable infant[71]; 2 to 3 times more Zn may be required during diarrhoea
Copper (Cu) µmol	1.6–3.1	3.1	0.32	0.32	PN intakes refer to stable infant[71]; do not administer iv Cu in cholestasis
Chromium (Cr)★ ★µmol			0.004	0.004	Do not supplement preterm enteral formulas routinely
Selenium (Se) µmol		0.13	0.025	0.025	Do not supplement preterm enteral formulas routinely
Manganese (Mn)★ ★µmol	0.04–0.24	0.3	0.018	0.018	1 µg (0.018 µmol)/kg/day induces positive Mn balance in infants without diarrhoea[71]; withhold iv Mn in cholestasis; monitor Mn status by serum levels[62] and MRI[72]
Molybdenum (Mo)★ ★µmol		0.015–0.05	0.003	0.003	Do not add Mo routinely to enteral formulas or short term PN regimens[71]
Iodine (I) µmol	0.09–0.58	0.39	0.008	0.008	Infants absorb extra iodine from topical disinfectants

★ Amounts not adjusted for absorption or excess loss of nutrient. a: amounts based on oral Reference Nutrient intakes (★★ or safe intake)[60], b: data from ESPGAN, 1987[64], c: data from Lucas, 1991[59], d: data from Yu, 1992[65], e: data from Greene *et al*, 1988[66], f: data from Poole 1983[67].

Table 20.5a – Recommended vitamin intakes in enteral and parenteral regimens★

	ENTERAL Adult (a) dose/day	PARENTERAL Adult (b) dose/day	Comments
Vitamin A µg (retinol equivalents)	700	3,300 IU/day	Increased losses in steatorrhoea, high losses in nephrotic syndrome, low storage in liver disease; enteral requirement in IF patients typically 3000–15,000 µg/day[1,2]
Vitamin D (cholecalciferol) µg	0–10	5	Increased losses in steatorrhoea, routine PN supplementation may induce hypercalcaemia and osteomalacia[2]; adult recommendations assume adequate sunlight exposure; IF patients need typically 4000 µg/day by enteral route
Vitamin E (alpha-tocopherol)★ µg	> 4000	10,000–50,000	Requirements depend on iv or enteral intake of PUFA, selenium supplementation decreases requirements; enteral requirements of IF patients typically 34,000 µg/day[2]
Vitamin K★★ µg	1 µg/kg/day	10 mg menadione/week	Increased losses in steatorrhoea, increased requirements in neonatal period and during broad spectrum antibiotic treatment
Vitamin B₁ (thiamine) µg	900 (males) 800 (females)	1,200–5,000	Increased requirements during high carbohydrate intake
Vitamin B₂ (riboflavine) µg	1,300 (males) 1,100 (females)	3,600	Contribution by colonic bacteria unquantified, accelerated flavoprotein breakdown in catabolic patients interferes with assessment of requirements
Niacin µg	6,600 µg (NE) per 1000 kcal	40,000	Low intakes of tryptophan, pyridoxine or riboflavine may increase requirements
Vitamin B₆ (pyridoxine) µg	1,400 (males) 1,200 (females) or 15 µg/g protein	4000	Malabsorbed in diseased/bypassed small intestine, requirements related to total amino acid metabolism (co-factor in transaminases, decarboxylases, etc)
Vitamin B₁₂ (cobalamin) µg	1.5	3	Malabsorbed in ileal resection or bypass, utilised by small intestinal bacteria which reduce its bioavailability
Folic acid µg	200	400	Sulfasalazine reduces absorption, alcoholism increases requirements
Vitamin C (ascorbic acid) µg	40,000	100,000	Enteral administration further increases risk of oxalate stones in SBS patients. Critically-ill patients probably need 500,000 µg/day iv
Panthotenic acid★ ★µg	3,000–7,000	15,000	
Biotin★ ★µg	10–200	60	Bioavailability of biotin synthesised by colonic bacteria unknown

★ Amounts not adjusted for absorption or excess loss of nutrient. a: amounts based on oral Reference Nutrient intakes (★★ or safe intake)[61] b: refers to patients without excess gi loss[61,62,63]

Table 20.5b – Recommended vitamin intakes in enteral and parenteral regimens★

	ENTERAL dose/day Preterm (b, c) dose/kg/day	ENTERAL Term (a) dose/day	PARENTERAL dose/day Preterm (d) dose/kg/day	PARENTERAL Term (d) dose/kg/day	Comments
Vitamin A µg (retinol equivalents)	99–248	350	500	700	Preterm infant invariably depleted at birth. PN-related toxicity reported in infants at doses above 1300 µg/day
Vitamin D (cholecalciferol) µg	up to 5.0	8.5	4	10	Concentration in preterm formulas should not exceed 3 µg/100 kcal
Vitamin E (alpha-tocopherol)★ µg	at least 660	400 µg/g PUFA	2,800	7,000	Preterm formulas should contain at least 0.9 mg/g PUFA. Large iv doses induced liver failure in preterm infants
Vitamin K★ ★µg	nil	10	80	200	Phytoquinolone recommended. Synthetic water-soluble preparation causes dose dependent toxicity. Preterm infants need 0.5–1.0 mg im at birth, then 2–3 µg/kg weekly till breast-fed
Vitamin B₁ (thiamine) µg	22–413	200	350	1,200	Supplementation of preterm breast milk (20 µg/100 kcal) only if milk is heat-treated
Vitamin B₂ (riboflavine) µg	66–990	400	150	1,400	Renal clearance of excess iv dose reduced in preterm infant
Niacin µg	90–800	3,000	6,800	17,000	Preterm formulas should contain at least 800 µg/100 kcal
Vitamin B₆ (pyridoxine) µg	39–413	200	180	1.0	Preterm formulas should contain at least 15 µg/g protein and/or 300 µg/100 kcal
Vitamin B₁₂ (cobalamin) µg	at least 0.17	0.3	0.3	1,000	Marked elevation of serum B₁₂ reported in preterm infants receiving 600 µg/kg/day iv
Folic acid µg	at least 66	50	56	140	Red cell folate levels adequate in preterm infants receiving 75 µg/kg/day iv
Vitamin C (ascorbic acid) µg	8,300–66,000	25,000	25,000	80,000	Preterm infants need lower doses than term infants to maintain normal plasma ascorbic acid levels (> 34 µmol/L)
Panthotenic acid★ ★µg	at least 330	1,700	2,000	5,000	Preterm formulas should contain at least 300 µg/100 kcal
Biotin★ ★µg		10–200	6.0	20	Preterm formulas should contain 1.5 µg/100 kcal

★ Amounts not adjusted for absorption or excess loss of nutrient. a: amounts based on oral Reference Nutrient intakes (★★ or safe intake)[61], b: data from ESPGAN, 1987[64], c: data from Lucas, 1991[59], d: data from Greene et al, 1988[66].

333

feeds. This is because only proportions of trace elements are absorbed. Prolonged excess administration of trace elements can lead to toxicity because the regulatory role of the gut is bypassed (e.g. the gut is the only major site regulating iron status within the body). Toxicity may also occur because of reduced excretion of trace elements in urine (e.g. when there is renal impairment) or in bile (e.g. of manganese when there is liver impairment).

In contrast to recommended parenteral trace element requirements, which are less than those of normal healthy people, the RIV for vitamins are often higher than those for health. This is partly because the requirements of many vitamins may increase with many diseases, especially acute inflammatory diseases, and partly because tissue stores may require repletion. In addition, excess vitamins may be necessary to counteract any losses that occur during preparation, storage and administration of PN solutions.

Chronic intestinal losses of divalent cations are worsened by the presence of fat in the diet,[35] and are not reversed by octreotide[36] or omeprazole.[37] Because 24-hour urinary magnesium drops before serum magnesium, additions to PN regimens can be based on both these parameters. Urinary calcium losses often parallel those of magnesium. Renal calcium reabsorption is lower during PN induced diuresis[38] and may also be influenced by poor vitamin D status resulting from malabsorption, which is associated with low intestinal levels of calcium-binding proteins.[39] It has long been known that the plasma phosphate concentration can drop precipitously during refeeding, especially with glucose (no fat) regimens, due to intracellular shifts, which partly result in the formation of intracellular high energy phosphate bonds. Fat emulsions supply some phosphorus as phosphatidylcholine and therefore reduce the risk of hypophosphataemia.

ENTERAL REGIMENS

The calculations for energy requirements are the same as for parenteral nutrition. The nitrogen supplied is quoted in grams of protein. Examples of typical commercial enteral feeds are shown in Table 20.6. Occasionally more sodium chloride (to bring the total sodium concentration to 100 mmol/L) is added to the feeds in patients with high output stomas or fistulae while trying to keep the osmolality near to 280–300 mOsm/kg.

Although early minimal enteral feeding (MEF) (e.g. 200 ml/day in adults) does not contribute significantly to nutrient requirements, it may help to reduce PN-associated intestinal atrophy and minimize trans-intestinal bacterial translocation. The addition of

Table 20.6 – Composition of typical enteral feeds

	Polymeric (ca 1 kcal/ml)* e.g. Enterae 400® (per 100 g)	Monomeric (ca 1 kcal/ml)† e.g. Peptide 2⁺® (per 100 g)	Elemental (ca 0.75 kcal/ml) e.g. Elemental 028® (per 100 g)
Energy (Kcal)	440	440	364
Fat: CHO: Protein energies (kcal)	38:49:13	38:49:13	17:71:12
CHO (g)	60 (maltodextrin)	59 (maltodextrin)	70
Lactose	0.17	0	0
Protein	13.8 (whey protein)	13.8 (peptides, 86% of MW<1000)	10.0 (as amino acids)
Gluten	Nil	Nil	Nil
Glutamine (g)	Nil	Nil	0.09
Fat (g)	18 (arachis oil)	18 (sunflower + MCT oils)	6.64 (arachis oil)
LCT:MCT	100:1	17:83	100:1
Fibre	Nil	Nil	Nil
Osmolality (mOsm/kg)	269	389	684

* IF patients with normal transit time and good pancreatic function may absorb LCT.
† Moderate osmolality, peptide content, and MCT supplementation are desirable properties in IF patients, fibre supplementation should be considered.

low-dose enteral feeding to intravenously fed rats has been reported to increase nitrogen retention and reduced bacterial translocation[40] and reduce PN-associated increases in macromolecular lactose permeability.[41] MEF increases neonatal gut motility and promotes the release of gut trophic hormones, such as gastrin and enteroglucagon. Enteral feeding has been reported to reverse PN-induced enterocyte atrophy in human volunteers[42] and to preserve intestinal mucosal integrity in PN-fed critically ill patients.[43] These effects have been ascribed to a variety of nutrients/physico-chemical properties of the feed, including its tonicity[44] and the presence of peptides,[45] which have higher intestinal transport rates and higher capacity for transport than that for free amino acids.[46] Enteral glutamine has been reported to improve splanchnic blood flow in rats[47] and to reduce small intestinal damage in dogs receiving therapeutic doses of radiation.[48] However, no benefits have been observed in adult human patients suffering from 5-FU-induced mucositis.[49]

Carbohydrate that is not absorbed in the small intestine (including fibre present in some enteral feeds) is fermented to short-chain fatty acids, which are subsequently absorbed for further metabolism in human tissues. Such a process can provide a substantial amount of energy (up to 4 MJ/day in a group of patient with IF)[50] and result in improved intestinal adaptation, as in rats with a short bowel.[51] LCT has also been reported to improve mucosal height and leucine balance in rat with a short bowel.[52] The theoretical advantages of arginine[53] or nucleotide[54] supplementation merit further clinical evaluation. Exposing the ileal remnant to fat[55] or starch[56] retards gastric emptying (the 'ileal brake')[57] through release of peptide YY.[58] Typical enteral regimens and their limitations are shown in Table 20.6.

Neonates requiring PN (e.g. sick pre-term infants, infants recovering from necrotizing enterocolitis) may be gradually started on mother's milk or a pre-term formula, fortified with phosphate and other additives as necessary, aiming to deliver daily 110–165 kcal/kg of energy and 0.46–0.64 g N/kg in protein for pre-term infants, and 115 kcal/kg and ~ 0.29 g N/kg for term infants.[59] When enteral feeds are not tolerated MEF (e.g. 1 ml of infant formula per hour) should be encouraged.

CONCLUSION

The fluid and electrolyte requirements in intestinal failure cannot only vary substantially between individuals, but also within individuals. For example, gastro-intestinal fluid losses may decrease with time, whilst an intestinal fistula heals or abdominal sepsis is eradicated. In contrast, the fluid losses usually increase when patients with a short bowel increase their food intake. The changes in food intake can obviously affect the intravenous requirements of nutrients. The increase in food intake that occurs in patients with resolving ileus suggests that it is time to contemplate weaning off parenteral nutrition. On the other hand, oral intake may slowly decrease with time while intravenous requirements increase, as in patients with progressive motility disorders or fibrosing conditions of the abdomen. In all these situations it is necessary to monitor the changes and adjust the intravenous intake appropriately.

REFERENCES

1. Robertson JD, Reid DD. Standards for the basal metabolism of normal people in Britain. *Lancet* 1952; **262**: 940–943.

2. Fleish PA. Le metabolism basal standard et sa determination au moyen du 'Metabocalculator'. *Helvetica Medica Acta* 1952; **1**: 23–43.

3. Harris JA, Benedict FG. A biometric study of basal metabolism in man. Carnegie Institute Publication No. 279. Carnegie Institute, Washington, 1919.

4. Pullicino E. Aspects of energy metabolism in hospitalised patients. CNAA, British Lending Library, Identification Number DX 96679, p. 59.

5. Bessey PQ, Wilmore DG. In: Kinney JM, Jeejeebhoy KN, Hill G, Owen O (eds) *Nutrition and Metabolism in Patient Care*. WB Saunders: Philadelphia, 1988, p. 676.

6. Elia M. Artificial nutritional support. In: Badenoch J. (ed) *Medicine International*, Oxon, UK, Medicine Group (UK) Ltd, 1990; **82**: 3392–3396, .

7. Kinney JM, Roe CF. Caloric equivalent of fever. *Ann Surg* 1962; **156**: 611–622.

8. Pullicino E, Coward A, Elia M. Total energy expenditure measured by the doubly labelled water technique. *Metabolism* 1993; **42**: 58–64.

9. Roberts SB, Young VR. Energy costs of fat and protein deposition in the human infant. *Am J Clin Nutr* 1988; **48**: 951–955.

10. Pullicino E, Goldberg G, Elia M. Energy expenditure and substrate metabolism measured by 24-hour whole-body calorimetry in patients receiving cyclic and continuous total parenteral nutrition. *Clin Sci* 1991; **80**: 571–582.

11. King RFGJ, McMahon MJ. Almond DJ. Evidence for adaptive diet-induced thermogenesis in man during intravenous nutrition with hypertonic glucose. *Clin Sci* 1986; **71**: 31–39.

12. Ashkanazi J, Carpentier YA, Elwyn DH, *et al.* Influence of total parenteral nutrition on fuel utilization in injury and sepsis. *Ann Surg* 1980; **191**: 40–46.

13. Lipsky CL, Spear ML. Parenteral nutrition in necrotizing enterocolitis. *Clin Perinatol* 1995; **22**: 389–409.

14. Jiang ZJ, Zhang S, Wang X, Yang N, Zhu Y, Wilmore D. A comparison of medium-chain and long-chain triglycerides in surgical patients. *Ann Surg* 1993; **217**: 175–184.

15. Bach AC, Frey A, Lutz O. Clinical and experimental effects of medium-chain triglyceride-based fat emulsion: a review. *Clin Nutr* 1989; **8**: 223–235.

16. Sedman PC, Sonners SS, Ramsden CW, Brennan TG, Guillou PJ. Effects of different lipid emulsions on lymphocyte function during total parenteral nutrition. *Br J Surg* 1991; **78**: 1396–1399.

17. Penn D, Ludwig B, Schmidt-Sommerfield E, Pascu F. Effect of nutrition and tissue carnitine concentration in infants of different gestational ages. *Biol Neonate* 1985; **47**: 130–135.

18. Baldermann H, Wicklmayer M, Rett K, Banholzer P, Dietze G, Mehner H. Untersuchungen zur Veranderung des Sonographiebefundes der Leber unter parenteraler Ehrnahrung mit LCT bzw. MCT/LCT Lipidlozungen. *Infusions Therapie* 1988; **15**: 140–147.

19. Elia M. The effects of nitrogen and energy intake on metabolism of normal, depleted and injured man.: considerations for practical nutritional support. *Clin Nutr* 1992; **1**: 173–192.

20. Saffle JR, Medina E, Raymond J, Westenskow D, Kravitz M, Warden G. Use of indirect calorimetry in the nutritional management of the burned patient. *J Trauma* 1985; **25**: 32–39.

21. Newsholme EA, Carrie AL. Quantitative aspects of glucose and glutamine metabolism by intestinal cells. *Gut* 1994; **35** (suppl 1): S13–S17.

22. Bai MX, Jiang ZM, Liu YW, Wang WT, Li DM, Wilmore DW. Effects of alanyl-glutamine on gut barrier function. *Nutrition* 1996; **12**: 793–796.

23. Hwang TL, O'Dwyer ST, Smith RJ, Wilmore DW. Preservation of the small bowel mucosa using glutamine-supplemented parenteral nutrition. *Surg Forum* 1986; **37**: 56–58.

24. Bai M, Jiang Z, Ma Y. Glutamine-enriched nutritional solutions attenuate bacterial translocation in rats after 60% intestinal resections. *Chung Hua I Hsueh Tsa Chih* 1996; **76**: 116–119.

25. Stehle P, Zander J, Mertes J, Albers S, Puchstein C, Lawin P, Furst P. Effect of parenteral glutamine peptide supplements on muscle glutamine after major surgery. *Lancet* 1989; **1**: 231–233.

26. Tremel H, Kienle B, Weilemann S, Stehle P, Furst P. Glutamine dipeptide-supplemented parenteral nutrition maintains intestinal function in the critically ill. *Gastroenterology* 1994; **107**: 1595–1601.

27. Hornsby-Lewis L, Shike M, Brown P, Pearlstone D, Brennan MF. L-glutamine supplementation in home total parenteral nutrition patients: stability, safety and effects on intestinal absorption. *J Parenter Enteral Nutr* 1994; **18**: 268–273.

28. Allen SJ, Pierro A, Cope L, Macleod A, Howard CV. Glutamine supplemented parenteral nutrition in a child with short-bowel syndrome. *J Paediatr Gastroenterol Nutr* 1993; **17**: 329–332.

29. Morlion B, Stehle P, Wachtler P, Sichoff HP, Koller M, Furst P, Puchstein C. Total parenteral nutrition with glutamine dipeptide after major abdominal surgery: a randomized, double-blind, controlled study. *Ann Surg* 1998; **227**: 302–308.

30. Ziegler TR, Young LS, Benfell K, *et al.* Clinical and metabolic efficacy of glutamine-supplemented parenteral nutrition after bone marrow transplantation. A randomized, double blind, controlled study. *Ann Int Med* 1992; **116**: 821–828.

31. Rassin DK. Protein requirements in neonates. In: Lebenthal E (ed) *Textbook of Gastroenterology and Nutrition in Infancy*. Raven Press: New York, 1989, p. 288.

32. Geggel HS, Ament ME, Heckenlively JR, Diedre A, Martin BS. Nutritional requirements for taurine in patients receiving long-term parenteral nutrition. *N Engl J Med* 1985; **312**: 142–146.

33. Bernardo JF, Murakami S, Branch RA, Sabra R. Potassium depletion potentiates amphotericin B-induced toxicity to renal tubules. *Nephron* 1995; **70**: 235–241.

34. Moore F. Energy and the maintenance of the body cell mass. *J Parenter Enteral Nutr* 1980; **4**: 228–260.

35. Ovesen L, Chu R, Howard L. The influence of dietary fat on jejunostomy output in patients with severe short bowel syndrome. *Am J Clin Nutr* 1983; **38**: 270–277.

36. Ladefoged K, Christensen KC, Hegnhopj J, Jarnum S. Effect of a long-acting somatostain analogue SMS 201–995 on jejunostomy effluents in patients with severe short bowel syndrome. *Gut* 1989; **30**: 943–949.

37. Nightingale JM, Lennard-Jones JE. The short bowel syndrome: what's new and old? *Dig Dis* 1993; **11**: 12–31.

38. Lipkin EW, Benedetti TJ, Chait A. Successful pregnancy outcome using total parenteral nutrition from the first trimester of pregnancy. *J Parenter Enteral Nutr* 1986; **10**: 665–669.

39. Staun M, Jarnum S. Measurement of 10 000–molecular weight calcium-binding protein in small-intestinal biopsy specimens from patients with malabsorption syndromes. *Scan J Gastroenterol* 1988; **23**: 827–832.

40. Sax HC, Illig KA, Ryan CK, Hardy DJ. Low dose enteral feeding is beneficial during parenteral nutrition. *Am J Surg* 1996; **171**: 587–590.

41. Illig KA, Ryan CK, Hardy DJ, Rhodes J, Locke W, Sax HC. Total parenteral nutrition induced changes in gut mucosal function: atrophy alone is not the issue. *Surgery* 1992; **112**: 631–637.

42. Buchman AL, Moukarzel AA, Bhuta S, *et al.* Parenteral nutrition is associated with intestinal morphologic and functional changes in humans. *J Parenter Enteral Nutr* 1995; **19**: 453–460.

43. Hadfield RJ, Sinclair DG, Houldsworth PE, Evans TW. Effects of enteral and parenteral nutrition on gut permeability in the critically ill. *Am J Respir Crit Care Med* 1995; **152**: 1545–1548.

44. Weser E, Babbitt J, Vandeventer A. Relationship between enteral glucose load and adaptive mucosal growth in the small bowel. *Dig Dis Sci* 1985; **30**: 675–681.

45. Cosnes J, Evard D, Beaugerie L, Gendre JP, Le Quintrec Y. Improvement in protein absorption with a small-peptide-based diet in patients with high jejunostomy. *Nutrition* 1992; **8**: 406–411.

46. Steinhard HJ. Comparison of enteral resorption rates of free amino acids and oligopeptides. *Leber Magen Darm* 1984; **14**: 51–56.

47. Houdijk AP, Van Leeuwen PA, Boermeester MA, *et al.* Glutamine-enriched enteral diet increases splanchnic blood flow in the rat. *Am J Physiol* 1994; **267**: G1035–1040.

48. Kemberg S, Souba W, Dolson D, Salloum R, Hautamaki R. Prophylactic glutamine protects the intestinal mucosa from radiation to injury. *Cancer* 1990; **66**: 62–68.

49. Jebb SA, Osborne RJ, Maugham TS, Mohideen N, Mack P, Shelley MD, Elia M. 5-Fluorouracil and folinic acid-induced mucositis: no effect of oral glutamine supplementation. *Br J Cancer* 1994; **70**: 732–735.

50. Nordgard I, Hansen BS, Mortensen PB. Importance of colonic support for energy absorbtion as intestinal-failure proceeds. *Am J Clin Nutr* 1996; **64**: 221–231.

51. Aghdassi E, Plapler H, Kurian R, *et al.* Colonic fermentation and nutritional recovery in rats with massive small bowel resection. *Gastroenterology* 1994; **107**: 637–642.

52. Vanderhoof JA, Grandjean CJ, Kaufman SS, Burkley KT, Antonson DL. Effect of high percentage medium chain triglyceride diet on mucosal adaptation following massive bowel resection in rats. *J Parenter Enteral Nutr* 1984; **8**: 685–689.

53. Cynober L. Can arginine and ornithine support gut functions? *Gut* 1994; **35**: S42–44.

54. Grimble GK. Dietary nucleotides and gut mucosal defence. *Gut* 1994; **35**: S46–51.

55. Pironi L, Stanghellini V, Miglioli M, *et al.* Fat-induced ileal break in humans: a dose-dependent phenomenon correlated to the plasma levels of peptide YY. *Gastroenterology* 1993; **105**: 733–739.

56. Layer P, Zinsmeister AR, Dimango EP. Effects of decreasing intraluminal amylase activity on starch digestion and post-prandial gastrointestinal function in humans. *Gastroenterology* 1986; **91**: 41–48.

57. Spiller RC, Trotman IF, Higgins BE. The ileal brake-inhibition of jejunal motility after ileal fat perfusion in man. *Gut* 1984; **25**: 365–374.

58. Savage AP, Adrian TE, Carolan G, Chatterjee VK. Bloom SR. Effects of peptide YY (PYY) on mouth to caecum intestinal transit time and on the rate of gastric emptying in healthy volunteers. *Gut* 1987; **28**: 166–170.

59. Lucas A. Feeding the pre-term infant. In: Ballabriga A, Brunser O, Dobbing J, Gracey M, Senterre J (eds) *Clinical Nutrition of the Young Child.* Raven Press: New York, 1991, **16**: 317–336.

60. Department of Health. Dietary reference values for food energy and nutrients for the United Kingdom, Report on Health and Social Subjects No. 41. HMSO: London, 1991.

61. Elia M. Special nutritional problems and the use of enteral and parenteral nutrition. In: Weatherall DJ, Ledingham JGG, Warrel DA (eds) *Oxford Textbook of Medicine.* Oxford University Press: New York, 1996, pp. 1314–1326.

62. Jeejeebhoy K. Nutrient requirements and deficiencies in GI diseases. In: Sleisenger S, Fordtran J (eds) *Gastrointestinal Disease: Pathophysiology/Diagnosis/Management,* 5th edn, Vol 2. WB Saunders: Philadelphia, 1993, pp. 2017–2047.

63. Shills M. Parenteral nutrition. In: Shils M, Olson J, Shike M (eds) *Modern Nutrition in Health and Disease,* 8th edn. Lea and Feibiger: Philadelphia, 1994, pp. 1430–1458.

64. Committee on Nutrition and Feeding of the Preterm Infant, European Society of Gastroenterology and Nutrition. Nutrition and feeding of the preterm infant. *Acta Paediatr Scand* 1987; Suppl 336: 3–14.

65. Yu V, Macmahon RA. Intravenous feeding in the preterm neonate. In: Yu V (ed) *Intravenous Feeding of the Neonate.* Edward Arnold: London, pp. 240–249.

66. Greene HL, Hambridge MK, Shanler R. Guidelines for the use of vitamins, trace elements, calcium, magnesium, and phosphorus in infants and children receiving total parenteral nutrition: report on the Subcommittee on Paediatric Parenteral Nutrient Requirements from Committee on Clinical Practice Issues of the American Society for Clinical Nutrition. *Am J Clin Nutr* 1988; **48**: 1324–1342.

67. Poole RL. Electrolyte and mineral requirements. In: Kerner JE (ed) *Manual of Paediatric Parenteral Nutrition*. John Wiley: New York, 1983, pp. 129–136.

68. Grinstead WC, Pak CY, Krejs GJ. Effect of 1,25-dihydroxyvitamin D3 on calcium absorption in the colon of healthy humans. *Am J Physiol* 1984: **247**: G189–192.

69. Freeman JB. Magnesium requirements are increased during parenteral nutrition. *Surg Forum* 1977; **28**: 61–62.

70. Abumrad NN. Molybdenum: is it an essential trace metal? *Bull NY Acad Med* 1984; **60**: 163–171.

71. Zlotkin S, Atkinson S, Lockitch G. Trace elements in nutrition for premature infants. *Clin Perinatol* 1995; **22**: 223–240.

72. Ono J, Harada K, Kodaka R, *et al*. Manganese deposition in the brain during long term total parenteral nutrition. *J Parenter Enteral Nutr* 1995; **19**(4): 311–312.

21

Formulation and administration of enteral feeds

Gil Hardy and Jackie Edington

*I*n considering the nutritional support of hospital patients the general, almost obligatory, rule that has been promulgated in recent years is 'if the gut works, use it'. This has led to the broad acceptance that nutrition given via the intestine (enteral nutrition (EN)) is better than parenteral nutrition (PN). Enteral nutrition is claimed to: be physiological, improve gastrointestinal function, prevent bacterial translocation and improve patient outcome while being safer and less expensive than parenteral nutrition. However, at present most of these assumptions are not evidence-based. There is no documented evidence for reduced bacterial translocation or improved intestinal function in humans, although there are animal data[1] which show that intestinal mass, mucosal weight, villus height and disaccharidase activity all decrease in animals fed with PN compared with EN. Although there is no direct evidence that patient outcome or safety are better, there are studies which show fewer complications with EN compared with PN. These include patients with pancreatitis,[2] following a total gastrectomy[3] and after hepatic resection.[4] There are fewer septic complications[2] and natural killer cell activity is higher in patients fed with EN compared with PN.[4] The frequently quoted paper in favour of EN, by Moore et al,[5] is a meta-analysis of eight studies (six are unpublished). Their analysis shows no difference between EN and PN in non-infectious complications, mortality rates or length of hospital stay. However, more septic complications were noted with PN in patients who had had abdominal trauma. A comprehensive review of published prospective randomized controlled trials (with over 70 references) by Lipman[6] concluded that with the exception of reduced septic morbidity in abdominal trauma (which was offset by an increased incidence of EN-related complications) the only significant difference between EN and PN was the lower cost of EN.

A balanced approach to the route of nutrition support is appropriate. It is important to consider the nutritional support requirements of each individual patient, then choose the most appropriate route of delivery for that patient. Guidelines, as proposed by Bell et al.,[7] for successfully feeding critically ill patients suggest giving both PN and EN simultaneously until nutritional goals can be met solely by EN (Table 21.1). Other authors claim that, if enteral feeding is started slowly and aspirates checked regularly, then it alone may be appropriate and feasible in critically ill patients.[8]

Table 21.1 – Guidelines for feeding critically ill patients[7]

1. Initiate PN and EN simultaneously
2. Establish nutrient intake goals that can be achieved by combining both therapies
3. Begin PN with 1.0–1.5 litres of a complete regimen until fluid status stabilizes
4. Begin EN with a full strength solution at around 10 ml/h
5. Advance EN to goal rate as patient tolerates more
6. Decrease PN as tube feeding rate increases whilst maintaining nutritional goals

HISTORY, INGREDIENTS AND MANUFACTURING

Various mixtures of milk, egg, beef or chicken broth, wine, brandy and pancreatic tissue have been administered to patients rectally since Ancient Egyptian times.[9] John Hunter in 1790 successfully used a 'tube' passed through the mouth into the stomach to feed a patient who was unable to swallow due to 'paralysis of the muscles of deglutition'. The 'tube', which was designed by a watchmaker, consisted of eel skin wrapped round a flexible whalebone and was attached to a pig's bladder which acted as a reservoir. Hunter recommended that jellies, eggs beaten with a little water, sugar and wine or milk should be given as food.[10]

Today whole protein feeds are made from milk components (e.g. calcium caseinates) or soya protein isolates as the predominant protein sources, various oils (e.g. soya, corn or safflower) as fat sources, and ingredients derived from corn starch (e.g. maltodextrin), sucrose, and glucose as sources of carbohydrate. Some have insoluble and/or soluble fibre added. The protein sources in semi-elemental feeds (peptide or elemental diets) are based upon the products of hydrolysis of milk components (caseinates, whey protein and lactalbumin) or soy protein, with some specific amino acids and medium-chain triglycerides added. Most feeds intended for use as sole source of nutrition, are fortified with essential vitamins, minerals and trace elements. Some also contain other nutrients such as choline, taurine, arginine and glutamine. Feeds can usually be stored at room temperature unopened for up to 1 year.

STABILITY

The stability of macro- and micro-nutrients depend upon the exposure of the feed to heat, pH, light and air (Table 21.2). Heat processing to produce a sterile liquid feed can destroy some vitamins (e.g. all B vitamins especially thiamine and vitamin B_6, folic acid and pantothenic acid) and heat-sensitive amino acids (e.g. glutamine and cysteine). Hence glutamine and cysteine are absent from most commercial feeds. The amount of vitamin and amino acid lost will depend on the time for which heat is used to destroy harmful organisms. Thiamine is more stable to heat at low pH, but when the pH is high, losses are considerable. Riboflavin is unstable at high pH and is light-sensitive. Vitamin A losses can occur if light and air are not rigorously excluded. Vitamin C is the least stable of all the vitamins, it is readily oxidized in air, a process which is catalysed by heat, high pH and the presence of copper and/or iron. Whilst vitamin C is partially protected by the addition of bisulphite, thiamine destruction is accelerated. Vitamin E is relatively stable to heat but oxidized in the presence of air. However, manufacturers generally fortify feeds to levels designed to compensate for losses, which occur during processing. In addition, most manufacturers have rigorous quality assurance programmes designed to test levels of all nutrients during the 'quarantine' period after products are manufactured, but before they are released for sale, to ensure that nutrient levels, which are listed on the labels, are accurate. Most companies also conduct routine stability trials to determine the average levels of nutrients over the shelf-life of the product. These average label claims are those which are declared on the label.

Table 21.2 – Vitamin and amino acid stability in enteral feeds

Heat
Vitamins
B vitamins (especially thiamine and B_6), folic acid and pantothenic acid
Amino acids
Cysteine and glutamine
Light
Vitamin A and riboflavin
pH
Riboflavin and thiamine at high (alkaline) pH
Air
Vitamins A, C and E all oxidize

Most liquid, ready-to-use feeds are filled aseptically into cartons, plastic containers or glass bottles. These are then subjected to ultra high temperatures (UHT) to kill any bacteria present. A temperature of about 143 to 152°C is maintained for 5–10 seconds. The resultant sterile feed will keep for several months but variable losses of vitamin C and folic acid may occur during storage. It is difficult to give precise values for expected losses, and they will be accentuated when the containers are opened and exposed to air. However, if they are kept in the closed carton in which they are transported, the contents will be protected from light and oxygen.

The process of freeze drying has been used for over 50 years, and was refined during World War II in order to supply huge quantities of dried plasma and penicillin to the armed forces. It is now used extensively in the pharmaceutical industry as one of the best methods for preserving biological materials and for protecting heat-sensitive drugs. It has also been successfully adopted for producing EN feeds (e.g. Protina G® or GlutaminOx®) which contain glutamine.

FORMULATIONS

The type of EN formulation used, as for PN, is directly dependent on the nutrient needs and goals of therapy for the patient.[11] Enteral feeds fall into two different categories:

Oral (or sip) feeds

Most prescribable sip feeds are nutritionally complete and most can be used as sole source of nutrition; however, in general they should only be used to supplement a patient's diet. There is a wide range of 'ready-to-use' commercial sip feeds (e.g. Ensure Plus®, Fresubin® and Fortisip®).

Tube feeds

Tube feeds may be administered via a nasoenteric tube or via a percutaneous endoscopic gastrostomy (PEG) or jejunostomy, are nutritionally complete and can be safely given as the sole source of nutrition. These include whole protein feeds for patients with 'normal' gut function, peptide feeds often used for jejunal feeding, and elemental feeds (free amino acids hence hyperosmolar) to treat some patients with Crohn's disease. Some of the nutritional considerations relating to enteral feeds are shown in Table 21.3. Many tube feeds are available (e.g. Osmolite®, Jevity®, Nutrison®, Fresubin®).

Table 21.3 – Nutritional considerations for feed constituents

1. Protein source (intact protein, peptides or amino acids)
2. Carbohydrate content and source (e.g. lactose free)
3. Fat content and source (long-chain triglycerides (LCT) vs medium-chain triglycerides (MCT))
4. Energy density
5. Energy distribution (i.e. % of energy supplied by protein, carbohydrate and fat)
6. Fibre content and source
7. Renal solute load
8. Electrolyte composition
9. Lactose/gluten content
10. Vitamin and mineral content (i.e. volume required to supply RNI)
11. Osmolality
12. Viscosity
13. Palatability and patient acceptance

A more comprehensive list of prescribable enteral feeds (classified as 'Borderline Substances') is to be found in the British National Formulary (BNF). Unlike in the USA, very little EN 'compounding' is carried out in UK pharmacy departments. The EN products can be classified into seven groups (Table 21.4).

Table 21.4 – Classification of prescribable enteral products★

1. Oral supplements (sip feeds) – to provide greater nutritional value and/or energy density to the diet
2. Polymeric tube feeds – nutritionally complete feeds with whole protein, maltodextrin, LCT, fat and often fibre
3. Elemental/peptide feeds for sip and/or tube feeding – mono/oligo-peptides and mono/oligo-saccharides which may be more easily digested and absorbed (but have a high osmolality, especially the elemental diet)
4. Disease-specific formulae – for cardiopulmonary, liver or renal failure
5. Modular diets (e.g. powdered carbohydrate or protein supplements – to individualize a patients diet)
6. Feeds for inborn errors of metabolism (e.g. phenylketonuria)
7. Infant formulae (e.g. lactose free feeds or those which do not contain cows milk)

★ This list is not exhaustive and does not include gluten-free foods or low protein foods.

Protein

It is common to refer to protein requirements for enteral feeding and nitrogen requirements for parenteral feed-ing. The eight essential amino acids (EAA) (in adults: isoleucine, leucine, lysine, methionine, phenylalanine, threonine, tryptophan and valine) cannot be manufactured by the body but can be used to make the non-essential amino acids (NEAAs), which provide most of an individuals metabolic need for nitrogen. The quality of protein is as important as the quantity. Whilst chemical scores based on reference standards for egg or milk proteins provide useful data, they do not take into account imbalances in protein amino acid patterns, different digestion rates and absorption of specific amino acids and losses during processing. Published data based on actual protein and EAA requirements for humans that accommodate age and lifestyle factors, allow reasonably accurate amounts to be determined.[12] Nevertheless, most enteral and parenteral products have a lower protein quality value when compared to egg or milk.

Glutamine

A potential problem related to the increasing use of EN, supplemented with novel amino acids such as glutamine, is that the content of glutamine in protein- and peptide-based enteral feeds is not accurately known. The amount of glutamine, which is heat labile, will depend upon the protein source and manufacturing conditions. Whole protein diets based on casein, whey or soy protein will differ in their glutamine content. Partially hydrolysed protein (peptide diets) will contain little free glutamine as it is converted to glutamate and ammonia during processing and storage. An estimation of the amount of protein-bound glutamine in over 30 feeds has been described by Swails et al.[13] Using this calculation method most whole protein feeds theoretically contain between 3.5 and 5.0 g glutamine per 1000 kcal (4200 kJ). A more accurate analytical determination involves the conversion of protein-bound glutamine to L-2,4-diaminobutyric acid, which is then measured by high performance liquid chromatography (HPLC).[14] Analysis of ten protein-based and four peptide-based feeds confirms that glutamine content is usually overestimated by theoretical computations. The actual amount provided by whole protein diets corresponds to 6–8 g per day and peptide diets provide only 1–5 g glutamine per day. These fall far short of the 20–25 g per day supplementation used in clinical studies that have demonstrated improved outcome for the critically ill.[15–17]

Arginine

In times of severe stress or trauma, plasma and tissue levels of both glutamine and arginine can fall below normal. Endogenous supplies of these 'conditionally essential' amino acids may then be insufficient to meet the increased protein turnover and energy requirements of the immune system. Supplementation by the enteral or parenteral routes has therefore been advocated.

Arginine is stable to heat processing and can therefore be formulated into EN regimens. All protein-based enteral feeds contain theoretically between 3 and 5 g arginine per 1000 kcal (4200 kJ) whilst some have been further enriched with additional free amino acid (Impact®, Perative® and Alitraq®). Lower infection rates and reduced hospital stays have been reported with these arginine-enriched diets,[18] but it remains difficult to interpret the potentially beneficial effects of arginine supplementation because of its co-administration with other immunostimulating nutrients during these trials.

Nucleotides

An increased requirement for dietary sources of nucleotides to improve immune function, small intestinal development and other processes involving rapid cell growth, especially in infants has recently been recognized. Although a number of manufacturers have incorporated nucleotide sources into infant feeding formulas in various parts of the world, and at least one enteral feed (Impact®) is enriched with nucleotides (together with arginine and fish oils), caution has been advised over their routine use.[19]

Carbohydrate

Carbohydrate is an essential component of enteral feeds, however Recommended Nutrient Intakes (RNIs) have not been published.[20] Most enteral feeds are designed to supply a non-protein calorie to nitrogen ratio of between 94:1 and 154:1. These proportions of energy and protein help to ensure that the carbohydrate in the feed is used for energy while 'sparing' protein for other functions (e.g. wound healing and immunocompetence). The form of the carbohydrate is important since it influences osmolality, palatability and glycaemic response.

Fat

Fats are included in most enteral feeds as a concentrated energy source that helps to meet energy requirements and to minimize endogenous protein catabolism. Unlike carbohydrate and protein, lipids do not contribute to osmolality. All enteral feeds contain the omega-6 and omega-3 fatty acids, linoleic and linolenic acids, which must be supplied in the diet as they cannot be synthesized *de novo*.

In some peptide feeds, fractionated coconut oil is used as a source of medium-chain triglycerides. These are absorbed directly into the lymphatic system and so may minimize steatorrhoea in patients with malabsorption.

Vitamins and Minerals

All sip and tube feeds which are intended for use as sole source of nutrition are fortified with essential vitamins, minerals and trace elements to supply the RNI in volumes which are generally between 1 and 2 litres, although in more energy-dense feeds this volume will be lower. The RNIs are dietary guidelines for healthy subjects and therefore it cannot be assumed that they are representative of the micronutrient requirements of stressed patients who have increased requirements for all nutrients due to changes in metabolism. Some feeds, therefore, contain higher levels of some micronutrients, which are known to benefit patients in order to account for increased requirements.

Phosphate

With modern PN regimens the problem of hypophosphataemia has been virtually eliminated. Similarly, most EN products contain sufficient phosphate to meet a patient's normal requirements. However, cases of hypophosphataemia during feeding of patients with Crohn's disease, chronic alcoholism, vitamin D deficiency or anorexia nervosa have been described.[21,22] Thus, it is advisable to monitor serum phosphate levels regularly during the first days/weeks of nutritional support, and when necessary provide additional enteral or occasionally parenteral supplementation.

Trace elements

Few reported trace element deficiencies have been associated with enteral feeding. However in one study, 15 of 19 patients receiving home enteral feeding had a trace element or vitamin deficiency (in six of these there were multiple deficiencies).[23] Infants fed proprietary formulas may have low plasma selenium levels compared to those receiving human milk. Selenium is a co-factor for the activity of the enzyme glutathione peroxidase, which is involved in the disposal of free radicals. The amount and form in which selenium is given, and interactions with other components of the feed, are important in determining a patient's selenium (and glutathione) status.[24] Selenite, a less stable form than selenate, may be reduced to elemental selenium which is not bioavailable. The organic forms of selenium (e.g. selenomethionine) may be preferentially used and stored in the body, but all forms of selenium increase glutathione peroxidase activity in subjects with poor selenium status.[25]

Copper deficiency is very unusual in patients receiving EN or PN. A case of microcytic anaemia and neutropenia due to copper deficiency during long-term enteral nutrition with a defined formula diet has been reported from Japan.[26] Complete restoration of the patient's haematological abnormalities was achieved by supplementing the feed with a standard (PN) trace element supplement providing 14 μmol/day of additional copper.

The likelihood of interactions between trace elements and vitamins with the other constituents of EN is theoretically just as great as that in PN. Indeed UHT heat treatment of most EN feeds could potentially accentuate the interactions compared to room temperature compounding of PN. The manufacturers of enteral feeds are required to comply with food law and the ingredients listed on the label must represent average nutrient levels over the shelf-life of these products. Therefore, manufacturers' quality assurance processes are designed to ensure that the quantities of nutrients listed on the labels are accurate throughout the specified life of the products.

Osmolality

Enterally administered hyperosmolar solutions may cause altered nutrient absorption,[27] hypertonic dehydration[28] and intestinal ischaemia.[29] In patients with a jejunostomy they cause large stomal water and sodium losses. In enterally fed pre-term infants they may cause necrotizing enterocolitis. The American Academy of Pediatrics recommends that for 'normal' infants the osmolarity of EN feeds should not exceed 400 mOsm/L (equivalent to 450 mOsm/kg).[30] The joint working party of the Paediatric Group and the Parenteral and Enteral Nutrition Group of the British Dietetic Association recommends that whole protein enteral feeds should be isotonic and that peptide feeds should have an upper limit for osmolality of 400 mOsm/kg water.[31] These figures may or may not be applicable to adults but at present

it seems advisable to adhere to these guidelines for critically ill patients.

Whilst many commercial products now state osmolality on their labels or accompanying literature, the addition of other medications, energy supplements, vitamins, glutamine etc. will automatically increase osmolality and needs to be taken into account. The Department of Pharmacy Services at the Children's Hospital of Philadelphia have measured the osmolality and published data on almost 100 oral medications and enteral formulas.[32]

Unfortunately there are currently no feeds available with a sodium content of about 100 mmol/L and a total osmolality about 300 mOsm/kg that would be suitable for patients with a jejunostomy, or a high output fistula or ileostomy. Enteral feeds for these patients need to have sodium chloride added to the feed before they are given.

FEEDING ROUTES/ ADMINISTRATION

The choice of feeding route is determined by alimentary tract function, previous gastrointestinal surgery (e.g. gastrectomy), accessibility of the gastrointestinal tract (GIT), practicality of using the GIT and patient preference. In patients who are able to eat, but unable to meet their nutritional requirements with everyday food and drink, fortified foods or sip feeds can help to increase intake of energy, protein and other nutrients.

In those who are unable to eat, but have a functioning GIT, tube feeds may be administered via a nasogastric tube in the short-term, or a gastrostomy or jejunostomy in the long-term. Nasogastric feeding is the most common form of tube feeding, and can be used to meet total nutritional requirements, or to complement oral or parenteral nutrition. A gastrostomy (most commonly a PEG) or jejunostomy is used for patients who are expected to require tube feeding for longer than about 3 weeks. Jejunostomy feeding is used when the stomach cannot be used (e.g. if patient has had a gastrectomy) and the patient has otherwise a functioning GIT. Jejunostomy feeding has been successfully used to feed patients after liver transplantation.[33] In patients who do not have adequate functioning gut, or whose nutritional goals cannot be met by EN, parenteral feeding is indicated.

Delivery techniques

For most tube-fed patients, a feeding pump is used to deliver the feed. Pump controlled feeding can be continuous or intermittent. In the hospital setting, continuous feeding is the most common. For patients who require feeding at home, intermittent feeding allows more flexibility and freedom. In addition, when feeding is stopped for 4 or more hours each day, the gastric pH drops to below 2.5 and this has the additional advantage of having an antibacterial effect. Gravity or bolus feeding, which supplies 100–400 ml of feed over 10–30 minutes several times a day, can be used with stable patients who may find it better psychologically. However, if not introduced carefully, it can increase the incidence of diarrhoea, cramps, nausea, bloating and/or abdominal discomfort[34] (Chapter 31).

Tube blockage

Tube blockage can occur in enterally fed patients and may lead to the feeding tube needing to be replaced. Protein coagulation, which occurs at low pH, is usually the cause of blockage and may be aggravated by the administration of medications through the tube. To avoid tube blockage, the tube should be flushed with water before and after feeding, and some advocate every 4 hours during feeding. Tubes should also be flushed before and after any medication is administered and medications should never be mixed with feeds as this may cause feeds to become unstable, thus increasing the potential for the tube to become blocked. Along with other measures (Chapter 31), a suspension of pancreatic enzymes and bicarbonate can prevent tube blockage and decreases the rate of tube occlusion tenfold[35] (e.g. a Creon® capsule dissolved in 10 ml 8.4% sodium bicarbonate).

Diarrhoea

Much research has been undertaken to understand and define the pathogenesis of enteral feeding-related diarrhoea. Factors such as antibiotics, high osmolality feed, lactose intolerance, contaminated feeds, laxatives and overflow incontinence have all been implicated (Chapter 31). There are anecdotal reports that glutamine- or fibre-containing feeds alleviate diarrhoea, but these have not been supported by controlled clinical trials. In a canine model, intestinal transit in the upper small intestine was slowed with fibre but it had little impact on bowel function.[36] Administration of *Saccharomyces bonlardi* decreased the frequency of diarrhoea in a multi-centred study of critically ill patients, by 25% compared to placebo.[37] Further studies in a broader selection of patients are needed to substantiate this interesting and low cost measure.

Concomitant drug therapy, the solubilizing agents used for some drugs, medications containing sorbitol, antacids and quinidine used in association with EN have all been responsible for diarrhoea.[38] Polyethylene glycol and propylene glycol are commonly used as water-miscible solvents in products, such as lorazepam, and are associated with diarrhoea. There was a prompt resolution of diarrhoea in a patient with adult respiratory distress syndrome, who was receiving Pulmocare®, when crushed lorazepam tablets were substituted for lorazepam solution.[39]

COMPATIBILITY OF DRUGS

Mixing drugs with feeds is generally discouraged in favour of direct enteral bolus administration. Most published data relating to the compatibility/stability of additives to EN feeds emanate from hospital or academic pharmacy departments in the USA.

A pH-dependent precipitation of protein from the feed, accompanied by phase separation, was observed after morphine addition (2 mg/ml) to three standard feeds. This phenomenon was not observed when a more concentrated morphine solution (20 mg/ml) was used.[40]

A dilemma exists regarding the alleged interaction between phenytoin and EN feeds. This was first reported in 1982 by Bauer[41] but the study has been criticized and two well-controlled scientific investigations in normal volunteers found no significant interaction.[42,43] However, in many clinical situations associated with EN feeding, reductions in serum phenytoin have been documented.[44] To minimize such a drug–nutrient interaction, tube feeding is either stopped 1 hour before and 1 hour after each oral phenytoin dose,[45] or phenytoin is given 2 hours after stopping the tube feeding.[46] Serum phenytoin levels should be routinely monitored, especially for patients on an intensive therapy unit.

Guidance needs to be provided to clinicians and nurses so that 'enteral' medications are administered in the same manner. The nutrition team pharmacist should study the pharmacokinetic profiles for phenytoin and other drugs during artificial feeding.

FEED CONTAMINATION

EN feeds may become contaminated with micro-organisms during preparation and administration and might be a source of nosocomial infection.[47] It is assumed that micro-organisms present in a feed administered into the gut (especially the stomach), in the same way as food taken orally, will be destroyed by gastric acid and digestive enzymes. Thus infection control procedures have remained less stringent for EN than those for PN. Contamination of a feed may not be clinically relevant unless a patient is immuno-suppressed, is taking drugs to inhibit gastric acid production, is being fed directly into the small bowel or if there is an enteropathic organism in the feed. As such patients may not be immediately identified, it is recommended that feeds are always prepared and administered using an aseptic technique.

Microbial contamination of EN can occur during preparation, decanting and assembly of mixed or ready-to-use products, or more commonly during the subsequent manipulation of the feeding system.[48] The risk and magnitude of contamination is directly related to the type and number of manipulations of the system and the use (or non-use) of aseptic techniques.[49] Several policies and procedures intended to minimize EN contamination have been published in USA and Europe and are based on tradition rather than controlled experimental findings.

Anderton et al.[50] published guidance notes prepared for the British Dietetic Association in 1986 and recommended that at no time should any internal part of the nutrient container or giving set be allowed to come into contact with hands, clothes or surrounding surfaces. Nurses often do not wash their hands before handling EN systems but micro-organisms detected in patient's feeds can be transferred from nurses' hands or from patients themselves.[51,52] Typical organisms isolated from feeds include the skin contaminants *Staph. epidermidis* and Gram-negative bacilli.[53] Retrograde spread of organisms from the patient, via the giving set, to the EN container have been reported.[54] Contamination is more likely in patients on an intensive therapy unit if feeds are reconstituted with non-pasteurized water rather than with sterile water.[55] Microbiological contamination of EN tubes may be due to the practice of flushing the tube with tap water.[56] Two studies have reported no difference in the incidence of contamination of ready-to-use feeds compared with those prepared from powders.[57,58] Major reductions in bacterial counts for EN prepared in the pharmacy occurred after improvements in aseptic techniques, the use of sterile water for reconstitution and/or rinsing and the incorporation of a preservative (potassium sorbate) into the feed.[59]

The practice of flushing and rinsing giving sets when changing EN containers is common in the USA, but rinsing may be unnecessary if the sets are changed at least every 24 hours.[60] Historically, hang-time for paediatric formulas has been only 4 hours, but by use of meticulous preparation procedures hang times may be extended up to 24 hours, providing the EN preparation starts without significant contamination.[61]

It is important to have an ongoing quality assurance programme. The team approach to quality assurance with the key participation of the pharmacist and/or microbiologist has been previously advocated by Anderton.[62] She has proposed an adaptation of the food industry's Hazard Analysis Critical Control Point (HACCP) system for the preparation and administration of enteral feeds (Table 21.5).[63]

Table 21.5 – Adaptation of the food industry's Hazard Analysis Critical Control Point (HACCP) system for the preparation and administration of enteral feeds[63]

1. Analysis of the entire process from raw materials to consumption
2. Identification and assessment of the potential hazards involved with handling
3. Identification of points where control over a hazard can be achieved
4. Specification and implementation of monitoring and control procedures

Implementation of procedures akin to HACCP for EN has so many similarities to the quality assurance procedures already long followed by pharmacists compounding PN. The possibility to adapt and transfer the aseptic quality assurance procedures from PN therapy to EN therapy in order to improve the stability, compatibility and safety of all nutrition support products seems logical and cost-effective. With their background training in pharmacokinetics and microbiology, the pharmacist is best qualified to take on this responsibility as the guardian of quality assurance for the nutrition support team.

REFERENCES

1. Levine GM, Deren JJ, Steiger E, Zinno R. Role of oral intake in maintenance of gut mass and disaccharidase activity. *Gastroenterology* 1974; **67**: 975–982.

2. Kalfarentzos F, Kehagias J, Mead N, Kokkinis K, Gogos CA. Enteral nutrition is superior to parenteral nutrition in severe acute pancreatitis: results of a randomized prospective trial. *Br J Surg* 1997; **84**: 1665–1669.

3. Sand J, Luostarinen M, Matikainen M. Enteral or parenteral feeding after total gastrectomy: prospective randomised pilot study. *Eur J Surg* 1997; **163**: 761–766.

4. Shirabe K, Matsumata T, Shimada M, *et al.* A comparison of parenteral hyperalimentation and early enteral feeding regarding systemic immunity after major hepatic resection – the results of a randomized prospective study. *Hepatogastroenterology* 1997; **44**: 205–209.

5. Moore FA, Feliciano DV, Andrassy RJ, *et al.* Early enteral feeding compared with parenteral reduces post-operative septic complications. The results of a meta analysis. *Ann Surg* 1992; **216**: 172–183.

6. Lipman TO. Grains or veins: is enteral nutrition really better than parenteral nutrition? A look at the evidence. *J Parenter Enteral Nutr* 1998; **22**: 167–182.

7. Bell SJ, Borlase BC, Swails W, Dascoulias K, Ainsley B, Forse RA. Experience with enteral nutrition in a hospital population of acutely ill patients. *J Am Diet Assoc* 1994; **94**: 414–419.

8. Adam S, Armstrong RF, Bullen C, Cohen SL, Scott A, Singer M, Webb AR. Critical Care Algorithm: Enteral and parenteral nutrition. *Clin Intens Care* 1991; **2**: 252–255.

9. The history of enteral nutrition. In: Randall HT, Rombeau JL, Caldwell MD (eds) *Clinical Nutrition: Enteral and Tube Feeding*, 2nd edn. WB Saunders: Philadelphia, 1990.

10. Hunter J. A case of paralysis of the muscles of deglutition cured by an artificial mode of conveying food and medicines into the stomach. *Trans Soc Improvement Med Chir Know* 1793; **1**: 182–188.

11. Randall HT. Enteral nutrition: tube feeding in acute and chronic illness. *J Parenter Enteral Nutr* 1984; **8**: 113–136.

12. Dubin S, McKee K, Battish S. Essential amino acid reference profile affects the evaluation of enteral feeding products. *J Am Diet Assoc* 1994; **94**: 884–887.

13. Swails WS, Bell SJ, Borlase BC, Forse RA, Blackbum GL. Glutamine content of whole proteins: Implications for enteral formulas. *Nutr Clin Pract* 1992; **7**: 77–80.

14. Kuhn KS, Stehle P, Fürst P. Glutamine content of protein and peptide-based enteral products. *J Parenter Enteral Nutr* 1996; **20**: 292–295.

15. Jones C, Palmer TEA, Griffiths RD. Randomised clinical outcome study of critically ill patients given glutamine-supplemented enteral nutrition. *Nutrition* 1998; **14**: *Nutrition* 1999; **15**: 108–115.

16. Jensen G, Miller RH, Talabiska D, Fish J, Gianferante L. A double-blind prospective randomised study of glutamine enriched compared with standard peptide-based feeding in critical ill patients. *Am J Clin Nutr* 1996; **64**: 615–621.

17. Houdijk AP, Rijnsburger ER, Jansen J, *et al.* Randomised trial of glutamine-enriched enteral nutrition on infectious morbidity in patients with multiple trauma. *Lancet* 1998; **352**: 772–776.

18. Daly JM, Liberman MD, Goldfine J. Enteral nutrition with supplemented arginine, RNA and omega-3 fatty acids in patients after operation: immunologic, metabolic and clinical outcome. *Surgery* 1992; **112**: 56–67.

19. Rudolph FB, Van Buren T. The metabolic effects of enterally administered ribonucleic acid. *Curr Opin Clin Nutri Met Care* 1998; **1**: 527–530.

20. Department of Health. Dietary Reference Values for Food Energy and Nutrients for the United Kingdom. HMSO: London, 1992, p. 41.

21. Maier-Dobersberger T, Lochs H. Enteral supplementation of phosphate does not prevent hypophosphatemia during refeeding of cachectic patients. *J Parenter Enteral Nutr* 1994; **18**: 182–184.

22. Payne-James JJ, Rees RG, Newton MA, *et al.* Acute respiratory failure in association with hypophosphatemia after refeeding in anorexia nervosa. *J Clin Nutr Gastroenterol* 1988; **3**: 67–68.

23. McWhirter JP, Hambling CE, Pennington CR. The nutritional status of patients receiving home enteral feeding. *Clin Nutr* 1994; **13**: 201–211.

24. McGuire MK, Burgert SL, Milner JA, *et al.* Selenium status of infants is influenced by supplementation of formula or maternal diets. *Am J Clin Nutr* 1993; **58**: 643–648.

25. Selenium: biochemical actions, interactions and some human health implications. In: Levander OA, Prasad AS (eds) *Clinical, Biochemical, and Nutritional Aspects of Trace Elements.* Alan R. Liss: New York, 1982, pp. 345–368.

26. Tamura H, Hirose S, Watanabe O, Arai K, Murakawa M, Matsumura O, Isoda K. Anaemia and neutropenia due to copper deficiency in enteral nutrition. *J Parenter Enteral Nutr* 1994; **18**: 185–189.

27. Lifschitz CH, Carrazza F. Effect of formula carbohydrate concentration on tolerance and macronutrient absorption in infants with severe chronic diarrhoea. *J Pediatr* 1990; **117**: 378–383.

28. Abrams CA, Phillips LL, Berkowitz C. Hazards of over concentrated milk formula: hyperosmolality, DIC and gangrene. *JAMA* 1975; **232**: 1136–1140.

29. Wilcox DT, Fiorello AB, Glick PL. Hypovolemic shock and intestinal ischemia: a preventable complication of incomplete formula labelling. *J Pediatr* 1993; **122**: 103–104.

30. American Academy of Pediatrics Committee on Nutrition. Commentary on breastfeeding and infant formula, including proposed standards for formulas. *Pediatrics* 1976; **57**: 278.

31. Russell C, Micklewright A, Scott D, *et al. Paediatric Enteral Feeding Solutions and Systems.* British Dietetic Association: Birmingham, 1994, p. 1.

32. Jew RK, Owen D, Kaufman D, Balmer D. Osmolality of commonly used medications and formulas in the neonatal intensive care unit. *Nutr Clin Pract* 1997; **12**: 158–163.

33. Wicks C, Somasundaram S, Bjarnason I, *et al.* Comparison of enteral feeding and total parenteral nutrition after liver transplantation. *Lancet* 1994; **344**: 837–840.

34. Methods of artificial nutritional support. In: Todorovic VE, Micklewright A. *A Pocket Guide to Clinical Nutrition*, 2nd edn. British Dietetic Association: Birmingham, 1997, pp. 5.1–5.10.

35. Sriram K, Jayanthi V, Lakshmi RG, George VS. Prophylactic locking of enteral feeding tubes with pancreatic enzymes. *J Parenter Enteral Nutr* 1997; **21**: 353–356.

36. Lin HC, Zhao XT, Chu AW, Lin YP, Wang L. Fibre-supplemented enteral formula slows intestinal transit by intensifying inhibitory feedback from the distal gut. *Am J Clin Nutr* 1997; **65**: 1840–1844.

37. Bleichner G, Bléhaut H, Mentec H, Moyse D. *Saccharmyces boulardii* prevents diarrhoea in critically ill tube-fed patients. A multicentre, randomised, double-blind placebo-controlled trial. *Intens Care Med* 1997; **23**: 517–523.

38. Lutomski DM, Gora ML, Wright SM, Martin JE. Sorbitol content of selected oral liquids. *Ann Pharmacother* 1993; **27**: 269–274.

39. Shephard MF, Felt-Gunderson PA. Diarrhoea associated with Lorazepam solution in a tube-fed patient. *Nutr Clin Pract* 1996; **11**: 117–120.

40. Udeani GO, Bass J, Johnston TP. Compatibility of oral morphine sulfate solution with enteral feeding products. *Ann Pharmacotherap* 1994; **28**: 451–455.

41. Bauer LA. Interference of oral phenytoin absorption by continuous nasogastric feedings. *Neurology* 1982; **32**: 570–572.

42. Krueger KA, Garnett WR, Comstock TJ, Fitzsimmons WE, Karnes HT, Pellock JM. Effect of two administration schedules of an enteral nutrient formula on phenytoin bio-availability. *Epilepsy* 1987; **28**: 706–712.

43. Marvel ME, Bertino JS Jr. Comparative effects of an elemental and a complex enteral feeding formulation on the absorption of phenytoin suspension. *J Parenter Enteral Nutr* 1991; **15**: 316–318.

44. Stockley IH. Anticonvulsant drug interactions. In: *Drug Interactions*, 4th edn. The Pharmaceutical Press: London, 1996, pp. 304–364.

45. Hatton J, Magnuson B. Therapeutic options. *Nutr Clin Pract* 1996; **11**: 30–31.

46. Gilbert S. How to minimise interaction between phenytoin and enteral feedings: a strategic approach. *Nutr Clin Pract* 1996; **11**: 28–30.

47. Fagerman KE, Paauw JD, McCamish MA. Effects of time, temperature and preservative on bacterial growth in enteral nutrient solutions. *Am J Hosp Pharm* 1984; **41**: 1122–1126.

48. Anderton A. Microbiological aspects of the preparation and administration of nasogastric and nasoenteric tube feeds in hospitals. *Hum Nut App Nutr* 1983; **3 7A**: 426–440.

49. Anderson KR, Norris DJ, Godfrey LB. Bacterial contamination of tube feeding formulas. *J Parenter Enteral Nutr* 1984; **8**: 673–678.

50. Anderton A, Howard JP, Scott DE. Microbiological control in enteral feeding. Summary of guidance document prepared on behalf of the Committee of the Parenteral and Enteral Nutrition Group of the British Dietetic Association. *Hum Nut App Nutr* 1986; **40A**: 163–167.

51. Kohn CL. The relationship between enteral formula contamination and length of enteral delivery set usage. *J Parenter Enteral Nutr* 1991; **15**: 567–571.

52. Thurn J, Crossley K, Gerdts A, Maki M, Johnson J. Enteral hyperalimentation as a source of nosocomial infection. *J Hosp Infect* 1990; **15**: 203–217.

53. Schroeder P, Fisher D, Volz M, Paloucek J. Microbial contamination of enteral feeding solutions in a community hospital. *J Parenter Enteral Nutr* 1983; **7**: 364–368.

54. Payne-James JJ, Rana SK, Bray MJ, McSwiggan DA, Silk DBA. Retrograde (ascending) bacterial contamination of enteral diet administration systems. *J Parenter Enteral Nutr* 1992; **16**: 369–373.

55. Ottoviani D, Vazquez JA, Centa P, Davidson LJ, Janson D, Graham TO. Contamination of enteral formula in hospitalised patients. *J Parenter Enteral Nutr* 1996; **20**: 28S.

56. Bussy V, Marechal F, Nasca S. Microbial contamination of enteral feeding tubes occurring during nutritional treatment. *J Parenter Enteral Nutr* 1992; **16**: 552–557.

57. Nugent M, Hansell DT, Gray GR. Bacterial contamination of reconstituted and commercially prepared enteral feeds. *Clin Nutr* 1987; **6**: 21–24.

58. Navajas M, Chacon DJ, Solvas JF, Vargas RG. Bacterial contamination of enteral feeds as a possible risk of nosocomial infection. *J Hosp Infect* 1992; **21**: 111–120.

59. Fagerman KE. Limiting bacterial contamination of enteral nutrient solutions: 6–year history with reduction of contamination at two institutions. *Nutr Clin Pract* 1992; **7**: 31–36.

60. Kohn-Keeth C, Shott S, Olree K. The effects of rinsing enteral delivery sets on formula contamination. *Nutr Clin Pract* 1996; **11**: 269–273.

61. Amold T, Fidanza SJ, Smith S, Krebs NF, Wedemeyer H, Childress L, James JF. Enteral feeding contamination in a paediatric hospital. *Nutr Clin Pract* 1997; **12**: 93.

62. Anderton A. Bacterial contamination of enteral feeds and feeding systems. *Clin Nutr* 1993; **12**: S16–S32.

63. Anderton A. What is the HACCP (hazard analysis critical control point) approach and how can it be applied to enteral tube feeding? *J Hum Nutr Dietet* 1994; **7**: 53–60.

22

Formulation of parenteral feeds

Martin J. Lee and Michael C. Allwood

*T*his chapter outlines the components of a parenteral nutrition solution, shows some of the preparations available and describes some features relating to the stability and compatibility of the parenteral nutrition (PN) solution.

COMPONENTS OF A PN SOLUTION

When PN first became a treatment option, many separate infusions were given from bottles of high strength glucose, protein hydrolysates or amino acids and fat emulsion; to some of these vitamins and minerals were added on the ward by nursing staff. Infusion systems comprised multiple lines with two- or three-way taps, connected to the central line. The risk of the line becoming infected was high due to contamination from changing infusion containers and handling the administration lines. The risk of extrinsic contamination of PN mixtures was found to be significantly reduced if they were compounded under strict aseptic conditions. Thus, an all-in-one system for PN was developed and introduced in the late 1970s.[1-3]

As the clinical benefits of the all-in-one system were increasingly recognized by clinicians, the demand for more complex mixtures and bags with shelf-lives greater than 24 hours produced new challenges for pharmacists, who needed to ensure the stability and compatibility of these complete complex PN admixtures. Some admixtures can contain more than 50 different components. This means that careful formulation and strict mixing protocols must be followed during compounding. Pharmacy-operated compounding services, either commercial companies or hospital-based, were introduced into the UK in the early 1980s and have made a major impact on reducing infection risks in patients receiving PN. Most adult patients can be supported nutritionally with a range of standardized regimens that essentially are designed to mimic a 'normal diet'. Parenteral nutrition supplies: nitrogen as amino acids, energy as carbohydrate alone or in combination with lipid, water, electrolytes and micronutrients. The British National Formulary contains a table listing the different solutions available for parenteral feeding and their contents.[4]

Nitrogen

Currently available amino acid solutions containing synthetic L-amino acids supply all the traditionally termed 'essential' and 'non-essential' amino acids. However, not all amino acids are included because of potential stability problems (e.g. glutamine and cysteine). Commercial sources of nitrogen include Aminoplex®, Synthamin®, Aminosteril® and Vamin®. Amino acid solutions are available with electrolytes minimized or eliminated. Higher strength solutions with nitrogen contents greater than 18 g/L are available allowing more concentrated formulations to be compounded when administration volume is important (e.g. Hyperamine 30®, Aminoplex 24®, Intrafusin 22®).

Recently, dipeptide solutions have become available as a vehicle for less soluble heat-labile amino acids, e.g. glutamine. Glamin® is a solution of free amino acids and dipeptide glycyl-L-glutamine, which is chemically stable and hydrolysed to free glutamine and glycine in plasma and tissues, and dipeptide glycyl-L-tyrosine, which is hydrolysed to glycine and tyrosine. Dipeptiven® contains N(2)-L-alanyl-L-glutamine. These solutions can be used for hypercatabolic or hypermetabolic states.

The newer paediatric preparations such as Primene® and Vaminolact® contain the aminosulfonic acid taurine. Aminosteril® is the only adult amino acid solution containing taurine and may alleviate taurine deficiency which has been implicated in the hepatic problems of some patients receiving long-term PN.

Energy

The type of energy substrate is important both for optimizing the efficiency of energy utilization and minimizing metabolic complications. Amino acids are a metabolically important but expensive source of energy, thus carbohydrates and lipids are the two main sources of energy in parenteral feeds.

It is conventional, though illogical, to describe the energy given in PN as non-protein energy. This means that only energy derived from carbohydrate and lipid is quoted. The protein (nitrogen) energy is not usually stated. This contrasts to enteral nutrition where the total energy content of a feed is indicated. In parenteral feeds the protein content is usually quoted in grams of nitrogen.

There is still debate as to which energy source should be used during parenteral nutrition. Some advocate the use of glucose alone with fat emulsion administered weekly to provide essential fatty acids. More commonly energy is provided as a mixture of glucose and lipid together. Providing the administered substrate is adequately utilized, there is no difference in the efficacy of glucose or fat with regards to nitrogen sparing.

Carbohydrate

Glucose is generally the carbohydrate of choice for parenteral nutrition and is available, either alone in a range of concentrations of 5–70% w/v, (weight/volume) or in combination with electrolytes. The energy value of glucose is approximately 4 kcal/g (Table 22.1).

Advantages:

- Inexpensive and readily available
- Effectively metabolized in the presence of insulin
- Stimulates insulin release so encouraging nitrogen retention in muscles.

Disadvantages:

- Concentrated solutions are hypertonic so preventing peripheral infusion
- Hyperglycaemia and glycosuria may occur
- Essential fatty acid deficiency can occur if used as the only energy source.

Table 22.1 – Glucose concentration and energy level

Glucose conc. w/v	Approx. energy content per litre (kcal)
5%	200
10%	400
15%	600
20%	800
40%	1600
50%	2000

Although glucose is the most commonly used carbohydrate source in PN, fructose and sorbitol are also used in some countries. Sorbitol, which is largely converted to fructose, gained popularity because fructose was considered not to need insulin for it's metabolism. However, this is not so as 70% of infused fructose is converted to glucose.[5] A fructose infusion may also result in hyperuricaemia and a metabolic acidosis – the latter occurring because about 30% of

fructose is metabolized to lactate and pyruvate. In addition, fructose and sorbitol are dangerous to the rare patients with hereditary fructose intolerance.[6] These alternative carbohydrate sources do not offer any advantages over glucose.

Lipid

Most commercial lipid emulsions consist of soya bean long-chain triglycerides (LCT) emulsified with, and in effect surrounded by, egg-derived phospholids to mimic the structure of chylomicrons. They are available as 10 and 20% w/v concentrations (e.g. Intralipid®, Lipofundin®, Ivelip® and Lipovenos®). Intralipid® is also available as a 30% w/v concentration (Table 22.2).

The calorific value of lipid is approximately 9 kcal/g allowing large amounts of calories to be administered in a relatively small volume of low osmolality.

Advantages:

- High energy content
- Isotonic allowing peripheral infusion
- Source of essential fatty acids and vitamin E.

Disadvantages:

- Expensive compared to glucose
- Lipid droplets may interfere with routine blood tests
- Some patients may have reduced ability to clear lipid
- Risk of catheter occlusion with complex compounded solutions
- Pharmaceutical limitations on stability and shelf life.

Table 22.2 – Commercial lipid emulsions

Lipid conc. w/v	Volume (ml)	Approx. energy content (kcal)
10%	500	550
20%	500	1000
30%	330	1000

The fatty acids in LCT emulsions have chain lengths of 16–20 carbon atoms. Fat emulsions are available as a mixture of LCTs and medium–chain triglycerides (MCTs) in a ration of 1:1 (w/v). MCTs have chain lengths of 6–10 carbon atoms; they enter portal bloodstream rather than lymphatic system, enter cells via a carnitine-independent fatty acid transport system and are less immunosuppressive than tri-glycerides. These LCT/MCT mixtures are cleared from the plasma faster than LCT alone[7] and are of benefit in multiple trauma.[8,9]

Structured MCT/LCTs, n-3 fatty acids and short-chain fatty acids (SCFA) are currently being investigated as potential substrates.

Electrolytes

Salts are available either as product licensed or un-licensed injections for inclusion into feeding bags. Examples are sodium (as chloride or acetate), potassium (as chloride or phosphate), phosphate (as mono- and dibasic potassium salts), magnesium (as sulphate or chloride) and calcium (as chloride or gluconate). Commercially available amino acid and carbohydrate solutions may contain some electrolytes and trace elements and so reduce the number of additions required when a formulation is com-pounded.

Calcium injections, particularly calcium gluconate, may be contaminated with aluminium, which may be a problem for patients with renal impairment and pre-term infants.[10,11]

Organic phosphate injections, which are not currently licensed in the UK, such as glucose-1 phos-phate, glycero-phosphate and fructose-1,6-diphos-phate reduce the possibility of calcium phosphate precipitation in PN mixtures. The phosphate group on these compounds is covalently bonded to an organic structure (glucose, glycerol or fructose) and thus is not ionized, hence does not precipitate with calcium to form inorganic calcium phosphate.

Micro-nutrients

Trace elements

The provision of precise amounts of trace elements is difficult due to uncertainty about how much to give and in what chemical form. In addition, the amino acid and other solutions may be contaminated with trace elements. They are usually provided as standard commercial preparations as combinations of trace elements, which provide a daily-recommended amount (e.g. Additrace®). The amounts in these preparations generally prevent clinical deficiency states occurring except selenium.[12,13]

Extra amounts of selected trace elements are sometimes added to supplement the commercially available products. The acute phase of response to injury or infection is associated with alteration in dynamics of many trace elements, particularly iron, zinc and copper. The fall in serum iron and zinc and rise in serum copper are brought about by changes in the concentration of specific tissue cytokines, tumour necrosis factor and interleukin 6. The metabolic rate after elective surgery may increase by 10–20% and with severe sepsis by up to 50%. When the metabolic rate is increased there is a greater requirement for trace elements partly because all essential trace elements are involved in enzyme-catalysed reactions, many of which are central to intermediary metabolism, and because there are multiple sites from which trace elements can be lost (e.g. patients with fistulas or diarrhoea loose large amounts of Cu, Mn and Zn).

Vitamins

A number of multivitamin preparations for parenteral use are available which provide the recommended daily requirements of vitamins (e.g. Cernevit®, Solivito N®, Vitlipid N Adult®). Solivito N® is a lyophilized mixture of water-soluble vitamins requir-ing reconstitution. Vitlipid N Adult® is an oil in water emulsion containing the fat-soluble vitamins A, D_2, E and K_1 in the oil phase of the emulsion with a com-position corresponding to that of Intralipid 10%. Cernevit® consists of a combination of water- and fat-soluble vitamins, excluding phytomenadione, for use in adults and children over 12 years. Multibionta® contains a high level of vitamin A, which may be a problem in patients with liver disease. Parentrovite® because of its higher thiamine content may be advan-tageous when thiamine deficiency is anticipated or when a relatively carbohydrate-rich feeding regime is used.

A major problem is the loss of vitamins from PN mixtures after compounding, whether due to chemical degradation, by exposure to ultraviolet light, adsorption onto the surface of the infusion bag or administration sets. Therefore, the fact that the patient has theoretically received an adequate vitamin intake according to the prescription, does not ensure maintenance of vitamin status because of these chemical losses.

Water

Water makes up most of a parenteral feeding bag with the quantity varying according to a patient's needs. If large amounts are needed this is usually given in conjunction with sodium chloride, which is usually lost from the body with water.

PERIPHERAL NUTRITION FORMULATIONS

PN via the peripheral veins when the central route is not suitable or available has been used routinely for years throughout Europe. The most common complication with the use of the peripheral route is thrombophlebitis. The osmolality of solutions used in glucose-based PN can be so high that they have to be infused into central veins because if used peripherally they cause painful thrombophlebitis. The isotonicity of fat emulsions enables them to be given peripherally with a minimal risk of thrombophlebitis. Some nutrition mixtures of glucose and lipid may be infused peripherally with a reduced incidence of thrombophlebitis. This may be partly because glucose concentrations can be reduced when lipids are included, which reduces osmolality, and partly because lipid emulsions seem to have a protective influence on vascular endothelium.[14] The development of thrombophlebitis is believed to be greater when the infusate osmolality rises above 600 mosm/L. A more recent study by Timmer and Schipper[15] has shown that the 'osmolality rate' (osmolality × infusion rate) correlates more with peripheral vein thrombosis than osmolality alone. Greater incidence has been noted with increasing electrolyte content, especially potassium in PN bags. The addition of heparin and hydrocortisone to infusions has been used to reduce the incidence of peripheral vein thrombophlebitis.

STABILITY AND COMPATIBILITY OF PN SOLUTIONS

Since PN solutions are highly complex mixtures of chemicals, it is inevitable that chemical reactions can occur following compounding. These can be divided into two categories: physical incompatibility leading to precipitation, and chemical degradation leading to loss of nutritional or pharmacological efficacy, and possibly enhanced toxicity due to hazardous degradation products.

Both of these reactions can take place in compounded PN mixtures. Avoiding precipitation and minimizing degradation requires an understanding of the major reasons why they occur in a complex mixture like PN. The chemical composition and physical properties of PN mixtures vary greatly between regimens. This will depend on the commercial amino acid source, the particular electrolyte salts used, the relative concentrations of ingredients and the final volume. The presence of fat emulsion is also important. In describing the potential chemical and physical interactions that can take place, it is important to realize that each regimen is chemically unique. Extrapolation of stability data from one to another regimen requires a full understanding of all the factors that can influence stability.

Physical incompatibility

Electrolytes

The most common cause of precipitation in PN mixtures is due to calcium phosphate insolubility.[16–19] The factors influencing the solubility of calcium phosphate in PN mixtures are multi-factorial, but the most important variable is pH.[16]

The final pH of a mixture is influenced by the following factors:

The commercial amino acid used[17]. These vary from around 5 to pH's greater than 7. For example, Vamin® products have a pH around 5.2 while Aminoplex 12® is close to pH 7. These differences can be very important because the amino acids, due to their strong buffering capacity, are the major controllers of the pH in the final mixture.[17]

The inorganic phosphate source[19]. These are again strong buffers yet differ markedly between products. In particular, potassium dihydrogen phosphate injection (acid phosphate) has a very low pH. Because phosphate salts form very strong buffering systems, the choice of phosphate injection has a marked effect on final pH of the PN mixture.[20]

The buffering capacity of amino acids and inorganic phosphate[17]

The chemical equilibrium for inorganic phosphate salts in water is shown in Figure 22.1. Note that pH is the controlling factor for which phosphate species actually predominate in any particular solution. In PN mixtures, we are interested in pHs between 5 and 7. As already discussed, the actual pH of any PN mixture will depend in the amino acid source, final concentration and phosphate source. At pH 5, the dihydrogen-phosphate salt predominates, while at pH 7, the predominate salt is the mono-phosphate species.[21]

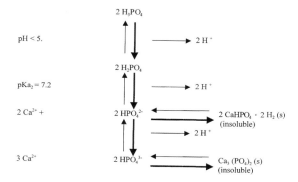

Figure 22.1 – Speciation of phosphate salts in parenteral nutrition mixtures.

Calcium mono-hydrogen phosphate is 60 times less soluble than the dihydrogen salt.[17] As the pH increases, there is an increasing likelihood of precipitation. Thus precipitation of calcium phosphate is less likely in Vamin®-containing mixtures, using acid phosphate injection as the phosphate source.

Unfortunately, it is more complicated. Since the most important cause of precipitation in PN mixtures is the formation of insoluble calcium phosphate, the calcium source needs to be considered.[19] Calcium injections come in two forms: calcium chloride injection which is fully ionized in aqueous solution, or calcium gluconate injection which is only partially ionized in aqueous solution. These, therefore, behave differently in PN mixtures, and precipitation is most likely with the chloride salt.[19] So calcium gluconate is preferred to reduce the risk of precipitation in PN mixtures. But there is another complication. The degree of ionization of calcium gluconate is only slightly influenced by pH, but is substantially effected by temperature.[17] Raising the temperature increases the dissociation of calcium gluconate. So paradoxically,

PN mixtures containing calcium gluconate stored in the refrigerator are less likely to precipitate, compared with PN mixtures at room temperature. More important, however, is the possible risk of precipitation in the line, as the infusion warms to body temperature, especially within the canopy of a neonatal cot. (Note also the concerns about high aluminium levels in calcium gluconate injection as previously indicated.)

Other factors can also effect calcium phosphate solubility in PN mixtures. These are summarized in Table 22.3.

In summary, the greatest risk of precipitation is from forming calcium phosphate salts. In clinical practice, it is normally possible to achieve adult requirements without running the risk of calcium phosphate precipitation. But in neonates and small children, because of their far greater needs for these essential compounds, it is very difficult to formulate parenteral nutrition mixtures without creating an incompatible mixture. This means that compounding and administration must also be carefully controlled.

Other possible causes of precipitation

There are some other possible causes of precipitation but all are far less likely than calcium phosphate. All are associated with trace elements. These differ also from calcium phosphate because they usually take many days before they are evident. (In contrast, calcium phosphate precipitates will appear within 24 hours of compounding.)

There are two significant trace element – PN mixture interactions which can cause precipitation: copper and sulphide (a degradation product of cysteine is only found in Vamin® and Vaminolact® products in the UK)[24] and iron and phosphate (only reported with certain Synthamin®-containing PN mixtures).[25]

Fat emulsions

Before leaving physico-chemical problems, it is important to consider fat emulsions. A fat emulsion is formed by a long period of homogenization to form a very fine emulsion. Each fat particle is kept separate by the fact that the surface is covered in the negative charges of the phospholipid 'tails' protruding around its surface. So charge repulsion maintains the emulsion in a stable state.

The average fat globule size is around 400 nm (0.4 μm), small enough to pass through the smallest

Table 22.3 – Factors that effect calcium phosphate solubility in PN mixtures

Factor	Likely effect	Reason for effect
Magnesium concentration	Reduces likelihood of precipitation	Magnesium phosphate more soluble than calcium phosphate salts[22]
Amino acid source	May decrease or increase precipitation	Some amino acids specifically bind calcium and reduce salt formation[17]
Amino acid	Increase may improve solubility	Enhanced binding capacity and solubility
Organic phosphate	Removes risk of calcium precipitation	Phosphate is in organic covalent form (e.g. glucose phosphate) and so phosphate does not precipitate[23]

capillaries. So the essential requirement of any fat emulsion after being added to a PN mixture, is that this size does not increase to the extent that it might block these capillaries. This forms the basis for deciding if the fat emulsion remains within acceptable limits.

The fat emulsion is mixed with a whole range of compounds, which, crucially, include electrolytes, in particular, cations. These can neutralize the negative surface charges of the oil globules. The particles start to come together as aggregates and form small clumps. Since oil is lighter than water, these aggregates tend to float to the surface and form a 'cream' layer ("just like the top-of-the-milk"). Shaking can disperse these clumps. Therefore, the formation of a cream layer is not normally considered hazardous because the particles remain discreet. However, if the particles start to coalesce to form larger oil globules, this is more hazardous. This can usually only be detected by careful particle-size analysis.

In fact, it requires relatively large concentrations of cations to significantly reduce these surface charges, but divalent cations are much more efficient charge neutralizers. So, in practice it is the concentration of divalent cations, which is most important.[26] There has been some attempt to quantify this effect, by applying colloid theory to fat emulsions in PN mixtures. Unfortunately, the relatively simple equations used in colloid science cannot be applied because of the complexity of PN mixtures. So our approach to predicting the stability of 'all-in-one' PN mixtures is far more empirical. There are some rules we can use:[26]

a. Destabilize fat emulsions

- HIGH concentrations of calcium and magnesium
- LOW pH

- LOW relative volumes of fat emulsion
- HIGH ratio of acidic to basic amino acids

b. Stabilize fat emulsions

- HIGH glucose concentrations.

The commercial amino acid used will have a major impact on fat emulsion stability. Stability information should never be extrapolated between PN mixtures with different commercial sources of amino acids.

CHEMICAL DEGRADATION

Most ingredients are remarkably stable after compounding, at least during the normal shelf lives of PN mixtures, and in particular the 4-week shelf life most commonly used in practice.[27–32] There are three possible chemical mechanisms for the degradation of specific PN ingredients (Table 22.4).

Table 22.4 – Chemical mechanisms for PN degradation

Reaction	Most important candidate(s)
1. Oxidation	Vitamin C (ascorbic acid)
2. Reduction	Vitamin B_1 (thiamine)
3. Photodegradation	Vitamin A (retinol)
	Vitamin E (tocopherol)

Note firstly that these are all vitamins, so it is the addition of vitamins that subsequently limits the shelf life of PN mixtures. It is important to consider stability at two stages, during storage after compounding and during administration.

Vitamin C (ascorbic acid) degradation

The degradation pathway for ascorbic acid is shown in Figure 22.2. There are two important things to note. First, the first stage in the reaction is reversible; this is important because dehydro-ascorbic is equally biologically functional. Second, the reaction involves oxygen which can originate from:

1. Infusions and additives – glucose, electrolytes, water for reconstituting vitamins, but not amino acid infusions or fat emulsion, both of which are usually nitrogen–overlaid

2. Air in the bag after compounding, if not removed prior to sealing

3. Air which dissolves in the infusions during the filling process especially as they pass through the filling lines

4. Oxygen permeating through the bag wall during storage.

Oxygen reacts with ascorbic acid rapidly, catalysed by copper ions.[33,34] Within an hour or two, the oxygen will have reacted to reduce ascorbic acid to dehydro-ascorbic acid.[34] This in turn is further oxidized and/or hydrolysed to keto-gulonic acid. So the amount of

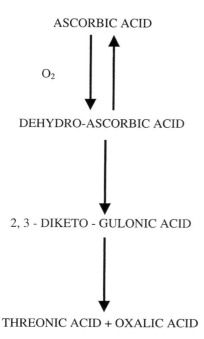

ASCORBIC ACID

O_2

DEHYDRO-ASCORBIC ACID

2, 3 - DIKETO - GULONIC ACID

THREONIC ACID + OXALIC ACID

Figure 22.2 – Ascorbic acid degradation pathway.

ascorbic acid degraded depends almost entirely on the amount of oxygen present in the PN mixture and bag after compounding and sealing.

As an example, it can be expected that the quantity of ascorbic acid degraded after compounding a typical adult formulation will amount to 40–60 mg.[34] In addition, degradation will continue as oxygen permeates through the EVA wall of the bag accounting for a further 10–15 mg per day.[34] This can be improved by using multi-layered bags, which are almost impermeable to oxygen. The secondary degradation stage is eliminated in these bags.[34] A comparison of ascorbate (AA + DHAA) degradation in EVA and multi-layered bags is illustrated in Figure 22.3. Note how degradation is initially rapid, but then the rate of losses level off to almost zero, after a few hours. This is accounted for by the initial reaction with dissolved oxygen in the PN infusion. Once all the oxygen has reacted, no further degradation of ascorbic acid takes place.

Ascorbic acid is the least stable ingredient in any PN mixture and some loss is inevitable. The amount the patient receives depends on the quantity of oxygen in the infusion and bag, and on the type of bag used. If an EVA bag, the maximum shelf life is only 3–5 days, because of the high oxygen permeability of EVA. In a multi-layered bag, the shelf life after compounding can be up to 4 weeks, provided the initial compounding is undertaken efficiently to avoid excess amounts of oxygen being present.[34,35]

Vitamin B₁ (thiamine) reduction

Thiamine is degraded by a reduction reaction with sodium metabisulphite.[33] Some amino acid infusions contain sodium metabisulphite as a reducing agent to prevent oxidation of amino acids during manufacture and storage. In fact, only one commercial product in the UK contains metabisulphite and that is Freamine III®. The likely losses in a PN mixture are illustrated in Figure 22.4. Note how degradation falls over time. Thiamine is stable for at least 28 days in other mixtures.[36]

Vitamin A (retinol) photodegradation

The most light-sensitive ingredient of any PN mixture is retinol (vitamin A).[28,37] But note the following important points:

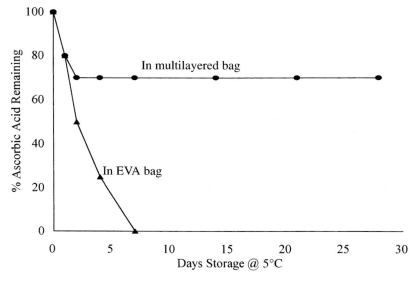

Figure 22.3 – Degradation of ascorbate in PN mixture during storage.

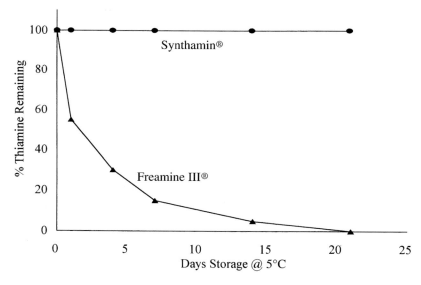

Figure 22.4 – Degradation of thiamine (added as Cernavit®) in a PN mixture containing Freamine III® or Synthamin®.

- Since degradation is caused by exposure to ultra-violet light (below 350 nm wavelength), therefore only daylight degrades retinol[38]

- Artificial light contains no UV emission

- Photodegradation will proceed both in the bag and in the administration set as the solution is infused.[37]

Many factors can influence the rate of retinol degradation during PN administration, including the time of day, the position with respect to the window, volume in bag, infusion rate, the presence of fat which reduces degradation, and the light protecting cover over bag.[28,37]

The practical outcomes for administration are that exposure to direct sunlight must be avoided, protecting the bag content with a cover is essential, not protecting the set will lead to some losses, administration at night or well away from a window will reduce losses substantially. Finally, the fat emulsion in 'all-in-one' mixtures offers some protection.[28]

DRUG ADDITIONS TO PN MIXTURES

It is generally recommended that drugs should only be added to PN mixtures if absolutely necessary. Evidence is available which identifies the compatibility and stability of specific drugs in particular mixtures.

H₂ antagonists

Cimetidine is stable in PN regimens, and shelf lives of up to 28 days have been indicated in certain mixtures.[39] In contrast, ranitidine is far less stable. Half-lives of only a few days are indicated in many regimens, although it is possible to extend this in multi-layered bags, as degradation is by oxidation.[40,41]

Heparin

Heparin is commonly added to mixtures for neonates, but great care is necessary to avoid destabilizing the fat emulsion, either in 'all-in-one' mixtures, or when non-fat mixtures mix with fat emulsion in the administration line. Standard heparin interacts with the emulsifying agent in fat emulsions, in the presence of calcium ions, to form calcium–heparin bridges.[42] The emulsion rapidly destabilizes and cracks within a few minutes. This risk can be avoided by using low molecular weight heparin.[42]

Hydrocortisone

Hydrocortisone – this drug is compatible, but relatively unstable in PN mixtures, and a shelf life of only a few days is indicated by studies.[42]

SUMMARY

This has been a summary of the major stability issues concerning PN compounding and administration. Losses of key ingredients will occur, although strategies can be adopted to minimize such losses. It is possible to assign extended shelf lives to some complete PN mixtures.

REFERENCES

1. Solassol C, Joyeux H, Etco L, Pujol H, Romieu C. New techniques for long term intravenous feeding: an artificial gut in 75 patients. *Ann Surg* 1974; **179**: 519–522.

2. Solassol C, Joyeux H, Etco L, Pujol H, Romieu C. Long-term parenteral nutrition: an artificial gut. *Int Surg* 1976; **61**: 266–270.

3. Hardy G. Ten years TPN with 3 litre bags. *Pharm J* 1987; H526–528.

4. British National Formulary: British Medical Association and Royal Pharmaceutical Society of Great Britain.

5. Pennington CR. Parenteral nutrition. In: Therapeutic Nutrition. Chapman and Hall Medical: Cambridge, 1988, p. 124.

6. Keller U. Zuckerersatzstoffe fructose und sorbit: ein unnotiges Risiko in der parenteralen. *Emhrung Schweiz Med Wochenschr* 1989; **119**: 101–106.

7. Richelle M, Deckelbaum RJ, Vanwyenberg V, Carpentier Y. Lipoprotein metabolism during and after a 6-h infusion of MCT/LCT vs LCT emulsion in man. *Clin Nutr* 1997; **16**:119–123.

8. Jeevanandum M, Holaday N, Voss T, Buier R, Peterson S. Efficiency of a mixture of MCT (75%) and LCT (25%) fat emulsions in nutritional management of multiple-trauma patients. *Nutrition* 1995; **11**: 275–283.

9. Adolph M, Hailer S, Eckart J. Serum phospholid fatty acids in severely injured patients on TPN with MCT/LCT emulsions. *Ann Nutr Metab* 1995; **39**: 251–260.

10. Hayes P, Martin T, Pybus J. Aluminium content of intravenous solutions, additives and equipment used to prepare parenteral nutrition mixtures. *Aust J Hosp Pharm* 1992; **22**(5): 353–359.

11. Bishop N, Morley R, Day J, Lucas A. Aluminium neurotoxicity in preterm infants receiving IV feeding solutions. *N Engl J Med* 1997; **22**: 1557–1558.

12. Shenkin A, Fell GS, Halls DJ, Dunbar PM, Holbrook IB, Irving MH. Essential trace element provision to patients receiving home intravenous nutrition in the United Kingdom. *Clin Nutr* 1986; **5**: 91–97.

13. Davis AT, Franz FP, Courtnay DA, Ullrey DE, Scholten DJ, Dean RE. Plasma vitamin and mineral status in home parenteral nutrition patients. *J Parenter Enteral Nutr* 1987; **11**: 480–485.

14. Pineault M, Chessex P, Piedboeuf B, Bisaillon S. Beneficial effect of co-infusing a lipid emulsion on venous patency. *J Parenter Enteral Nutr* 1989; **13**: 637–640.

15. Timmer JG, Schipper HG. Peripheral venous nutrition: the equal relevance of volume load and osmolarity in relation to phlebitis. *Clin Nutr* 1991; **10**: 71–75.

16. Eggert LD, Rusho WJ, MacKay MW, Chan GM. Calcium and phosphorus compatibility in parenteral nutrition solutions for neonates. *Am J Hosp Pharm* 1982; **39**: 49–53.

17. Durham B, Marcuard S, Khazanie PG, Meade G, Craft T, Nichols K. The solubility of calcium and phosphorus in neonatal total parenteral nutrition solutions. *J Parenter Enteral Nutr* 1991; **15**: 608–611.

18. Poole RL, Rupp CA, Kemer JA. Calcium and phosphorus in neonatal pameteral nutrition solutions. *J Parenter Enteral Nutr* 1983; **7**: 358–360.

19. Henry RS, Jurgens RW, Strugeon R, Athaniker N, Welco A, van Leuvan M. Compatibility of calcium chloride and calcium gluconate with sodium phosphate in a mixed TPN solution. *Am J Hosp Pharm* 1980; **37**: 673–674.

20. Allwood MC. The compatibility of calcium phosphate in paediatric TPN infusions. *J Clin Pharm Ther* 1987; **12**: 293–301.

21. Driscoll DF, Newton DW, Bistrion BR. Precipitation of calcium phosphate from parenteral nutrient fluids. *Am J Hosp Pharm* 1994; **51**: 2834–2836.

22. Kaminiski MV, Harris DF, Collin CF, Sommers GA. Electrolyte compatibility in a synthetic amino acid hyperalimantation solution. *Am J Hosp Pharm* 1974; **1**: 244–266.

23. Ronchera-Oms CL, Jimenez NV, Peidro J. Stability of parenteral nutrition admixtures containing organic phosphates. *Clin Nutr* 1995; **14**: 373–380.

24. Bates CG, Greiner G, Gegenheimer A. Precipitate in admixtures of new amino acid injection. *Am J Hosp Pharm* 1984; **41**: 1316.

25. Allwood MC. The compatibility of four trace elements in total parenteral nutrition infusions. *Inter J Pharmaceutics* 1983; **16**: 57–63.

26. Hardy G, Ball P, McElroy B. Basic principles for compounding all-in-one parenteral nutrition admixtures. *Clin Nutr Metab Care* 1998; **1**: 291–296.

27. Allwood MC. Stability of vitamins in TPN solutions stored in 3 L bags. *Br J Intraven Ther* 1982; **3**: 22–26.

28. Billion-Rey F, Guillaumont M, Frederich A, Aulanger G. Stability of fat-soluble vitamins A(retinol palmitate), E(tocopherol acetate) and Kl(phylloquinone) in total parenteral nutrition at home. *J Parenter Enteral Nutr* 1993; **17**: 56–60.

29. Dahl GB, Svensson L, Kinnander NJG, Zander M, Bergstrom UK. Stability of vitamins in soybean oil fat emulsion under conditions simulating intravenous feeding of neonates and children. *J Parenter Enteral Nutr* 1994; **18**: 234–239.

30. Dahl GB, Jeppson RI, Tengbom HJ. Vitamin stability in a TPN mixture stored in an EVA plastic bag. *J Clin Hosp Pharm* 1986; **11**: 271–279.

31. Schmutz CW, Martinelli E, Muhlebach S. Stability of vitamin KI assessed by HPLC in total parenteral nutrition. *Clin Nutr* (Suppl) 1992; **12**: 169.

32. Chen MF, Boyce W, Triplett L. Stability of B vitamins in mixed parenteral nutrition solution. *J Parenter Enteral Nutr* 1983; **7**: 462–464.

33. Allwood MC. Factors influencing the stability of ascorbic acid in total parenteral nutrition infusions. *J Clin Hosp Pharm* 1984; **9**: 75–85.

34. Allwood MC, Brown PE, Ghedini C, Hardy G. The stability of ascorbic acid in TPN mixtures stored in a multilayered bag. *Clin Nutr* 1992; **11**: 284–288.

35. Proot P, De Pourco L, Raymakers AA. Stability of ascorbic acid in a standard total parenteral nutrition mixture. *Clin Nutr* 1994; **13**: 273–279.

36. Keamey MJ, Allwood MC, Neal T, Hardy G. The stability of thiarnine in total parenteral nutrition mixtures stored in EVA and multilayered bags. *Clin Nutr* 1995; **14**: 295–301.

37. Allwood MC. The influence of light on vitamin A degradation during administration. *Clin Nutr* 1982; **1**: 63–70.

38. Allwood MC, Plane JH. The wavelength-dependent degradation of vitamin A exposed to ultraviolet light. *Inter J Pharmaceutics* 1986; **31**: 1–7.

39. Allwood MC, Martin H. The long term stability of cimetidine in total parenteral nutrition. *J Clin Pharm Ther* 1996; **21**: 19–21.

40. Allwood MC, Martin H. The stability of ranitidine in TPN mixtures. *Clin Nutr* 1995; **14**: 171–176.

41. Baumgartner TG, Henderson GN, Fox J, Gondi U. Stability of ranitidine and thiamine in parenteral nutrition solutions. *Nutrition* 1997; **13**: 547–553.

42. Wong C, Allwood MC, Everett NJ, McMahon MJ. Physical stability of a series of adult peripheral all-in-one admixtures containing heparin and hydrocortisone. *BAPEN Proc* 1993; 5–6.

23

Nursing and psychological aspects of care

Susanne Wood

The loss of a major organ's function challenges the integrity of the whole person. Although the primary changes may be physical they have an impact on how the person thinks and feels and this can limit future enjoyment of life.

Some patients with intestinal failure experience only a short illness before complete recovery, others such as those with an entero-cutaneous fistula may have longer periods of illness, possibly being left with a stoma or open wound. A few are left permanently disabled requiring long-term enteral and/or parenteral nutritional/fluid support. All patients require the same level of attention to their needs. Even those who appear to have responded well to treatment and achieved an excellent clinical outcome may be left with disabling fears resulting from their experiences.

Hospital admissions are often prolonged and the external world shrinks to that around the bedside, with the healthcare team, particularly nurses who usually spend most time with the patient, becoming the focus of social contact. Interactions take place while the nurse is giving personal care and treatment. As progress is commonly very slow and the care required arduous, for example changing a fistula appliance, nursing such patients can be physically and emotionally demanding.

Support systems to maintain the well-being of nurses, enabling them cope with the stress resulting from the care of patients with intestinal failure, need to be built into departmental organization. This can be achieved through strong leadership from an expert clinical nurse, staff development programmes, an open environment where feelings can be shared and the use of a model of care which provides a framework for safe, effective practice during hospital care, rehabilitation and ongoing treatment at home.

THE PATIENTS' UNDERSTANDING OF INTESTINAL FAILURE

Some of the features of intestinal failure which may include pain, nausea, diarrhoea, the effects of fistulas, difficult stomas, electrolyte imbalance and under-nutrition undermine the patients' dignity and sense of self-worth. There may be frequent, prolonged hospital admissions and numerous operations, each one being more difficult to face as the patients' experience of perioperative problems increase.

During acute illness feelings of helplessness are common and realistic. There is little the patient can control and events appear as an assault on the body and mind challenging the patients' belief in themselves as autonomous adults. For example, an inability to control the bowel and possibly seeing, and smelling, faeces draining from an abdominal wound may evoke primitive feelings about bowel function and being controlled by others in early life. Open wounds are often in a position where the patient can look into the body and see physical evidence of degeneration.

For the patient who develops chronic intestinal failure there is the daunting task of learning how to manage the condition at home, of becoming re-integrated into the family and society, and adapting expectations of daily life to one which may be different from that of other people and from their pre-morbid life.

THE BASIS, AIMS AND STRUCTURE OF NURSING CARE

In addition to the problems perceived by the patient are those arising from the pathology of the underlying disease and the physiological changes associated with intestinal failure. Some of these are life-threatening. Rapid alterations in water, electrolyte and glucose balance, the immediate risks of sepsis or haemorrhage and the long-term problems of undernutrition require close monitoring with medical and nursing interventions aimed at preventing them. For the patient needing home parenteral nutrition (HPN) the aims have to be adapted and made feasible for a community setting.

These problems impose physical and emotional constraints, which limit the patients' freedom to make choices about how they live and express their individuality. The extent of the restrictions depends equally upon the severity of the disease and the patients' tolerance of individual symptoms. The way in which a patient feels about different aspects of their condition is unique and commonly the weighting that they give to symptoms is at variance with that ascribed by health professionals. Patients often become frustrated or confused when an issue, which they believe important, receives little attention from doctors and nurses. Hence a barrier to communication may be created, and the patients' confidence in professional carers undermined.

The care of these patients is a dynamic process requiring regular re-assessment of their needs as life events occur or the disease progresses. For example, a teenager having HPN, living with their parents may have problems with establishing their identity as an adult. Likewise a person with a diagnosis of scleroderma, at first able to perform HPN unaided may, with time and disease progression, lose the ability to do so as their manual dexterity deteriorates. Future re-assessments should also take into account developments in medical practice and possibly the availability of intestinal transplantation.

Recognizing the patients' need to retain autonomy in the face of challenges to both the inner-being from anxiety, pain, the mental effects of dehydration, under-nutrition, drugs and anaesthetics, and the outer from changes in body image, physical weakness, alterations in relationships and social status creates an understanding of the patients' dilemma and forms a humane principle on which to base nursing care.

Treating patients with intestinal failure is a complex process requiring the skills of many disciplines; physicians, surgeons, nurses, dietitians, pharmacists, social workers and others. Each takes a part in replacing those functions which have been lost, supporting the patient through times when severe illness denies any self-determination, helping them make sense of what has happened and looking to the future during rehabilitation. Long-term care requires professionals to adopt a partnership role.

Nurses need to work collaboratively with other professionals to try to maximize the remaining gut function so reducing the disabling effects of the underlying disease, intestinal failure and invasive nutritional therapy, while at the same time helping the patient develop appropriate ways of coping.

An adaptation of Maslow's hierarchy of needs (Fig. 23.1) provides a realistic and workable method of organizing nursing care[1] and provides the structure for the rest of this chapter. It takes account of the requirement to achieve physiological stability before higher needs can be met. With the principles outlined above underpinning this framework, the nurse is provided with a model which can help to ensure the delivery of safe, effective and meaningful care.

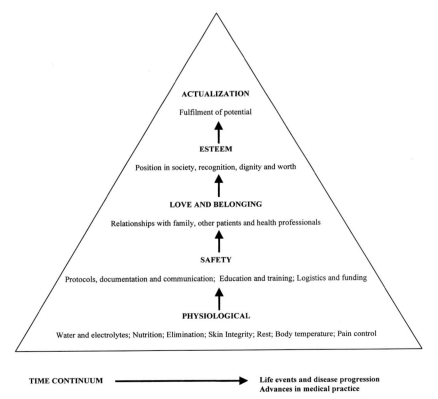

ACTUALIZATION

Fulfilment of potential

ESTEEM

Position in society, recognition, dignity and worth

LOVE AND BELONGING

Relationships with family, other patients and health professionals

SAFETY

Protocols, documentation and communication; Education and training; Logistics and funding

PHYSIOLOGICAL

Water and electrolytes; Nutrition; Elimination; Skin Integrity; Rest; Body temperature; Pain control

TIME CONTINUUM ⟶ **Life events and disease progression**
Advances in medical practice

Figure 23.1 – A model for the nursing care of patients with intestinal failure. Using a modification of Maslow's hierarchy of needs.[1]

PHYSIOLOGICAL NEEDS

Obtaining and maintaining physiological stability takes priority over other aspects of care because the physiological consequences of intestinal failure can threaten survival and impair other functions, such as the ability to think clearly, understand and learn (Table 23.1). Monitoring should be based on a sound understanding of how normal physiological processes have been altered in the individual patient. In order to achieve this, knowledge of current intestinal anatomy and the pathological effects of the underlying disease are essential.[2] Techniques and frequency of monitoring will depend on the clinical situation, the less stable, hospital-based patient, needing a greater intensity than the long-term patient living at home.

The analysis of monitoring records and development and implementation of a treatment plan is best performed collaboratively by all the professionals involved in the patient's care. This should be done through specially designed documentation and/or regular review meetings that are included in the organizational structure.

Water and electrolytes

Water, sodium and magnesium depletion cause most concern. Small bowel effluent contains approximately 100 mmol of sodium per litre[3] and excessive losses may occur if reabsorption is prevented by massive ileo-colonic resection, the presence of a jejunal stoma or a high small bowel fistula. The jejunal mucosa allows rapid flux of both water and sodium in order to maintain this concentration. In these patients, stomal/stool sodium losses are further increased by the oral intake of hypotonic, low sodium fluids.

A rapid increase in intestinal losses can lead to vascular collapse, hence the need for scrupulous records of fluid balance and daily body weight in the acutely sick or unstable patient. A fall in systolic blood pressure from lying to standing of more than 10 mmHg suggests water and sodium depletion. When total body sodium levels fall, conservation of sodium by the kidney helps to prevent further losses. Measuring the amount of sodium in a random specimen of urine is a helpful monitoring technique and values below 20 mmol/L indicate sodium depletion.[4] The frequency of clinical and biochemical assessments varies with the individual patient. Some patients with chronic negative water and sodium balance can gradually develop renal impairment.

Maintaining water and electrolyte balance

Those patients being treated for acute intestinal failure due to obstruction or entero-cutaneous fistula will usually receive water and electrolytes as part of an intravenous nutrition regimen, during a period of

Table 23.1 – Nursing aspects of physiological monitoring

Measurement	Target	
Volume of intestinal losses Speed of food transit	Effect of:	The disease process Dietary manipulation Medication to slow transit and reduce secretions.
Body weight	Daily:	Changes in fluid balance (1 kg = 1 L)
		Long-term changes in nutritional status
Records of fluid intake and output		Water and electrolyte balance
Clinical observation		
Thirst, lethargy, cramps, sunken dark ringed eyes, rapid low volume heart rate, dizziness on standing	Water and sodium status	
Lying and standing blood pressure		
Awareness of the urine concentration of sodium (aim > 20 mmol/L)		
Poor mental concentration, paraesthesia, tetany, cardiac arrhythmia, convulsions. Awareness of serum levels of magnesium aim for 0.7–1.0 mmol/L	Magnesium status	
Oedema, physical stamina, muscle mass, fat stores, signs of specific nutrient deficiencies	Nutritional status	
Awareness of serum albumin level aim for 35–45 g/L		

therapeutic bowel rest. Safe, reliable venous access is essential to ensure that the prescribed infusion is delivered on time.

Careful attention to mouth care will maintain good oral hygiene and may help to ameliorate some of the mental discomfort resulting from the lack of oral intake. If there are no medical contraindications, fruit juice mouthwashes or ice cubes can provide oral stimulation.

As thirst is one of the early symptoms of sodium depletion, it is important for the nurse to ensure that the patient understands the danger of drinking large amounts of water, tea, squashes, water and other hypotonic fluids, which will literally flush sodium from the body. If oral intake is possible, in addition to restricting hypotonic fluids, an oral rehydration solution, made from glucose 20 g (110 mmol), sodium chloride 3.5 gm (60 mmol), sodium bicarbonate 2.5 g (or sodium citrate 2.9 g) (30 mmol) diluted in 1 litre of water, may be prescribed to replace water and sodium losses. The solution is rather unpalatable and is best sipped, chilled and possibly slightly flavoured with fruit juice. Patients needing to continue this treatment at home should learn how to make the solution. The pharmacist will provide either the measured ingredients mixed ready for adding to water or measuring scoops for the individual ingredients. The patient is less dependent on the pharmacy with the latter method.[5]

Separating solids and liquids in the diet may slow gastrointestinal transit, so promoting the absorption of nutrients and reducing water and electrolyte losses. The effect of withholding fluids for approximately 45 minutes before and after a meal can be monitored by recording the time taken for food to pass through the gut (by asking the patient) and the volume of intestinal fluid losses.

For patients with very high intestinal losses, persistently greater than 2 litres a day, it is likely that parenteral supplementation of electrolytes will be required. If needs are limited to sodium chloride infusions, the subcutaneous route may be selected. Otherwise intravenous infusions of sodium chloride, magnesium and occasionally potassium may be prescribed to be administered alone or with other nutrients as part of a HPN regimen.

Magnesium

While there is commonly a high level of awareness about the importance of water and sodium balance, deficiency of magnesium may not be appreciated until clinical signs occur. These are often first observed by the nurse. Realizing the significance of rather jerky movements, paraesthesiae and occasionally tetany (if also hypocalcaemic), and timely reporting them to the clinician can avoid progression to fits.

Nutrition

Failure of the main function of the intestine, to digest and absorb nutrients increases the risk of undernutrition. Even if large amounts of food are eaten the reduction of intestinal absorptive capacity may lead to severe weight loss. This can be very difficult for the patient and others to understand and can be the cause of great distress. The nurse should discover patients' beliefs about their condition, correct any misunderstandings and provide explanations for patients and, if requested by the patient, to any family or friends. Otherwise fantasies may develop as the result of inaccurate interpretation of symptoms and confusion occurring during patient teaching.

Weight loss combines with other factors, such as the presence of stomas, wounds, tubes entering the body and fluids leaving it, to distort body image. It is easy for professionals to forget that the thin sick person they see may have an internal picture of a healthy wellnourished young-looking self. Dressing in clothes, which are now too big, and seeing the reflection in mirrors confirms these differences to the patient and the nurse needs to be sensitive to the effect this has on self-esteem. All members of the professional team need to be aware of the way in which they approach the patient, addressing the inner person not the outer image.

The effects of undernutrition due to intestinal failure are the same as those due to other causes. Muscle weakness, impaired immune competence, delayed wound healing and psychological disturbances are not only potentially life-threatening but also add to the difficulty of dealing with the condition. Feelings of hopelessness and loss of motivation are realistic in the face of trying to manage a high output stoma or fistula or profuse diarrhoea when lack of energy limits physical stamina and flattens any emotional response.

Maintaining nutritional status

The aim of care is to achieve a body weight, which provides strength, energy and appearance, acceptable to the patient. For patients other than those with a fistula or obstruction, being treated by therapeutic bowel rest and parenteral nutrition, every attempt is made to promote the enteral absorption of nutrients through manipulation of the diet and measures to maximize remaining intestinal function.

Food

The ideal diet for a patient with intestinal failure is variable and depends upon remaining bowel anatomy (Chapter 22). In general, foods which appear to increase the volume of stomal/stool output and the speed at which it occurs (e.g. those high in fibre, lactose and fat) are generally avoided. However, food restrictions must be balanced against the need to ensure a high nutrient intake, this is particularly important for fat which has a high energy density. In practice the foods tolerated by a patient are variable and cannot always be predicted. Some well-tolerated foods may suddenly, for no obvious reason, temporarily cause high gut losses, which later may return to their previous acceptable amount.

For the nurse it is important to ensure the patient receives the appropriate diet and that the effect is carefully monitored, by recording the volume of intestinal losses and/or the speed of food transit, and communicating these results to the doctor and dietitian. Prescribed medication, such as loperamide and codeine phosphate, designed to control transit and H_2 antagonists to control secretions are administered approximately 45–60 minutes prior to meals. Loperamide may need to be tipped out of its capsule. Within the hospital a self-medication programme should be considered, as this therapy is likely to continue at home.

Liquid supplements and tube feeding

In order to increase nutrient intake, liquid supplements may be prescribed and sipped between meals. Sometimes this is extended to overnight tube feeding, so using the gut 24 hours a day. If it is anticipated that the treatment will need to continue long-term the naso-gastric route may be used initially to test therapeutic benefit and patient tolerance before conversion to a gastrostomy. However, the choice between nightly self-naso-gastric intubation and a gastrostomy should be the patient's, following discussion with the nutrition team. Details of discharge planning for enteral tube feeding at home are described in Table 23.2.

Parenteral nutrition

Hospital-based patients with intestinal failure due to fistula or obstruction will often have nutritional status

Table 23.2 – Home enteral tube feeding – discharge planning

Enteral access	
Naso-gastric tube	Check supply in community, identify who has skills and is available to replace tube if it becomes displaced or blocked
Gastrostomy or jejunostomy	Provide information on care of the stoma site, how to prevent blockage and how to obtain and replace a damaged hub
Feed	Identify who will be prescribing and providing the feed and when the first delivery will be made. On discharge supply sufficient feed to ensure uninterrupted therapy Provide information on appropriate nutritional monitoring in the home and who will perform dietetic follow-up
Pump and equipment	Arrangements for the supply of the pump and equipment must be in place before discharge

maintained by parenteral nutrition, administered according to a standard hospital protocol. In chronic intestinal failure, when the enteral absorption of nutrients is inadequate to support life and health, parenteral nutrition at home will be needed either as a supplement, or less commonly as the sole source of nutrition.

While it is possible for HPN to maintain a normal for the patient body weight, this is at the expense of a therapy, which requires a high level of commitment by the patient to ensure success, and even with careful planning does restrict daily life.

Venous access When an intravenous device is inserted for parenteral nutrition, consideration should be given to whether it will be needed for treatment at home. Ensuring the catheter is accessible to the patient and in a position where it will not be visible when clothing is worn is of equal importance to selecting a device suitable for long-term use. The choice between a catheter with an external segment (Broviac or Hickman type) and a totally implanted access port should only be made following discussions with the patient (Table 23.3). Both are safe for HPN in motivated, competent patients.[6]

Intravenous regimen The volume and frequency of infusions are determined by calculating the water,

Table 23.3 – Selecting a venous catheter

Catheters with an external segment

Advantages
  Easy to handle and repair
  Possible to sterilize if it becomes infected

Disadvantages
  Visible evidence of the disability
  Requires dressings
  Possible infection risk when wet

Implanted ports

Advantages
  Not visible
  No dressing when not in use
  Freedom to bathe or swim

Disadvantages
  Need for repeated needle stick
  Difficult to sterilize if it becomes infected

electrolyte and nutrient requirements (Chapter 18). High stomal and fistula losses usually require daily intravenous replacement of water and sodium. If the colon is in continuity with the small bowel water and sodium absorption, and the salvaging of energy from the bacterial fermentation of carbohydrate, may reduce the need for daily replacement. In this case HPN patients can choose the infusion nights, giving a sense of freedom and control over their treatment.

The infusion rate is dependent on the individual patient's tolerance of the fluid volume, potassium and glucose content. When increasing flow rates to change from a 24-hour to an overnight infusion, the rate should be reduced to 50 ml/h for the last 30 minutes of the infusion period to prevent hypoglycaemia due to the sudden cessation of a high glucose intake.

Volumetric pumps used in hospital may be inappropriate for the patient at home. Infusions of greater than 10–12 hours can severely limit domestic and social life and an ambulatory system should be provided. Even the patient having infusions only during the period of sleep may have difficulty moving a stand, pump and large container of feed when making frequent visits to the bathroom to pass urine due to the rapid infusion rate. Care is needed in the selection of a safe, lightweight pump: with provision for repair or replacement within 12 hours of a fault occurring and a 6-monthly service, and a stable stand which can be wheeled over carpets.

Elimination

Management of a high output stoma or fistula requires detailed stoma care (Chapter 4). Preventing leakage is important not only to avoid sore skin but also to reduce the patient's anxiety and ensure accurate measurement of the effluent. Planned appliance changes should take place when the output is lowest, usually in the morning before eating and drinking, with adequate privacy. If the output is very high, the aid of a suction machine may help to draw the fluid away from the stoma while the adhesive flange is applied to the skin. The stoma spout should be prominent enough to permit a close seal.

When the bowel is in continuity frequent, profuse diarrhoea with urgency can make the patient's life a misery. The liquid nature of the stool often leads to incontinence, with problems of peranal soreness and malodour. Such patients may be referred to a continence service for advice on the selection of pads, but unfortunately remedies are often far from satisfactory.

To reduce intestinal losses, patients often avoid eating and drinking before leaving home and take care to always be close to a public toilet.

Skin integrity

The effects of poor nutrition on wound healing may be direct through dehydration, reduced nutrient availability, or indirect in the development of infection from impaired immune competence. Furthermore lack of mobility due to weakness may contribute to pressure sore development.

In addition to good wound management, maintaining adequate nutrition and hydration are fundamental in promoting wound healing. Patients dependent on enteral support may require additional vitamin and zinc supplementation. Occasionally these may cause nausea and the nurse should discuss any symptoms and possible alternatives with the pharmacist.

Rest

Obtaining adequate rest in hospital is difficult for many reasons. Anxiety, noise, light, frequent disturbance for treatment all play a part in exhausting the patient. Treatment should be planned to reduce disturbance, for example by connecting a high output stoma or fistula appliance to a continuous drainage system to avoid the need for frequent emptying and reduce the risk of leakage.

When patients are discharged home, especially those receiving HPN, the anxiety about leaving the hospital and the sense of achievement at managing the treatment is often followed within several weeks by depression as the reality of future life becomes evident. In addition to informing the patient that this may happen, advice should be given about conserving energy, by taking short rests in the day, in order to cope with the emotional work needed during this period of change.

Arrangements should be made for the patient to easily contact named professionals in whom they have confidence when these or other problems occur. Encouraging an activity, within physical capacity, which gives pleasure and expresses individuality helps to provide continuity with the past life and anchors the patient to the present.

Body temperature/infection risks

Undernourished patients may feel the cold and easily develop hypothermia (Chapter 13) thus they need adequate warmth in hospital and at home.

There is a constant risk of infection, particularly from wounds and invasive devices such as intravenous lines. Infection control policies for the management of both should be clear and realistic. This is most important for patients receiving HPN in whom unnecessarily complex procedures may limit observance. Teaching principles – disinfection of the catheter entry site and hub with chlorhexidine 0.5% in 70% ethyl alcohol,[7] the use of sterile gloves when handling connections and to avoid touching inner parts of the connections – provides a sound basis for practice.

Protocols should also be in place for actions to be taken by the patient, general practitioner and hospital staff should the patient notice a temperature or rigors at home.

Pain control

Pain may arise from physical or emotional causes. The anxiety surrounding dependence on others, frequent medication and artificial support systems; the sight of open wounds and experience of painful dressings; loss of control over bowel function combine together to create what can become an intractable problem. Professionals may become frustrated by an inability to control the pain adding to the patient's anxiety, and resort to increasing doses of powerful analgesia. A pain

control team can provide expert advice and external support for both patient and professional carers. Poor outcomes have been identified in patients receiving HPN dependent on opiates and sedatives.[8]

SAFETY

Protocols, documentation and communication

Standard hospital protocols for the management of parenteral nutrition should be tailored to the needs of the individual who requires HPN (Table 23.4).

Table 23.4 – Home parenteral nutrition – factors influencing protocol design

Physical condition	Dexterity Stamina Sensory perception
Motivation	Prognosis Psychosocial adaptation
Home conditions	Hand basins, stairs, doorways and carpets Space for performing procedures and storing equipment
Family and social life	Time to perform procedures Possibility of travel

Organizing HPN can seem a daunting task, but through methodical planning a smooth transition from hospital to home can be achieved (Table 23.5). Particular care is needed when communicating with those healthcare professionals who may have little experience of HPN, the general practitioner, the medical and pharmaceutical advisors to the commissioning authority responsible for funding and community nursing teams. Clear information is essential to promote confidence and develop good relationships between, the patient, primary care team and hospital staff.

Education and training

Anxiety, pain, poor concentration due to water and electrolyte imbalance, weakness, unfamiliar equipment and language, distractions in the environment are all barriers to learning. To avoid the effect of different teaching styles one nurse should take responsibility for

Table 23.5 – Home parenteral nutrition – discharge protocol and documentation in UK

1. Assess patient's nursing needs	*Nursing care plan*
2. Achieve clinical and nutritional stability	*Prescription form*
3. Draw up list of equipment (including pump and refrigerator)	*Equipment list*
4. Arrange funding (if no established contract)	*Health Authority (HA) information pack*
Contact the health commissioning authority of the patient's residence for details of their preferred provider.	
If HA has no preferred provider, select one (usually a commercial home care company)	
5. Send HPN prescription and equipment list to designated provider	
6. Contact general practitioner (GP)	*GP information pack*
7. Agree provisional discharge date with patient, family, hospital team, GP and HPN provider	
8. Teach knowledge/skills for HPN while above are taking place	*Patient information pack, Teaching plan including learning goals*
If nursing assistance needed to perform procedures at home, discuss with district nurses	
9. Establish protocol for 24-hour telephone emergency contact access	*Emergency contact card*
10. Refer to medical social worker for social security benefits advice	*Benefit claim forms*
11. Inform about support group.	*PINNT application form*
Arrange for patient to meet a suitable HPN patient (if they wish)	
12. When learning goals are achieved confirm discharge date and arrange for delivery of feed and equipment to home, before discharge if possible	
13. On discharge provide the patient with equipment for 3 days HPN, medication to take home, copy of the feed prescription, equipment list and details of first out-patient visit	
14. Arrange to telephone the patient at a specified time in the evening after the feed has been connected for the first time	
15. Visit the patient at home soon after discharge. Meet the GP if possible.	*Post discharge visit checklist*

an individual patient, using a structured programme (Table 23.6).

It should be recognized that learning HPN can be exhausting. Practical procedures require the patient to walk to a hand basin, wash the hands according to protocol, prepare the sterile surface, perform the procedure, clear the equipment and, with the teaching nurse, reflect upon and modify practice.

Logistics and funding

Arrangements for the funding of HPN, supply of feed and equipment and follow-up care must be in place before the patient leaves hospital. This high cost, rare (approximately 300 cases in the UK in 1997[9]) treatment is currently funded by the authority responsible for commissioning health care in the patients area of residence. Often a commercial supplier will be contracted to provide the feed, equipment and sometimes specialist nursing care, being paid either directly by the commissioning authority or via the discharging hospital who can better monitor the service.

The equipment supplied at home may be from a different manufacturer and look different to that used in hospital. Assembling all the requirements, from hospital stock, for the first few days' therapy at home allows the patient time to become accustomed to the new equipment and can help to reduce anxiety.

Only in exceptional circumstances should a patient be discharged immediately before or during a weekend or public holiday when health services are limited.

LOVE AND BELONGING

Relationships with family, other patients and health professionals

It is easy for patients receiving HPN to feel isolated, even within their own family. Everyone deals with these feelings in their own way. For some, membership of a support group, such as Patients on Intravenous and

Table 23.6 – Home parenteral nutrition – patient learning goals

1. The principles of normal intestinal function
2. How gut function has changed in themself and the need for home parenteral nutrition
3. How to minimize the effects of the intestinal changes and those of the underlying disease
4. The principles of parenteral nutrition
5. The principles of asepsis
6. How to: Manage the catheter entry site
       Make additives to the feed
       Connect the infusion to the catheter
       Manage an infusion pump, recognize and respond to alarms
       Disconnect the infusion
       Irrigate the catheter
       Protect the catheter from seat belts and during swimming
7. How to prevent, recognize and respond to:
       Fever
       Central venous occlusion
       Catheter occlusion
       Catheter fracture
       Hyper/hypoglycaemia
       Fluid and sodium imbalance
8. How to store and check nutrient solutions and how they will be delivered
9. How to store and order equipment and how it will be delivered
10. How to obtain expert help 24 hours a day
11. The details of follow-up arrangements
12. The existence of a patient support group (PINNT)
13. The social security benefits to which they may be entitled
14. How to explain their condition to others
15. Know to take antibiotics (like a patient with a prosthetic heart valve) before dental or medical procedures

Naso-gastric Nutrition Therapy (PINNT) in the UK, can be helpful. Others prefer to keep their feelings private. Professional carers need to create an environment in which the patient is able to share their experiences and receive compassionate support.

For some patients the problems are too complex to cope with, producing a range of overt and covert manifestations of emotional distress. This in no way implies failure on the patient's part but requires the professional carers to provide a more supportive framework, which might include counselling and psychotherapy.

ESTEEM

Position in society, recognition, dignity and worth

Living as a disabled person in a society prejudiced against disability leads to a variety of responses. Many patients with chronic intestinal failure needing HPN look well only because they have faced the difficulties of their daily life and committed themselves to the struggle needed to maintain their health. They share the frustrations experienced by people living with other hidden illnesses in that they wish to feel and look well, not be pitied but have the reality of their situation acknowledged.

SELF-ACTUALIZATION

Fulfilment of potential

Most individuals aspire to, rather than achieve, full potential. The way in which a patient chooses to live is unique to that person and the nurse should respect that right and avoid value judgements. Working with patients who face great difficulties, yet are able to create and enjoy a satisfying life, challenges professionals to consider their own belief systems.

REFERENCES

1. Maslow AH. Toward a Psychology of Being, 2nd edn. Van Nostrand Reinhold: New York, 1968.

2. Wood SR. Nutrition and the short bowel syndrome. In: Myers C (ed) *Stoma Care: A Patient-centred Approach.* Edward Arnold: London, 1996.

3. Davis GR, Santa Ane CA, Morawsli SG, Fordtran JS. Permeability characteristics of human jejunum, ileum, proximal colon and distal colon: results of potential difference in measurements and unidirectional fluxes. *Gastroenterology* 1982; **83**: 844–850.

4. Ladefoged K, Olgaard K. Fluid and electrolyte absorption and renin angiotensin-aldosterone axis in patients with severe short bowel syndrome. *Scand J Gastroenterol* 1979; **14**: 729–735.

5. Lennard-Jones JE. Oral rehydration solution in short bowel syndrome. *Clin Ther* 1990: **12** (Suppl A): 129–137.

6. Howard L, Claunch C, McDowell R, Timchalk M. Five years of experience in patients receiving home nutrition

7. support with the implanted reservoir: a comparison with the external catheter. *J Parenter Enteral Nutr* 1988; **13**: 478–483.

7. Rannem T, Ladefogel K, Hegnhoj J, Hylander Moller E, Bruun B, Jarnum S. Catheter related sepsis in long term parenteral nutrition with Broviac catheters. An evaluation of different disinfectants. *Clin Nutr* 1990; **9**: 131–136.

8. Richards DM, Scott NA, Shaffer JL, Irving M. Opiate and sedative dependence predicts poor outcome for patients receiving home parenteral nutrition. *J Parenter Enteral Nutr* 1997; **21**: 336–338.

9. British Artificial Nutrition Survey 1997; The British Association for Parenteral and Enteral Nutrition.

24

Management of a high-output jejunostomy

J. M. D. Nightingale

*M*ost of the classical work published about patients with a short residual length of intestine has related to those with jejunum in continuity with colon.[1-3] An increasing number of patients with a jejunostomy are being managed, mainly because the colon is often removed during the surgical treatment of Crohn's disease. These patients have immediate and serious problems because of large intestinal losses of water, sodium and magnesium. The residual bowel length may not have been measured and such patients are often categorized as having ileostomy diarrhoea. The management of patients with a jejunostomy, ileostomy diarrhoea or a high-output enterocutaneous fistula is the same. This chapter outlines the medical problems caused by the large volumes of fluid lost from the stoma or fistula and, using data from balance studies, discusses treatments. Information about stoma care is found in Chapter 4.

PRESENTATION OF PATIENTS WITH A JEJUNOSTOMY

The problem of fluid loss from a jejunostomy is apparent immediately after the surgery that removes the bowel. The fasting stomal output may be 2 or more litres in 24 hours, and it will rise when food and drink are consumed to as much as 8 or more litres a day. This results in dehydration, sodium depletion and hypomagnesaemia which must be recognized and treated. These patients are dependent on their treatment; if they miss a day of treatment, they become very unwell from dehydration.

Patients with a jejunostomy do have problems of protein–energy undernutrition but these develop slowly over several weeks and are usually attended to at the same time as the fluid balance problems. The nutritional problems should be predicted and treated before the patient becomes undernourished.

BALANCE STUDIES

Balance studies have provided the most useful information about the problems and the management of patients with a jejunostomy. They are easier to perform in patients with a jejunostomy than in patients with a short bowel and a preserved colon as a 1–3-day run-in period is not required, and the stomal bag allows for easier collection.

Patients with a short bowel may not feel hungry, and those with a jejunostomy are often just in positive water and sodium balance, so cannot abruptly stop treatments that are maintaining their equilibrium. Patients who suddenly stop taking codeine phosphate when they have been taking it for several months or years are likely to develop the symptoms and signs of opiate withdrawal, which include diarrhoea, manifested as a rise in stomal output. Balance studies are rarely done in the ideal experimental setting with the patient taking no drugs.

There are three possible ways to study intestinal balance in patients with a short bowel. With each, a duplicate oral intake is made and assayed.

1. Test meal

A standardized meal containing a non-absorbable marker (e.g. polyethylene glycol) is given and the stool or stomal output is collected for a fixed period while nothing else is taken orally. Rodrigues *et al.* showed that over 90% of a non-absorbable marker in a liquid test meal was recovered from jejunostomy fluid in the 6 hours after the meal.[4,5] This technique is not appropriate for patients with a retained colon as the time taken for the food residue to be passed in the stool may be 2–3 days.

2. Investigator-selected diet

For each 24-hour period, the investigator specifies the exact composition and amount and the time at which food and drink are to be consumed by the patient. This is an experimental ideal but patients with a short bowel are fastidious eaters who often feel full very quickly, and such a study is difficult to perform in practice. Studies have been done, however, in which the proportion and total amount of macronutrients and fluid are fixed.[6] A 2-day collection is adequate for patients with a jejunostomy, but if the colon has been retained a run-in period of at least 2 days is needed, so that remnants of other meals will have been passed in the stool.

3. Patient-selected diet

Patients select a diet freely on the first study day and eat and drink whatever is normal for them. They keep an accurate record of the food and drink, the amount and the time at which it is consumed. On all subsequent study days they consume exactly the same food and drink in the same amounts and at exactly the same times as on the first day. All studies by Nightingale *et al.* use this method for 2 paired control days and 2 further paired test days when a therapy is given.[7]

The way in which stool, ileostomy or jejunostomy output is analysed is important. When jejunostomy output is centrifuged, three layers are seen: fat at the top, fluid in the middle and solid at the bottom. In general, the higher the output the larger the middle layer of fluid; if the output is low (less than 1 litre daily) then it may not be possible to see a fluid layer, and the fatty layer and the solid component merge together. Most studies perform all analyses on an aliquot of the total mixed output (e.g. Nightingale *et al.*). This involves freeze-drying a sample for bomb calorimetry and determination of the energy content, mixing with acid and filtering for some electrolyte measurements (e.g. sodium and potassium), and ashing and mixing with acid for others (e.g. calcium and magnesium). It is simpler to aspirate the fluid layer, filter it, and assay for electrolytes; however this can only be done when there is a large liquid output and when the patient is taking little or no solid food. It is often difficult in publications to determine on which part of the output the assay has been performed.

REASONS FOR THE HIGH VOLUME OF JEJUNOSTOMY OUTPUT

A stoma may produce a high output if there is intra-abdominal sepsis, enteritis (e.g. Clostridium or Salmonella), partial or intermittent bowel obstruction, recurrent disease in the remaining bowel (e.g. Crohn's disease or irradiation) or sudden stopping of drugs (steroids or opiates). If these are not present, there are three potential reasons for the high volume of output: loss of the normal daily secretions produced in response to food, gastric acid hypersecretion, and rapid gastrointestinal transit.

Loss of normal daily intestinal secretions

The most important reason for a large volume of stomal output is that the normal daily intestinal secretions produced in response to food and drink (about 4 litres/day) cannot be reabsorbed in the short length of bowel remaining, so are lost through the stoma. In most normal subjects, about 6 litres of chyme pass the duodeno-jejunal flexure daily and the meal is still just diluted by intestinal secretions 100 cm distal from the duodeno-jejunal flexure.[8,9] When the small bowel length is less than this, more emerges from the stoma than is taken in by mouth. Even in the fasting state there is an obligatory loss of intestinal secretions produced with the migrating myoelectric complex (MMC).[10]

Gastric acid hypersecretion

There is some evidence to suggest, at least in the short term, that loss of intestinal phase negative feedback inhibition results in hypergastrinaemia[11,12] and gastric acid hypersecretion, which may all contribute to the high output from a jejunostomy (Ch. 12). In man, gastric acid hypersecretion has only been demonstrated in the immediate postoperative period in patients with a retained colon.[13] It is unclear whether this phenomenon persists beyond the first weeks, but a low pH (<6) in the fresh stomal effluent when it exceeds 1 litre daily is suggestive.

Rapid gastrointestinal transit

Rapid gastric emptying of liquid occurs and may increase the stomal output[14] (Fig. 24.1). The gastric emptying rate is fastest in those with the shortest lengths of residual jejunum. Small bowel transit time for liquid and solid is also very rapid.[14] Both of these effects may be mainly due to low serum levels of peptide YY[12] and, to a lesser extent, low levels of GLP-2.[15]

THE PROBLEM OF HIGH-VOLUME JEJUNOSTOMY OUTPUT

Water and sodium losses

Balance studies in patients with a jejunostomy, using a patient-selected diet, showed that the daily weight of stomal output was about 6–8 kg/d in those on parenteral nutrition with added saline and about 2 kg/d among those receiving oral supplements. The intestinal output is mostly water (mean 92%, range 85–96%) and there is a good correlation between stomal output weight and its sodium content (Fig. 24.2). The mean jejunostomy sodium concentration is 88 mmol/L, being lower in patients with a shorter remaining length of jejunum and higher in those with

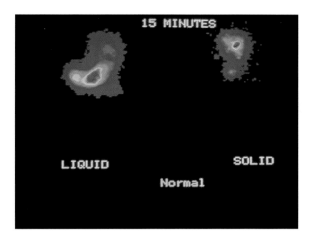 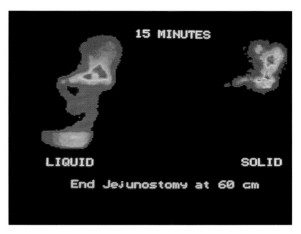

Figure 24.1 – Gastric emptying of liquid and solid in a normal subject (a) and in a patient (b) with a jejunostomy 30 cm from the duodeno-jejunal flexure 15 minutes after starting to eat a meal of a pancake and orange juice.

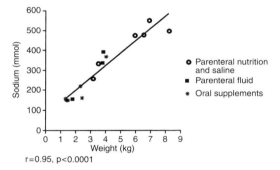

r=0.95, p<0.0001

Figure 24.2 – Wet weight and sodium content of jejunostomy output for 15 patients with less than 200 cm remaining jejunum. (r=0.96, p<0.0001). The mean sodium concentration was 88 mmol/L (range 60–118 mmol).

more. The sodium concentration in the terminal ileum may be nearer to that of plasma (140 mmol/L).

Type of patient with a jejunostomy

Classification of patients with a jejunostomy is based upon balance studies using a patient-selected diet. The weight and sodium content of the diet is compared to the weight and sodium content of the stomal output. The patients can be divided into one of two groups, either net 'secretors' or net 'absorbers', according to intestinal water and sodium balance. This balance depends upon the degree of dilution of food and drink

by digestive juices and the net absorption that has occurred[7] (Fig. 24.3).

'**Absorbers**' tend to have more than 100 cm of residual jejunum and can absorb more water and sodium from their diet (which may have been modified to have an increased amount of sodium) than they take orally. Their daily jejunostomy output is usually about 2 kg or less in 24 hours, thus they can be managed with oral sodium and water supplements and parenteral fluids are not needed.

'**Secretors**' tend to have less than 100 cm of residual jejunum and lose more water and sodium from their stoma than they take by mouth. Usual daily stomal output may be 4–8 kg. These patients cannot convert from negative to positive water and sodium balance by taking a modified diet or sodium supplements and they need long-term parenteral supplements.[7] These requirements change very little with time.[16] The jejunostomy output from a net 'secretor' increases during the daytime in response to food and decreases at night, thus any drug therapy that aims to reduce the output must be given prior to food (Fig. 24.4).

A clinician, unlike a research worker, is unlikely to be able to perform accurate balance studies, in which case the classification can be predicted from knowledge of the residual jejunal length. The change from a net secretory state to a net absorptive state in terms of intestinal water and sodium balance occurs at a jejunal length of about 100 cm.

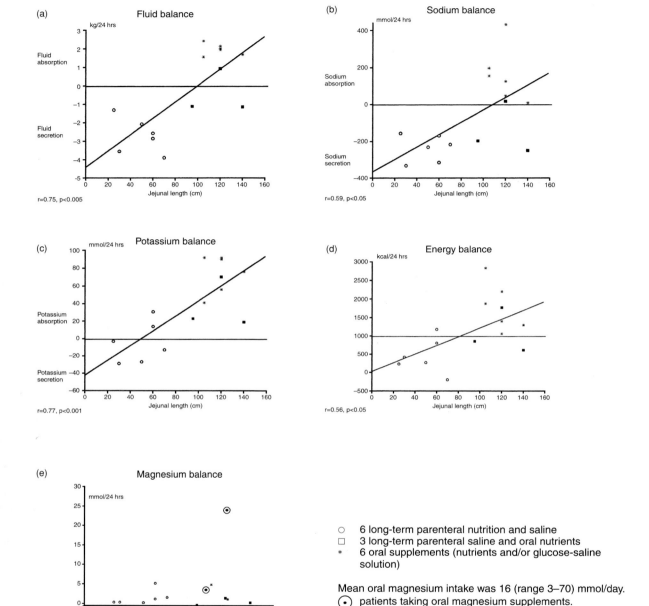

Figure 24.3 – Balance studies using the patient-selected diet performed for 2 days on 15 patients with a jejunostomy who were all maintaining fluid, electrolyte and nutritional status. Six needed long-term intravenous nutrition, 3 required long-term intravenous fluids but maintained their nutrition with an oral diet, and 6 took oral fluid and nutrient supplements.[7] (a) Total weight, (b) sodium, (c) potassium (d) energy and (e) magnesium. Note that positive intestinal fluid and sodium balance is achieved at 100 cm jejunum, potassium at 50 cm, and there was no relationship with magnesium balance.

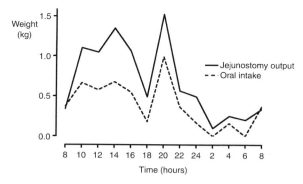

Figure 24.4 – Oral intake (kg) and stomal output measured every 2 hours in a patient who has 30 cm of residual jejunum and shows net secretion.

Potassium deficiency

The effluent from a jejunostomy or ileostomy contains relatively little potassium (about 15 mmol/L).[7,17,18] Values are higher in patients with a colostomy as the colon secretes potassium. Potassium problems are unusual and the potassium intake rarely needs to be greater than normal. Net loss through the stoma occurs only when less than 50 cm of jejunum remains[7] (Fig. 24.3c).

Low serum potassium levels do not usually reflect gut losses, but may occur when a patient is sodium depleted and thus has secondary hyperaldosteronism. The high aldosterone levels cause renal conservation of sodium at the expense of potassium, which is excreted in the urine in greater amounts than normal.[17–19]

Hypomagnesaemia causes dysfunction of many of the potassium transport systems (e.g. the Na^+/K^+-ATPase pump) and increases renal excretion of potassium; thus hypomagnesaemia can cause a hypo-kalaemia, which is resistant to potassium treatment.[20]

Before hypokalaemia can be corrected in patients with a high-output stoma, sodium and water depletion must be corrected and the serum magnesium brought into the normal range.

Magnesium deficiency

Patients with a jejunostomy are often in precarious magnesium and calcium balance,[21,22] and the balance does not correlate with residual jejunal length (Fig. 24.3e). Magnesium deficiency is common: 70% of patients who were not receiving parenteral nutrition needed magnesium supplements.[16] It may cause fatigue, depression, irritability, muscle weakness, tetany

if there is associated hypocalcaemia, and, if very severe, convulsions. High aldosterone levels increase urinary magnesium losses and a high–fat diet binds to magnesium to increase the amount in the stomal output[23] (Ch. 12).

Nutrient malabsorption

In the long term, parenteral nutrition with additional fluids is always needed if a patient absorbs less than one-third of the oral energy intake[4,7] and is usually needed when less than 75 cm of jejunum remain. In some young people with high-energy requirements, parenteral nutrition may be needed even when absorption is 35–60%.

MANAGEMENT OF HIGH-VOLUME OUTPUT FROM A JEJUNOSTOMY

1. Exclude other causes of a high output

Intra–abdominal sepsis, enteritis, partial or intermittent bowel obstruction, recurrent disease or sudden stopping of drugs need to be excluded. An Addisonian crisis can cause a high stomal output in a patient who has been on steroids for a long time when the drugs are suddenly stopped at the time of surgery. This must be recognized immediately, blood taken and plasma frozen for a cortisol level, and intravenous hydro-cortisone given.

2. Define the problem

Clinical assessment

The initial assessment of water and sodium deficiencies involves asking the patient about feeling dry, thirsty, lethargic, faint or having muscle weakness and cramps. Examination may detect dry mucous membranes, reduced skin turgor and postural systolic hypotension. A rapid fall in body weight and negative fluid balance with a low urine volume are important guides. In general, patients who have a stomal output of more than 2 litres daily fasting or when they eat are likely to require water and sodium supplements.

If dehydration is severe, serum creatinine and urea will rise. Urinary electrolytes are usually more useful than serum measurements because the normal physiological homeostatic mechanisms preserve serum electrolyte concentrations until the late stages of depletion. A low random urinary sodium concentration (< 5 mmol/L) is the best indicator of maximal sodium conservation and therefore sodium deficiency, even if serum estimations are normal. When interpreting a urinary sodium result it is important to check that the patient is not receiving diuretics or intravenous/subcutaneous saline.

Bowel length measurement

Predictions about the outcome can be made if the residual length of small intestine from the duodenojejunal flexure has been measured at surgery or radiologically from a small bowel meal film using an opisometer.[24,25] The remaining small bowel length is often unknown. Estimates made from the length of bowel resected are unreliable as the normal small intestinal length is so variable (Ch. 2).

Patients with a very short length of residual intestine are liable to water and sodium deficiency; this may result in loss of extracellular fluid volume, hypotension and pre-renal failure.

Monitoring

Accurate daily measurements of body weight, fluid balance (especially stomal effluent) and postural blood pressure are important. Serum electrolyte (creatinine, potassium and magnesium) and urinary sodium estimation may be done every 1–2 days initially but once or twice weekly when the patient is stable. The aims are to maintain hydration and body weight and a daily urine volume of at least 800 ml with a sodium concentration greater than 20 mmol/L.

3. Treat

Total jejunal loss of sodium increases in a linear relationship with volume (at a concentration of about 90 mmol/L) so the clinician can predict with reasonable accuracy that an effluent volume of 3 litres contains 270 mmol of sodium (Fig. 24.2). The concentration of sodium in the output remains constant whatever treatment is given. While there is a small obligatory stomal loss when fasting, the greatest increase in stomal output is after food or drink (Fig. 24.4). Consideration should be given to attempting to reduce stomal output, even in patients with a jejunostomy requiring parenteral nutrition, as this may well reduce the amount or frequency of intravenous fluid replacement and the social difficulties in managing the stoma.

Restrict oral fluids

Jejunal mucosa is 'leaky' and rapid sodium fluxes occur across it. If water or any solution with a sodium concentration of less than 90 mmol/L is drunk there is a net efflux of sodium from the plasma into the bowel lumen[26] until a luminal sodium concentration of 90–100 mmol/L is reached. In a patient with a jejunostomy this fluid is then lost in the stomal output. It is a common mistake for patients to be encouraged to drink oral hypotonic solutions to quench their thirst, but this literally washes sodium out of the body.[26–30]

Treatment for the high output from a jejunostomy, ileostomy or high fistula begins with the patient restricting the total amount of oral hypotonic fluid (water, tea, coffee, fruit juices, alcohol or dilute salt solutions) to less than 500 ml daily. To make up the rest of the fluid requirement the patient is encouraged to drink a glucose–saline replacement solution. Many patients at home with marginally high stomal outputs (1–1.5 litres) will be helped by a combination of oral fluid restriction (less than 1.5 litres per day) and the addition of salt to their diet.

If there is marked sodium and water depletion and severe thirst, it is often difficult to replace previous losses with an oral regimen; intravenous normal saline, 2–4 litres/day, is then given to correct the deficit. Great care must be taken not to give too much fluid as this will readily cause oedema, partly due to the high circulating aldosterone levels.[17–19,30] Sometimes, admitting patients with a high output, giving intravenous saline and keeping them 'nil by mouth' will demonstrate to them that their output is driven by their oral intake. Intravenous fluids are gradually withdrawn over 2–3 days while food and oral fluids are reintroduced.

Patients are often advised to take liquids and solids at different times (no liquid for half an hour before and after food), however there is no published evidence that this reduces stomal output or increases absorption of macro- or micronutrients.[31]

Drink oral glucose–saline solution

Patients with stomal losses of less than 1200 ml daily can usually maintain sodium balance by adding extra salt to the limit of palatability at the table and when cooking. When stoma losses are in the range 1200–2000 ml, or sometimes more, it is possible for a patient to maintain sodium balance by taking a glucose–saline solution or salt capsules.[28] In hot weather, patients with a stoma are more likely to have problems of dehydration because of water and sodium loss in sweat.

As the sodium content of jejunostomy (or ileostomy) effluent is relatively constant at about 90 mmol/L and as there is coupled absorption of sodium and glucose in the jejunum,[32–34] patients are advised to sip a glucose–saline solution with a sodium concentration of at least 90 mmol/L throughout the day. The World Health Organization (WHO) cholera solution has a sodium concentration of 90 mmol/L[35] and is commonly used (without the potassium chloride):

Sodium chloride	60 mmol (3.5 g)
Sodium bicarbonate (or citrate)	30 mmol (2.5 g) (2.9 g)
Glucose	110 mmol (20 g)
Tap water	1 litre

The concentration of sodium in this solution is much higher than that of many commercial preparations used to treat infective or traveller's diarrhoeas. Patients can prepare this solution at home using simple measuring scoops. There is no evidence that the sodium bicarbonate adds to the effectiveness of this solution[34] and it may be more palatable if sodium bicarbonate is replaced by sodium citrate. If the sodium concentration is increased further (e.g. to 136 mmol/L), absorption of sodium and water is improved.[36] Another oral rehydration solution that is more concentrated and simpler is made up as follows:

Sodium chloride	120 mmol (7.0 g)
Glucose	44 mmol (8 g)
Tap water	1 litre

Although taste perception changes in patients who are depleted in salt and water, they may find this solution, which tastes like 'sweet dilute seawater', too salty to drink.

A glucose-polymer (55 g Maxijul®) may be substituted for glucose to increase the energy intake by a mean of 115 kcal/d.[28] An oral rehydration solution based on rice powder can further increase the amount of energy absorbed: one study has shown that if there is a functioning terminal ileum, the sodium concentration in this solution can be reduced to 60 mmol/L.[37] The glucose-polymer/rice-based solution can be especially useful in diabetic patients as it causes less extreme changes in blood glucose than glucose-based solutions.

The patient should be encouraged to sip a total of one litre or more of one of these solutions in small quantities at intervals throughout the day. As compliance is often a major problem, patients need to understand the need for the solution. The solution may be chilled and/or flavoured with fruit juice to improve palatability.

Sodium chloride capsules (500 mg each) are effective when taken in large amounts (14/24 h), but can cause some patients to feel sick and even vomit.[28] If an enteral feed is given, sodium chloride needs to be added to make the total sodium concentration of the feed 100 mmol/L while keeping the osmolality near to 300 mOsm/kg.

Some patients cannot be maintained with an oral regimen (usually if jejunal length is less than 100 cm) and regular parenteral saline supplements are needed. Most such patients also need oral or parenteral nutritional supplements, but a few need only one or two litres of parenteral saline daily, often with added magnesium sulphate (14 mmol/L). This may be given as a regular infusion at home.

Drug therapy of high-volume output from a jejunostomy

If restricting oral fluids and giving a glucose–saline solution to drink are not adequate treatment, drugs may be needed. The intestinal output, especially in net 'secretors' rises after meals (Fig. 24.4), and it is therefore important to give the drugs before food. Drugs used to reduce jejunostomy output act to reduce either intestinal motility or secretions.

Antimotility (antidiarrhoeal) drugs

Opiate drugs such as codeine phosphate have been used for many years to treat diarrhoea but are sedative and, in the long term, addictive. Synthetic drugs were manufactured with the aim that they should be free of opiate-like activity upon the central nervous system. Diphenoxylate (Lomotil®) was the first to be used in clinical practice but has largely been replaced by loperamide (Imodium®) which has no central nervous system effects. Loperamide is preferred to codeine phosphate as it does not sedate and is not addictive. Codeine phosphate increases the output of stomal fat;[38,39] loperamide does not,[39,40] although it does reduce post-prandial pancreaticobiliary secretion of trypsin and bilirubin in patients with a short bowel and preserved colon.[41]

Loperamide and codeine phosphate reduce intestinal motility and thus decrease water and sodium output from an ileostomy by about 20–30%.[38,39,42] Oral loperamide, 4 mg taken four times a day, was more effective in reducing the weight and sodium content of ileostomy fluid than codeine phosphate 60 mg taken four times a day,[39] but the effect of both together may be greater.[43] Loperamide circulates through the enterohepatic circulation, but this is severely disrupted in these patients, and small bowel transit may be rapid. Thus high doses of loperamide (e.g. 12–24 mg) at a time) may be needed, as in patients who have had a vagotomy and pyloroplasty.[44] These drugs are effective in most patients with a jejunostomy,[5] particularly net 'absorbers'. A combination of both of these drugs, taken before food, a glucose–saline solution and other fluid restriction can liberate some patients from dependence on parenteral saline supplements.[43]

Antisecretory drugs

Food and drink are diluted by digestive juices, thus the volume of stomal effluent can be reduced in 'secretors' by drugs that reduce the secretions from the stomach, liver and pancreas. Drugs that reduce gastric acid secretion, such as the H_2 antagonists or proton pump inhibitors or the somatostatin analogue octreotide, are most commonly used.

H_2 antagonists/proton pump inhibitors

Cimetidine (400 mg orally or intravenously four times a day) reduced the output from a jejunostomy/ileostomy when the daily output exceeded 2 litres daily.[45,46] This beneficial effect is likely to be due to the reduction in normal daily gastric acid secretion or to a reduction in gastric acid hypersecretion.

Omeprazole, 40 mg orally once a day, reduced the stomal output by a mean of 0.7 kg/24 h in 7 patients with a net secretory output.[47] (Fig. 24.5a) Omeprazole, 40 mg given intravenously twice a day, reduced the jejunostomy output in patients whose output exceeded 2.6 kg/24 h.[48] Omeprazole is readily absorbed in the duodenum and upper small bowel, but if less than

50 cm of jejunum remains it may need to be given intravenously. Giving omeprazole orally dissolved in bicarbonate may improve absorption enough for it to be successful. Omeprazole has little beneficial effect in patients who are net absorbers.

Oral omeprazole, 40 mg once daily, gave an equivalent reduction in stomal output to oral ranitidine, 300 mg twice daily, in one patient.[7,47] Intravenous omeprazole, 40 mg twice daily, was more effective than intravenous ranitidine 150 mg twice daily, probably because the dose of ranitidine was too low.[48] Oral omeprazole, 40 mg once daily, was shown in two patients to be equivalent to intravenous octreotide 50 µg twice daily.[7,47]

Omeprazole, ranitidine and cimetidine reduce jejunostomy output in those with the highest outputs (net 'secretors') while often having no effect on net 'absorbers'. They may need to be given intravenously if less than 50 cm of jejunum remains. They do not change the absorption of energy, carbohydrate, lipid, nitrogen and divalent cations[45–48] and do not reduce jejunostomy output sufficiently to prevent the need for parenteral fluid and electrolyte replacement.

Somatostatin and octreotide

Somatostatin and octreotide reduce salivary, gastric and pancreatico-biliary secretions, slow small bowel transit, and may delay gastric emptying; for these reasons they may be expected to reduce the intestinal output from a jejunostomy in both net 'secretors' and 'absorbers'. Somatostatin has a serum half-life of 3 minutes so is given by continuous infusion, whereas that of octreotide is 90 minutes so it is usually given as regular (two or three times daily) subcutaneous injections before food.

Somatostatin. Four patients with more than 100 cm of small intestine remaining (one also had some residual colon) were given a continuous infusion of somatostatin, 4 µg/min for 24 hours. Mean daily intestinal output reduced from 1.9 kg to 1.2 kg, however magnesium, nitrogen and fat absorption were unchanged.[49]

Octreotide.

Effect of octreotide upon water, sodium and magnesium balance. A case report in 1984 first demonstrated that 50 µg of octreotide given subcutaneously twice a day allowed a patient with ileostomy diarrhoea to stop intravenous fluids.[50] Several studies in adults have shown octreotide to reduce ileostomy diarrhoea and

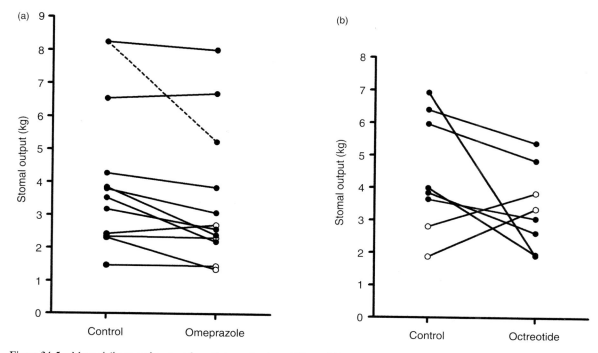

Figure 24.5 – Mean daily stomal output from 2 day collections. Effect of (a) omeprazole (40 mg orally once a day), and (b) octreotide (50 μg given intravenously twice a day) except ○ when 100 μg given subcutaneously three times a day into net 'absorbers' upon jejunostomy output. The dotted line shows the effect of intravenous omeprazole given to one patient with 30 cm jejunum after there was no response to an oral dose.

large-volume jejunostomy outputs (Table 24.1).[5,51–58] The greatest reductions in intestinal output have occurred in net 'secretors', (Fig. 24.5b) and many patients have been able to reduce the volume of parenteral supplements needed.[54,58] Although some patients have achieved positive intestinal fluid balance, they have rarely been able to stop parenteral fluids completely.[54,58] All studies have shown a reduction in sodium output which parallels that of the intestinal output.[5,51–58] Stomal output has been reported as reduced[56] in 2 and increased[55] in 2 jejunostomy patients classified as net 'absorbers'.[56] However, in one study in which all patients had mild ileostomy diarrhoea (0.8–1.3 kg/24 h) and were thus net absorbers, the output reduced by 0.3 kg/24 h.[52] Octreotide, 20–100 μg/24 h, has been used successfully to reduce ileostomy diarrhoea in 2 children aged 3 months and 5 years.[59] In 3 patients, an intravenous dose of 50 μg octreotide twice a day was as effective in reducing the intestinal output as 100 μg three times a day.[53] Magnesium balance has not been changed by octreotide.[53,56]

The effect of octreotide is maintained in the long term.[51,53,54,56,58] After a year's continuous therapy with 50 μg intravenous octreotide twice daily, the reduction in stomal output was the same as at the start of treatment.[54,58]

Somatostatin and octreotide both reduce the output from a high fistula and appear to accelerate the rate of spontaneous closure.[60,61]

Effect of octreotide upon nutrient absorption. Although octreotide reduces stimulated gastric acid and pancreatic enzyme secretion and reduces the splanchnic uptake of amino acids,[62] it does not significantly change total energy[54,57,58] or nitrogen absorption.[51,53,56–58] As pancreatico-biliary secretion is reduced, it would be expected that fat absorption would be reduced.[51] However, it is usually unchanged.[56–58]

Problems of octreotide therapy. A subcutaneous injection of octreotide may be painful, especially in the very thin, while an intravenous injection may cause flushing, nausea and headache.[54] Blood glucose generally remains within the normal range.[56] Patients with a jejunostomy have a very high prevalence of gallstones (45%),[16] and long-term octreotide therapy may further increase this.[63] Although hypoglycaemia may occur,[59] there is no evidence that octreotide

Table 24.1 – Octreotide to treat high-volume ileostomy or jejunostomy output

Author	Number	Dose	Days	Stomal output (l or kg/24 h)	
				Control	Octreotide
Ileostomy diarrhoea					
Cooper *et al.*[51] 1986	5	25 µg/h infusion	3	5.3	4.2
Kusuhara *et al.*[52]★ 1992	12	100 µg t.d.s.	5	1.0	0.7
High-output jejunostomy					
Shaffer *et al.*[53] 1988	6(?)	50–150 µg/24 h s.c.	3	4.0	2.4
Rodrigues *et al.*[5] 1989★★	4(4)	50 µg s.c.	6 h	0.9/6 h†	0.4/6 h†
Nightingale *et al.*[54,55] 1989	6(6)	50 µg b.d. i.v.	2	5.0	2.8
	2(0)	100 µg t.d.s.			
Ladefoged *et al.*[56] 1989	6(4)	25 µg/h infusion	2	–	1.1 less
	5(4)	50 µg b.d. s.c.	2	–	1.4 less
Lemann *et al.*[57] 1993	7(7)	100 µg t.d.s. s.c.	10 h	1.6/10 h†	1.0/10 h†
O'Keefe *et al.*[58] 1994	10(10)	100 µg t.d.s. s.c.	3	8.1†	4.8†

★Defunctioning ileostomy above 'ileoanal anastomosis'.
( ) number of net 'secretors'.
s.c. = subcutaneous; i.v. = intravenous; b.d. = twice daily; t.d.s. = three times a day.
All had normal meals except ★★ in which a liquid meal was given.
Median results except †, where means are presented.

causes diabetes or hypothyroidism after prolonged usage. Increasing the consistency of the small bowel contents could increase the risk of developing small bowel obstruction if there are adhesions.[58]

Mechanism of action of octreotide. Octreotide increases total intestinal transit time.[5,51,57,58] This probably reflects an increase in small bowel transit time as the rate of gastric emptying remains normal.[51,57] This slowing of transit may be the mechanism whereby some net 'absorbers' respond to octreotide therapy. In net 'secretors', the reduction in jejunostomy output was similar to that achieved with omeprazole, hence the suggestion that, in these patients, octreotide acts mainly by reducing the volume of gastric acid secreted in response to food.[64] A reduction in pancreatico-biliary secretion may explain why fat malabsorption increases in some patients[51] and it may be this that increases the intestinal output in some net 'absorbers'.[64,65]

Octreotide at a dose of 50 µg twice daily given subcutaneously or intravenously reduces intestinal water and sodium losses in most patients with a jejunostomy, and in some with ileostomy diarrhoea or a high small intestinal fistula. This effect is greatest in patients with the highest net 'secretory' output and is maintained long-term without tolerance developing. The reduction in output may reduce, but rarely avoids, the need for parenteral fluids. Some patients use these preparations, particularly octreotide, before meals to diminish the social inconvenience of a profuse jejunostomy output after food. In these patients octreotide does not affect the absorption of magnesium or nutrients.

Steroids

The distal ileum, with its tight intracellular junctions, can concentrate the intraluminal contents. This ability develops from 2 to 16 weeks after the formation of an ileostomy.[66,67] This capacity for sodium absorption may partly relate to high aldosterone levels[18,19] and can be induced by mineralocorticoids (e.g. 2 mg oral fludro-cortisone or 2 mg intravenous D-aldosterone)[68-70] or high-dose hydrocortisone.[71] Although intraluminal hydrocortisone does increase jejunal water, sodium and glucose absorption in normal subjects,[72] mineralo-corticoids do not usually reduce ileostomy output. However, studies have only been performed in patients with a relatively normal ileostomy output. Studies of patients with a high-output ileostomy or jejunostomy are awaited, but it would not be surprising if these were disappointing, as high circulating aldosterone levels may have already maximized sodium absorption.

Desmopressin

Desmopressin, an analogue of antidiuretic hormone, has no effect upon ileal fluid or electrolyte loss in man.[73]

MAGNESIUM SUPPLEMENTS

Dehydration and sodium depletion cause secondary hyperaldosteronism, which leads to renal magnesium loss; correction of these conditions may help to treat magnesium depletion. In addition, a diet relatively low in fat reduces stool or stomal magnesium losses[23] (Ch. 16).

Serum magnesium levels can usually be improved by oral supplements, however the data about the magnesium absorption from different preparations are often derived from normal volunteer studies and studies of patients with a short bowel and retained colon (Ch. 12). Tablet dissolution and magnesium availability may be very different in patients with a jejunostomy than in normal subjects and patients with a short bowel and retained colon. Most magnesium salts are poorly absorbed. Magnesium oxide is a commonly used preparation, although magnesium diglycinate (chelate) is absorbed equally well and as an intact dipeptide in the proximal jejunum.[74] Magnesium oxide may be given to a total of 12–24 mmol daily. Oral magnesium treatment, such as three gelatine capsules each of 4 mmol (160 mg of MgO), is usually given at night when intestinal transit is assumed to be slowest and hence there is more time for absorption. This regimen increases magnesium absorption[21] and does not appear to increase stomal output.

If oral magnesium supplements do not bring the magnesium level into the normal range, oral 1α-hydroxycholecalciferol in a gradually increasing dose (every 2–4 weeks) of 1–9 µg daily has been shown to improve magnesium balance in patients with a retained colon.[21,75] This action occurs by increasing both intestinal and renal magnesium absorption.[75] As hypomagnesaemia will have caused both a failure of parathormone release and a resistance to its action, 1α-hydroxycholecalciferol cannot be made in the kidney in adequate amounts. Thus it is important that the 1α preparation is given (Ch. 12).

Magnesium can occasionally be given as: a subcutaneous injection of 4 mmol magnesium sulphate every 2 or more days, but this can cause skin ulceration; an intramuscular injection of 10 mmol/L, but this is painful; or a regular intravenous infusion of 12 or more mmol, usually in a litre of saline over 1–2 hours, though this can cause a flushing sensation.

NUTRIENT ABSORPTION

Need for enteral or parenteral nutrition

Most patients with less than 75 cm of jejunum remaining need long-term parenteral nutrition; most in the range 75–100 cm need parenteral saline (sometimes with added magnesium) but manage to maintain nutritional status with an enteral regimen even though they may only absorb about 50–60% of their oral energy intake.

All patients wish to eat food so as to feel normal and to maintain social relationships. In patients maintained on parenteral nutrition, an oral intake is detrimental as it increases jejunostomy losses (Fig. 24.4). Patients taking an oral regimen need to consume more energy than a normal person to compensate for malabsorption. Most patients can achieve this by eating more high-energy food. Oral sip-feeds may be given in addition to food, preferably taken between meals and at bedtime. By these means, a patient may increase energy intake by at least 1000 kcal/d. If oral sip-feeds during the day fail to achieve weight gain or maintain nutrition, a nasogastric or gastrostomy tube may be inserted and a feed given at night so that the short residual length of intestine is used at a time when it is usually inactive. There are rarely any problems inserting a percutaneous endoscopic gastrostomy (PEG) in patients with Crohn's disease provided that there is no distal obstruction.[76]

Once weight is regained, the daily energy requirement may decrease so that a nocturnal feed can be reduced or stopped and sip-feeds during the day may become adequate. Only if these measures fail and the patient continues to lose weight, or fails to regain lost weight, is parenteral nutrition given.

Type of food

Patients with a jejunostomy absorb a constant proportion of the nitrogen, energy and fat from their diet.[6,23,77] Increasing fat in the diet raises fat excretion but does not usually increase stomal output, nor make the output offensive.[6,23,77] One study showed that increasing fat in the diet increased the loss of the divalent cations Mg and Ca,[23] but this was not the case in another.[77] There is no advantage in giving a diet of small molecules (e.g. an elemental diet); this causes a feed to be hyperosmolar[77] and usually contains little sodium, so potentially increasing the losses of water and sodium from the stoma. A peptide diet still has the problem of a relatively high osmolality and thus can increase stomal output.[78] Little advantage comes from taking a diet of water-soluble medium-chain tri-glycerides in place of normal fat.[79] The addition of glutamine, 15 g, to a litre of rehydration solution in patients with a jejunostomy resulted in no additional benefit in terms of water or sodium absorption.[80] The fibre content of the diet plays only a minor role in determining jejunal output.[39]

A synthetic bile acid resistant to bacterial deconjugation and dehydroxylation, cholylsarcosine (4 g taken three times a day), was given to 3 patients with a jejunostomy and resulted in an improvement in fat (18%, 37% and 51%) and calcium absorption but did not affect the volume of stomal output[81,82] (Ch. 25).

Thus jejunostomy patients need a large total oral energy intake of a polymeric, iso-osmolar (300 mOsm/kg) diet that is relatively high in fat with added salt (sodium concentration 100 mmol/L). The volume of the stomal output may become so high with a normal diet or with extra feeding that it is a major social disability. If this is the case, parenteral feeding may be needed to enable oral intake to be reduced.

DRUGS GIVEN FOR OTHER CONDITIONS

Many drugs are incompletely absorbed by patients with a short bowel and may be needed in much higher amounts than usual (e.g. thyroxine, warfarin and digoxin[83]) or may need to be given intravenously.

CHANGES IN JEJUNOSTOMY OUTPUT WITH TIME

Patients with a normal terminal ileostomy experience a decrease in stomal output from about day 5 to 16 weeks after its formation.[84] Hill *et al.* showed, in patients with an 'ileostomy' following an ileal resection, that there was no decrease in ileostomy water, sodium and potassium losses from 11 days after the resection to 6 months.[85] There is no structural

change in distal duodenal mucosa in patients with an established jejunostomy.[62] Thus there is no evidence for any structural or functional adaptive changes occurring in patients with a jejunostomy (Ch. 16). The fluid and nutrients needed change very little with time and are likely to be the same for as long as the jejunostomy remains.[7]

FUTURE TREATMENTS

Plasma levels of GLP-2 which causes villus growth, and peptide YY which slows upper gastrointestinal transit, are low, and future treatments may be directed at correcting these (Ch. 16). GLP-2 has been given with some success to patients with a jejunostomy,[86] and peptide YY agonists are available but have yet to be used.[87]

No unabsorbed carbohydrate has been found which increases the viscosity of a liquid supplement and, by decreasing the rate of gastric emptying, improves nutrient absorption. The ideal nutrient solution with an osmolality of 300 mOsm/kg and a sodium concentration of 100 mmol/litre has yet to be marketed.

SUMMARY

Patients with a stomal output in excess of oral fluid intake ('secretors'), usually more than 2 litres daily, require at least prolonged parenteral saline therapy and usually antisecretory drugs (e.g. omeprazole 40 mg daily). If the output is in the range of 1–2 litres/day and less than the oral intake (net 'absorbers'), then a reduction of oral fluid intake, taking a glucose–saline solution and using drugs that reduce gut motility (e.g. loperamide 4 mg four times a day before food) may be all that is necessary. Magnesium depletion is common and may be treated with magnesium oxide capsules, correction of dehydration, and 1α-hydroxychole-calciferol. Food needs to have extra salt added. Cholylsarcosine is a promising way of improving lipid absorption. GLP-2 or PYY agonists may provide a means in the future of increasing absorption.

REFERENCES

1. Flint JM. The effect of extensive resections of the small intestine. *Bull Johns Hopkins Hosp* 1912; **23**: 127–144.

2. Haymond HE. Massive resection of the small intestine: an analysis of 257 collected cases. *Surg Gynecol Obst* 1935; **61**: 693–705.

3. Booth CC. The metabolic effects of intestinal resection in man. *Postgrad Med J* 1961; **37**: 725–739.

4. Rodrigues CA, Lennard-Jones JE, Thompson DG, Farthing MJG. Energy absorption as a measure of intestinal failure in the short bowel syndrome. *Gut* 1989; **30**: 176–183.

5. Rodrigues CA, Lennard-Jones JE, Walker ER, Thompson DG, Farthing MJG. The effects of octreotide, soy polysaccharide, codeine and loperamide on nutrient, fluid and electrolyte absorption in the short bowel syndrome. *Aliment Pharmacol Ther* 1989; **3**: 159–169.

6. Nordgaard I, Hansen BS, Mortensen PB. Colon as a digestive organ in patients with short bowel. *Lancet* 1994; **343**: 373–376.

7. Nightingale JMD, Lennard-Jones JE, Walker ER, Farthing MJG. Jejunal efflux in short bowel syndrome. *Lancet* 1990; **336**: 765–768.

8. Borgström B, Dahlqvist A, Lundh G, Sjövall J. Studies of intestinal digestion and absorption in the human. *J Clin Invest* 1957; **36**: 1521–1536.

9. Fordtran JS, Locklear TW. Ionic constituents and osmolality of gastric and small intestinal fluids after eating. *Am J Dig Dis* 1966; **11**: 503–521.

10. Vantrappen GR, Peeters RL, Janssens J. The secretory component of the interdigestive migrating motor complex in man. *Scand J Gastroenterol* 1979; **14**: 663–667.

11. Buxton B. Small bowel resection and gastric acid hypersecretion. *Gut* 1974; **15**: 229–238.

12. Nightingale JMD, Kamm MA, van der Sijp JRM, Walker ER, Ghatei MA, Bloom SR, Lennard-Jones JE. Gastrointestinal hormones in the short bowel syndrome. PYY may be the 'colonic brake' to gastric emptying. *Gut* 1996; **39**: 267–272.

13. Windsor CWO, Fejfar J, Woodward DAK. Gastric secretion after massive small bowel resection. *Gut* 1969; **10**: 779–786.

14. Nightingale JMD, Kamm MA, van der Sijp JRM *et al*. Disturbed gastric emptying in the short bowel syndrome. Evidence for a "colonic brake". *Gut* 1993; **34**: 1171–1176.

15. Jeppesen PB, Hartmann B, Hansen BS, Thulesen J, Holst JJ, Mortensen PB. Impaired stimulated glucagon-like peptide 2 response in ileal resected short bowel patients with intestinal failure. *Gut* 1999; **45**: 559–563.

16. Nightingale JMD, Lennard-Jones JE, Gertner DJ, Wood SR, Bartram CI. Colonic preservation reduces the need for parenteral therapy, increases the incidence of renal stones but does not change the high prevalence of gallstones in patients with a short bowel. *Gut* 1992; **33**: 1493–1497.

17. Ladefoged K, Ølgaard K. Fluid and electrolyte absorption and renin–angiotensin–aldosterone axis in patients with severe short-bowel syndrome. *Scand J Gastroenterol* 1979; **14**: 729–735.

18. Ladefoged K, Ølgaard K. Sodium homeostasis after small-bowel resection. *Scand J Gastroenterol* 1985; **20**: 361–369.

19. Kennedy HJ, Al-Dujaili EAS, Edwards CRW, Truelove SC. Water and electrolyte balance in subjects with a permanent ileostomy. *Gut* 1983; **24**: 702–705.

20. Whang R, Whang DD, Ryan MP. Refractory potassium repletion. A consequence of magnesium deficiency. *Arch Intern Med* 1992; **152**: 40–45.

21. Selby PL, Peacock M, Bambach CP. Hypomagnesaemia after small bowel resection: treatment with 1 alpha-hydroxylated vitamin D metabolites. *Br J Surg* 1984; **71**: 334–337.

22. McIntyre PB, Fitchew M, Lennard-Jones JE. Patients with a jejunostomy do not need a special diet. *Gastroenterology* 1986; **91**: 25–33.

23. Ovesen L, Chu R, Howard L. The influence of dietary fat on jejunostomy output in patients with severe short bowel syndrome. *Am J Clin Nutr* 1983; **38**: 270–277.

24. Nightingale JMD, Bartram CI, Lennard-Jones JE. Length of residual small bowel after partial resection: Correlation between radiographic and surgical measurements. *Gastrointest Radiol* 1991; **16**: 305–306.

25. Carbonnel F, Cosnes J, Chevret S *et al*. The role of anatomic factors in nutritional autonomy after extensive small bowel resection. *J Parenter Enteral Nutr* 1996; **20**: 275–280.

26. Newton CR, Gonvers JJ, McIntyre PB, Preston DM, Lennard-Jones JE. Effect of different drinks on fluid and electrolyte losses from a jejunostomy. *J Roy Soc Med* 1985; **78**: 27–34.

27. Griffin GE, Fagan EF, Hodgson HJ, Chadwick VS. Enteral therapy in the management of massive gut resection complicated by chronic fluid and electrolyte depletion. *Dig Dis Sci* 1982; **27**: 902–908.

28. Nightingale JMD, Lennard-Jones JE, Walker ER, Farthing MJG. Oral salt supplements to compensate for jejunostomy losses: comparison of sodium chloride capsules, glucose electrolyte solution and glucose polymer electrolyte solution (Maxijul). *Gut* 1992; **33**: 759–761.

29. Rodrigues CA, Lennard-Jones JE, Thompson DG, Farthing MJG. What is the ideal sodium concentration of oral rehydration solutions for short bowel patients? *Clin Sci* 1988; **74(suppl 18)**: 69.

30. Newton CR, Drury P, Gonvers JJ, McIntyre P, Preston DM, Lennard-Jones JE. Incidence and treatment of sodium depletion in ileostomists. *Scand J Gastroenterol* 1982; **74(suppl)**: 159–160.

31. Woolf GM, Miller C, Kurian R, Jeejeebhoy KN. Nutritional absorption in short bowel syndrome. Evaluation of fluid, calorie and divalent cation requirements. *Dig Dis Sci* 1987; **32:** 8–15.

32. Olsen WA, Ingelfinger FJ. The role of sodium in intestinal glucose absorption in man. *J Clin Invest* 1968; **47:** 1133–1142.

33. Sladen GE, Dawson AM. Interrelationships between the absorptions of glucose, sodium and water by the normal human jejunum. *Clin Sci* 1969; **36:** 119–132.

34. Fordtran JS. Stimulation of active and passive sodium absorption by sugars in the human jejunum. *J Clin Invest* 1975; **55:** 728–737.

35. Avery ME, Snyder JD. Oral therapy for acute diarrhoea. The underused simple solution. *N Engl J Med* 1990; **323:** 891–894.

36. Beaugerie L, Cosnes J, Verwaerde F, Dupas H, Lamy P, Gendre J-P, Le Quintrec Y. Isotonic high-sodium oral rehydration solution for increasing sodium absorption in patients with short-bowel syndrome. *Am J Clin Nutr* 1991; **53:** 769–772.

37. Bodemar G, Sjodahl R. Rice and glucose oral rehydration solutions in patients with high ileostomal fluid output. *Lancet* 1992; **340:** 862.

38. Newton CR. Effect of codeine phosphate, Lomotil and Isogel on ileostomy function. *Gut* 1978; **19:** 377–383.

39. King RFGJ, Norton T, Hill GL. A double-blind crossover study of the effect of loperamide hydrochloride and codeine phosphate on ileostomy output. *Aust NZ J Surg* 1982; **52:** 121–124.

40. Tytgat GN, Huibregtse K, Dagevos J, van den Ende A. Effect of loperamide on fecal output and composition in well-established ileostomy and ileorectal anastomosis. *Dig Dis* 1977; **22:** 669–676.

41. Remington M, Fleming CR, Malagelada J-R. Inhibition of postprandial pancreatic and biliary secretion by loperamide in patients with short bowel syndrome. *Gut* 1982; **23:** 98–101.

42. Tytgat GN, Huibregtse K. Loperamide and ileostomy output – placebo-controlled double-blind crossover study. *Br Med J* 1975; **2:** 667–668.

43. Nightingale JMD, Lennard-Jones JE, Walker ER. A patient with jejunostomy liberated from home intravenous therapy after 14 years; contribution of balance studies. *Clin Nutr* 1992; **11:** 101–105.

44. O'Brien JD, Thompson DG, McIntyre A, Burnham WR, Walker ER. Effect of codeine and loperamide on upper intestinal transit and absorption in normal subjects and patients with postvagotomy diarrhoea. *Gut* 1988; **29:** 312–318.

45. Aly A, Barany F, Kollberg B, Monsen U, Wisen O, Johansson C. Effect of an H_2-receptor blocking agent on diarrhoeas after extensive small bowel resection in Crohn's disease. *Acta Med Scand* 1980; **207:** 119–122.

46. Jacobsen O, Ladefoged K, Stage JG, Jarnum S. Effects of cimetidine on jejunostomy effluents in patients with severe short bowel syndrome. *Scand J Gastroenterol* 1986; **21:** 824–828.

47. Nightingale JMD, Walker ER, Farthing MJG, Lennard-Jones JE. Effect of omeprazole on intestinal output in the short bowel syndrome. *Aliment Pharmacol Ther* 1991; **5:** 405–412.

48. Jeppesen PB, Staun M, Tjellesen L, Mortensen PB. Effect of intravenous ranitidine and omeprazole on intestinal absorption of water, sodium, macronutrients in patients with intestinal resection. *Gut* 1998; **43:** 763–769.

49. Dharmsathophorn K, Gorelick FS, Sherwin RS, Cataland S, Dobbins JW. Somatostatin decreases diarrhoea in patients with the short bowel syndrome. *J Clin Gastroenterol* 1982; **4:** 521–524.

50. Williams NS, Cooper JC, Axon ATR, King RFGJ, Barker M. Use of a long acting somatostatin analogue in controlling life threatening ileostomy diarrhoea. *Br Med J* 1984; **289:** 1027–1028.

51. Cooper JC, Williams NS, King RFGJ, Barker MCJ. Effects of a long acting somatostatin analogue in patients with severe ileostomy diarrhoea. *Br J Surg* 1986; **73:** 128–131.

52. Kusuhara K, Kusunoki M, Okamoto T, Sakanoue Y, Utsunomiya J. Reduction of the effluent volume in high-output ileostomy patients by a somatostatin analogue, SMS 201-995. *Int J Colorectal Dis* 1992; **7:** 202–205.

53. Shaffer JL, O'Hanrahan T, Rowntree S, Shipley K, Irving MH. Does somatostatin analogue (201-995) reduce high output stoma effluent? A controlled trial. *Gut* 1988; **29:** A1432–1433.

54. Nightingale JMD, Walker ER, Burnham WR, Farthing MJG, Lennard-Jones JE. Octreotide (a somatostatin analogue) improves the quality of life in some patients with a short intestine. *Aliment Pharmacol Ther* 1989; **3:** 367–373.

55. Nightingale JMD. The Sir David Cuthbertson Medal Lecture. Clinical problems of a short bowel and their treatment. *Proc Nutr Soc* 1994; **53:** 373–391.

56. Ladefoged K, Christensen KC, Hegnhoj J, Jarnum S. Effect of a long acting somatostatin analogue SMS 201-995 on jejunostomy effluents in patients with severe short bowel syndrome. *Gut* 1989; **30:** 943–949.

57. Lémann M, de Montigny S, Mahé S *et al*. Effect of octreotide on water and electrolytes losses, nutrient absorption and transit in short bowel syndrome. *Eur J Gastroenterol Hepatol* 1993; **5**: 817–822.

58. O'Keefe SJD, Peterson ME, Fleming R. Octreotide as an adjunct to home parenteral nutrition in the management of permanent end-jejunostomy syndrome. *J Parenter Enteral Nutr* 1994; **18**: 26–34.

59. Lamireau T, Galperine RI, Ohlbaum P, Demarquez JL, Vergnes P, Kurzenne Y, Hehunstre JP. Use of a long acting somatostatin analogue in controlling ileostomy diarrhoea in infants. *Acta Paediatr Scand* 1990; **79**: 871–872.

60. Nubiola P, Badia JM, Martinez-Rodenas F, Gil MJ, Segura M, Sancho J, Sitges-Serra A. Treatment of 27 postoperative enterocutaneous fistulas with the long half life somatostatin analogue SMS 201-995. *Ann Surg* 1989; **210**: 56–58.

61. Scott NA, Finnegan S, Irving MH. Octreotide and post-operative enterocutaneous fistulae: a controlled prospective study. *Acta Gastroenterol Belg* 1993; **56**: 266–270.

62. O'Keefe SJD, Haymond MW, Bennet WM, Oswald B, Nelson DK, Shorter RG. Long-acting somatostatin analogue therapy and protein metabolism in patients with jejunostomies. *Gastroenterology* 1994; **107**: 379–388.

63. Dowling RH, Hussaini SH, Murphy GM, Wass JAH. Gallstones during octreotide therapy. *Digestion* 1993; **54(suppl 1)**: 107–120.

64. Nightingale JMD, Walker ER, Burnham WR, Farthing MJG, Lennard-Jones JE. The short bowel syndrome. *Digestion* 1990; **45(suppl 1)**: 77–83.

65. Camilleri M, Prather CM, Evans MA, Andresen-Reid ML. Balance studies and polymeric glucose solution to optimise therapy after massive intestinal resection. *Mayo Clin Proc* 1992; **67**: 755–760.

66. Wright HK, Cleveland JC, Tilson MD, Herskovic T. Morphology and absorptive capacity of the ileum after ileostomy in man. *Am J Surg* 1969; **117**: 242–245.

67. Ladas SD, Isaacs PET, Murphy GM, Sladen GE. Fasting and postprandial ileal function in adapted ileostomates and normal subjects. *Gut* 1986; **27**: 906–912.

68. Goulston K, Harrison DD, Skyring AP. Effect of mineralocorticoids on the sodium/potassium ratio of human ileostomy fluid. *Lancet* 1963; **ii**: 541–543.

69. Levitan R, Goulston K. Water and electrolyte content of human ileostomy fluid after d-aldosterone administration. *Gastroenterology* 1967; **52**: 510–512.

70. Kramer P, Levitan R. Effect of 9 α-fludrocortisone on the ileal excreta of ileostomized subjects. *Gastroenterology* 1972; **62**: 235–241.

71. Feretis CB, Vyssoulis GP, Pararas BN, Nissiotis AS, Calaitzopoulos JD, Apostolidis NS, Golematis BCH. The influence of corticosteroids on ileostomy discharge of patients operated for ulcerative colitis. *Am Surg* 1984; **50**: 433–436.

72. Sandle GI, Keir MJ, Record CO. The effect of hydrocortisone on the transport of water, sodium and glucose in the jejunum. Perfusion studies in normal subjects and patients with coeliac disease. *Scand J Gastroenterol* 1981; **16**: 667–671.

73. Sutters M, Carmichael DJS, Unwin RJ *et al*. 'Low sodium' diuresis and ileal loss in patients with ileostomies: effect of desmopressin. *Gut* 1991; **32**: 649–653.

74. Schuette SA, Lashner BA, Janghorbani M. Bioavailability of magnesium diglycinate vs magnesium oxide in patients with ileal resection. *J Parenter Enteral Nutr* 1994; **18**: 430–435.

75. Fukumoto S, Matsumoto T, Tanaka Y, Harada S, Ogata E. Renal magnesium wasting in a patient with short bowel syndrome with magnesium deficiency: effect of 1α-hydroxyvitamin D_3 treatment. *J Clin Endocrinol Metab* 1987; **65**: 1301–1304.

76. Nightingale JMD. Gastrostomy placement in patients with Crohn's disease. *Eur J Gastroenterol Hepatol* 2000; **12**: 1073–1075.

77. McIntyre PB, Fitchew M, Lennard-Jones JE. Patients with a jejunostomy do not need a special diet. *Gastroenterology* 1986; **91**: 25–33.

78. Bosaeus I, Carlsson NG, Andersson H. Low-fat versus medium-fat enteral diets. Effects on bile salt excretion in jejunostomy patients. *Scand J Gastroenterol* 1986; **21**: 891–896.

79. Jeppesen PB, Mortensen PB. The influence of a preserved colon on the absorption of medium-chain fat in patients with small bowel resection. *Gut* 1998; **43**: 478–483.

80. Beaugerie L, Carbonnel F, Hecketsweiler B, Dechelotte P, Gendre J-P, Cosnes J. Effects of an isotonic oral rehydration solution, enriched with glutamine, on fluid and sodium absorption in patients with a short bowel. *Aliment Pharmacol Ther* 1997; **11**: 741–746.

81. Gruy-Kapral C, Little KH, Fortran JS, Meziere TL, Hagey LR, Hofmann AF. Conjugated bile acid replacement therapy for short-bowel syndrome. *Gastroenterology* 1999; **116**: 15–21.

82. Weinand I, Hofmann AF, Jordan A. Cholylsarcosine use for bile acid replacement in short bowel syndrome. *Gastroenterology* 1999; **116**: G0441.

83. Ehrenpreis ED, Guerriero S, Nogueras JJ, Carroll MA. Malabsorption of digoxin tablets, gel caps, and elixir in a patient with an end jejunostomy. *Ann Pharmacother* 1994; **28:** 1239–1240.

84. Crawford N, Brooke BN. Ileostomy chemistry. *Lancet* 1957; **i:** 864–867, 64, 65.

85. Hill GL, Mair WSJ, Goligher JC. Impairment of 'ileostomy adaptation' in patients after ileal resection. *Gut* 1974; **15:** 982–987.

86. Jeppesen PB, Hartmann B, Thulesen J *et al.* Treatment of short bowel patients with glucagon like peptide-2 (GLP-2), a newly discovered intestinotrophic, anti-secretory, and transit modulating peptide. *Gastro-enterology* 2000; **118:** A178–A179.

87. Litvak DA, Iseki H, Evers M *et al.* Characterization of two novel proabsorptive peptide YY analogs, BIM-43073D and BIM-43004C. *Dig Dis Sci* 1999; **44:** 643–648.

25

Dietary Treatment of Patients with a Short Bowel

Palle Bekker Jeppesen and Per Brøbech Mortensen

*P*atients with a short bowel present challenging management problems. By manipulating the diet and maximally utilizing the remaining intestine, some patients can maintain or improve their nutritional status thus avoiding the needing for parenteral supplements, and others may be able to reduce the amount of parenteral nutrition they need. In healthy subjects, with normal small and large intestines, more than 95% of ingested energy is retained and only 5% is lost in the faeces. The stomal/stool losses are much greater in patients with a short bowel and dietary advice aims to maximize the absorption of nutrients, without increasing the stomal/stool volume.

BALANCE STUDIES

Intestinal balance studies done with patients eating their habitual diet provide the simplest and most useful measure of residual intestinal absorptive capacity (Chapter 24), it is not always possible to perform these in the clinical setting. The results of balance studies may identify those patients with severe malabsorption who are likely to have irreversible intestinal failure, and those whose balance is 'borderline' in whom dietary manipulation may prevent the need for parenteral supplements. From balance studies, patients with a short bowel can be defined as either having problems with energy or fluid (sodium and water) balance or both (Fig. 25.1). Some patients (area 1) have problems with sodium and water losses, these are likely to be patients with a jejunostomy and 85–200 cm jejunum remaining.[1] Some patients (area 4) have problems with macronutrient absorption; these are often patients with very short jejunum in continuity with a functioning colon. Other patients (area 3) have problems with sodium, water and energy balance, these could be patients with a jejunostomy and less than 85 cm jejunum or patients who have had colonic resections and have very little remaining jejunum. In some of patients with diseases in the remaining bowel (e.g. Crohn's disease or radiation enteritis), the lengths of remaining bowel may correlate poorly with residual function.

It is a clinical ideal to measure macronutrient absorption with bomb calorimetry on freeze-dried samples[2,3] and to measure the amount of nitrogen, carbohydrate, fat, electrolytes and water in faeces, urine and a duplicate diet. However, it is rarely clinically possible to obtain these figures, and measurements of patient weight, stomal output or stool weight and fat content, serum biochemistry and urinary sodium excretion may be adequate.

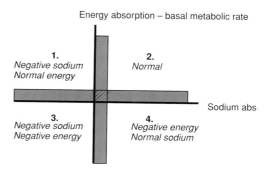

Figure 25.1 – Characterization of intestinal failure. The *x*-axis crosses the *y*-axis at the value 1 (energy absorption/basal metabolic rate = 1) and the *y*-axis crosses the *x*-axis at the value 0 (sodium absorption = 0). ▓: sodium needed to cover non gastrointestinal losses (urine/sweat); ▓: energy needed for physical activity.

ENERGY REQUIREMENTS

The energy requirements of a patient are those needed to maintain health, growth and an 'appropriate' level of physical activity (Chapter 18). In undernourished patients with a short bowel there is a fall in the basal metabolic rate (BMR) mainly due to a reduction of lean body mass. The largest component of energy expenditure is the BMR, which is affected by age, sex and body weight.[4]

ANATOMICAL AND PHYSIOLOGICAL CONSIDERATIONS

When considering the dietary management of patients with a short bowel, clarification of the remaining intestinal anatomy can predict the outcome. The outcome depends on the length, function and type of the residual small bowel and on the presence of a functioning colon.[5] The recognition of the colon, not only as an organ for fluid an electrolyte absorption, but also as a potential energy-salvaging organ has altered the dietary recommendations for patients with a short bowel and a remaining functional colon.[6]

Problems of an ileal resection

In normal humans, digestion and absorption of most nutrients occur in the duodenum and jejunum.[7,8] Intubation experiments have shown that most carbohydrate and protein are absorbed in the upper 200 cm of the jejunum.[7] Fat is absorbed over a longer length of the intestine, a distance that increases as oral intake rises.[8] Thus after a distal small intestinal resection fat malabsorption would be expected to be a problem before that of carbohydrate and protein malabsorption. Unabsorbed fatty acids will bind to divalent cations (calcium and magnesium) potentially to cause their loss in the stomal output/stool. In patients with a short bowel, nutrient absorption correlates with residual jejunal length.[1,2,9]

There is back diffusion of sodium through leaky jejunal intracellular junctions; this means that the jejunal contents are always isotonic. Thus patients with remaining jejunum will loose water if hyperosmolar solutions are given (e.g. an elemental diet), or sodium if water without added salt is given. A diet of relatively large molecules, thus of low osmolality, and added sodium chloride will help make an iso-osmolar chyme. These consequences of jejunal physiology are largely overcome if a functioning colon remains. In the ileum there are tight intercellular junctions, which allow the luminal contents to become hyperosmolar, thus the type of diet consumed is not critical.

Transit time is slower in the ileum than in the jejunum, thus if an ileal remnant remains, more absorption is possible due to more contact time between nutrients and the absorptive surface than if a jejunal remnant of similar length remains.

The ileum has a high capacity for adaptation and can assume most of the absorptive functions of the jejunum if the jejunum has been resected. This is not the case if ileum has been resected for the remaining jejunum has little capacity for adaptation (Chapter 16).

The terminal ileum is the selective site for active absorption of vitamin B_{12} and for the reabsorption of bile acids. In this respect removal of more than 100 cm ileum will lead to bile acid malabsorption.[10] Although hepatic biosynthesis of bile acids can increase 10- to 20-fold, bile acid secretion into the intestine decreases progressively throughout the day with subsequent impaired fatty acid and monoglyceride absorption, and thus steatorrhoea.[11]

Advantages of colonic preservation

In patients with a preserved colon there is an increased load of nutrients, water and electrolytes arriving in the colon. The colon can absorb up to 5 litres of fluid daily.[12] If carbohydrate is not absorbed in the remaining small intestine, the colonic microflora, in an anaerobic environment, break them down (fermenta-

tion) to short-chain fatty acids (SCFAs). The lack of oxygen within the colon stops the complete oxidation of SCFAs to carbon dioxide and water. Unabsorbed protein in the colon is degraded by bacteria to amino acids and peptides, which either are incorporated into bacterial protein or deaminated to form ammonia, carbon dioxide and SCFAs.

The total concentration of SCFAs in the small bowel is low, they are highest in the caecum and fall by 10–30% towards the distal part of the colon/rectum. In the colon and faeces they are the predominant anions (60–130 mmol/L). Thus, pH is lowest in the caecum, particularly after a high carbohydrate meal which is associated with a high rate of fermentation, and the pH rises distally in the colon as the contents are buffered. Three SCFAs made in the colon, butyrate, proprionate and acetate having 4, 3 and 2 carbon atoms respectively. The colonic mucosal cells preferentially metabolize much butyrate; proprionate and acetate are transported to the liver in the portal blood (in which their concentrations are lower than those in the colonic lumen). The liver extensively takes up butyrate and propionate and only negligible amounts appear in peripheral blood. Although there is a substantial hepatic clearance of acetate, some does reach the peripheral blood to be utilized by peripheral tissues. In healthy individuals the production of SCFAs contributes to about 5–10% of the energy absorbed, which is much less than in plant-eating animals.[13-15]

The role of SCFAs as nutrients has been neglected in human physiology. However, it is due to this process that many patients have survived after a major small bowel resection. Studies have demonstrated the importance of colon in salvaging energy in short bowel patients with a colon and severe malabsorption.[16-18] In these patients colonic fermentation may provide up to 1000 kcal (4.2 MJ) each day.[19] There is evidence that this formation of SCFAs causes structural small bowel adaptation, for when metronidazole is given to rats that have had an 80% small intestinal resection to stop fermentation, the residual small intestine does not adapt.[20]

GENERAL NUTRITIONAL CONSIDERATIONS

The total amount of energy absorbed by a patient with a short bowel is not surprisingly reduced and depends upon the amount of bowel remaining. Woolf et al. found a mean energy absorption of 62% (range 52–76) after a 10-day study in eight patients with a short bowel, three had a remaining colon and two were receiving long-term parenteral nutrition.[21] Rodrigues *et al.* showed median energy absorption after a liquid test meal to be 87% (range 82–92) in five ileostomists, 67% (range 59–78) in seven patients with a jejunostomy who normally received oral nutrient supplements and 27% (range 2–63) in five short bowel patients (one had a colon remaining) who normally received parenteral nutrition.[2] Messing *et al.* showed an overall energy absorption of 67% (range 41–85) after a 3-day balance study in ten patients with a short bowel, all but one had some retained colon and five received parenteral nutrition.[22]

Thus if a patient with a short bowel is to be maintained upon an oral diet they may need to consume twice as much food as a normal person. It is fortunate that most patients with a short bowel compensate for their absorptive handicap by increasing their oral intake (hyperphagia).[23–25] This may not be adequate, and protein–energy malnutrition may still occur if energy absorption falls below 40–50%; if so a nocturnal enteral feed or supplemental parenteral nutrition may be needed.

Most studies of absorption following a small bowel resection have stressed the importance of fat mal-absorption. The proportion of fat absorbed from different diets remains constant[19,26] and increasing amounts of fat in the diet leads to greater amounts of fat in the stool/stomal output. There is a positive linear relationship between the lipid concentration in the luminal aqueous phase and the proportion absorbed by the normal small intestine.[27,28] A high-carbohydrate, low-fat diet decreases the concentration of dietary fat offered to the intestine, and thus patients with a short bowel may not fully utilize their remaining small intestine for fat absorption. Much of the dietary advice given to patients with a short bowel has traditionally centred on fat intake.

Studies that have investigated the effect of dietary manipulation are summarized in Table 25.1.

DIETARY TREATMENT FOR PATIENTS WITH JEJUNUM IN CONTINUITY WITH A FUNCTIONING COLON

Carbohydrate

The importance of the colon in the fluid and electro-lyte absorption and its role in ileal-resection diarrhoea is well recognized.[29] The awareness that the colon is important in the digestion of carbohydrates and proteins, and hence in salvaging energy in patients with short bowel and a preserved colon, is recent. In many hindgut fermenting herbivorous and omnivorous animals, this bacterial degradation of carbohydrates to the easily absorbed SCFAs contribute to more than 50% of their maintenance energy requirements. In humans, Bond *et al.* studied the absorption of sucrose in patients with jejunal by-pass, and showed that an appreciable fraction of carbohydrate was removed during colonic transit.[16] Royall *et al.* also described the colonic fermentation and suggested the energy-salvaging role of the colon.[17,18] Nightingale *et al.* found that patients with a short bowel did better, not only in respect to fluid absorption but also with regard to the needs for parenteral nutrition, if they had at least half of the colon retained. They estimated that, in terms of the need for parenteral nutrition, colonic preservation was equivalent to about 50 cm of small intestine.[30]

Nordgaard *et al.* compared the clinical effect of a high-fat (60%) low-carbohydrate (20%) diet with a high-carbohydrate (60%) low-fat (20%) diet in patients with a preserved colon.[6] Eight patients on two different 4-day periods received two isocaloric diets of 2557 kcal/day (10.7 MJ/day). The high-carbohydrate low-fat diet reduced faecal energy loss by 478 kcal/day (2.0 MJ/day) compared with the low-carbohydrate high-fat diets. Energy absorption was significantly greater on the high-carbohydrate low-fat diet (69%) compared with the low-carbohydrate high-fat diet (49%). The faecal carbohydrate content was low and not influenced by the amount of carbohydrate consumed, whereas the amount of faecal fat was dependent upon the amount of fat ingested. There was no change in the faecal volume between the two study periods, but the amount of water consumed with the high-carbohydrate diet was a litre more than with the high-fat diet, suggesting that a high-carbohydrate diet results in more water absorption.

Messing *et al.* showed overall 67% (range 41–85) energy absorption after a 3-day balance study in ten patients (all but one had a retained colon and five received parenteral nutrition) of a 3107 kcal/day diet (13.0 MJ/day) containing 31% fat, 46% carbohydrate and 23% protein. The absorption of fat, carbohydrate and protein was 52, 79 and 61% respectively.[22] Whether the patients were receiving parenteral nutrition or not there was no difference in oral intake.

A high carbohydrate diet tends to be very bulky and the increased load of carbohydrate into the colon and

Table 25.1. – Studies of diet composition on nutrient absoption in patients with a short bowel

Reference	No. and type of patients	Small bowel lengths	Diet composition	Effect on energy absorption	Effect on water and sodium absorption	Effect on divalent cation absorption
Jejunostomy						
McIntyre et al.[66]	7 Jejunostomy	<150 cm remaining	Chemically defined vs polymeric diet. Three solid diets of variable fat/fibre	None	None	None for Ca and Mg
Nordgaard et al.[6]	6 Jejunostomy	100–250 cm	20 vs 60% fat 60 vs 20% CHO	None	None	–
Ovesen et al.[65]	5 Jejunostomy	35–125 cm	30% vs 60% fat Polyunsaturated to saturated fatty acid ratio 1:1 or 1:4	–	None	High fat diet increased stomal Ca, Mg, Cu and Zn losses
Jeppesen et al.[59]	6 Jejunostomy 3 Ileostomy	Mean 203 cm	60% LCT vs 30% MCT+ 30% LCT	None	None	–
Woolf et al.[64]	5 Jejunostomy 3 Jejunum-colon	–	60% vs 20% fat	None	None	None
Jejunum-colon						
Nordgaard et al.[6]	6 Jejunum-ileum-colon 2 Jejunum-colon	50–245 cm	20 vs 60% fat 60 vs 20% CHO	High-carbohydrate/low-fat diet Increased energy absorption	None	–
Andersson et al.[67]	10 Jejunum-colon 1 Ileostomy 2 active Crohn's without resection	Mean 90 cm small intestine resected	100 g fat vs 40 g fat	–	Reduced water and sodium excretion in low-fat diets.	–
Hessov et al.[54]	7 Jejunum-colon 2 active Crohn's without resection	Mean 145 cm ileum resected	100 g fat vs 40 g fat	–	–	High-fat diet increased divalent cation loss
Jeppesen et al.[59]	2 Jejunum-colon 8 Jejunum-ileum-colon	Mean 143 cm	60% LCT vs 30% MCT+ 30% LCT	MCT diet increased energy absorption	None	–

subsequent fermentation may lead to an increased production of gases. Patients tend to find their own balance, maximizing energy intake and absorption, reducing the social disability of bloating and the bulky offensive stools provoked by carbohydrates and fats respectively.

In patients with a retained colon, 20 grams of lactose from milk or yogurt are adequately fermented and absorbed by the colon without causing diarrhoea, so these do not need to be restricted.[31]

D-lactic acidosis

Although conservation of the colon in short bowel patients is highly desirably, its presence is associated with the extremely rare occurrence of D-lactic acidosis. D-lactic acidosis is only seen in patients with a short bowel and a preserved colon. Lactic acid produced and utilized by mammalian cells is the L(+) isomer but colonic bacteria produce both the L(+) and the D(–) isomers, which do not usually accumulate, may be converted to each other by a racemase, and may further degrade to SCFAs. In rare conditions, however, the colonic flora have the capacity to very rapidly degrade a surplus of easily fermentable carbohydrate to D(–) and L(+) lactate, which may accumulate in the colon resulting in absorption and elevated concentrations in blood and urine. Although man has some enzymes that degrade D(–) lactate, most is excreted in the urine[33] and a metabolic acidosis results and is probably the cause of clinical symptoms. However, the infusion of the sodium salt of D(–) and L(+) lactate to cause plasma concentrations of D(–) lactate comparable to those found in symptomatic patients with D(–) lactate acidosis appears to be harmless.[34]

D(–) lactic acidosis can cause ataxia, blurred vision, ophthalmoplegia and nystagmus, slurred speech, aggressiveness, inappropriate behaviour and stupor, which may progress to coma.[35] It is suspected when a patient is found to have a metabolic acidosis with a large anion gap, and confirmed by increased concentrations of D(–) lactate in blood and urine. The measurement may need to be repeated due to hourly fluctuations in blood levels.[36] The finding of moderate amounts of D(–) lactate in the faeces is common and rarely associated with elevated blood concentrations.

Several conditions have been suggested to be necessary for the development of D(–) lactic acidosis, which is not common as fewer than 40 cases have been reported in the literature during the past 20 years, many of whom had had intestinal by-pass surgery for obesity.[37] Small intestinal malabsorption and the presence of a bacterial fermentation chamber (the colon) are required. The type of food ingested may play a role as a diet rich in mono- and oligosaccharides, and rapidly digestible starch may result in D-lactic acid accumulation.[38] A change in colonic flora with a reduction in Gram-negative anaerobes and a predominance of Gram-positive anaerobes, especially *Lactobacillus*, *Eubacterium* and *Bifidobacterium*, has been found[39] and leads to an increased chance of lactate formation.[40] The treatment of D-lactic acidosis is focused on ways to reduce the formation of colonic lactate. The diet is changed so that simple carbohydrates (mono- and oligosaccharides)[41] are restricted and more slowly digestible polysaccharides (starch) encouraged and thiamine may be given. If very severe the patient may need to fast and be given parenteral nutrition. Bacterial production of lactate is reduced by giving broad-spectrum antibiotics (neomycin or vancomycin). Medium-chain triglycerides (MCTs) may be omitted.[42] Patients who have had intestinal by-pass surgery may need to have small bowel continuity restored.

Fat

Long-chain fatty acids (LCFAs) are absorbed only in the small intestine, whereas carbohydrates and protein are absorbed in both the small and large intestine. Diarrhoea associated with steatorrhoea has been associated with the production of hydroxy fatty acids from unsaturated fatty acids in the colon.[43] These hydroxy fatty acids, as well as fatty acids and their soaps, accelerate transit time in the colon, causing diarrhoea.[44–48] Unabsorbed LCFAs in the colon may worsen diarrhoea by reducing water and sodium absorption[46] and increasing the colonic transit rate.[48] They are toxic to bacteria, thereby reducing the amount of carbohydrate fermented.[49,50] They bind to calcium and magnesium, increasing the stool losses, and they increase oxalate absorption.

Both unabsorbed fatty acids and unabsorbed bile acids in the colon inhibit colonic mucosal absorption, thereby contributing to diarrhoea.[10,51,52]

Theoretically, a low-fat diet is recommended in the symptomatic treatment of patients after a small bowel resection,[53] especially in the early months. However, in practice, it is hard to implement. Fat yields twice as much energy as comparable weights of carbohydrate and it makes food palatable. A balance has to be achieved between maintaining weight and strength, and worsening steatorrhoea. However, the overall effect of a high-fat diet on the already large stool volume is probably small (Table 25.1). A low-fat diet may increase calcium, magnesium and zinc absorption.[54]

MCTs are an alternative source of energy and are absorbed from the small and large bowel.[55] Replacement of normal fat with MCT has been advocated but the effect on energy absorption and stool volume has not been fully evaluated.[56-58] Jeppesen et al.[54,59] have shown, in patients with a preserved colon, that the absorption of C8–C18-fatty acids gradually decreases as the length of the fatty acid chain increases. Faecal excretion of medium-chain fatty acids (MCFAs) was negligible and MCT absorption was almost complete even when long-chain triglycerides (LCT) were malabsorbed. Patients with a colon absorb C8–C10-fatty acids better than patients without a colon. In contrast, a preserved colon does not improve the absorption of long-chain C14–18-fatty acids. On average, a 30% MCT diet increased fat (MCT+LCT) absorption from 23% to 58% ($P < 0.001$) in patients with a colon, and increased energy absorption from 46% to 58% ($P < 0.05$). The mechanism is probably by colonic absorption of the water-soluble MCFAs, in a similar fashion to that of SCFAs.

The combination of low-fat diets and fat malabsorption may result in low concentrations of plasma essential fatty acids and lowered absorption of fat-soluble vitamins, and these patients may need supplements by the enteral or parenteral route.[60] Some units rub sunflower oil onto the skin, which may be an effective way of ensuring the absorption of the essential fatty acids[61]

Calcium oxalate renal stones

Renal stone formation may occur in patients who are chronically dehydrated and pass low volumes of concentrated urine. When there is malabsorption of fat and the colon is present, increased urinary excretion of oxalate is an additional risk factor (Chapter 15). Symptomatic calcium oxalate renal stones occurred in one-quarter of a series of patients with less than 200 cm of jejunum anastomosed to colon, whereas no renal stones were diagnosed in a comparable group of patients with an end jejunostomy.[30] A low-oxalate diet is recommended (little or no spinach, parsley, rhubarb, beetroot, cocoa and tea). As calcium may precipitate with fatty acids to form soaps, thus leaving oxalate free to be absorbed, the fat in the diet may be reduced.[62] In our experience renal stone formation has become less common, as we prevent chronic dehydration from occurring by infusing saline at home.

DIETARY TREATMENT FOR PATIENTS WITH A JEJUNOSTOMY

As protein and carbohydrate are absorbed to a greater extent in the upper small intestine than fat, it may be expected that a high-carbohydrate low-fat diet would be most beneficial, however a diet high in carbohydrate is likely to be hyperosmolar and thus to increase fluid losses from the stoma. A high-fat diet may have the advantage of being of lower osmolality, but unabsorbed fatty acids may bind divalent cations increasing their losses. As the stomal sodium losses are about 100 mmol/L, any diet will need added sodium chloride. The following review of the studies looks at the evidence for the dietary advice.

The 1869 kcal/day (7.8 MJ/day) diet used by Woolf et al. for a 10-day randomized, controlled cross-over study, contained 46% fat, 32% carbohydrate and 22% protein and the respective absorption of these was 54, 61 and 81%.[21] They noted that fluid intake with meals did not affect nutrient absorption. Although many clinicians advise no liquid to be taken with a meal and for half an hour afterwards there is no published evidence in terms of energy or fluid balance to suggest that this is beneficial.

Fat and divalent cations

Simko et al. showed that increasing dietary fat from 64 to 200 g/day increased fat absorption from 44 to 133 g/day without increasing stool weight. This increase was not due to any changes in transit time. A decrease in bile salt excretion was noted.[63]

Woolf et al. studied, in a randomized cross-over study, the effect of a high-fat (60%) versus a low-fat diet (20%) of about 1649 kcal/day (6.9 MJ/day) on eight patients, five of whom had jejunostomies and three had jejuno-transverse anastomoses (four patients received parenteral nutrition).[64] Faecal water and dry weight were not different during the two study periods. The faecal fat excretion was three times higher on high-fat than on low-fat diets, but the proportion of ingested fat absorbed was not different between the two diets. There were no significant differences in the mean total energy and in percentage of fat, protein and carbohydrate absorbed, between the high- and low-fat diets. The absorption of fat and non-fat energy was similar and averaged 65% of intake. There was no significant difference in the absorption of calcium, magnesium or zinc between the diets.

Nordgard *et al.* also studied the effect of a high-fat (60%) versus a low-fat diet (20%) on faecal excretion and energy absorption in six short bowel patients with a jejunostomy (two received parenteral supplements) in a randomized cross-over design.[6] Mean energy intake was 2533 kcal/day (10.6 MJ/day). Faecal water and dry weight were not different during the two study periods and absorption of dietary energy was approximately 50% in both periods. A trend towards a reduced faecal energy excretion during the low-fat diet was noted. Absorption of divalent cations was not measured.

Ovesen *et al.* compared the effect of three iso-energetic diets on jejunostomy output of fluid, fat sodium, potassium, calcium, magnesium, zinc and copper in five patients receiving HPN.[65] One was low in fat (30%) but high in complex carbohydrate (55%), and two were high in fat (60%) but low in carbo-hydrate (25%). The polyunsaturated/saturated fatty acid ratios of the two high fat diets were 1:4 and 1:1. Diets were eaten for 9 days each with collections of excreta the last two. Mean energy intake was approxi-mately 1912 kcal/day (8.0 MJ/day). Although increas-ing the percentage of fat in the diet increased the amount of steatorrhoea, altering the polyunsaturated/saturated fatty acid ratio had no clearly beneficial effect on the amount of fat absorbed. Neither the amount of fat, nor the type of fat, had any consistent influence on jejunostomy volume. The sodium and potassium con-centration of the jejunostomy fluid stayed constant and hence monovalent cation losses reflected jejunostomy volume rather than the fat or carbohydrate content of the diet. The high-fat diet increased the stomal losses of divalent cations; calcium, magnesium, zinc and copper. In most cases a net divalent cation secretion on the high-fat diet was converted into a net absorption on the low-fat high-carbohydrate diet. An increased fat malabsorption, and thus binding of divalent cations in these patients, may explain the difference from the study by McIntyre *et al.*[66] Altering the poly-unsaturated/saturated fatty acid ratio had no consistent effect on divalent cation losses.

In contrast to patients with a retained colon jejunostomy, patients do not significantly benefit from MCFAs. Although fat absorption increased from 37% to 46% ($P = 0.05$) overall energy absorption did not improve because malabsorption of carbohydrate and protein increased ($P < 0.05$).[55,59]

Large or small molecules

McIntyre *et al.* compared the absorption of a liquid diet consisting of small peptides, oligosaccharides and little fat (half of which was MCTs) with the absorption of a polymeric diet in patients with a jejunostomy (< 150 cm).[66] They also studied three solid diets with various amounts of fibre and fat. They found no difference in nitrogen, fat and energy absorption between the liquid and the polymeric diets and no difference among the solid diets. None of the diets significantly changed the weight of stoma effluent. A high-fat diet led to increased fat excretion though a constant amount was absorbed, but not to increased jejunostomy effluent or mineral (calcium and magnesium) losses. Those patients who absorbed more than 50% of their total oral energy intake sustained normal health by an increased nutrient intake, whereas two of the three patients with energy absorption below 40% needed parenteral supplements.

Based on these studies, a low-fat diet has no benefit in terms of energy, fluid or monovalent electrolyte absorption in patients with a jejunostomy. A constant proportion of dietary fat is absorbed, and more is absorbed when more is consumed. Dietary fat provides essential fatty acids[60] and increases both diet palatability and energy density. The increased fat content in stomal output is not usually malodorous and thus not a social problem. Two studies have shown fatty acids to increase the stomal output of divalent cations[54,65] and another two found no effect[64,66] (Table 25.1).

Conjugated bile acid treatment

As fat malabsorption in both types of patient with a short bowel may be partly due to bile acid depletion, there is interest in the use of cholylsarcosine. Cholylsarcosine, a synthetic bile acid resistant to bacterial deconjugation and dehydroxylation, does not itself cause colonic secretion so does not usually cause diarrhoea. When 4 grams are taken three times a day, there is variable improvement in fat and calcium absorption in patients with a short bowel with or without a retained functioning colon. It occasionally causes nausea.[68–70]

SUMMARY

The use of balance studies to measure residual intestinal absorption is ideal to determine the dietary treatment of an individual patient with a short bowel (Table 25.2). Patients can be categorized as having problems with sodium or protein–energy balance, or both. These studies enable the physician to identify the

Table 25.2 – Dietary recommendations in short bowel patients according to intestinal anatomy

Dietary content	Jejunostomy or ileostomy	Jejuno-ileal or jejunocolic anastomosis
Energy	High	High
Long-chain triglycerides	Normal	Low
Medium-chain triglycerides	Normal	High
Carbohydrate	Normal★	High†
Oxalate	Normal	Low
Sodium chloride	Extra needed	Normal

★ Polysaccharides in preference to mono/disaccharides to keep osmolality low.

† Polysaccharides in preference to mono/disaccharides to reduce the extremely rare occurrence of D(−) lactic acidosis.

patients with irreversible intestinal failure, either due to sodium or energy malabsorption, and those in whom dietary manipulations are likely to be beneficial. Dietary recommendations are dependent upon the remaining intestinal physiology. In patients with a preserved colon a high-carbohydrate, low-LCT diet is recommended, and MCTs may be of benefit. Manipulation of the fat:carbohydrate ratio does not affect energy absorption in patients with a jejunostomy and the use of MCTs does not improve overall energy absorption. Patients with a jejunostomy do need a diet with added sodium chloride.

The consequences of dietary manipulations, not only on nutrient, electrolyte and fluid absorption, but also on overall quality of life and patient autonomy, needs to be taken into consideration. The manipulations may affect diet palatability, satiety, abdominal discomfort, bloating and passing of wind, faecal consistency and incontinence. Some patients cope with the hyperphagia, large stool volumes, fatigue and chronic dehydration in order to avoid a life dominated by having a central line and needing to give parenteral supplements. Others see parenteral supplements as a place of refuge escaping the demands of constant hyperphagia, large stool volumes and abdominal discomfort. Balance studies are not only tools for studying intestinal physiology, but also they allow a patient the opportunity to experience the effects of different diets upon their fluid and energy absorption and on their well-being.

Optimal nutritional care, guidance and support is of vital importance in the long-term management of patients with a short bowel.

REFERENCES

1. Nightingale JM, Lennard Jones JE, Walker ER, Farthing MJ. Jejunal efflux in short bowel syndrome. *Lancet* 1990; **336**: 765–768.

2. Rodrigues CA, Lennard Jones JE, Thompson DG, Farthing MJ. Energy absorption as a measure of intestinal failure in the short bowel syndrome. *Gut* 1989; **30**: 176–183.

3. Heymsfield SB, Smith J, Kasriel S, Barlow J, Lynn MJ, Nixon D, Lawson DH. Energy malabsorption: measurement and nutritional consequences. *Am J Clin Nutr* 1981; **34**: 1954–1960.

4. Schofield WN. Predicting basal metabolic rate, new standards and review of previous work. *Hum Nutr Clin Nutr* 1985; **39 (Suppl 1):** 5–41.

5. Carbonnel F, Cosnes J, Chevret S, *et al.* The role of anatomic factors in nutritional autonomy after extensive small bowel resection. *J Parenter Enteral Nutr* 1996; **20**: 275–280.

6. Nordgaard I, Hansen BS, Mortensen PB. Colon as a digestive organ in patients with short bowel. *Lancet* 1994; **343**: 373–376.

7. Borgström B, Dahlqvist A, Lundh G, Sjövall J. Studies of intestinal digestion and absorption in the human. *J Clin Invest* 1957; **36**: 1521–1536.

8. Booth CC, Alldis D, Read AE. Studies on the site of fat absorption: 2. Fat balances after resection of varying amounts of the small intestine in man. *Gut* 1961; **2**: 168–174.

9. Hylander E, Ladefoged K, Jarnum S. Nitrogen absorption following small-intestinal resection. *Scand J Gastroenterol* 1980; **7**: 853–858.

10. Hofmann AF, Poley JR. Role of bile acid malabsorption in pathogenesis of diarrhea and steatorrhea in patients with ileal resection. I. Response to cholestyramine or replacement of dietary long chain triglyceride by medium chain triglyceride. *Gastroenterology* 1972; **62**: 918–934.

11. Fordtran JS, Bunch F, Davis GR. Ox bile treatment of severe steatorrhea in an ileectomy-ileostomy patient. *Gastroenterology* 1982; **82**: 564–568.

12. Debongnie JC, Phillips SF. Capacity of the human colon to absorb fluid. *Gastroenterology* 1978; **74**: 698–703.

13. McNeil NI. The contribution of the large intestine to energy supplies in man. *Am J Clin Nutr* 1984; **39**: 338–342.

14. McNeil NI. Nutritional implications of human and mammalian large intestinal function. *World Rev Nutr Diet* 1988; **56**: 1–42.

15. Stephen AM, Haddad AC, Phillips SF. Passage of carbohydrate into the colon. Direct measurements in humans. *Gastroenterology* 1983; **85**: 589–595.

16. Bond JH, Currier BE, Buchwald H, Levitt MD. Colonic conservation of malabsorbed carbohydrate. *Gastroenterology* 1980; **78**: 444–447.

17. Royall D, Wolever TM, Jeejeebhoy KN. Evidence for colonic conservation of malabsorbed carbohydrate in short bowel syndrome. *Am J Gastroenterol* 1992; **87**: 751–756.

18. Royall D, Wolever TM, Jeejeebhoy KN. Clinical significance of colonic fermentation. *Am J Gastroenterol* 1990; **85**: 1307–1312.

19. Nordgaard I, Hansen BS, Mortensen PB. Importance of colonic support for energy absorption as small-bowel failure proceeds. *Am J Clin Nutr* 1996; **64**: 222–231.

20. Aghdassi E, Plapler H, Kurian R, *et al*. Colonic fermentation and nutritional recovery in rats with massive small bowel resection. *Gastroenterology* 1994; **107**: 637–642.

21. Woolf GM, Miller C, Kurian R, Jeejeebhoy KN. Nutritional absorption in short bowel syndrome. Evaluation of fluid, calorie, and divalent cation requirements. *Dig Dis Sci* 1987; **32**: 8–15.

22. Messing B, Pigot F, Rongier M, Morin MC, Ndeindoum U, Rambaud JC. Intestinal absorption of free oral hyperalimentation in the very short bowel syndrome. *Gastroenterology* 1991; **100**: 1502–1508.

23. Cosnes J, Gendre JP, Evard D, Le Quintrec Y. Compensatory enteral hyperalimentation for management of patients with severe short bowel syndrome. *Am J Clin Nutr* 1985; **41**: 1002–1009.

24. Cosnes J, Lamy P, Beaugerie L, Le Quintrec M, Gendre JP, Le Quintrec Y. Adaptive hyperphagia in patients with postsurgical malabsorption. *Gastroenterology* 1990; **99**: 1814–1819.

25. DiCecco S, Nelson J, Burnes J, Fleming CR. Nutritional intake of gut failure patients on home parenteral nutrition. *J Parenter Enteral Nutr* 1987; **11**: 529–532.

26. Booth CC. The metabolic effects of intestinal resection in man. *Postgrad Med J* 1961; **37**: 725–739.

27. Borgström B. Studies on intestinal cholesterol absorption in the human. *J Clin Invest* 1960; **39**: 809–815.

28. Hofmann AF, Borgström B. The intraluminal phase of fat digestion in man: The lipid content of the micellar and oil phases of intestinal content obtained during fat digestion and absorption. *J Clin Invest* 1964; **43**: 247–257.

29. Cummings JH, James WP, Wiggins HS. Role of the colon in ileal-resection diarrhoea. *Lancet* 1973; **1**: 344–347.

30. Nightingale JM, Lennard Jones JE, Gertner DJ, Wood SR, Bartram CI. Colonic preservation reduces need for parenteral therapy, increases incidence of renal stones, but does not change high prevalence of gall stones in patients with a short bowel. *Gut* 1992; **33**: 1493–1497.

31. Arrigomi E, Marteau P, Briet F, Pochart P, Rambaud J-C, Messing B. Tolerance and absorption of lactose from milk and yogurt during short-bowel syndrome in humans. *Am J Clin Nutr* 1994; **60**: 926–929.

32. Oh MS, Uribarri J, Alveranga D, Lazar I, Bazilinski N, Carroll HJ. Metabolic utilization and renal handling of D-lactate in men. *Metabolism* 1985; **34**: 621–625.

33. de Vrese M, Koppenhoefer B, Barth CA. D-Lactic acid metabolism after an oral load of DL-lactate. *Clin Nutr* 1990; **9**: 23–28.

34. Connor H, Woods HF, Ledingham JGG. Comparison of the kinetics and utilisation of D(–)- and L(+)-sodium lactate in normal man. *Ann Nutr Metab* 1983; 481–487.

35. Dahlquist NR, Perrault J, Callaway CW, Jones JD. D-Lactic acidosis and encephalopathy after jejuno-ileostomy: response to overfeeding and to fasting in humans. *Mayo Clin Proc* 1984; **59**: 141–145.

36. Hove H, Mortensen PB. Colonic lactate metabolism and D-lactic acidosis. *Dig Dis Sci* 1995; **40**: 320–330.

37. Thurn JR, Pierpont GL, Ludvigsen CW, Eckfeldt JH. D-Lactate encephalopathy. *Am J Med* 1985; **79**(6): 717–721.

38. Editorial. The colon, the rumen, and D-lactic acidosis. *Lancet* 1990; **336**: 599–600.

39. Stolberg L, Rolfe R, Gitlin N, Merritt J, Mann L Jr, Linder J, Finegold S. D-Lactic acidosis due to abnormal gut flora: diagnosis and treatment of two cases. *N Engl J Med* 1982; **306**: 1344–1348.

40. Hove H, Mortensen PB. Colonic lactate metabolism and D-lactic acidosis. *Dig Dis Sci* 1995; **40**: 320–330.

41. Mayne AJ, Handy DJ, Preece MA, George RH, Booth I. Dietary management of D-lactic acidosis in short bowel syndrome. *Arch Dis Child* 1990; **65**: 229–231.

42. Jover R, Leon J, Palazon JM, Dominguez JR. D-lactic acidosis associated with the use of medium-chain triglycerides. *Lancet* 1995; **346**: 314.

43. Kellock TD, Pearson JR, Russell RI, Walker JG, Wiggins HS. The incidence and clinical significance of faecal hydroxy fatty acids. *Gut* 1969; **10**: 1055.

44. Binder HJ. Editorial: Fecal fatty acids-mediators of diarrhea? *Gastroenterology* 1973; **65**: 847–850.

45. Ammon HV, Phillips SF. Inhibition of ileal water absorption by intraluminal fatty acids. Influence of chain length, hydroxylation, and conjugation of fatty acids. *J Clin Invest* 1974; **53**: 205–210.

46. Ammon HV, Phillips SF. Inhibition of colonic water and electrolyte absorption by fatty acids in man. *Gastroenterology* 1973; **65**: 744–749.

47. James AT, Webb JPW. The occurrence of unusual fatty acids in faecal lipids from human beings with normal and abnormal fat absorption. *Biochem J* 1961; **78**: 333–339.

48. Spiller RC, Brown ML, Phillips SF. Decreased fluid tolerance, accelerated transit, and abnormal motility of the human colon induced by oleic acid. *Gastroenterology* 1986; **91**: 100–107.

49. Knapp H R, Melly MA. Bactericidal effects of poly-unsaturated fatty acids. *J Infect Dis* 1986; **154**: 84–94.

50. Thompson L, Edwards RE, Greenwood D, Spiller RC. Inhibitory effect of long-chain fatty acids (LCFAs) on colonic bacteria. *Gut* 1990; **31**: A1167.

51. Chadwick VS, Gaginella TS, Carlson GL, Debongnie JC, Phillips SF, Hofmann AF. Effect of molecular structure on bile acid-induced alterations in absorptive function, permeability, and morphology in the perfused rabbit colon. *J Lab Clin Med* 1979; **94**: 661–674.

52. Mekjian HS, Phillips SF, Hofmann AF. Colonic secretion of water and electrolytes induced by bile acids: perfusion studies in man. *J Clin Invest* 1971; **50**: 1569–1577.

53. Andersson H. The use of a low-fat diet in the sympto-matic treatment of ileopathia. *World Rev Nutr Diet* 1982; **40**: 1–18.

54. Hessov I, Andersson H, Isaksson B. Effects of a low-fat diet on mineral absorption in small-bowel disease. *Scand J Gastroenterol* 1983; **18**: 551–554.

55. Jeppesen PB, Mortensen PB. Colonic digestion of medium-chain fat in patients with short bowel. *Gastroenterology* 1997; **112**: A882.

56. Bochenek W, Rodgers JB Jr, Balint JA. Effects of changes in dietary lipids on intestinal fluid loss in the short-bowel syndrome. *Ann Intern Med* 1970; **72**: 205–213.

57. Zurier RB, Campbell RG, Hashim SA, Van Itallie TB. Use of medium-chain triglyceride in management of patients with massive resection of the small intestine. *N Engl J Med* 1966; **274**: 490–493.

58. Tandon RK, Rodgers JB Jr, Balint JA. The effects of medium-chain triglycerides in the short bowel syndrome. Increased glucose and water transport. *Am J Dig Dis* 1972; **17**: 233–238.

59. Jeppesen PB, Mortensen PB. The influence of a preserved colon on the absorption of medium-chain fat in patients with small bowel resection. *Gut* 1998; **43**: 478–483.

60. Jeppesen PB, Christensen MS, Høy C-E, Mortensen PB. Essential fatty acid deficiency in patients with severe fat malabsorption. *Am J Clin Nutr* 1997; **65**: 837–843.

61. Press M, Hartop PJ, Prottey C. Correction of essential fatty-acid deficiency in man by cutaneous application of sunflower-seed oil. *Lancet* 1974; **ii**: 597–599.

62. Earnest DL, Johnson G, Williams HE, Admirand WH. Hyperoxaluria in patients with ileal resection: an abnor-mality in dietary oxalate absorption. *Gastroenterology* 1974; **66**: 1114–1122.

63. Simko V, McCarroll AM, Goodman S, Weesner RE, Kelley RE. High-fat diet in a short bowel syndrome. Intestinal absorption and gastroenteropancreatic hormone responses. *Dig Dis Sci* 1980; **25**: 333–339.

64. Woolf GM, Miller C, Kurian R, Jeejeebhoy KN. Diet for patients with a short bowel: high fat or high carbo-hydrate? *Gastroenterology* 1983; **84**: 823–828.

65. Ovesen L, Chu R, Howard L. The influence of dietary fat on jejunostomy output in patients with severe short bowel syndrome. *Am J Clin Nutr* 1983; **38**: 270–277.

66. McIntyre PB, Fitchew M, Lennard Jones JE. Patients with a high jejunostomy do not need a special diet. *Gastroenterology* 1986; **91**: 25–33.

67. Andersson H, Isaksson B, Sjögren B. Fat-reduced diet in the symptomatic treatment of small bowel disease. *Gut* 1974; **15**: 351–359.

68. Gruy-Kapral C, Little KH, Fortran JS, Meziere TL, Hagey LR, Hofmann AF. Conjugated bile acid replace-ment therapy for short-bowel syndrome. *Gastro-enterology* 1999; **116**: 15–21.

69. Weinand I, Hofmann AF, Jordan A. Cholylsarcosine use for bile acid replacement in short bowel syndrome. *Gastroenterology* 1999; **116**: G0441.

70. Heydorn S, Jeppesen PB, Mortensen PB. Bile acid replacement therapy with cholylsarcosine for short-bowel syndrome. *Scand J Gastroenterol* 1999; **34**: 818–823.

Section 6

Outcome of intestinal failure

26

Home enteral and parenteral nutrition in adults

B. Messing, X. Hébuterne and J. Nightingale

INTRODUCTION

*T*he administration at home of enteral (HEN) and parenteral nutrition (HPN) has improved over the last 25 years. HEN is used mainly for patients with oral failure (OF); these are patients in whom there is an inappropriate and involuntary reduction in the oral intake below the minimal amount necessary to maintain protein–energy equilibrium. This occurs predominantly in patients with dysphagia. HPN is almost exclusively used for patients with acute or chronic intestinal failure (IF), when oral or enteral nutrition is temporarily or permanently impossible or where absorption is insufficient. Patients with OF or IF may not only be in a negative nutrient balance but also in a negative fluid balance. OF is often unrecognized, partly because it is not thought of and partly because these patients are looked after by a myriad of medical specialties. IF is usually recognized because these patients tend to be under the care of appropriate specialists and have more immediate problems. It is paradoxically more difficult to recognize and treat the problems of OF than IF.

In 1970, Scribner, followed in the same year by Shils, reported patients being treated with parenteral nutrition at home.[1,2] Over the next 20 years there were many reports of patients being treated at home with parenteral nutrition and with few complications.[3–17] This chapter describes the incidence and prevalence, underlying reasons for and outcomes of patients receiving HEN and HPN, with the greater emphasis upon HPN.

REGISTERS AND SPECIALIST CENTRES

In several European countries, North America and Japan, the indications for and results of HEN and HPN are recorded in national registers.[18–23] In addition to many centres in the USA, centres throughout the world have reported.[24–28] In France, agreed centres collect data on more than 90% of patients needing long-term HPN.[26,29] In the United Kingdom, data are derived from the British Artificial Nutrition Survey (BANS).[30] In the USA, information comes primarily from the Oley-American Society for Parenteral and Enteral Nutrition Information System (OASIS) and from Medicare. Medicare covers 48% of HEN patients and 27% of HPN patients.[18,21] In Canada, the UK, Ireland, France and Belgium, patients are followed in hospital/university centres, the organization being run in conjunction with their National Health Services.[19] There is great variation between and within countries of the number of patients receiving HEN and HPN.[31]

A nutrition team is essential in the implementation of parenteral nutrition, especially if it is to be carried out at home.[19,32] Nursing staff, dietitians, pharmacists, doctors, social and psychiatric workers and psychologists all play essential roles. The team must be competent in managing both enteral and parenteral nutrition. Many patients referred to specialist centres for HPN (e.g. intestinal failure units) can be more appropriately given HEN. A specialist referral centre has the role of evaluating, training, following up and re-evaluating patients who predominantly need HPN;[19,33,34] it should offer excellent specialist nutritional and gastroenterological care. The efficiency and the safety of HPN may be gauged by the incidence of catheter-related sepsis. There is usually an inverse relationship between the rate of catheter-related sepsis and the number of catheters inserted.[34–36] The HPN centres usually offer logistical facilities (e.g. supply of nutrients directly to the patient's home) and can obtain cost reductions because of the large volume of orders.[19] The centre must have a specialist nurse or doctor on call 24 hours a day to answer problems from patients at home. A centre should continually carry out audits on aspects of its care and ideally be actively involved in clinical research.[34,36–39]

The provision by an HPN centre of a multidisciplinary approach and the facility for patients to meet others with similar problems help to prevent the individual patient feeling isolated. In addition, there are patient support groups in some countries (e.g. Patients on Intravenous and Naso-gastric Nutrition Therapy, PINNT, in the UK and the Oley Foundation in the USA); these produce excellent information leaflets and discuss relevant topics (e.g. body image, not eating, tube/skin care, travel, pumps, treatment options, etc.).[40]

DATA PRESENTATION

There is no standardization in the way that prevalence and outcome data are presented, though most prevalence data are presented per 10^6 inhabitants (or population). In Europe, prevalence is quoted as one-day or point prevalence, while a yearly (also called annual occurrence) or, rarely, a 3-yearly prevalence is quoted in the USA. Thus USA prevalence figures are 3–4 times higher than European figures.[41] Data about the complications of nutritional support are often given as the proportion of patients developing a specified complication; however this alone is not adequate and a time denominator must be included. Complication rates are usually quoted in terms of episodes per patient per measure of time. At home, the number of episodes per patient per year is often quoted whereas, in hospital, episodes per patient per 100 days (or months) is commonly used. Occasionally, the less preferred measure of one episode per number of catheter days is given. In addition, other outcome data include an assessment of nutritional status and quality of life, details of the number stopping HEN/HPN, mortality (due to disease or treatment) and hospital readmission rates (with duration).

INCIDENCE AND PREVALENCE

In most countries there are 10 or more times the number of patients receiving HEN than HPN. In the UK, the one-day prevalence of HEN in 1998 was 200–267 patients/10^6 inhabitants and for HPN it was 6–8 patients/10^6 inhabitants.[30] Between 1994 and 1996 in the region of Nice in the south of France, the annual incidence of HEN was 99 patients/10^6 inhabitants compared with 8 patients/10^6 inhabitants for HPN.[42] The overall reported incidence of HPN in Europe ranges from 0.4 to 3.0 patients/10^6 inhabitants/year and the one-day prevalence from 0.7 to 12.7 patients/10^6 inhabitants.[23]

Between 1989 and 1992, in the USA, the annual prevalence of HEN was estimated at 415 patients/10^6 inhabitants and HPN at 120 patients/10^6 inhabitants.[21] The annual incidence of patients starting HPN is about 10 times greater than in Europe and the number requiring HEN and HPN has been increasing each year.[21,42,43] The reasons for such a large number of HPN patients in the USA are partly the calculation of annual prevalence rather than one-day prevalence and partly the fact that patients go home early with conditions that do not need HPN for more than 3 months (e.g. patients needing terminal care). It is cheaper for patients to be at home than in hospital, and there is good organization for HPN.[21,41,43]

It is interesting that the incidence of patients in France being treated with HEN, unlike HPN, was growing between 1990 and 1994 but has subsequently become stable. The ways in which the patient population being treated with HPN is changing can be seen from looking at the annual incidence of HPN

in France (Table 26.1). The reduction in the incidence of non-cancer non-HIV intestinal illnesses from 2.73 to 2.39/10^6 from 1993 to 1995 is mainly explained by a reduction in the occurrence of radiation enteritis.[26] During the same period there was an increase in patients with cancer and HIV infection. These trends are observed in most countries.

Table 26.1 – Incidence/prevalence of HPN in France per 10^6 adults[26]

	1993	1994	1995
Point prevalence	3.54	3.59	4.40
Incidence			
Total	3.72	3.61	3.93
Intestinal disease	2.73	2.37	2.39
HIV	0.28	0.52	0.71
Cancer	0.71	0.73	0.83

INDICATIONS FOR HOME ENTERAL NUTRITION

There are three major reasons for HEN to be needed: dysphagia, anorexia and intestinal failure. Dysphagia and anorexia cause a reduced intake, and intestinal failure results in reduced absorption. Some patients may have several reasons for needing HEN (e.g. anorexia and moderate intestinal failure). Of 500 patients followed in France for six years, HEN was given for dysphagia, anorexia, and 'moderate' intestinal failure in 58%, 30%, and 12% of patients, respectively (Hébuterne X and Schneider SM unpublished data). The underlying diagnoses of 162 adults and 21 children treated with HEN for a mean of 231 days were neurological diseases (44%), digestive disease (20%), head and neck cancer (13%), anorexia (9%), trauma (4%), AIDS (3%), and other (7%).[42] The reasons for enteral tube feeding in the UK are given in Table 26.2: 64% of adults have disease of the central nervous system (most are strokes in the elderly), 21% of gastrointestinal tract, 9% of genitourinary system, 3% of respiratory system and 1% have cardiac disease.[30] In the USA, 42% of HEN patients have cancer and 31% dysphagia, 1% Crohn's disease, 1% radiation damage and 1% AIDS.[21]

Dysphagia

Dysphagia is the major reason for a patient to receive HEN (77% in the UK).[30] It may be secondary to a

Table 26.2 – Underlying disease for which HEN is given to adults and children in the UK (BANS)[30]

	n=8832	
Cerebrovascular disease	2466★	(28)
Oesophageal cancer	1086	(12)
Cerebral palsy	451†	(5)
Motor neurone disease	393	(4)
Multiple sclerosis	369	(4)
Cystic fibrosis	324	(4)
Congenital handicap	281	(3)
Cerebral trauma	257	(3)
Crohn's disease	216	(2)
Oropharyngeal cancer	188	(2)
Parkinson's disease	143	(2)
Dementia	129	(1)
Congenital malformation	112	(1)
Gastric cancer	87	(1)
Other	2330	(26)

Most common reason: ★ in the elderly, † in children.

neurological problem (usually cerebrovascular disease), a vegetative state, a head and neck cancer, or a rare benign cause. In most cases dysphagia will remain a permanent problem; in some cases it is temporary, for example, during radiation therapy or chemotherapy or prior to removal of an upper gastrointestinal cancer. HEN is most commonly administered through a percutaneous gastrostomy which has either been placed at endoscopy (PEG)[44] or, less commonly, fluoroscopically. Aspiration is less likely to occur with a PEG than with a nasogastric feeding tube.[45]

It may be difficult, for ethical and legal reasons, to propose the insertion of a PEG for HEN.[46] In the UK there are two documents that give advice.[47,48] They differentiate medical treatment (giving drugs, enteral or oral fluid or nutrition) from basic care (hygiene functions which include warmth, toileting, washing and offering oral nutrition and hydration, and compassionate functions such as relieving distressing symptoms such as pain, vomiting or breathlessness). Medical treatment can be refused by the patient and can be withheld or withdrawn by the doctor acting in the patient's best interest; basic care, however, must be provided for all patients unless they actively resist it. The doctor, although ultimately responsible, is wise to discuss the situation with the patient, family and/or carers and to obtain their agreement in any decisions about providing artificial nutrition support. If a patient has previously expressed his or her wishes or has made a living will, these must be respected. An algorithm for

the decision to give HEN to a patient with dysphagia is given in Figure 26.1.

Anorexia

Anorexia represents a growing indication for HEN and defines a patient without dysphagia who cannot take adequate nutrition by mouth to meet his or her nutritional requirements. Some patients may have associated increased energy requirements (AIDS or cancer patients). Anorexia is generally found in very old patients, is secondary to an acute or chronic illness (surgery, infection, dementia or psychological disorder) and is associated with the problems of undernutrition. Active dietetic support is needed for these patients; if sip-feeds are unsuccessful, enteral feeding in the hospital may be given for 3–4 weeks. If voluntary intake improves significantly during this time, enteral nutrition can be stopped; if not, there is a high chance that long-term HEN will be needed.[49]

Intestinal failure

In the case of intestinal failure, oral intake is insufficient regardless of the gastrointestinal problems that have led or will lead to undernutrition. A patient with chronic diarrhoea may be a candidate for enteral rather than parenteral nutrition if the daily stool weight is less than 500 g and the daily faecal fat less than 20 g (72 mmol). There are many diagnoses responsible for maldigestion (e.g. chronic pancreatitis or previous gastrectomy) or malabsorption (e.g. short bowel, small bowel dysfunction or HIV/AIDS). Patients with more than 200 cm of small intestine remaining and a functioning colon may need a period of enteral support. Long-term enteral support may be needed in patients with a jejunostomy and 100–200 cm of remaining small intestine.[50]

Persistent vegetative state

Persistent vegetative state (PVS) is a clinical condition of complete unawareness of self and the environment, accompanied by sleep–wake cycles, with either complete or partial preservation of hypothalamic and brain stem autonomic functions;[51] there is no interaction between the patient and others, and the patient is doubly incontinent.[47] Some authors argue that physicians are not obliged to provide nutritional support in this condition because there is no clinical benefit although physiological functions can be maintained.[52] Others strongly disagree with this attitude on the basis that every human being has the right to food and water, even in situations in which medical inter-

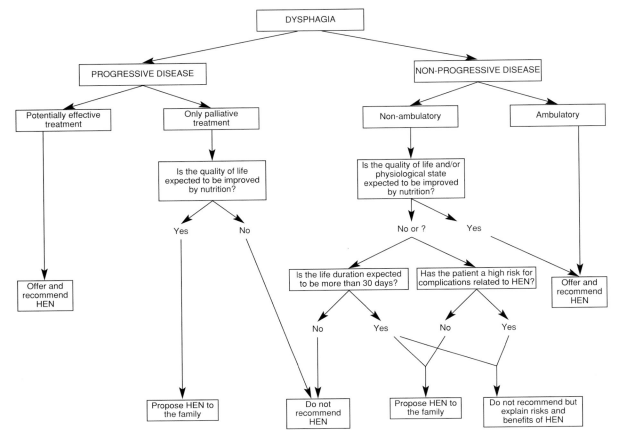

Figure 26.1 – Algorithm for starting HEN.

ventions can be ethically withheld.[53] The physician needs to explain all outcomes to the family and then, in some countries, let them decide. In the UK, an application to stop the feeding has to be made to the High Court. If the family wish to care for their family member at home, it can be argued that the medical profession must provide both the means by which food and water can be given, and the feed itself.

The criteria for giving HEN are summarized in Box 26.1. The success of HEN depends on patient selection, safe placement of a feeding tube/device, suitable nutrients and administration system, adequate education about enteral feeding, and regular monitoring.

Box 26.1 – Criteria for proposing that a patient be started on HEN

Oral failure
A functional/usable gastrointestinal tract
Ability to tolerate enteral nutritional therapy in the hospital (for at least 7 days)
No other medical or surgical problems – ready to be discharged
A clean and safe home
Patient or carer able to perform all enteral procedures safely

OUTCOME OF HOME ENTERAL NUTRITION

The overall HEN-related complication rate needing hospital admission was 0.3–0.4 per patient per year (with little difference between the diagnoses); this was half that of patients receiving HPN[21] (Ch. 31).

The quality of life for most patients in the UK receiving HEN was poor. In East Anglia, 40% were unable to walk, 39% were unable to speak, and 20% were housebound; only 29% could speak normally, 29% could walk unaided, and 21% left their home daily without aid; 53% took laxatives and 31% antidiarrhoeal drugs. Nine per cent of patients receiving gastrostomy tube feeding developed aspiration pneumonia and in this event most needed hospital admission.[54] While the health-related quality of life for patients with gastrostomy tubes is poor (usually due to severe physical disability) compared to that of the general population, the majority of patients and carers rated the gastrostomy 'positively'.[55]

The outcome of patients on HEN at one centre in France is represented in Table 26.3; the overall probability of survival was 44% at one year and 29% at 5 years.[42] In the UK overall, 22% died by 1 year, and 14% returned to oral feeding. There was a low mortality for cerebral palsy, cystic fibrosis and multiple sclerosis. Patients with motor neurone disease, dementia and malignancy had a high mortality of 30–60% in the first year. Patients who had a cerebrovascular accident and were over 75 years were 3–4 times more likely to die while on HEN than those patients aged less than 65. Fourteen per cent of those who had had a stroke returned to oral feeding, thus it is important to assess continually a patient's ability to swallow as it may improve and allow tube feeding to be stopped.[30]

It is estimated that 10% of nursing home residents in the USA are receiving HEN.[40] In the USA, after one year of HEN therapy, the outcome for neurological patients with dysphagia was that 48% had died, 25% were continuing, and 19% had stopped and resumed full oral nutrition; of all these patients, 71% had 'minimal rehabilitation' (i.e. were barely ambulatory). The outcome for cancer patients at one year was that 59% had died, 6% were continuing on HEN, and 30% had stopped and resumed full oral nutrition.[21] Patients with small bowel malabsorption needing HEN are uncommon, but at one year 82% were alive, 43% had 'complete rehabilitation', and 45% had stopped HEN and resumed an oral intake.[40]

Readmission to hospital in the USA for non-HEN problems was less common for patients with neuromuscular disorders of swallowing (0.9/year), than with cancer or small bowel disease (both 2.7/year).[40]

INDICATIONS FOR HOME PARENTERAL NUTRITION

HPN is needed for patients with acute or chronic intestinal failure in whom nutritional and/or water and electrolyte balance cannot be corrected by oral or enteral feeding, and for whom PN is feasible at home. PN may be short- or long-term depending upon whether the intestinal failure is reversible or irreversible.

In adults, there are four main diagnostic indications for non-HIV patients needing HPN; these are Crohn's disease, mesenteric infarction, radiation enteritis and cancer (gastrointestinal or gynaecological) (Table 26.4). The distribution of these diagnostic groups varies between countries. Cancer is now the most common underlying diagnosis in all reporting countries except

Table 26.3 – Outcome of patients on HEN (follow-up 18–65 months)[42]

	Full oral nutrition n=51	Continued HEN n=19	Died n=93	Stopped for other reasons n=20
Neurological disease	16%	13%	65%	6%
Head and neck cancer	33%	5%	54%	8%
Digestive disease	49%	3%	26%	22%
Post-traumatic dysphagia	14%	43%	0%	43%
Anorexia (elderly)	30%	6%	58%	6%
AIDS	0%	0%	100%	0%
Other	50%	25%	17%	8%

Table 26.4 – Underlying disease for which HPN is given to adults

	Europe[23]	USA[21]	Japan[20]
Year(s)	1997	1989–1992	1990
Number (M:F)	494 (0.7)	5357 (equal)	231 (1.6)
Age at start (years)	Most 41–60	Mean 41	Mean 46
Underlying disease (%)			
Cancer	39★	41	40
Crohn's disease	19	11	20
Vascular disease	15	6	19
Radiation enteritis	7	3	2
AIDS	2	5	–
Other	18	34	19

★ 78% in Germany and 80% in Sweden.

the UK, France and Denmark.[18–20,22,23,32,56–58] In the USA, cancers represented 16% of patients in 1984, 39% in 1987, and 41% in 1992. The percentage of patients in the USA receiving HPN for HIV was 2% at the end of the 1980s and 4% at the start of the 1990s.[18,21] The number of patients with diagnoses other than cancer or HIV is remaining relatively constant.

The most common anatomical reasons for patients to receive HPN in Europe are a short bowel (35%), intestinal obstruction (28%), fistula (7%) or pseudo-obstruction (7%).[23]

Short bowel

Problems of having a short bowel may occur when less than 1.5–2.0 metres of small intestine remain.[50,59] The most common reasons for this are resections for mesenteric ischaemia (volvulus, trauma, arterial or venous occlusion), Crohn's disease and radiation enteritis. Patients with a short bowel represent about 25% (range 10–30%) of all reasons for HPN[19] and 55% (range 52–68%) of the non-cancer non-HIV reasons.[19,29,32,33,60] Of those patients who need HPN for more than 2 years, about three-quarters have a short bowel.[29,33,58]

Functional causes of intestinal failure

Intestinal obstruction and/or fistulae

The group of patients with intestinal obstruction and/or fistulae contains most patients with a 'surgical' potentially reversible cause of acute intestinal failure.

In the first multicentre European study of non-cancer non-HIV causes, small bowel obstruction accounted for 20–30% and intestinal fistulae for 20% of patients.[19] Intestinal obstruction is especially common in patients with radiation enteritis and Crohn's disease.[19] Intestinal obstruction was present in 40% of HPN cancer patients and 10% of HPN patients with an abdominal fistula.[26,57] Intestinal obstruction is important as its presence precludes oral/enteral feeding. There may be an increase in complications related to the enforced resting of the digestive system, and vomiting may result in a reduction in the quality of life. The prognosis for all non-malignant diagnoses is worse when intestinal obstruction is also present.[29]

Crohn's disease

PN may be beneficial in patients with Crohn's disease as a treatment for concomitant undernutrition (which, if rectified, slows disease progression) or by providing complete bowel rest in patients who have not responded to conventional medical treatments.[19,60] In addition, it may be necessary to give nutritional and/or fluid replacement in patients who have had bowel resections leaving a short bowel. PN may be given for a period of 1–2 months prior to definitive surgery for intestinal obstruction or fistulae. Most patients with active small bowel Crohn's disease will need immunosuppressive and/or surgical treatment in addition to HPN.[19,60]

Radiation enteritis

Radiation enteritis is more commonly treated with HPN in France than in other countries. Between 1993 and 1995, however, the proportion of patients treated with HPN for this reason reduced from 15% to 8%, while other non-cancer, non-HIV indications remained the same. Providing the underlying malignancy has been eradicated, this severe, often multifocal enteritis can be treated with HPN. PN is often given prior to elective surgery (often for chronic obstruction); this allows the surgery to be carefully planned and performed when the inflammatory process has become quiescent and the nutritional state as near to normal as possible.[19]

Chronic intestinal pseudo-obstruction

Chronic intestinal pseudo-obstruction may result in undernutrition caused by both nausea/vomiting and malabsorption; thus HPN is needed, often with extra fluid[19,61] (Ch. 8).

Other medical indications

Some patients with severe malabsorption resistant to medical treatments or with intestinal lymphangectasia will benefit from HPN. Other patients who may benefit from HPN are those with villus atrophy resistant to a gluten-free diet (e.g. with common variable immunological deficiencies) or those non-compliant to the gluten-free diet for whom the slightest deviation from the gluten-free regimen causes total small bowel villus atrophy. A Shilling test with intrinsic factor may be done after 3 months of HPN to monitor the response to a gluten-free diet;[62] however, care must be taken to exclude a small bowel lymphoma (small bowel biopsies with lymphocyte typing).

In the USA, 23% of Medicare patients received HPN during renal dialysis.[21,43]

Other surgical indications

Some patients need HPN because of severe post-operative intestinal adhesions (frozen peritoneum) or jejuno–ileal exclusion by fistulae and/or temporary enterostomies.[21,57] According to circumstances, a delay of 3–6 months offers the best chance of a wound or fistula healing and of fewer postoperative complications.[19,32]

Controversial indications

There is much ethical debate about whether patients with active incurable cancer or HIV should receive HPN. HPN may improve nutritional status, but there is little convincing evidence that it prolongs life or improves the quality of life,[21,63–66] although some reports appear encouraging at first.[67–70] World-wide, however, active incurable cancer is the single most common reason for giving HPN (Table 26.4). The American Society for Parenteral and Enteral Nutrition (ASPEN) has issued a consultative document about the indications for giving HPN to these patients.[19,44] It may not be appropriate to give HPN to patients in whom recent progression of the underlying illness might cause a situation of total dependence and a mediocre quality of life.[32,61,64] For every HPN patient, an explicit agreement between patient, family and medical staff is necessary to ascertain the aims and the appropriate means of treatment for the individual patient. Prospective controlled trials may help to indicate who will benefit most from HPN.

HIV. Severe undernutrition in patients with HIV may be partly due to anorexia, resistant vomiting, infection, diarrhoea and/or malabsorption (Ch. 6). HPN may be considered after any opportunistic infections have been controlled and if enteral feeding has proved unsuccessful.[37,66,70,71] HPN may be most appropriate for those who, in the absence of persistent infection, are capable of learning the procedures, do not vomit after food and have had one or no episode of diarrhoea due to parasites (e.g. cryptosporidiosis, microsporidiosis or enteropathic HIV).[37,66] HIV infection has become a rare indication for starting HPN since the introduction of the antiprotease drugs in 1995–1996.

Cancer. Cancer as a reason for starting HPN varies in frequency from country to country (0–80%).[19–21,22,23,26,32,57] This variation is the result of the absence of a medical consensus that takes cultural, ethical and financial considerations into account.[21,63] The most common underlying cancers are those of the large bowel (17%), ovary (13%), stomach (8%) or pancreas (8%).[72] Intestinal obstruction and vomiting is the most common reason for giving HPN to a patient with cancer (45–65%), though some have a short bowel (22%).[26,57,69] Anorexia (12%), diarrhoea and malabsorption (11%), malnutrition (3%) and enterocutaneous fistula (3%) account for most other reasons for starting HPN.[69] Some patients receive chemotherapy in association with HPN.[26,63] Patients who have been 'cured' of cancer may need HPN because of residual short bowel or radiation damage.

MATERIALS AND METHODS FOR HOME PARENTERAL NUTRITION

The aim of PN at home is to transfer the techniques used in hospital to the home and to create conditions that allow the patient to lead an active and fulfilling life; at the same time, HPN should be cost-effective. The ideal features of a company supplying a patient at home with equipment and nutrition are listed in Box 26.2. HPN is administered via a central vein catheter to give a nutritious all-in-one feed of about 3 litres and is usually given for a mean of 5 (range 3–7) nights per week. Since the 1970s the equipment and techniques for HPN have improved in terms of vascular access, nutritional mixtures, and the application of cyclical PN. There has been encouragement, when appropriate, for oral or enteral nutrition.

Box 26.2 – Ideal features of a home care company

1. Supply and maintain a variety of equipment and feeds

Ancillaries
Equipment (hardware)   :
- pump (12-monthly servicing)
- portable pump available
- drip stand
- procedure trolley
- refrigerator and thermometer

Consumables (dry goods):
- dressing packs, towels, gloves, cleaning solutions, needles/filter straws, clamps, syringes, connection devices, sharps bin, etc.

Parenteral nutrition
Shelf life greater than 1 week
Flushes (heparin or saline)

2. Delivery
Delivery staff in uniform and carrying identification (notification given of change of driver)
Unpack and store supplies, even when patient is out
Delivery arrives on time (± 2 hours – needs to come from geographically near depot)
Parenteral nutrition bags every 2 weeks (depending upon stability)
Consumables every 4 weeks
Deliver all over home country and abroad

3. 24-hour telephone contact
Patient phoned about stock levels (at least every 4 weeks)

4. Replace damaged equipment (pump and fridge) within 24 hours

5. Remove sharps (and if necessary clinical waste)

6. 24-hour nursing support

7. Train patients or staff in the techniques in hospital or at home

8. Fast and easy change of prescription/details

9. Provide patient information booklet

10. Maintain contact with GP and hospital

11. Remove all equipment after feeding stops (within a week)

12. Proven track record

Vascular access

A central venous access catheter made of silicone or polyurethane is placed so that its tip lies at the junction of the superior vena cava and right atrium.[35] There is no difference between the two materials in complication rates, except that some types of polyurethane catheter may be more prone to fracture.[73] The administration set (about 150 cm) is linked at one end to the external end of the catheter and at the other to the all-in-one nutrient mixture. The administration set passes through a programmable pump that has several alarms.

The catheter most frequently used for HPN (80%) is one with a subcutaneous cuff that stops external migration and an external end that can be capped off. In 20% a catheter with an implantable port is used; this gives a better cosmetic appearance, makes bathing and swimming easier, and does not require a dressing. Ports were initially used by patients requiring chemotherapy.[19,26,57,65] They have the disadvantages that the self-sealing septum has a finite life (about 2000 punctures), that a needle has to be put through skin for each feed, and that they cannot be repaired and need to be removed surgically if problems occur. Of patients with experience of both a port and an external catheter, 80% prefer the port.[74] A port is most appropriate for those patients who do not feed every night.

Feeding bag/regimen issues

In the home, a place must be reserved to store materials, a fridge is needed in which to keep the nutrient bags[19] and, for some patients, an area to sterilize the connections for the feeding line is necessary.

Feed composition

The nutrient mixture volume is 1.5–4.0 litres; the requirements are greater if all or most of the colon has been removed[59,75] or if there is a discharging stoma or fistula. A patient's needs are likely to vary with time. Usually, 0.6–1.2 g/kg of protein (0.1–0.2 g/kg of nitrogen), 150–350 g of glucose and less than 1 g/kg of lipid are given each day[38,76] (Ch. 20). Most patients (except those with radiation damage or pseudo-obstruction) take an amount of food orally that exceeds their resting energy expenditure (by 170–200%), however little energy is absorbed.[77]

The amount of minerals needed by each patient varies. Some patients, most commonly those with a jejunostomy,[30] only need supplements of water, electrolytes and micronutrients (magnesium).[78] The amounts of most trace elements and vitamins are calculated according to the recommendations of the American Medical Association. When there are large gastrointestinal fluid losses, there is a need for extra zinc (5–10 mg/d) and selenium (50–100 μg/d). Cholestasis reduces the need for manganese, copper and iron.[58,79] Metal contaminants (e.g. aluminium and manganese[80]) have been found in excess in some nutrient mixtures. Essential fatty acid deficiency is common in HPN patients who have less than 100 cm small bowel remaining.[81] Lipid emulsions have a variable content of vitamin K, which may need to be taken into account if a patient is taking warfarin. Vitamin E requirements rise if there are significant gastrointestinal losses and/or if there is a plentiful supply of polyunsaturated fatty acids, as contained in most lipid emulsions.[19] The requirement for vitamin D (cholecalciferol) is estimated at between 0 and 200 IU per day,[65,79] depending upon sunlight exposure. The stability of some vitamins is limited, which is why many nutrient mixtures have a shelf life of less than 10 days. Shelf life is much longer if the solution does not contain lipid or vitamins[65] (Ch. 21).

Single bag vs. multiple glass bottles

Parenteral administration of different intravenous nutrients from multiple glass bottles was gradually replaced in the 1980s by a single all-in-one disposable bag made of ethyl vinyl acetate.[19] A study in Europe in 1986 showed that 90% of HPN patients used a single bag compared with 10% who used multiple containers.[19] In the USA, patients preferred the single bag system to that of multiple containers.[19] The single bag mixture is given by a single administration set and pump; this reduces the number of times the feeding line is handled (particularly at night) and thus reduces the chance of septicaemia occurring.[19,35] Bags with two (or more) compartments are now available in which lipids are stored separately but are mixed with the other nutrients just before the infusion begins; this increases the shelf life of the whole bag.

Timing and frequency of PN

Since cyclical (intermittent or discontinuous) PN was first described in 1976 in a hospital setting, several studies have demonstrated psychological, physical and metabolic advantages of cyclical nocturnal PN (10–16 hours in 24 hours) compared to continuous feeding.[82] In practice, PN is often administered continuously in hospital, while since 1970 it has almost always been given at night-time at home.[19] HPN given at night, although not physiological, allows total freedom of movement during the day but usually means that the patient must get up one or more times at night to pass urine. Multicentre European studies have shown that 87–90% of patients feed at night, 2–5% during the daytime, and 5–11% continuously.[57] Patients prefer cyclical PN to continuous PN,[19] though portable pumps may make daytime HPN more attractive as well as physiological. The perfusion is delivered at 150–300 ml/h, with a two-fold decline in rate over the last hour to avoid rebound hypoglycaemia.[35,82]

The metabolic and nutritional status of the patient is best optimized by prescribing the minimum number of nutrient perfusions, and it is desirable to achieve one or more days without PN. It is better for a patient to feed on 5 or 6 of 7 nights with more energy in each bag than to feed every night. This goal, and even discontinuation of PN, may be achieved within 2–6 weeks in some patients (e.g. those with a short bowel and a preserved colon) when and if compensatory hyperphagia occurs,[83,84] although intravenous electrolytes (3–6 litres a week),[59] mineral and/or micronutrient supplements (e.g. oral zinc or magnesium and intramuscular B$_{12}$) may still need to be continued. PN can sometimes be discontinued in patients with a jejunostomy if their treatment is optimized (Ch. 24).

Additional oral or enteral nutrition

Resting the digestive tract and giving total PN has demonstrated the importance of specific intestinal substrates, such as glutamine, short-chain fatty acids and nucleotides,[60] which are not at present included in routine PN mixtures. An oral intake reduces biliary sludge[85] and cholestasis (and possibly steatosis)[85,86] and promotes intestinal adaptive mechanisms.[59] A patient will be much less socially disadvantaged if he or she can eat some food at meal times. Therefore, with some clinical exceptions (e.g. Crohn's disease or fistulae), it is better in the absence of obstruction to continue HPN with some oral complementary nutrition.[65] In addition, hyperphagia is one of the most important components in promoting intestinal adaptation and thus weaning patients off HPN.[84]

EDUCATION OF PATIENTS ABOUT HOME PARENTERAL NUTRITION

The length of the hospital stay, which allows optimal treatment of the underlying illness, the attainment of a stable medical condition, and education in PN techniques, is between 3 weeks and 3 months.[19] The main aim of the education, usually carried out by a nurse, is to bring the patient from a situation of passive dependence to one of active independence. An average 3 of weeks is needed to acquire completely the HPN techniques.[19,57] Models, booklets and audio-visual techniques are used to achieve this. The stress of being in hospital is reduced by this education.[19] Successful patient education requires the patient to have an understanding of his or her illness, self-confidence after acquiring the techniques necessary to perform HPN, and a good relationship with the nutrition team. It is helpful to the training for the patient to meet other self-sufficient patients.

Complete autonomy is necessary for long-term HPN patients,[32,36] as they will have fewer septic complications.[36] Partial autonomy is acceptable when the envisaged duration of HPN is less than 3 months (i.e. malignant disease).[26,57] Of long-term HPN patients, 95% are totally autonomous; this does not relate to the patient's age.[19,87]

COMPLICATIONS OF HOME PARENTERAL NUTRITION

A patient at home may be expected to need one hospital admission a year for a septic, mechanical, thrombotic or metabolic complication relating to the HPN.[32] The frequency of HPN complications necessitating admission was 32% dehydration or an electrolyte problem, 27% catheter-related sepsis, 17% blocked catheter, 12% exit site infection, 10% positional problems and 5% liver abnormalities.[88]

Complications of HPN (catheter sepsis, thrombosis/embolisms and/or a severe hepatopathy) are responsible for the death of 3–7% of patients (8–30% of all causes of death).[21,29,32] The association of liver disease with intestinal insufficiency is an indication for transplanting both small bowel and liver together.[89] The international register shows that 40–50% of patients having a small bowel transplant have also needed a liver transplant, and the probability of graft survival is no worse than for small bowel transplant alone.[90]

Catheter-related sepsis

The incidence of catheter-related sepsis is related not to the type of catheter used but to the strictness of the aseptic technique used during manipulations of the catheter (especially its hub connection).[35] The frequency of infections is an indication of the competency of the nutrition team, who can significantly reduce catheter-related sepsis by educating their patients. Catheter sepsis rates (Denmark, France, USA and UK) vary between 0.33 and 0.70/catheter/year.[27,32,36,91,92] A subgroup of patients (30–50%) present many times with infected catheters. Patients who are dependent upon opiates or sedatives have an increased frequency of catheter-related sepsis and other complications,[93] and patients with a stoma have a higher rate of catheter-related sepsis than those without a stoma.[27] Recurrent episodes of catheter-related sepsis can arise from diseased teeth,[94] urinary tract infections or bacterial overgrowth in the small bowel. Catheter-related sepsis is rarely fatal.[21,29] The annual rate of catheter-related sepsis is significantly higher in HIV patients (1.20–1.50/patient/year of HPN) than in non-HIV patients.[36,37,70] This increase may be partly secondary to acquired immunodeficiency, but mostly results from the use of the feeding line for non-nutritional treatments.

The diagnosis of a catheter-related infection is suspected if a fever occurs shortly after starting a nutrient infusion and is likely if peripheral and catheter cultures or cultures from an endoluminal brush[95] show appropriate organisms. It is confirmed after removal of the catheter and culture of its tip. An infection of the catheter does not usually necessitate its removal, but there are two essential measures: the PN must be stopped for 48–72 hours, and, after blood cultures have been taken, an antibiotic is given via the line.[35,96] Some insert urokinase into the line after giving the antibiotic. These measures permit sterilization of the catheter and continuation of PN via the same catheter in 95% of cases.[96] Infections associated with an entry site or the subcutaneous course of a catheter, and those occurring on an implanted port generally mean that the catheter has to be removed.[96]

Catheter obstruction

Obstruction of the catheter may occur secondary to a reflux of blood back up into the catheter. A fibrin sheath can be treated by giving one or more injections of antifibrinolytic drugs into the line.[19,34] Blockage can be caused by a progressive build-up of lipid, especially in those patients who have lipid regularly incorporated into their feeding bag rather than given separately. It can be cleared by putting ethanol down the line and may be prevented by a daily infusion down the line of physiological serum (20–50 ml).[19] In adults, line blockage is rarely due to the precipitation of calcium and phosphate; hydrochloric acid may clear this (Ch. 32).

Venous thrombosis

Catheter-induced venous thrombosis and pulmonary emboli may occur with an incidence of 0.06/year,[32] but this is likely to be an underestimate.[35] There is an increased risk in cancer patients and those with a primary coagulation deficiency (i.e. mesenteric infarction) or abnormalities of platelet function (i.e. Crohn's disease). The use of anticoagulation (preventative or curative) is often justifiable and reduces the risk of thrombosis with a central catheter. Treatment with heparin, then warfarin, for catheter-induced venous thrombosis may avert the need to remove the catheter.[35]

Mechanical problems

Mechanical problems occur with an incidence of 0.44/year.[32] Damage to the external segment of a catheter (catheter tear or cracking of the hub) is most common in children/adolescents.[97] Before a Dacron cuff was used this could result in intravascular displacement of the catheter, which could embolize to the lungs. A damaged catheter can allow an air embolism to occur. Damage to a catheter can usually be repaired using special repair kits, but the risk of infection is always high. Portacaths may leak, especially if the needle has been passed through the same spot of the membrane and not rotated. This causes local pain and erythema, which becomes more intense on starting the infusion.

Metabolic complications

Metabolic problems occur with an overall incidence of about 0.12/year.[32]

Micronutrients

Thirty-three per cent of HPN patients may have a micronutrient deficiency (most commonly of iron) but this rarely causes clinical problems.[98] Nutrient mixtures include trace elements and fat- and water-soluble vitamins so that deficiencies are less likely.[65] The main deficiencies and surpluses of micronutrients were described often for the first time in HPN patients.[58,65,79] A poor sodium supply leads to hyperaldosteronism with hypokalaemia. An insufficient

supply of magnesium may lead to hypocalcaemia, which is resistant to vitamin D, and hypokalaemia.[99] Micronutrient deficiencies can be fatal (e.g. cardiomyopathy from severe selenium deficiency) or lead to a major functional problem (e.g. neuropathy with or without a cerebellar syndrome from a deficiency of vitamin E, which is more likely if a lipid emulsion is rich in polyunsaturated acids).

Problems of excessive amounts of micronutrients occur partly because HPN short-circuits absorption and the metabolic filtering functions of the liver. Thus some components, especially metals, accumulate in the tissues.[58,65,79] Aluminium contamination has been implicated as one of the factors in hepatopathy and osteopathy.[19,65,100] Intracerebral manganese has been detected in patients receiving HPN and in patients with a portacaval shunt using magnetic resonance imaging: this shows a T_2 hypersignal in the brain central grey matter cells. Manganese deposition may be responsible for the occurrence of encephalopathy and extrapyramidal signs.[101]

Hepatic complications

Abnormal liver function tests or liver disease associated with PN may relate to the underlying illness, its treatment (e.g. surgery/bowel resection) and nutritional factors.[85,86] In the acute setting, abdominal sepsis, renal failure, pre-existing liver disease and blood transfusions are more commonly related to abnormal liver histology than parenteral nutrition.[102]

Chronic cholestasis, as defined by two of three tests (γ-glutamyl transferase, alkaline phosphatase and conjugated bilirubin) being more than 1.5 times the upper limit of normal for more than 6 months, was documented in 65% of patients receiving long-term HPN.[38] HPN-related liver disease (portal fibrosis or cirrhosis or any clinical features of chronic liver disease) occurred in 42%, and 22% of all deaths were due to liver disease.[38] Data from the USA showed that 15% of adult patients receiving HPN developed end stage liver disease, and this was most common in those with a very short bowel and chronic inflammation.[103] Tumour necrosis factor, released by chronic inflammation, may be partly responsible.[104]

Cholestasis. Resting of the entire digestive system (total PN) is the main factor responsible for increased biliary sludge formation and cholelithiasis, which occurs at 1.5 months and 4.0 months respectively.[85,86] Following an ileal or colonic resection there is a major lack of bile acids, especially those combined with taurine conjugates, and there is an increase in production of secondary bile acids and/or lithocolic acid.[58,86] Since bile is more prone to form sludge if mixed with solutions lacking in taurine or methyl donors (S adenosyl methionine) and is restored in experimental models by giving them, it is logical to propose that HPN patients receive an amino acid solution enriched with taurine.[58] Stimulation of gallbladder contraction by maintaining a minimal oral intake of food (protein and long-chain triglycerides), which causes cholecystokinin release, is a way of preventing the formation of biliary sludge. Ursodeoxycholic acid is an effective medical prophylaxis/treatment for chronic cholestasis in patients receiving HPN.[85,86] Automatic cholecystectomy following surgery that results in a short bowel can be questioned (Ch. 14).

In two decades of HPN the frequency of biliary complications has decreased from 40% to less than 15%,[19] and may now be no different to that of patients with ileal disease or who have had an ileal resection.[19]

Hepatocellular steatosis. Although a fatty liver, shown on ultrasound or biopsy (steatosis), does occur, the liver function test abnormalities that this causes are often of a cholestatic nature.

Excess nutrients. When parenteral nutrition was first used, excessive amounts of energy (more than 2000 kcal daily or more than 5 g glucose, 2 g lipid and 2 g amino acids/kg/d) were often given and resulted in steatosis (fatty liver). This meant that either an increase in triglyceride manufacture or a failure of triglyceride oxidation was occurring. Abnormalities are more apparent if there is any degree of glucose intolerance.[85] Excessive supplies of macronutrients, proteins and/or lipids all cause a chronic cholestatic picture on standard liver function tests.[85,86,105] Apart from these circumstances, a multivariate analysis on a series of 90 HPN patients has shown that a supply of 20% lipid emulsions rich in ω6 polyunsaturated fatty acids was associated with chronic cholestasis and, when more than 1 g lipid/kg/day was given, with severe hepatopathy.[38] Patients should therefore be given less than this.

Cholestatic abnormalities on liver function tests can be associated with a disorder of the liver, spleen and bone marrow (cytopenias).[65] Polyunsaturated fatty acids and phospholipids may accumulate, especially in the Kupffer cells (macrophages), in patients receiving HPN.[58] This causes a microvacuole steatosis which, unlike macrovacuole steatosis, often goes unnoticed unless specific stains are used on liver biopsy material (e.g. oil red O). Sea-blue histiocytes, shown with Giemsa staining, may be seen on bone marrow examination when HPN that includes a lipid emulsion rich in polyunsaturated fatty acids has been given for a median of 5 years.[76] The finding in an adult receiving HPN of thrombocytopenia causing a haemorrhagic tendency, pulmonary infiltrates, itching, hepatosplenomegaly with or without portal hypertension, and sea-blue histiocytes on examination of the bone marrow is termed Silverstein syndrome.[76,106] In children, Silverstein syndrome is associated with fever, jaundice, thrombocytopenia, and disseminated intravascular coagulation.[18] Development of this syndrome makes it essential to stop intravenous lipids; the itching will recede over several months but the patient should not be exposed to the risk of essential fatty acid deficiency.[58]

Glutamine has been shown in animals to protect against steatosis.[104]

Lack of nutrients. It is not surprising that the greatest problems with liver disease occur in those with the shortest length of remaining bowel who are dependent for all their nutritional needs upon the parenteral nutrition solution infused. It is this group that has the greatest degree of cholestasis and fibrosis and the highest mortality from HPN-induced liver disease.[103,107] Essential fatty acid deficiency will cause steatosis.[104] Choline deficiency is a rare reversible cause of liver function test abnormalities.[108] Low plasma levels of lysine, which in the liver and kidneys makes carnitine, have been observed in patients receiving HPN. Carnitine is responsible for the transfer of long-chain fatty acids into the mitochondria for oxidation. Low plasma carnitine levels associated with low lysine levels have been found in patients with a raised alkaline phosphatase and a low serum albumin, as is characteristic of steatosis.[109]

Bowel bacteria. When part of the intestine has been removed there is a change in the intestinal bacterial flora. If the intestinal mucosa is damaged, intestinal bacteria, particularly those in defunctioned or blind-ending bowel, may translocate across the mucosa and cause a release of tumour necrosis factor which can cause hepatic steatosis.[85,86]

Osteopathy

When HPN is begun, osteopenia and/or osteomalacia have been found in about 50% of patients; this is the result of immobility and chronic malabsorption causing negative calcium, magnesium and vitamin D balance.[19,110]

Patients receiving HPN for more than 6 months may develop a progressive osteopathy of the lower limb long bones with associated joint pains, hypercalciuria and a low bone formation rate (serum osteocalcin, a measure of bone turnover, is low).[19,65,111–116] This is a restructuring osteopathy in which the rate of trabecular bone resorption exceeds that of formation.[65] Patients may also complain of loose teeth or of them actually falling out soon after starting parenteral nutrition; this may relate to a loss of alveolar bone.[117] PN osteopathy is different from that caused by the other well-recognized risk factors for osteoporosis, although these factors may also be present, namely increasing age, female gender, smoking, alcohol, reduced exercise, reduced sunlight exposure, and treatment with steroids, loop diuretics or heparin. In some reports serum vitamin 1,25 hydroxy-vitamin D levels have been reduced while 25 hydroxy-vitamin D levels were normal,[118,119] but in more recent reports both have been within the normal range.[115] Reports of parathormone levels are very variable (usually low) and the normal diurnal nocturnal rise of parathormone is prevented by PN.[114]

Factors that may be responsible include aluminium or vitamin D toxicity, amino acid infusions, acidity, hypomagnesaemia, a reduced parathormone response, hypercalciuria and cytokine effects. In the past, aluminium contamination of feeds in adults caused pain in the long bones and weight-bearing joints, a decreased rate of bone formation and patchy osteomalacia on bone biopsy;[100,116,120] the aluminium loading was reduced and bone disease improved by changing from a casein hydrolysate solution to a balanced crystalline amino acid solution.[121] Vitamin D administration has been associated with bone disease[122] and in those with depressed parathormone levels it can be corrected by removing vitamin D from the feed. After the removal of vitamin D the serum levels of parathormone and 1,25 hydroxy-vitamin D increased towards normal.[119] Intravenously infused amino acids increase urinary calcium loss[123] and intravenous phosphate reduces it.[124] An amino acid infusion of more than 2 g/kg caused more calcium to be lost in urine than was infused.[123] Hypomagnesaemia, which is common in patients with a short bowel, reduces the secretion and function of parathormone. Renal conservation of calcium is therefore reduced and 1,25 hydroxy-vitamin D is not made in adequate amounts, thus calcium and magnesium are not adequately absorbed from the gut (Ch. 12); this may further contribute to bone disease. Cytokines, such as inter-leukins 1 and 6 and tumour necrosis factor alpha, can all increase bone resorption.[125]

Oral calcium supplements, vitamin D, oestrogen in women, sunlight exposure, a small amount of fluoride and/or biphosphonates may be used depending upon regular bone density measurements.[126] A 10-day course of calcitonin may be helpful in relieving pain from the osteopathy. Vitamin D should be stopped if the serum parathormone or 1,25 hydroxy-vitamin D levels are low and the 25 hydroxy-vitamin D level is normal.[119]

OUTCOME OF HOME PARENTERAL NUTRITION

Most reports indicate maintenance of or gain in body weight and gain in muscle strength (grip or peak flow)[10,25,92] with HPN; it is not usually stated whether patients achieved their former, ideal or desired weight. Patients with a short bowel receiving HPN can usually have their weight gradually increased to whatever they choose and most will ultimately have a body mass index within the normal range.[50] It is often easier to regulate a patient's weight with parenteral rather than enteral nutrition as the ability to increase energy intake enterally may be limited by gastrointestinal symptoms.

Quality of life

Many publications have shown a relatively good quality of life for patients receiving HPN.[21,32,50,88,127–132] In non-cancer non-AIDS patients, HPN increases survival adjusted for quality of life by 3.3 years in comparison with intermittent PN in hospital.[19,56,64] The improvement in quality of life results from social and professional reintegration.[19]

The UK and European multicentre studies evaluated social reintegration according to the degree of dependency by classifying patients into four categories: I, at full-time work or looking after home and family unaided; II, at work part-time or looking after home and family with help; III, unable to work but able to cope with own treatments unaided and able to go out occasionally; IV, housebound and needing major assistance with HPN).[19,32] Of patients less than 65 years old (93% of the HPN population) 52–66% were stage I or II, and 1–8% stage IV. The majority of stage III patients presented a partial incapacity relating to an underlying pathology or the existence of a stoma.[19] These good results depended on a satisfactory weight gain (observed in 95% of patients) and a rare need for re-admission to hospital.[19,21] In the USA, complete functional rehabilitation is observed in 49–83% of patients within the first year of HPN, with the exception of patients having encapsulating peritonitis (23%), cancer (29%) or AIDS (8%).[21] Psychological problems encountered during HPN are not different to those met with other chronic illnesses.[19,64]

After a period of adaptation to HPN of 6 months to 2 years, 75% of non-cancer non-HIV patients achieved individual rehabilitation objectives of 7–10, as measured on a 10-point scale with 1 being no rehabili-tation and 10 perfect rehabilitation.[19] Pregnancies have been brought successfully to term in patients receiving HPN.[19,64,133,134]

After 2 months of PN given to patients with HIV infection, body weight and lean body mass increased[37,70] and the quality of life (Karnowsky index) improved by 9%.[70] It is difficult to distinguish those who will respond to HPN,[37] except that those who do best will usually also have had an underlying infection treated.

Fifty-eight per cent of patients receiving HPN said that their sleep was disrupted by frequent urination, 40% complained of cramps in their hands or feet, and 27% complained of dry scaly skin.[88] Noisy pumps and the bright lights on the pumps interrupt the sleep of most patients having HPN at night.[135]

Chance of stopping HPN

The chance of stopping HPN depends upon the underlying diagnosis. In the USA, 52% were able to stop HPN by one year for all non-cancer non-AIDS reasons,[21] which is a similar result to that in Europe.[23] In the Franco-Belgian study, 46% of patients remained on HPN for more than 2 years; 87% of these patients had a short bowel.[29,39,58] In Denmark, only 19% were able to stop PN, and in a quarter of these cases this was because intestinal continuity was restored.[27]

The probabilities of ceasing HPN in patients with a short bowel are affected by the presence of residual disease in the remaining intestine, upon the length and type of disease-free small bowel and the amount of functional colon, possibly the presence of a functional ileocaecal valve, and the degree to which adaptation has occurred.[39] The outlook is much better if the colon has been preserved (jejuno-colic or jejuno-ileal anastomosis); in such cases, if more than 50–100 cm of small bowel remains, the patient is likely to stop parenteral nutrition.[39,50,75,136] Unabsorbed protein and carbohydrate arriving undigested and unabsorbed in the colon can be fermented by bacteria to short-chain fatty acids that can be absorbed and provide a source of energy of up to 1000 kcal per day.[60,83,137] The colon can be considered for nutrient absorptive purposes as having an absorptive value equivalent to 30–70 cm of small intestine.[39,50,59,137] A patient with a jejunostomy sited less than 100–115 cm from the duodeno-jejunal flexure is likely to need long-term HPN or parenteral water and electrolytes.[39,78,136] For a patient with a short bowel to be able to stop PN requires the restitution and the maintenance of a satisfactory nutritional state;[59] for this to happen hyperphagia needs to have developed to compensate for malabsorption.[83,84] The majority of patients with a short bowel absorb at least 30% of oral lipids and more than 50% of oral protein, and mono/disaccharides during free oral hypercaloric nutrition.[59,84,138] Patients with a short bowel who are able to stop HPN (25%) usually do so within the first 2 years (range 3–24 months). If unable to stop within 2 years, the patient has less than a 5% chance of ever being able to stop.[33,39]

Survival

In non-actuarial analysis, it is estimated that around 25% of patients die while on HPN (Table 26.5). However, 80–90% of these deaths are attributable to the progress of the underlying disease and the remaining 10–20% from the septic, mechanical, thrombotic or metabolic complications of HPN.[21,29] Death resulted from non-PN causes in 51% or the primary disease in 30%.[29] PN-related deaths (11%) were from sepsis, superior vena cava thrombosis with pulmonary emboli, or liver failure. Patients with chronic intestinal obstruction had a higher mortality and most of these died from sepsis.[29] Patients older than 65 years have a 'reasonably good' outcome[87] and should not be precluded from starting HPN. In Denmark, 25% of patients will have died at 5 years. There is no relation-ship between the sex of the patient and survival.[39]

Non-cancer, non-HIV patients

Survival depends upon patient age, underlying diag-nosis, presence of chronic intestinal obstruction, and the experience of the unit managing the patient. In the USA, survival at 1 year was 87%; this is comparable to data from Canada and Europe.[21,29] In France at the end of the 1980s, the probability of surviving for 5 years was 75%; this survival depended upon the progression of the original illness,[29] and other studies have given a survival figure of 62%. At 1 year, the probability of survival with HPN (for Crohn's disease, ischaemia or

Table 26.5 – Mortality of HPN patients in Belgium/France and USA

Year(s) studied	Belgium/France[29] 1980–1989			USA[21] 1989–1992
Mortality (years)	*1*	*3*	*5*	*1*
	%	%	%	%
Overall	9	30	38	16
Cancer★	–	–	–	63
Crohn's disease	2	16	18	2
Vascular disease	4	70	44	19
Radiation enteritis	18	65	48	22
Motility disorder	–	72	–	21
AIDS★	–	–	–	73

★ Cancer and AIDS were excluded from the Franco-Belgian study, hence the lower 1-year mortality figures.

pseudo-obstruction) was 90–95% up to the age of 18 and from 35 to 55, while it was 64–73% for those older than 65.[21] Of those with radiation enteritis or elderly men with a mesenteric infarct, 40–42% survive 5 years, compared with 75% of patients with Crohn's disease.[18,19] In the Franco-Belgian study a better prognosis was recognized in patients aged less than 40, whatever the diagnosis providing there was not chronic intestinal obstruction.[29] Prognosis is dependent upon the experience of the centres: in France and Belgium it was better in 1987–1989 than in 1980–1983, which corresponded to the starting of the HPN programmes.[29]

The predicted increase in numbers of patients needing HPN makes it necessary to try to develop alternative treatments to long-term HPN for irreversible intestinal insufficiency.

Cancer or HIV patients

The probability of survival on HPN for cancer is of the order of 60% at 6 months and 33% at 1 year;[58,60,69,72] 25% of patients will have stopped HPN at 1 year.[21] Thus HPN is only justifiable if the patient's quality of life is improved. As with HIV, studies of cost and efficiency related to survival and quality of life are particularly difficult to conduct, and large multicentre studies have yet to be done.[21] Patients with inoperable bowel obstruction given HPN had a median survival of only 53 days, but 82% of patients and their families perceived this to be beneficial.[67]

The average length of treatment with HPN for patients with AIDS does not usually exceed 4 months, and the probability of survival is around 40% at 6

months and 20% at 1 year.[21,26,57] Undernutrition correlates with the stage of the illness: although the restoration of nutritional status did not confer any short-term survival benefit,[70] it did in the long term.[71] However, with new antiretroviral therapies, in particular antiproteases, reduction in the viral potency can reduce the incidence and severity of infections by the partial restoration of CD4 levels; thus HPN may be considered periodically as an adjuvant therapy.[66] Currently, 30% of AIDS patients on HPN regain complete oral autonomy after 1 year.[21]

Hospital readmissions

Readmission to hospital occurs most commonly for disease-related problems; a third of such admissions of patients receiving HPN were for PN-related problems.[20] The readmission rate is higher if a patient has a fistula.[92] For patients with Crohn's disease receiving HPN, an admission occurred every 133 days and occupied an average of 16% of the patient's time.[14] Patients with Crohn's disease receiving HPN had 50% fewer hospital admissions than similar patients who were not receiving PN.[10]

About 50% of patients receiving HPN for HIV infection will be readmitted to hospital during the period when the HPN is being given.[37]

ECONOMIC ASPECTS

For most countries the total national cost of HPN is about the same as that for HEN even though there are a tenth the number of patients. The approximate annual cost in 2000 for a patient receiving HEN every day/night in UK was £5,000, France 73,000F, Canada CD$14,600 and USA $9–25,000. The average annual cost in 2000 for a patient receiving HPN every night in UK was £40,000, France 730,000F, Canada CD$40,000 and USA $40–100,000. The costs in the USA are very variable because there are different providers and commercial pharmacies in hospital competing in a free market. The cost of HPN in the USA is 35% of what it would be if the patient remained in hospital.[65] Analysis of cost/efficacy of the HPN program at Toronto General Hospital has shown that for non-cancer, non-HIV patients, there is a cost reduction of about 100,000F per patient per year by being at home. Similar results are reported from the USA.[56,64] The cost is greatest over the first 3 years of treatment and is substantially reduced in patients in whom the quality of life is good.[19,56]

In Canada, UK and France, the cost of treatment is undertaken almost totally by the National Health Services. In the USA private insurance generates around 80% of the cost.[18,19]

ALTERNATIVE THERAPIES TO HOME PARENTERAL NUTRITION

Patients receiving HPN for chronic irreversible intestinal failure may be helped by factors that stimulate small bowel growth (GLP-2) or delay gastro-intestinal transit (peptide YY), surgical reconstruction[139,140] or small bowel transplantation with or without liver.[90,141] For more details about therapies to reduce or remove the need for parenteral nutrition, see the relevant chapters.

Trophic, hormonal and nutritional factors

The administration over 4 weeks of a recombinant growth hormone with intravenous and oral nutrition enriched with glutamine, and a modified oral diet enriched with fermentable carbohydrate was reported to allow 40% of patients to stop HPN and another 40% to reduce the number of parenteral nutrition infusions. The uncontrolled study was of 47 adults with a short bowel (less than 100 cm of small intestine and no colon, or less than 50 cm and a colon) who had been receiving HPN for 6 years.[142]

This joint utilization of trophic hormonal and nutritional factors appeared very promising;[142] however, subsequent controlled studies have shown no such benefits[143,144] (Ch. 16).

Reconstructive surgery of the remaining bowel

An 8–12 cm long segment of small bowel may be turned round to make an antiperistaltic segment[139,140] (Ch. 33). This should slow transit, improve absorption, and play the role of a neo-ileocaecal valve. In 8 patients with a residual bowel length of 25–70 cm, in whom this procedure was performed and follow-up was for more than 4 years, cessation of PN was obtained in 4 patients, and in the other 4 patients the frequency of HPN was reduced.[140]

Intestinal transplantation

Transplantation may become an option for all patients with irreversible intestinal insufficiency.[90,141] The International Intestinal Transplantation Register has details of 180 transplants in 78 patients between 1985 and 1995 (55% were 10 years old and 10% were over 40). Sixty-four per cent of patients were transplanted for a short bowel, 13% for a malabsorption syndrome, 13% for a tumour, and 8% for chronic intestinal pseudo-obstruction.[90] Survival was better with immunosuppression by tacrolimus ($n=129$) than by cyclosporine ($n=49$). At 1 and 3 years the survival was 83% and 47% for intestine alone, 60% and 40% for intestine and liver, and 59% and 43% for multivisceral transplants. Among the 86 survivors (38%), 78% ceased PN, 12% had a reduction in the frequency of infusions, and 10% continued on HPN after the transplant was removed. Survival was similar after transplantation of the intestine alone compared to a combined graft of both intestine and liver. The majority of deaths were attributable to intense immunosuppression, thus it is important to remove a transplant early and return to HPN if the patient's life becomes in any way endangered[90] (Ch. 34).

HPN patients who are potential candidates for a transplant ideally have a remaining small intestinal length of less than 100 cm, are aged less than 60 years, and have a 90% probability of surviving for 2 years with their underlying illness.[29] Those currently referred for a transplant are patients in whom ongoing HPN carries an increased risk of death secondary to HPN complications (e.g. superior vena cava thrombosis, severe electrolyte abnormalities or cholestatic hepatopathy with evolving fibrosis).[89]

CONCLUSIONS

HEN is a valid and safe technique for nutritional support, providing nutrients mainly to patients with dysphagia who are not able to eat normally. HEN may also be provided for patients with moderate intestinal failure and for anorectic patients. The over-all clinical outcome of HEN patients is poor – the 1-year mortality rate is generally high – but not in those with intestinal failure. This poor clinical outcome suggests that better selection of candidates for HEN will be needed by studies focusing on the quality of life and prognostic factors. Each case needs to be carefully discussed with the patient and family, and there needs to be an awareness of the aims and potential benefits before a decision is made to start HEN.

HPN is a sophisticated and costly treatment given for acute or chronic intestinal failure. The prognosis for these patients is excellent: the majority achieve a normal nutritional state and complete reintegration into the community. The likelihood of ceasing HPN is around 50% and that of dying secondary to complications during treatment is less than 5%. More than 80% of deaths are secondary to complications from the original illness. The probability of survival after 5 years for non-cancer non-HIV causes is around 75%, taking all ages into account. These good results have been obtained because of technical and metabolic progress and the activity of nutrition teams. Patients with cancer or HIV may be given HPN as an adjuvant therapy but the probability of surviving 1 year is less than 20% and there is no good convincing evidence that it improves the quality of life.

Appropriate medical and surgical treatments, which include nutritional and/or hormonal trophic factors as well as reconstructive surgery of the remaining bowel, may help a patient to stop HPN. If, in spite of these treatments, there is severe irreversible intestinal failure necessitating long-term HPN and there are compli-cations from the HPN (poor venous access or hepatopathy), the patient and the nutrition team may consider small intestinal transplantation. It is currently safer, however, to remain on parenteral nutrition than to have a transplant unless there is severe fibrosing hepatopathy, when a combined small intestine and liver transplant may be considered.

REFERENCES

1. Scribner BH, Cole JJ, Christopher TG. Long-term parenteral nutrition; the concept of an artificial gut. *JAMA* 1970; **212:** 457–463.

2. Shils ME, Wright WL, Turnbull A, Brescia F. Long term parenteral nutrition through external arteriovenous shunt. *N Engl J Med* 1970; **283:** 341–343.

3. Broviac JW, Cole JJ, Scribner BH. A silicone rubber atrial catheter for prolonged parenteral alimentation. *Surg Gynecol Obstet* 1973; **136:** 602–606.

4. Jeejeebhoy KN, Zohrab WJ, Langer B, Phillips MJ, Kuksis A, Anderson GH. Total parenteral nutrition at home for 23 months, without complication, and with good rehabilitation. *Gastroenterology* 1973; **65:** 811–820.

5. Broviac JW, Scribner BH. Prolonged parenteral nutrition in the home. *Surg Gynecol Obstet* 1974; **139:** 24–28.

6. Shils ME. A program for total parenteral nutrition at home. *Am J Clin Nutr* 1975; **28:** 1429–1435.

7. Riella MC, Scribner BH. Five years experience with a right atrial catheter for prolonged parenteral nutrition at home. *Surg Gynecol Obstet* 1976; **143:** 205–208.

8. Jeejeebhoy KN, Langer B, Tsallas G, Chu RC, Kuksis A, Anderson H. Total parenteral nutrition at home: studies in patients surviving 4 months to 5 years. *Gastroenterology* 1976; **71:** 943–953.

9. Heizer WD, Orringer EP. Parenteral nutrition at home for 5 years via arteriovenous fistulae. *Gastroenterology* 1977; **72:** 527–532.

10. Fleming CR, McGill DB, Berkner S. Home parenteral nutrition as primary therapy in patients with extensive Crohn's disease of the small bowel and malnutrition. *Gastroenterology* 1977; **73:** 1077–1081.

11. Ladefoged K, Jarnum S. Long-term parenteral nutrition. *Br Med J* 1978; **2:** 262–266.

12. Milewski PJ, Gross E, Holbrook I, Clarke C, Turnberg LA, Irving MH. Parenteral nutrition at home in management of intestinal failure. *Br Med J* 1980; **1:** 1356–1357.

13. Fleming CR, Witzke DJ, Beart RW Jr. Catheter related complications in patients receiving home parenteral nutrition. *Ann Surg* 1980; **102:** 593–599.

14. Steiger E, Srp F. Morbidity and mortality related to home parenteral nutrition in patients with gut failure. *Am J Surg* 1983; **145:** 102–105.

15. Dudrick SJ, O'Donnell JJ, Englert DM *et al.* 100 patient-years of ambulatory home total parenteral nutrition. *Ann Surg* 1984; **199:** 770–781.

16. Mughal M, Irving M. Home parenteral nutrition in the United Kingdom and Ireland. *Lancet* 1986; **ii:** 383–387.

17. Stokes MA, Almond DJ, Pettit SH, Mughal MM, Turner M, Shaffer JL, Irving MH. Home parenteral nutrition: a review of 100 patient years of treatment in 76 consecutive cases. *Br J Surg* 1988; **75:** 481–483.

18. Howard L, Heaphey LL, Fleming CR, Lininger L, Steiger E. Four years of North American registry home parenteral nutrition: outcome data and their implications for patient management. *J Parenter Enteral Nutr* 1991; **15:** 384–394.

19. Messing B. Home parenteral nutrition. In: Payne-James J, Grimble G, Silk D (eds) *Artificial nutrition in clinical practice*. Edward Arnold, London, 1994, pp 365–379.

20. Takagi Y, Okada A, Sato T *et al*. Report on the first annual survey of home parenteral nutrition in Japan. *Surg Today* 1995; **25:** 193–201.

21. Howard L, Ament M, Fleming CR, Shike M, Steiger E. Current use and clinical outcome of home parenteral and enteral nutrition therapies in the United States. *Gastroenterology* 1995; **109:** 355–365.

22. de Francesco A, Fadda M, Malfi G, de Magistris A, da Pont MC, Balzola F. Home parenteral nutrition in Italy: data from the Italian national register. *Clin Nutr* 1995; **14(suppl 1):** 6–9.

23. Van Gossum A, Bakker H, Bozzetti F *et al*. Home parenteral nutrition in adults: a European multicentre survey in 1997. *Clin Nutr* 1999; **18:** 135–140.

24. Fletcher JP, Little JM, Mudie JM. Home parenteral nutrition: Westmead Hospital experience. *Aust NZ Surg* 1986; **56:** 897–900.

25. Stokes MA, Hill GL. Home parenteral nutrition at Auckland Hospital. *NZ Med J* 1991; **104:** 208–210.

26. Messing B, Barnoud D, Beau P *et al*. Données épidémiologiques 1993–1995 de la nutrition parentérale à domicile en centres agréés chez l'adulte en France. *Gastroenterol Clin Biol* 1998; **22:** 413–418.

27. Jeppesen PB, Staun M, Mortensen PB. Adult patients receiving home parenteral nutrition in Denmark from 1991–1996: who will benefit from intestinal transplantation? *Scand J Gastroenterol* 1998; **338:** 839–846.

28. Talaveron LJ, Roig JR, Molas TM, Casas VN, Merce PA, Masanes JR. Quality of the home parenteral nutrition program: 14 years of experience at a general university hospital. *Nutr Hosp* 2000; **15:** 64–70 (in Spanish).

29. Messing B, Lémann M, Landais P *et al*. Prognosis of patients with nonmalignant chronic intestinal failure receiving long-term home parenteral nutrition. *Gastroenterology* 1995; **108:** 1005–1010.

30. Elia M, Russell C, Shaffer J *et al*. *Report of the British Artificial Nutrition Survey – August 1999*. British Association of Parenteral and Enteral Nutrition.

31. Elia M. An international perspective on artificial nutritional support in the community. *Lancet* 1995; **345:** 1345–1349.

32. O'Hanrahan T, Irving MH. The role of home parenteral nutrition in the management of intestinal failure – report of 400 cases. *Clin Nutr* 1992; **11:** 331–336.

33. Ingham Clark CL, Lear PA, Wood S, Lennard-Jones JE, Wood RFM. Potential candidates for small bowel transplantation. *Br J Surg* 1992; **79:** 676–679.

34. Johnston DA, Richards J, Pennington CR. Auditing the effect of experience and change on home parenteral related complications. *Clin Nutr* 1994; **13:** 341–344.

35. Messing B, Matuchansky C. Review in depth. Techniques of providing parenteral nutrition. *Eur J Gastroenterol Hepatol* 1995; **7:** 507–513.

36. Nahon S, Crenn P, Alain S *et al*. Evaluation des complications infectieuses liées à la voie d'abord veineuse chez les patients en nutrition parentérale à domicile de 1993 à 1995. *Gastroenterol Clin Biol* 1997; **21:** A185.

37. Boulétreau P, Gérard M, Messing B *et al*. Home parenteral nutrition and AIDS. *Clin Nutr* 1995; **14:** 213–218.

38. Cavicchi M, Beau P, Crenn P, Degott C, Messing B. Prevalence of liver disease and contributing factors in patients receiving home parenteral nutrition for permanent intestinal failure. *Ann Intern Med* 2000; **132:** 525–532.

39. Messing B, Crenn P, Beau P, Boutron-Ruault MC, Rambaud JC, Matuchansky C. Long-term survival and parenteral nutrition dependence in adult patients with the short bowel syndrome. *Gastroenterology* 1999; **117:** 1043–1050.

40. Howard L, Patton L, Dahl RS. Outcome of long-term enteral feeding. *Gastrointest Endoscop Clin N Am* 1998; **8:** 705–722.

41. Howard L. Home parenteral nutrition: a transatlantic view. *Clin Nutr* 1999; **18:** 131–133.

42. Wehrlen-Martini S, Hébuterne X, Pugliese P, Pouget I, Volpei F, Mousnier A, Rampal P. 47 months activity of a center for home-enteral nutrition and long-term follow-up of the patients treated. *Nutr Clin Metab* 1997; **11:** 7–17.

43. Howard L. A global perspective of home parenteral and enteral nutrition. *Nutrition* 2000; **16:** 625–628.

44. American Gastrointestinal Association. American Gastrointestinal Association technical review on tube feeding for enteral nutrition. *Gastroenterology* 1995; **108:** 1282–1301.

45. Norton B, Homer-Ward M, Donnelly MT, Long RG, Holmes GKT. A randomised prospective comparison of percutaneous endoscopic gastrostomy and nasogastric tube feeding after acute dysphagic stroke. *Br Med J* 1996; **312:** 13–16.

46. Stewart JAD. Legal issues in the withdrawal of artificial nutrition and hydration. *CME Gastroenterol Hepatol Nutr* 2000; **3:** 7–9.

47. Lennard-Jones JE. *Ethical and legal aspects of clinical hydration and nutritional support.* British Association for Parenteral and Nutrition, London, 1998.

48. British Medical Association. *Withholding and withdrawing life-prolonging medical treatment.* BMJ Books, London, 1999.

49. Hébuterne X, Rampal P. Enteral nutrition of the elderly: an update. *Nutr Clin Metab* 1996; **10:** 19–29.

50. Nightingale JMD, Lennard-Jones JE, Gertner DJ, Wood SR, Bartram CI. Colonic preservation reduces the need for parenteral therapy, increases the incidence of renal stones but does not change the high prevalence of gallstones in patients with a short bowel. *Gut* 1992; **33:** 1493–1497.

51. The Multi-Society Task Force on PVS. Medical aspects of the persistent vegetative state. *N Engl J Med* 1994; **330:** 1499–1508, 1572–1579.

52. Rabeneck L, McCullough LB, Wray NP. Ethically justified, clinically comprehensive guidelines for percutaneous endoscopic gastrostomy tube placement. *Lancet* 1997; **349:** 496–498.

53. Rosner F. Guidelines for placement of percutaneous endoscopic gastrostomy tube. *Lancet* 1997; **349:** 958.

54. Parker T, Neale G, Elia M. Home enteral tube feeding in East Anglia. *Eur J Clin Nutr* 1996; **50:** 47–53.

55. Bannerman E, Pendlebury J, Phillips F, Ghosh S. A cross-sectional and longitudinal study of health-related quality of life after percutaneous gastrostomy. *Eur J Gastroenterol Hepatol* 2000; **12:** 1101–1109.

56. Detsky AS. Evaluating a mature technology: long-term home parenteral nutrition. *Gastroenterology* 1995; **108:** 1302–1304.

57. Van Gossum A, Bakker H, De Francesco A *et al*. Home parenteral nutrition in adults: a multicentre survey in Europe in 1993. ESPEN-Home Artificial Nutrition Working Group. *Clin Nutr* 1996; **15:** 53–59.

58. Messing B. Nutrition parentérale de longue durée chez l'adulte. *Nutr Clin Metab* 1996; **10:** 167–175.

59. Nightingale JMD. Clinical problems of a short bowel and their treatment. *Proc Nutr Soc* 1994; **53:** 373–391.

60. Fleming CR, Jeejeebhoy KN. Advances in clinical nutrition. *Gastroenterology* 1994; **106:** 1365–1373.

61. Miglioli M, Pironi L. Chronic intestinal pseudo-obstruction. *Clin Nutr* 1995; **14(suppl 1):** 21–23.

62. Messing B, Halphen M, Bitoun A, Modigliani R, Rambaud JC. Place et résultats de la nutrition parentérale dans le traitement de la maladie coeliaque de l'adulte. *Acta Gastroenterol Belg* 1986; **69:** 460–461.

63. Bozzeti F. Home parenteral nutrition in cancer patients. *Clin Nutr* 1995; **14(suppl l):** 36–40.

64. Pironi L, Tognoni G. Cost-benefit and cost-effectiveness analysis of home artificial nutrition: reappraisal of available data. *Clin Nutr* 1995; **14(suppl l):** 87–91.

65. Shils ME. Parenteral nutrition. In: Shils ME, Olson JA, Shike M (eds) *Modern nutrition in health and disease.* Lea & Febiger, London, 1994, pp 1430–1458.

66. Sukkar SG, Giacosa A. Home nutritional support in AIDS patients. *Clin Nutr* 1995; **14(suppl l):** 41–45.

67. August DA, Thorn D, Fisher RL, Welchek CM. Home parenteral nutrition for patients with inoperable malignant bowel obstruction. *J Parenter Enteral Nutr* 1991; **15:** 323–327.

68. King LA, Carson LF, Konstantinides N *et al*. Outcome assessment of home parenteral nutrition in patients with gynaecologic malignancies: what have we learned in a decade of experience? *Gynecol Oncol* 1993; **51:** 377–382.

69. Cozzaglio L, Balzola F, Cosentino F *et al*. Outcome of cancer patients receiving home parenteral nutrition. *J Parenter Enteral Nutr* 1997; **21:** 339–342.

70. Melchior J-C, Chastang C, Gelas P *et al*. for the French Multicenter Total Parenteral Nutrition Cooperative Group Study. Efficacy of 2-month total parenteral nutrition in AIDS patients: a controlled randomised prospective trial. *AIDS* 1996; **10:** 379–384.

71. Melchior J-C, Gelas P, Carbonnel F *et al*. Improved survival by home total parenteral nutrition in AIDS patients: follow-up of a controlled randomised prospective trial. *AIDS* 1998; **12:** 336–337.

72. Howard L. Home parenteral and enteral nutrition in cancer patients. *Cancer* 1993; **72:** 3531–3541.

73. Beau P, Matrat S. A comparative study of polyurethane and silicone cuffed-catheters in long-term home parenteral nutrition patients. *Clin Nutr* 1999; **18:** 175–177.

74. Howard L, Claunch C, McDowell R, Timchalk M. Five years of experience in patients receiving home nutritional support with the implanted reservoir: a comparison with the external catheter. *J Parenteral Enteral Nutr* 1989; **13:** 478–741.

75. Jeppesen PB, Mortensen PB. Significance of a preserved colon for parenteral energy requirements in patients receiving home parenteral nutrition. *Scand J Gastroenterol* 1998; **33:** 1175–1179.

76. Bigorgne C, Le Tourneau A, Messing B *et al*. Sea-blue histiocyte syndrome in bone marrow secondary to total parenteral nutrition including fat-emulsion sources: a clinicopathological study of seven cases. *Br J Haematol* 1996; **95:** 258–262.

77. DiCecco S, Nelson J, Burnes J, Fleming CR. Nutritional intake of gut failure patients on home parenteral nutrition. *J Parenter Enteral Nutr* 1987; **11:** 529–532.

78. Nightingale JMD, Lennard-Jones JE, Walker ER, Farthing MJG. Jejunal efflux in short bowel syndrome. *Lancet* 1990; **336:** 765–768.

79. Zazzo JF, Messing B. Nutrition artificielle et oligo-éléments chez l'adulte. In: Chappuis P, Favier A (eds) *Oligoéléments en nutrition et en thérapeutique.* Technique & Documentation – Lavoisier, Paris, 1995, pp 39–55.

80. Fitzgerald K, Mikalunas V, Rubin H, McCarthy R, Vanagunas A, Craig RM. Hypermagnesemia in patients receiving total parenteral nutrition. *J Parenter Enteral Nutr* 1999; **23:** 333–336.

81. Jeppesen PB, Hoy C-E, Mortensen PB. Essential fatty acid deficiency in patients receiving home parenteral nutrition. *Am J Clin Nutr* 1998; **68:** 126–133.

82. Matuchansky C, Messing B, Jeejeebhoy KN, Beau P, Béliah M, Allard JP. Cyclical parenteral nutrition. *Lancet* 1992; **340:** 588–592.

83. Briet F, Flourié B, Achour L, Maurel M, Rambaud JC, Messing B. Bacterial adaptation in patients with short bowel and colon in continuity. *Gastroenterology* 1995; **109:** 1446–1453.

84. Messing B, Pigot F, Rongier M, Morin MC, Ndeindoum U, Rambaud JC. Intestinal absorption of free oral alimentation in the very short bowel syndrome. *Gastroenterology* 1991; **100:** 1502–1508.

85. Quigley EMM, Marsh MN, Shaffer JL, Markin RS. Hepatobiliary complications of total parenteral nutrition. *Gastroenterology* 1993; **104:** 286–301.

86. Cano N, Messing B. Conséquences physio-pathologiques hépatobiliaires de la nutrition artificielle: influence de la voie d'administration entérale *versus* parentérale. *Nutr Clin Metab* 1994; **8:** 149–162.

87. Howard L, Malone M. Clinical outcome of geriatric patients in the United States receiving home parenteral and enteral nutrition. *Am J Clin Nutr* 1997; **66:** 1364–1370.

88. Herfindal ET, Bernstein LR, Kudzia K, Wong A. Survey of home nutritional support patients. *J Parenter Enteral Nutr* 1989; **13:** 255–261.

89. Quigley EMM. Small intestinal transplantation: reflections on an evolving approach to intestinal failure. *Gastroenterology* 1996; **110:** 2009–2012.

90. Grant D. Intestinal transplantation 1997 report of the international registry. *Transplantation* 1999; **67:** 1061–1064.

91. North American Home Parenteral and Enteral Nutrition Patient Registry. *Annual report with outcome profiles 1985–1992.* The Oley Foundation, Albany, New York, 1994.

92. Gouttebel MC, Saint-Aubert B, Jinquet O, Astre C, Joyeux H. Ambulatory home parenteral nutrition. *J Parenter Enteral Nutr* 1987; **11:** 475–479.

93. Richards DM, Scott NA, Shaffer JL, Irving M. Opiate and sedative dependence predicts a poor outcome for patients receiving home parenteral nutrition. *J Parenter Enteral Nutr* 1997; **21:** 336–338.

94. Nightingale JMD, Simpson AJ, Wood SR, Lennard-Jones JE. Fungal feeding-line infections: beware the eyes and teeth. *J Royal Soc Med* 1995; **88:** 258–263.

95. Kite P, Dobbins BM, Wilcox MH et al. Evaluation of a novel endoluminal brush method for in situ diagnosis of catheter related sepsis. *J Clin Pathol* 1997; **50:** 278–282.

96. Messing B, Thuillier F, Béliah M, Alain S, Peitra-Cohen S, Man F. Traitement par verrou local d'antibiotique des infections bactériennes liées au cathéter central en nutrition parentérale. *Nutr Clin Metab* 1991; **5:** 105–112.

97. Fleming CR, Witzke DJ, Beart RW. Catheter-related complications in patients receiving home parenteral nutrition. *Ann Surg* 1980; **192:** 593–599.

98. Forbes GM, Forbes A. Micronutrient status in patients receiving home parenteral nutrition. *Nutrition* 1997; **13:** 941–944.

99. Ducreux M, Messing B, de Vernejoule MC, Bouhnik Y, Miravet L, Rambaud JC. Calcemic response to magnesium or 1-alpha-hydroxycholecalciferol treatment in intestinal hypomagnesemia. *Gastroenterol Clin Biol* 1991; **15:** 805–811.

100. Klein GL, Alfrey AC, Miller NL, Sherrard DJ, Hazlet TK, Ament ME, Coburn JW. Aluminium loading during total parenteral nutrition. *Am J Clin Nutr* 1982; **35:** 1425–1429.

101. Reynolds N, Blumsohn A, Baxter J, Houston G, Pennington CR. Manganese requirement and toxicity in patients on home parenteral nutrition. *Clin Nutr* 1998; **17:** 227–230.

102. Wolfe BM, Walker BK, Shaul DB, Wong L, Ruebner BH. Effect of total parenteral nutrition on hepatic histology. *Arch Surg* 1998; **123:** 1084–1090.

103. Chan S, McCowen KC, Bistrian BR et al. Incidence, prognosis, and etiology of end-stage liver disease in patients receiving home total parenteral nutrition. *Surgery* 1999; **126:** 28–34.

104. Braxton C, Lowry SF. Parenteral nutrition and liver dysfunction – new insight? *J Parenter Enteral Nutr* 1995; **19:** 3–4.

105. Messing B, Colombel JF, Heresbach D, Chazouilleres O, Galian A. Chronic cholestasis and macronutrient excess in patients treated with prolonged parenteral nutrition. *Nutrition* 1992; **8:** 30–36.

106. Silverstein MN, Ellefson RD, Ahern EJ. The syndrome of the sea-blue histiocyte. *N Engl J Med* 1970; **282:** 1–4.

107. Stanko RT, Nathan G, Mendelow H, Adibi SA. Development of hepatic cholestasis and fibrosis in patients with massive loss of intestine supported by prolonged parenteral nutrition. *Gastroenterology* 1987; **92:** 197–202.

108. Buchman AL, Dubin MD, Moukarzel AA *et al.* Choline deficiency: a cause of hepatic steatosis during parenteral nutrition that can be reversed with intravenous choline supplementation. *Hepatology* 1995; **22:** 1399–1403.

109. Berner YN, Larchian WA, Lowry SF, Nicora RR, Brennan MF, Shike M. Low plasma carnitine in patients on prolonged total parenteral nutrition: association with low plasma lysine. *J Parenter Enteral Nutr* 1990; **14:** 255–258.

110. Epstein S, Traberg H, Levine G, McClintock R. Bone and mineral status of patients beginning total parenteral nutrition. *J Parenter Enteral Nutr* 1986; **10:** 263–264.

111. Lipkin EW, Ott SM, Chesnut CH, Chait A. Mineral loss in the parenteral nutrition patient. *Am J Clin Nutr* 1988; **47:** 515–523.

112. Foldes J, Rimon B, Meggia–Sullam M *et al.* Progressive bone loss during long-term home parenteral nutrition. *J Parenter Enteral Nutr* 1990; **14:** 139–142.

113. Saitta JC, Ott SM, Sherrard DJ, Walden CE, Lipkin EW. Metabolic bone disease in adults receiving long-term parenteral nutrition: longitudinal study with regional densitometry and bone biopsy. *J Parenter Enteral Nutr* 1993; **17:** 214–219.

114. Goodman WG, Misra S, Veldhuis JD, Portale AA, Wang H-J, Ament ME, Salusky IB. Altered diurnal regulation of blood ionised calcium and serum parathyroid hormone concentrations during parenteral nutrition. *Am J Clin Nutr* 2000; **71:** 560–568.

115. Pironi L, Zolezzi C, Ruggeri E, Paganelli F, Pizzoferrato A, Miglioli M. Bone turnover in short-term and long-term home parenteral nutrition for benign disease. *Nutrition* 2000; **16:** 272–277.

116. Klein GL, Ament ME, Coburn JW. Metabolic bone disease in total parenteral nutrition. *Lancet* 1981; **1:** 835.

117. Wright KB, Holan G, Casamassimo PS, King DR. Alveolar bone loss in two children with short-bowel syndrome receiving total parenteral nutrition. *J Periodontol* 1991; **62:** 272–275.

118. Klein GL, Horst RL, Norman AW, Ament ME, Slatopolsky E, Coburn JW. Reduced serum levels of 1-alpha, 25-dihydroxyvitamin D during long term total parenteral nutrition. *Ann Intern Med* 1981; **94:** 638–643.

119. Verhage AH, Cheong WK, Allard JP, Jeejeebhoy KN. Increase in lumbar spine bone mineral content in patients on long-term parenteral nutrition without vitamin D supplementation. *J Parenter Enteral Nutr* 1995; **19:** 431–436.

120. de Vernejoul MC, Messing B, Modrowski D, Bielakoff J, Buisine A, Miravet L. Multifactorial low remodelling bone disease during cyclic total parenteral nutrition. *J Clin Endocrinol Metab* 1985; **60:** 109–113.

121. Vargas JH, Klein GL, Ament ME *et al.* Metabolic bone disease of total parenteral nutrition: course after changing from casein to amino acids in parenteral solutions with reduced aluminium content. *Am J Clin Nutr* 1988; **48:** 1070–1078.

122. Shike M, Harrison JE, Sturtridge WC *et al.* Metabolic bone disease in patients receiving long-term total parenteral nutrition. *Ann Intern Med* 1980; **92:** 343–350.

123. Bengoa JM, Sitrin MD, Wood RJ, Rosenberg IH. Amino acid-induced hypercalciuria in patients on total parenteral nutrition. *Am J Clin Nutr* 1983; **38:** 264–269.

124. Wood RJ, Sitrin MD, Cusson GJ, Rosenberg IH. Reduction of TPN-induced urinary calcium loss by increasing the phosphorus in the TPN prescription. *J Parenter Enteral Nutr* 1986; **10:** 188–190.

125. Jeejeebhoy KN. Metabolic bone disease and total parenteral nutrition: a progress report. *Am J Clin Nutr* 1998; **67:** 186–187.

126. Delmas PD. Biphosphonates in the treatment of bone diseases. *N Engl J Med* 1996; **335:** 1336–1337.

127. Perl M, Hall RCW, Dudrick SJ, Englert DM, Stickney SK, Gardner ER. Psychological aspects of long-term home hyperalimentation. *J Parenter Enteral Nutr* 1980; **4:** 554–560.

128. Ladefoged K. Quality of life in patients on permanent home parenteral nutrition. *J Parenter Enteral Nutr* 1981; **5:** 132–137.

129. Robb RA, Brakebill JI, Ivey MF, Christensen DB, Young JH, Scribner BH. Subjective assessment of patient outcomes of home parenteral nutrition. *Am J Hosp Pharm* 1983; **40:** 1646–1650.

130. Smith CE. Quality of life in long-term total parenteral nutrition patients and their family caregivers. *J Parenter Enteral Nutr* 1993; **17:** 501–506.

131. Richards DM, Irving MH. Assessing the quality of life of patients with intestinal failure on home parenteral nutrition. *Gut* 1997; **40:** 218–222.

132. Jeppesen PB, Langholz E, Mortensen PB. Quality of life in patients receiving home parenteral nutrition. *Gut* 1999; **44:** 844–852.

133. Abboud P, Messing B, Quereux C, Napoléone C, Zeitoun P, Wahl P. Maladie de Crohn et grossesse: à propos de deux observations. *J Gynecol Obstet Biol Reprod* 1996; **25:** 608–611.

134. Kirby DF, Fiorenza V, Craig RM. Intravenous nutritional support during pregnancy. *J Parenter Enteral Nutr* 1988; **12:** 72–80.

135. Carter D, Wheatley C, Martin R *et al*. Nights of bright lights and noisy pumps – home parenteral feeding. *Proc Nutr Soc* 1996; **55:** 149A.

136. Carbonnel F, Cosnes J, Chevret S *et al*. The role of anatomic factors in nutritional autonomy after extensive small bowel resection. *J Parenter Enteral Nutr* 1996; **20:** 275–280.

137. Nordgaard I, Hansen BS, Mortensen PB. Importance of colonic support for energy absorption as small-bowel failure proceeds. *Am J Clin Nutr* 1996; **64:** 222–231.

138. Mahé S, Messing B, Thuillier F, Tomé D. Digestion of bovine milk proteins in patients with a high jejunostomy. *Am J Clin Nutr* 1991; **54:** 534–539.

139. Thompson JS. Surgical aspects of the short-bowel syndrome. *Am J Surg* 1995; **170:** 532–536.

140. Panis Y, Messing B, Rivet P *et al*. Segmental reversal of the small bowel as an alternative of intestinal transplantation in patients with short bowel syndrome. *Ann Surg* 1997; **225:** 401–407.

141. Goulet O, Brousse N, Révillon Y, Ricour C. Pathology of human intestinal transplantation. In: Grant R, Wood RFM (eds) *Small bowel transplantation*. Edward Arnold, London, 1993, pp 112–120.

142. Byrne TA, Persinger RL, Young LS, Ziegier TS, Wilmore DW. A new treatment for patients with short-bowel syndrome: growth hormone, glutamine and a modified diet. *Ann Surg* 1995; **222:** 243–255.

143. Scolapio JS, Camilleri M, Fleming CR *et al*. Effect of growth hormone, glutamine, and diet on adaptation in short-bowel syndrome: a randomized, controlled study. *Gastroenterology* 1997; **113:** 1074–1081.

144. Szkudlarek J, Jeppesen PB, Mortensen PB. Effect of high dose growth hormone with glutamine and no change in diet on intestinal absorption in short bowel patients: a randomised, double blind, crossover, placebo controlled study. *Gut* 2000; **47:** 199–205.

27

Home enteral and parenteral nutrition for children

S. Hill and S. Long

INTRODUCTION

Children (less than 16 years old) throughout the world are increasingly being given enteral and parenteral nutrition at home because they are unable to sustain normal growth and development when consuming their normal diet.[1–12] The severity and complications of a chronic disease are worse in those who are undernourished.[13] Long-term home treatment can maintain a good nutritional state and promote catch-up growth;[14] it is also preferable to a prolonged period in hospital. Nutritional support should be begun early (within 1–5 days) as children have less nutritional reserve than adults. Age, nutritional state and intestinal losses should be taken into account. It has been estimated that a small premature baby (1 kg) has sufficient reserves to survive only 4 days, a larger premature baby (2 kg) 12 days, a full-term baby (3.5 kg) 33 days and a 1-year-old child 45 days.[15] When enteral nutrition is not tolerated or is contraindicated, parenteral nutrition must be started within 1–2 days of the intake/absorption becoming inadequate in a neonate/infant, but can be delayed for up to 5–7 days in a well-nourished adolescent.

All children in hospital must be measured and weighed regularly and the result plotted on a height and weight growth centile chart. Head circumference should also be charted in children under 2 years, and in some children mid-arm muscle circumference is also useful. If a child's weight is consistently falling through the centiles, if it is of a low weight for height, or if weight is below the second centile, the child is probably failing to thrive. Failure to thrive may be caused by diseases that interfere with ingestion, digestion or absorption of nutrients. If there is no readily treatable medical cause after assessment in a specialist paediatric gastroenterology unit, the diet may be altered/supplemented or the method of feeding changed under dietetic guidance/monitoring. If, after these measures, the child still fails to sustain normal growth, then enteral feeding may be given. If enteral feeding fails or if there are severe problems with fluid balance and nutrient absorption, parenteral nutrition may be used. Every effort is made to establish enteral in preference to parenteral nutrition in children who are failing to thrive; not only is it the more physiological feeding method but also there is far less potential for life-threatening complications. In general, only children with severe intestinal failure are treated with parenteral nutrition.

The steps considered when nutritional support is begun or, indeed, when withdrawn, are shown in Figure 27.1.

PREVALENCE

An estimate of the number of children at home receiving artificial nutritional support in the United Kingdom is provided by the British Artificial Nutrition Survey (BANS), which has tried to compile data on all patients needing artificial nutritional support at home

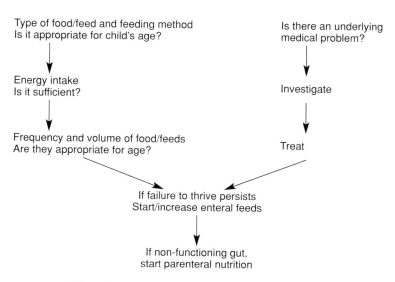

Figure 27.1 – Starting or withdrawing nutritional support.

since 1996. The point prevalence on December 31st, 1998, of children receiving home enteral nutrition (HEN) was 2832 (1821 were less than 4 years old); the prevalence of those receiving home parenteral nutrition (HPN) was 64 (most in the first decade).[16] Of all patients receiving HEN 26% and of those receiving HPN 18% were children, giving a prevalence estimate of 63 and 1–2 per million population respectively.

ENTERAL NUTRITION

As in adults, most children receiving long-term enteral nutrition have a normally functioning gut and only a few have a degree of intestinal failure (Tables 27.1, 27.2). Children with congenital abnormalities (i.e. those that date from birth but are not necessarily hereditary) are the largest group requiring both enteral and parenteral nutrition. Most have a mechanical problem with ingestion of nutrients, some a debilitating illness of a non-gastroenterological organ which

Table 27.1 – Reasons for home enteral nutrition in children in Scotland[2]

	n=156 (80 M) (%)
Neurological/cerebral palsy	46 (29)
Congenital/metabolic abnormalities	23 (15)
Cystic fibrosis	21 (13)
Chronic renal failure	17 (11)
Neoplastic disease	17 (11)
Gastrointestinal/hepatic disease	12 (8)
Failure to thrive	10 (6)
Cardiorespiratory disease	10 (6)

leads to loss of appetite and increased energy requirements (e.g. cardiac failure). Few have disorders of the gastrointestinal tract directly affecting digestion and absorption.

Mechanical problems ingesting nutrients

Neurological disease

Children with cerebral palsy are frequently unable to chew solid food; they may have abnormal swallowing mechanisms with risk of aspiration and also gastro-oesophageal reflux (usually worse with liquids). Oral intake can be maximized by giving pureed food. However, severely affected patients usually have a low weight for height and require high-calorie enteral feeding.[5] Feeds are usually best given as a continuous overnight infusion with daytime boluses, usually via a gastrostomy tube. Severe cerebral palsy is associated with a high incidence of epilepsy. Continuous feeding increases the possibility of aspiration in a child with poorly controlled epilepsy. Fluid intake must be carefully monitored in children who are unable to express thirst. Cerebral palsy patients are prone to constipation and frequently benefit from a fibre-containing feed. Feeding through a percutaneous endoscopic gastrostomy (PEG) usually results in normal growth and weight gain,[6] however ethical issues should be addressed before starting to give nutritional support.

Cleft lip/palate

Infants with a cleft lip or palate defect are often fed at home, most commonly via a nasogastric tube, until a surgical repair has been completed.[17]

Table 27.2 – Diagnostic categories of children in UK receiving home enteral tube feeding according to age on December 31st, 1998[15]

Diseases	0–4 yrs n=1821 %	5–9 yrs n=502 %	10–15 yrs n=509 %	Total <16 yrs n=2832 %
Central nervous system	35	49	41	39★
Genitourinary	29	22	15	25
Respiratory	6	14	26	11
Gastrointestinal	10	6	12	10
Cardiac	4	2	3	3
Other	16	7	3	12

★ 49% have cerebral palsy.

Malignancy

A gastrostomy tube may be used safely for patients with malignancy and can be inserted prior to radical chemotherapy or radiation treatment.[4]

Non-gastroenterological disease

Respiratory disease

Cystic fibrosis. Children with cystic fibrosis have malabsorption due to pancreatic enzyme insufficiency. In addition, energy requirements are increased up to 120% of predicted. The increase is partly the result of recurrent infections that are associated with loss of appetite and fatigue. There is a clear association between an improvement in nutritional state and lung disease.[18] Children are routinely given high-energy supplements, but many also need overnight enteral feeds, often given through a gastrostomy.[7] Gastro-oesophageal reflux is more common in children with cystic fibrosis and may be exacerbated by gastrostomy feeding.[19] Elemental/peptide preparations with medium-chain triglycerides may be given to bypass the need for pancreatic enzymes and so ensure maximum absorption.

Bronchopulmonary dysplasia. Growth failure is common in premature infants with bronchopulmonary dysplasia. The reasons are manifold and include poor appetite, abnormal sucking and swallowing mechanisms, poor gastric motility and gastro-oesophageal reflux. In addition, metabolic needs are increased.[20] Overnight enteral feeds may be needed for many months to supplement the daytime energy intake.

Renal disease

Failure to thrive is common in children with chronic renal disease, particularly when the onset is in infancy or early childhood. These children are commonly anorectic, a condition which may be exacerbated by gastro-oesophageal reflux. Many children continue to fail to thrive even when a diet or supplements of high energy content are given. Optimal growth is usually possible with an overnight enteral feed.[8] Most patients presenting early in life will have a gastrostomy inserted as soon as there is evidence of failure to thrive. A PEG does not appear to cause problems with peritoneal dialysis.

Congenital heart disease

Infants with congenital heart disease often have an increased energy requirement, but poor appetite, reduced absorption and, in severe right heart failure, a protein-losing enteropathy also contribute to undernutrition. An energy-dense formula is necessary when only a restricted fluid intake can be tolerated. Patients need to be in the best possible nutritional state before surgery. Significant catch-up weight gain can be achieved when a continuous overnight high-calorie feed is given.[21]

Gastrointestinal disease

Short bowel

Problems associated with a short bowel may occur following surgical resections when a neonate/infant/child has insufficient length of small bowel to absorb sufficient nutrients to maintain normal growth. The causes of a short bowel arising in the neonate/infant/child usually result in preservation of the colon and some terminal ileum (Ch. 7). In the neonate/infant the most common causes are necrotizing enterocolitis, multiple jejuno-ileal atresias, aganglionosis and gastroschisis; in the older child small intestinal (mid-gut) volvulus is a common cause.[22–28] These patients usually need a period of parenteral nutrition before they are weaned onto enteral feeding.

Children left with 30 cm small intestine or less are unlikely to survive without long-term parenteral nutrition; with more than this they may maintain their nutritional state by consuming a normal diet (ideally low in oxalate and high in polysaccharides – Ch. 25). In some studies a preserved ileocaecal valve does not affect survival or the type of nutritional support needed in the long term.[25,26] This is not the case in other studies,[22,27] probably because the preserved ileocaecal valve is also associated with preserved ileum and colon. Retention of the ileocaecal valve may reduce the chance of a bowel organism causing septicaemia[25] and it may reduce the time over which intestinal adaptation develops.[25,28]

In all cases, full use of the gut must be made in order to maximize absorptive ability. Overnight continuous enteral feeds may play an essential role, first in weaning the child off parenteral nutrition, then in the longer term at home. Overnight feeding allows maximal use of the remaining gut while enabling the child to attend school during the day. Intestinal function (if there is remaining ileum or colon) may continue to improve for 2 years or longer.

Crohn's disease

Crohn's disease is a relatively uncommon reason for children to need nutritional support, especially before the age of 10.[16]

Active disease. Liquid enteral feeds, usually taken at home, are the treatment of choice in children and teenagers with active Crohn's disease because the potential side-effects of steroids, particularly growth delay, may be avoided. The feed, in which the protein may be as single amino acids (elemental diet), peptides or whole protein (polymeric diet) plays a dual role in that it reduces intestinal inflammation as well as improving nutritional state, growth and development.[29] It is still not known for certain why the intestinal inflammation due to Crohn's disease resolves through improvement of nutritional status alone.[30–32] The change from a catabolic to an anabolic state and the removal of dietary allergens, bowel rest, change in gut flora and reduced synthesis of inflammatory mediators may all contribute. Sufficient liquid enteral feed is given to substitute the patient's whole diet, and solid food is withdrawn for a minimum period of 6 weeks. After the 6-week period, many children appear to benefit from continuing overnight feeds for several weeks or months as a dietary supplement is started. Some units gradually reintroduce foods, one or two at a time.[33] Gastrostomies are well tolerated and have few complications.[1] Some children will remain on enteral feeding through puberty and until they have completed their growth spurt. Children usually experience rapid catch-up weight gain and growth.[34]

Fibrotic strictures. A patient with small bowel strictures may have intermittent episodes of bowel obstruction (colicky abdominal pain, swelling, vomiting/constipation and later diarrhoea) caused by undigested solid food impacting at a stricture. The patient can be advised to consume a low residue/pureed diet or, if this fails, a completely liquid diet.

Other gastrointestinal disease

Some infants with gastro-oesophageal reflux fail to thrive even on adequate medication and thickened feeds. These patients can respond well to treatment with continuous overnight enteral feeds. If there is a poor response in spite of a good energy intake, other possible underlying diseases should be considered.

Children with protracted diarrhoea that is not readily amenable to treatment will need prolonged periods of enteral feeding. These children have more unusual enteropathies such as autoimmune enteropathy. Some patients with autoimmune enteropathy respond to treatment with immunosuppressive agents and exclusion of certain dietary antigens and cope without enteral feeds. Other children who may require continuous overnight feeds are those with motility disorders (e.g. intestinal pseudo-obstruction).

Protracted diarrhoea due to coeliac disease, disaccharide intolerance or cow's milk protein intolerance[35] or food-sensitive enteropathy usually responds to dietary modification although the child may need a period of enteral nutritional support. In pancreatic insufficiency, pancreatic supplements are needed as well as dietary changes and, in some cases, enteral support. The usual feeding regimen is an overnight continuous feed, possibly with daytime boluses. Most of these children will need semi-elemental or elemental feeds. In addition, they may tolerate small quantities of a limited diet. Children with coeliac disease should not need enteral feeds since there is usually a good response with catch-up weight gain and growth when gluten is withdrawn from the diet.

Methods and materials

The decision to start enteral feeding must be taken prudently as it may prove difficult to stop feeding enterally when it is no longer medically required. It can become a major psychological support for the parents and they may resist attempts to stop treatment.

The commercially prepared liquid formulations usually provide all nutritional needs (the correct balance of fluid, carbohydrate, fat, protein, minerals and vitamins) and may either supplement or completely replace a solid diet. Many patients requiring enteral feeds have specific nutritional requirements and these should be as simple as possible. Certain nutrients may improve intestinal function and thus are often added to feeds; for example, the amino acid glutamine, short-chain fatty acids and fibre (e.g. pectin which is metabolized to release short-chain fatty acids) may all improve intestinal adaptation.[36] Glutamine is the major amino acid source for enterocytes and many cells of the immune system. Short-chain fatty acids reduce inflammation.[37] Prebiotics (e.g. the non-digestible oligosaccharide chicory fructosoligosaccharide) are colonic microbial food substances that enhance the growth of probiotics (the beneficial bowel bacteria that ferment undigested carbohydrate/fibre). Fructosoligosaccharide acts as a dietary fibre, and may improve bioavailability of essential minerals; it also lowers the serum triglycerides.[38]

An enteral feed is usually administered via a naso-gastric tube in the short term or via a gastrostomy if needed for more than 2 months. Those with mild intestinal failure may have a continuous overnight enteral feed and a limited solid diet during the day. The complications associated with inserting a PEG appear to be greater in children than in adults, especially the development of symptomatic gastro–oesophageal reflux which can lead to aspiration pneumonia[39] (Chs 18, 31). Distress can be reduced in children aged 7 or over by good psychological preparation before insert-ing a nasogastric tube and subsequent support.[40] If gastric emptying is poor or there are symptoms of gastro–oesophageal reflux (with medical treatment), transpyloric feeding may be appropriate. A jejunal feeding tube is usually inserted at laparotomy. A percutaneous endoscopic gastrojejunostomy tube (PEGJ) can be inserted (see Ch. 18); experience with these has not been encouraging,[41] however the out-come may be better with the newer tubes. A jejunal feeding tube is of narrow bore and continuous rather than bolus feeds are usually given through it.

An experienced paediatric dietician should be involved in the management of enteral feeds to ensure that adequate energy is given in the best possible formulation and to supervise manipulation of feeds. The enteral feeds should gradually and regularly be manipulated to obtain maximal enteral absorption and, if at all possible, to ease transition to a normal diet.

Enteral feeding may also be given to children receiving parenteral nutrition to help maintain their protective small intestinal mucosal barrier. There must be a gradual structured training programme for children and carers (Box 27.1).

Organization of home enteral nutrition

Home enteral nutrition is considered for all children who will require treatment for at least 2–3 weeks. The feed may either be administered as boluses or con-tinuously with a pump, depending on the child's clinical condition. The home equipment (Box 27.2) is usually organized by nurses/dieticians in the com-munity. The family doctor usually prescribes the feed. A supply of feeds, tubes, giving sets and syringes is required, along with a pump for continuous overnight feeds. The pump should be capable of accurately administering small volumes of fluid. The manu-facturer or a home care company delivers the equip-ment to the home. The hospital nurses caring for the patient should ensure that the parents/carers are competent to administer the feeds. Members of the family need to be taught how to change the enteral feeding device/tube. If they do not wish to do this, provision needs to be made locally as to where and by whom the feeding device/tube is changed (both routinely and in emergencies). Once the child is at home the community paediatric nurse or the child's health visitor is contacted to offer additional support and expertise to the family. In most large centres there is a specialist dietician or nutrition nurse available to help with problems prior to discharge and those that arise at home.

Box 27.1 – Teaching plan for enteral feeding at home

Basic anatomy
Reason for enteral feeding
Tube care:
- securing
- verifying tip position
- flushing
- replacement

Equipment assembly
Preparation and administration of feed (includes storage and hanging times)
Pump operation
Cleaning equipment (includes feeding extensions, syringes and pump)
Complications (diarrhoea, blockage, leakage and alarms)
24-Hour contact numbers
Follow-up plans

Box 27.2 – Equipment required for home enteral nutrition

Tubes:
- nasogastric/gastrostomy

Feed
Administration set with reservoir
Pump:
- simple to use
- accurate for small volumes
- built in safety alarms
- preferably portable

Drip stand
Syringes, tape, litmus paper

PARENTERAL NUTRITION

Parenteral nutrition, in which nutrients are infused directly into the blood stream so bypassing the gut, is given to children with severe intestinal failure. Home parenteral nutrition is offered to children who are expected to require at least part of their nutrition parenterally for a minimum of 2–3 months. The alternative is prolonged hospitalization or withdrawal of treatment. Children receiving parenteral nutrition in hospital are at a much greater risk of septicaemia than they would be at home, provided home care is properly set up.[42] Other difficulties common to all chronically hospitalized children are those of psychosocial impairment and associated developmental delay. The major disruption of prolonged hospitalization is also an enormous burden for the family. Many parents have to cope with a regular job and other children in addition to the hospital visits. Home treatment improves the quality of life for the whole family although at first there may be difficulties in coping with the 'hi-tech' equipment.

Parenteral nutrition needs careful supervision from a multidisciplinary team that has a member available 24 hours a day to give advice and support. Most patients receiving long-term parenteral nutrition will continue to take some food orally; indeed some oral intake is beneficial and should be encouraged in order to prevent mucosal atrophy and to maintain the enterohepatic circulation.

Underlying disease

Most patients considered for home treatment have chronic severe intestinal failure. Other patients are terminally ill with a severe immunodeficiency or malignancy. They may only need home parenteral nutrition for a few weeks. Ethical issues should be carefully thought through before embarking on treatment of such patients. The patients with long-term chronic intestinal failure (Table 27.3) can be divided into three categories: those with a short bowel (Table 27.4), those suffering from an enteropathy, and those with a motility disorder. The children range in age from about 4 months to 16 years. It is unlikely that a child less than 4 months old could manage a home regimen that enabled the mother/carer to lead a reasonable life.

Methods and materials

The parents must be willing to be trained to administer the nutrition. They have to be competent at managing it before discharge. The specialist nutrition

Table 27.3 – Diagnosis of 64 children receiving HPN in UK on December 31st, 1998[15]

	N (%)
Pseudo-obstruction	11 (17)
Idiopathic intractable diarrhoea	8 (12)
Autoimmune enteropathy	5 (8)
Volvulus	3 (5)
Crohn's disease	2 (3)
Post necrotizing enterocolitis	1 (2)
Microvillus inclusion disease	1 (2)
Malignancy	1 (2)
Other gastrointestinal disease	24 (37)
Other diseases	8 (12)

Table 27.4 – Diagnosis of 60 children with a short bowel and receiving HPN in the United States[22]

	n=60 (40 M) (%)
Post necrotizing enterocolitis	24 (40)
Jejuno–ileal atresia	13 (22)
Aganglionosis	7 (12)
Mid-gut volvulus	6 (10)
Gastroschisis	5 (8)
Volvulus due to adhesions	4★ (7)
Trauma	1 (2)

★ 3 were undergoing surgery for retroperitoneal tumour.

nurse organizes a training programme with parents/carers which takes into account their abilities and the time available. Every effort is made to teach both parents so that care can be shared. Training is usually commenced within a month of planned discharge so that the techniques are fresh in the parents' minds when the child is discharged.

Venous access

Venous access is gained by a silicone rubber (Silastic) catheter placed via the subclavian vein (or occasionally the internal jugular vein) to have its tip positioned in the right atrium in a young child or at the superior vena caval/right atrial junction in an older one. The femoral veins can be used but are less suitable because the site is in the nappy area and so is susceptible to faecal contamination. A subcutaneous cuff fixes the line in place and prevents movement. The line should be dedicated to the infusion of parenteral nutrition only and can be expected to last for about 2 years. Growth may alter the position of the catheter tip, requiring it to be changed. In several children, central lines have remained in situ for as long as 8–10 years.

Infusion

A precisely formulated sterile bag of nutrients is infused into the child's blood stream. Two formulations are usually used for children on total parenteral nutrition: a glucose and amino acid preparation four or five nights a week, and a lipid-containing formulation for two or three nights. If fat is infused more frequently there is a high incidence of precipitation and deposits developing along the line and occluding it. Children on partial parenteral nutrition with sufficient enteral function to absorb their essential fatty acid requirement (estimated by a dietician) only need fat-free bags. It is important to devise a single-bag system to simplify its set-up and limit the chances of infection. The maximum infusion rate of glucose through a central vein should be 1.0–1.5 g/kg/h; if it is greater than this glycosuria may occur.[43]

The infant or child ideally receives all his or her parenteral nutrition in 12 hours (or at most 14 hours) overnight. It is unreasonable to expect a family to have a child attached to a pump for any longer than 12 hours and it would be difficult for a child of school age to pursue a reasonably normal lifestyle (even with a portable pump). The rate of infusion is constant for 11 hours then wound down for the final hour to prevent rebound hypoglycaemia when the infusion is stopped. The parenteral nutrition may be given as seldom as three nights a week. The child may also have an enteral feed, also infused overnight, and a limited diet. If at all possible, a minimum of two bolus feeds a day should be given to maintain enterohepatic circulation and intestinal mucosal integrity. The bolus volume can be as little as 20 ml/h.

Nutrients

Before going home, the child must be sufficiently stable to cope with the same nutrients being given for a week, which is the shortest reasonable time between prescription changes and delivery.

The nutrition is a commercially formulated preparation in which the nitrogen source is an amino acid preparation (75% of amino acids are converted into body protein[43]), carbohydrate is in the form of dextrose, and additional electrolytes and trace elements are added. Lipid is added to the feed two or three days

a week. If it is given more frequently there is a high risk of precipitation in the line with ensuing line occlusion (personal observation). Lipid should represent about 30% of non-protein energy, and linoleic acid should be 1–2% of total energy. The maximum lipid utilization rate is about 3.3–3.6 g/kg/d.[43] Many children receiving HPN can absorb sufficient essential fatty acids and fat-soluble vitamins from the gut (and skin) so that they do not need any parenteral lipid; they can manage with a formulation based upon amino acids and dextrose.

Stability data is available for up to 3 weeks for vitamins added to parenteral nutrition bags. There are problems with breakdown of vitamin A by ultraviolet light and loss of vitamin E. Most patients receiving long-term HPN have some intestinal function, and most vitamins (especially water-soluble ones) can be adequately absorbed from the gastrointestinal tract. Essential fatty acids can be absorbed from the skin of neonates if sunflower or safflower oil is applied daily.

Stability of the HPN formulation for children can be a major problem. They have high calcium and phosphate requirements and these two salts readily precipitate. The nutrition should be supplied by a licensed compounding unit that has access both to its own stability data and that available in specialist parenteral nutrition units elsewhere in the UK and Europe.

Organization of parenteral nutrition at home

All children with chronic severe intestinal failure should be assessed in a paediatric gastroenterology unit with an established multidisciplinary home parenteral nutrition service. Once such a unit has established that there is severe intractable intestinal failure and that the patient will almost certainly require parenteral nutrition for at least the next two months, home treatment should be planned.

Funding

A commercial home care company is usually contracted to supply the nutrients and equipment prescribed by the home parenteral nutrition team. The company is chosen according to a service specification, which may include pharmaceutical preparations, equipment requirements, patient liaison/back-up, quality and financial criteria. A larger home parenteral nutrition team can tender for one company to supply and deliver the nutrition/ancillaries to all its patients. This enables close and efficient working practices with a consistent system of care. Smaller units may tender for each individual patient but this creates much work.

The hospital team regularly audits the home care service and holds review meetings with them. From the patient's perspective, it is important to remain with one company so that a good relationship with the company and delivery drivers can be established. The company delivers the parenteral feeds, equipment and ancillaries (dry goods; Box 27.3).

Box 27.3 – Equipment required for home parenteral nutrition

Single items
Pump
Dispenser for handwash
Dressing trolley
Fridge
Fridge thermometer
Cool box and ice packs
Infusion pump and stand
Ambulatory pump and portable stand when appropriate
Scissors
Clamps
Central line repair kit

Items regularly replaced
Chlorhexidine gluconate hand scrub or Povidine iodine® handwash
70% Isopropyl alcohol hard surface disinfectant
Sterile wipes
Heparinized saline
Sodium chloride 0.9%
Pump administration sets appropriate for type of pump used and the system required
Sterile gloves
Sterile dressing pack
Sterile and non-sterile gauze swabs
Paper roll
Dressings
Tape
Ketodiastix®

Discharge planning

If home treatment is to be a success it is important to ensure that all aspects of care are well organized (Box 27.4). Once the hospital contracting department has

---

Box 27.4 – Discharge planning

Multidisciplinary ethical review (if necessary)
Agree funding with health authority
Specialist social worker and nutrition nurse interview parents
Home visit by nutrition nurse with/without social worker
Training programme
Discharge planning meeting

---

organized funding for home treatment, the specialist nutrition nurse and patient's social worker meet with the patient's parents/carers to discuss in detail what is involved with parenteral nutrition (PN) at home. The home PN prescription is worked out by the paediatrician and pharmacist and sent to the pharmacist at the home care company. The home PN paediatrician will arrange shared care with the local hospital paediatrician. The specialist nutrition nurse visits the home with a local community paediatric nurse. If any alterations to the home are required, the hospital social worker may need to discuss arrangements with the family and, if necessary, the local social worker.

A discharge planning meeting is held at the local hospital. Parents and most of the professionals involved (from the local hospital and community and specialist unit) are invited. It is essential that parents, nutrition nurse, the local paediatrician and paediatric gastroenterologist, local nurses and social workers are present. All aspects of care are addressed (e.g. which hospital admits the child for each potential problem, and a system for waste disposal).

Arrangements for practical support are tailored to the parents' wishes and to what can be made available. The parents are encouraged to accept any reasonable support offered. This may vary from help with housework during the day to a carer staying in the home overnight to provide practical help, for example changing nappies and attending to the pump if the alarm goes off. The parents are expected to connect and disconnect the line themselves every evening and morning to minimize the risk of septicaemia. Finally the child is discharged home, the specialist nutrition nurse being present for the first PN connection.

Continuing professional support

Specialist centre. The professionals from the specialist unit involved in care at home are the specialist nutrition nurse, paediatric gastroenterologist and dietician. The hospital social worker and psychologist provide other support and the pharmacist is involved in reviewing the PN regimen when necessary. A nutrition nurse should ideally be available during working hours, and a 24-hour on-call telephone service should be provided by the specialist unit.

The nutrition nurse has an extensive role and will be familiar with all aspects of care at home. He or she is usually the first point of contact with the hospital and liaises with other professionals as appropriate. In addition, the nurse visits the home when appropriate. The paediatric gastroenterologist liaises with the local hospital or general practitioner (GP) as necessary when medical problems arise. A dietician should continue to assess and ensure that the child receives adequate nutrition. A hospital pharmacist organizes changes to the home parenteral nutrition regimen with the home care company pharmacist. Families frequently need social work help and financial support.

Local services. Many professionals provide support. The most helpful professionals as perceived from a questionnaire survey were the GP (12 of 15) and paediatrician (10 of 15). All 11 children at school were well supported by school staff. Seven of the 15 were helped by a social worker and all children under 6 years had a supportive health visitor. A psychologist (3 clinical, 2 educational) helped 5 families, and 4 volunteered that the community nurses had helped.[44]

Long-term management

All children receiving long-term parenteral nutrition at home need to be regularly reviewed by the multi-disciplinary team in the specialist centre.

Growth and nutrition. Growth and development are monitored. Nutrition is adjusted as necessary. It is suggested that children receiving long-term PN should initially have weekly measurements of blood count, urea, sodium, potassium, calcium, magnesium, phosphate and liver function tests and monthly copper, zinc and selenium measurement. In a stable patient, however, all of these need only be measured every 2–3 months or even less often. Every 6 months measurements of the water-soluble (B and C) and fat-soluble (ADEK) vitamins are made and a liver/gall-bladder ultrasound is done. If previously normal, B group vitamins, vitamin D and thyroid function need only to be checked every 12 months. A lung perfusion scan and electrocardiogram are performed yearly.[43]

Underlying intestinal disease. The underlying intestinal disease and remaining intestinal function should be reviewed regularly and treatment appropriately adjusted. In most cases a yearly admission for observation and detailed review is helpful. Intestinal endoscopy can be repeated and drug treatment for the underlying disease altered as necessary. The aim is gradually to increase the enteral feed given.

Complications

Catheter-related complications (sepsis and thrombo-embolism) followed by cholestasis are the main problems experienced by neonates/infants and children receiving parenteral nutrition.[12,27,45,46]

Venous access

One complication that occurs particularly in smaller children is lack of venous access. Major vessels can become occluded with thrombus after they have been used for a central venous catheter. The usual course of events is that they re-canalize, but only after several months or years. It is common in children on long-term PN for all the usual sites for venous access to become thrombosed. Various other sites (e.g. the renal or azygos veins) can be used in some patients.

The lives of children with severe chronic intestinal failure depend on venous access for infusion of nutrients. It is therefore essential that every effort be made to maintain line patency. Lack of venous access is one of the indications for referral for assessment for intestinal transplant.

Catheter-related complications

Although survival on treatment and the chances of resuming full oral therapy are better for children than adults, children have more frequent admissions to hospital with catheter-related sepsis.[46] Catheter-related sepsis is the most common complication of home parenteral nutrition in children, occurring in 2–29%.

Deep vein thrombosis may be present in as many as 67% of children with a central feeding line at home.[47] Catheter occlusion can be caused by a calcium phosphate precipitate or by fibrin or lipid. One possible mechanism is the formation of antiphospho-lipid antibodies and a resulting hypercoagulable state with a form of antiphospholipid syndrome.[48] Intralipid contains phospholipids that can be immunogenic. Children with antiphospholipid or cardiolipin antibodies or with any evidence of thrombus formation are given long-term prophylactic anticoagulant treatment.[49]

If a parenteral feed is being given into a superficial vein (for example following removal of a central line when managing intractable septicaemia) the total concentration of glucose should be less than 15% to keep the osmolality low and reduce the chance of thrombophlebitis.

Cholestasis

Cholestasis is related to overfeeding, prematurity, sepsis and, rarely, surgery. It can progress to cirrhosis. Bacterial infection early in life occurs most commonly in the neonates that develop cholestasis; cholestasis usually starts within 2 weeks of the infection[50] and may be related to a breakdown in the gut mucosal barrier. Enteral feeding, even if it provides less than 10% of the total energy intake, is the most important factor in preventing/reversing cholestasis. Ursodeoxycholic acid, which reduces bile synthesis and secretion, solubilizes cholesterol and increases bile flow, may be beneficial. Small bowel stasis causes bacterial overgrowth with the manufacture of the less soluble, more hepatotoxic secondary bile acid lithocholate; oral antibiotics, for example, metronidazole, can prevent this. A deficiency of taurine, a conditionally essential amino acid, results in less of the more soluble taurine conjugated bile acids being made; this can be prevented/reversed by giving a taurine-enriched feed. Other factors that may contribute to hepatic damage are the phytosterols in lipid emulsions that may inhibit bile acid secretion, and copper and manganese which are usually excreted in bile but become hepatotoxic in cholestatic patients.[43] (Chs 26 and 32)

Nutrient abnormalities

Manganese toxicity. A minority of children on long-term parenteral nutrition have developed movement disorders and cholestatic liver disease in association with high blood manganese levels (reference range 73–350 nmol/l).[51] Magnetic resonance imaging has detected changes consistent with manganese deposition in the cerebral basal ganglia of these children and other asymptomatic children with high blood manganese levels above 600 nmol/l (616–1840 nmol/l) after 2–16 months of PN treatment.[51] They were receiving 0.8–1.0 μmol/kg/24 h.

Blood levels fell to 300–1171 nmol/l after reducing or stopping manganese in parenteral nutrition. The cholestatic liver disease and neurological damage improved as blood levels of manganese fell. Following this discovery manganese supplementation was routinely reduced to 0.018 μmol (1.0 μgm) Mn/kg/24 h as recommended by the Committee of Clinical Practice Issues of the American Society of Clinical Nutrition.[52]

Nutrient deficiencies. The nutritional complications of parenteral nutrition have gradually decreased as the composition of nutrient solutions has been improved. Selenium is one of the most recent additions to parenteral nutrition solutions. Prior to its addition there were case reports of deficiency.[53] Solutions are still free of iodine. Some patients acquire low circulating thyroxine levels secondary to iodine deficiency. In these patients, who tend to have severe intestinal failure, Betadine® can be applied to the skin.

Many patients are given oral vitamins in preference to adding vitamins to the parenteral solutions. Some vitamins have poor stability in parenteral nutrition solutions. They are best added to the solutions at home, but this increases the risk of sepsis. It is possible to add vitamins to the solutions at source, but blood levels need to be carefully monitored.

Outcome

Survival

Home treatment has developed over the past 15 years. The Hospital for Sick Children, Great Ormond Street, pioneered home parenteral nutrition in the UK. HPN was originally set up for children who could have a good quality of life on home treatment with a good life expectancy. More recently, children with a short life expectancy have also been discharged home on treatment. Altogether, about 60 children have been discharged home from Great Ormond Street Hospital, London, UK. The number of children on treatment has increased steadily from 10 in 1990 to about 30 in 2000. Approximately 40% are still on treatment and almost a quarter have died. Survival rates are continuing to improve. Children have normal growth and development, attend school and go on family holidays, including foreign travel. Long-term survival is possible: the oldest child is now aged 16.

In children with good life expectancy, the survival rates are 92% (34 of 37) 2-year survival and 77% (17 of 22) 5-year survival.[54] All 17 children who have survived 5 years on HPN are still alive up to 14 years later, with a mean and median survival of 9 years. Children grow and develop normally on parenteral nutrition. None of the children has developed liver disease once established on parenteral nutrition at home. In addition, liver function has improved in many children in whom it was abnormal on discharge.

Stopping parenteral nutrition

One-third of the patients discharged from Great Ormond Street Hospital on HPN have been weaned off treatment. Children with a short gut are usually able to tolerate increasing volumes of feed and may even be weaned off parenteral nutrition over several months or years. Most patients have been weaned off treatment from 6 months to 3 years (mean 2.5 years) after discharge.[54]

In neonates, small bowel length and percentage of energy taken by the enteral route at 12 weeks of life (adjusted age) related to the duration of parenteral nutrition. However, gestational age, presence of the ileocaecal valve and development of cholestasis were not related.[55] Of the children surviving with 10–30 cm remaining small bowel, 63% were able to stop parenteral nutrition after a mean 320 days (range 148–506) of parenteral nutrition. If less than 10 cm small bowel remained, PN was always needed but long-term survival was possible.[56]

Weaning a child off parenteral nutrition can be one of the most complex aspects of management. Even with extensive investigation and assessment of intestinal function, it can remain uncertain whether a child has adequate intestinal function to tolerate full enteral feeding. The parenteral treatment can be reduced while the volume of overnight enteral feed is increased and the child carefully observed. Many children can initially absorb sufficient energy but are unable to maintain fluid and electrolyte homeostasis. They may need intravenous saline infusions alone during a transition period from parenteral to enteral nutrition. Weaning from parenteral to enteral nutrition usually takes place at home. Patients and their families are rarely happy to undergo hospitalization when the child is well at home. They would often prefer to continue with the parenteral nutrition, despite the potential for life-threatening complications, than give up a treatment that has saved the child's life. If weaning from parenteral nutrition is to take place at home, it must be done gradually with regular outpatient review.

Quality of life on home parenteral nutrition

The aim of home parenteral nutrition is to enable children discharged from hospital to lead a good quality of life at home. The child reintegrates into normal childhood activities, such as attending school. The family can enjoy being complete again. They can enjoy holidays together as a family, both in the UK and abroad. Families have travelled from the UK to North America and Singapore.

An enormous burden of care is placed upon families when parents take on the responsibility for administering highly technical care at home. There is both emotional and physical stress. For the parents there is the physical stress of disturbed nights. The alarm on the nutrition infusion pump may sound. Nappies may need changing several times a night since virtually all the fluid intake takes place during the night. In addition, there is emotional stress from the knowledge that life-threatening complications such as septicaemia may develop at any time. Parents' response to a recent psychosocial questionnaire highlighted the fear of septicaemia as a major source of stress.[44]

Home parenteral nutrition has a major effect on the flexibility of the family. Parents felt that the family lifestyle had become rigid with loss of potential for spontaneous activities. The most difficult time for 9 of 15 families was the first few months at home. This finding was similar to that in adults on parenteral nutrition, who had a better quality of life when they had been on treatment for many months.[57] The treatment inhibited the parents' social lives and affected older siblings and in some cases the peer relationships of school-age children; for example, sleepovers (an important aspect of socialization for school children) were not possible.

All the families on our home programme have at least one other child, most have three children, and one has five. Despite the stresses of PN at home, most families have successfully incorporated PN into their lifestyle.[44]

Ethical issues

The three groups of patients for whom parenteral nutrition at home is likely to fail are: (1) medically unstable patients with significant variations in fluid and electrolyte requirements; (2) those with co-existing severe chronic disease involving other organs; (3) those in chaotic family circumstances. Giving parenteral nutrition in these situations probably causes, rather than relieves suffering, and administering HPN can be an intolerable burden of care for the family. As a result, some members of the nutrition team (paediatrician and nutrition nurse specialist) may need to take on an ethical role, informing the medical team directly involved in the child's care of the most likely long-term prognosis and prompting a full ethical review.

Patients are often started on parenteral nutrition in hospital with the expectation of both professionals and parents that it will only be needed for a few days or weeks. Once treatment has been started, the underlying disease may deteriorate and PN needs to be continued for longer. Some patients, particularly neonates, may develop significant disease involving other organs, for example neurological disease, that may not have been recognized prior to starting PN or developing after it started. The result may be a child who would not have been commenced on 'high-tech' treatment if the disease in other organs had been appreciated earlier. Major psychological difficulties, as the aims and objectives of the patient's management are dramatically altered, will occur in both parents and staff, especially if treatment is to be withdrawn. Withholding treatment in the beginning is easier, but it is often not possible in children with progressive disease to anticipate that treatment will be futile.

We set up a multidisciplinary working party to explore ethical and legal issues surrounding withholding or withdrawing treatment. The outcome was that the medical treatment of nutritional support can be withheld if: (a) the patient is dying; (b) death will be delayed without improving quality of or potential for life; (c) treatment will impose such severe suffering on the child and family that it would be unreasonable to expect them to bear it. These criteria were subsequently identified in the framework document on withdrawal and withholding treatment published by the Royal College of Paediatrics and Child Health.[58]

In children with other disabling chronic disease besides intestinal failure, ethical issues are dealt with by holding a multidisciplinary meeting. People involved have included the medical team caring for the patient, parents (with a lay advocate if wished), the child when appropriate, the paediatric gastroenterologist on the home parenteral nutrition team, and a paediatrician with ethical training. The aims and objectives of treatment are discussed and a management plan within a specific time frame is made.

Transplantation

Small bowel transplantation, often with liver, may be appropriate treatment for patients with no venous access or coexisting severe liver disease (Ch. 34). However, techniques for gaining venous access, even through thrombosed vessels, are improving and in our experience liver disease is not developing in patients on long-term treatment at home.

SUMMARY

A good nutritional state is a prerequisite for normal growth and development in childhood. The effects of inadequate nutrition in early life may have lifelong consequences (poor growth and intellectual development) in addition to worsening systemic illness. Children who need enteral nutrition usually have an underlying problem with ingesting or digesting sufficient energy, while patients needing parenteral nutrition have intestinal failure with a problem in absorption. Survival is now possible with a good quality of life, even in children with severe intestinal failure, but at a cost.

REFERENCES

1. Israel DM, Hassall E. Prolonged use of gastrostomy for enteral hyperalimentation in children with Crohn's disease. *Am J Gastroenterol* 1995; **90:** 1084–1088.

2. McCarey DW, Buchanan E, Gregory M, Clark BJ, Weaver LT. Home enteral feeding of children in the west of Scotland. *Scott Med J* 1997; **41:** 147–149.

3. Behrens R, Lang T, Muschweck H, Richter T, Hofbeck M. Percutaneous endoscopic gastrostomy in children and adolescents. *J Pediatr Gastroenterol Nutr* 1997; **25:** 487–491.

4. Pedersen AM, Kok K, Petersen G, Nielsen OH, Michaelsen KF, Schmiegelow K. Percutaneous endoscopic gastrostomy in children with cancer. *Acta Paediatr* 1999; **88:** 849–852.

5. Smith SW, Camfield C, Camfield P. Living with cerebral palsy and tube feeding: a population-based follow-up study. *J Pediatr* 1999; **135:** 307–310.

6. Brant CQ, Stanich P, Ferrari AP Jr. Improvement of children's nutritional status after enteral feeding by PEG: an interim report. *Gastrointest Endoscop* 1999; **50:** 183–188.

7. Rosenfeld M, Casey S, Pepe M, Ramsey BW. Nutritional effects of long-term gastrostomy feedings in children with cystic fibrosis. *J Am Diet Assoc* 1999; **99:** 191–194.

8. Ledermann SE, Shaw V, Trompeter RS. Long-term enteral nutrition in infants and young children with chronic renal failure. *Pediatr Nephrol* 1999; **13:** 870–875.

9. Bisset WM, Stapleford P, Long S, Chamberlain A, Sokel B, Milla PJ. Home parenteral nutrition in chronic intestinal failure. *Arch Dis Child* 1992; **67:** 109–114.

10. Huang FC, Chang MH, Chen CC. Home parenteral nutrition in children. *J Formos Med Assoc* 1996; **95:** 45–50.

11. Ksiazyk J, Lyszkowska M, Kierkus J, Bogucki K, Ratynska A, Tondys B, Socha J. Home parenteral nutrition in children: the Polish experience. *J Pediatr Gastroenterol Nutr* 1999; **28:** 152–156.

12. Koehler AN, Yaworski JA, Gardner M, Kocoshis S, Reyes J, Barksdale EM Jr. Coordinated interdisciplinary management of pediatric intestinal failure: a 2-year review. *J Pediatr Surg* 2000; **35:** 380–385.

13. Shepherd RW, Chin SE, Cleghorn GJ *et al.* Malnutrition in children with chronic liver disease accepted for liver transplantation: clinical profile and effect on outcome. *J Paediatr Child Health* 1991; **27:** 295–299.

14. Kang A, Zamora SA, Scott RB, Parsons HG. Catch-up growth in children treated with home enteral nutrition. *Pediatrics* 1998; **102:** 951–955.

15. Heird WC, Driscoll JM, Schullinger JN, Grebin B, Winters RW. Intravenous alimentation in paediatric patients. *J Paediatr* 1972; **80:** 351–372.

16. Elia M, Russell C, Shaffer J *et al. Report of the British Artificial Nutrition Survey – August 1999.* British Association of Parenteral and Enteral Nutrition.

17. Oliver RG, Jones G. Neonatal feeding of infants born with cleft lip and/or palate: parental perceptions of their experience in south Wales. *Cleft Palate Craniofac J* 1997; **34:** 526–532.

18. Shepherd R, Cooksley WGE, Domville-Cooke WD. Improved growth and clinical, nutritional and respiratory changes in response to nutritional therapy in cystic fibrosis. *J Pediatr* 1980; **97:** 351–357.

19. Scott RB, O'Loughlin EV, Gall DG. Gastro-esophageal reflux in cystic fibrosis. *J Pediatr* 1985; **106:** 223–227.

20. Kursner SI, Garg M, Bautsia DB, Bader D, Meritt RJ, Warburton D, Keens TG. Growth failure in infants with bronchopulmonary dysplasia: nutrition and elevated resting metabolic expenditure. *Pediatrics* 1988; **81:** 379–384.

21. Schwarz SM, Gewitz MH, See CC *et al.* Enteral nutrition in infants with congenital heart disease and growth failure. *Pediatrics* 1990; **86:** 368–373.

22. Pilling GP, Cresson SL. Massive resection of the small intestine in the neonatal period. *Pediatrics* 1957; **19:** 940–948.

23. Wilmore D. Factors correlating with a successful outcome following extensive intestinal resection in newborn infants. *J Pediatr* 1972; **80:** 88–95.

24. Grosfeld JL, Rescoria FJ, West KW. Short bowel syndrome in infancy and childhood. Analysis of survival in 60 patients. *Am J Surg* 1986; **151:** 41–46.

25. Goulet O J, Revillon Y, Dominique J *et al.* Neonatal short bowel syndrome. *J Paediatr* 1991; **119:** 18–23.

26. Weber TR, Tracy T Jr, Connors RH. Short bowel syndrome in children. Quality of life in an era of improved survival. *Arch Surg* 1991; **126:** 841–846.

27. Anagnostopoulos D, Valioulis J, Sfougaris D, Maliaropoulos N, Spyridakis J. Morbidity and mortality of short bowel syndrome in infancy and childhood. *Eur J Pediatr Surg* 1991; **1:** 273–276.

28. Galea MH, Holliday H, Carachi R, Kapila L. Short-bowel syndrome: a collective review. *J Pediatr Surg* 1992; **27:** 592–596.

29. Griffiths AM, Ohlsson A, Sherman PM, Sutherland LR. Meta-analysis of enteral nutrition as a primary treatment of active Crohn's disease. *Gastroenterology* 1995; **108:** 1056–1067.

30. Harries AD, Jones LA, Danis V, Fifield R, Heatley RV, Newcombe RG, Rhodes J. Controlled trial of supplemented oral nutrition in Crohn's disease. *Lancet* 1983; **i:** 887–890.

31. Aiges H, Markowitz J, Rosa J, Daum F. Home nocturnal supplemental naso-gastric feedings in growth-retarded adolescents with Crohn's disease. *Gastroenterology* 1989; **97:** 905–910.

32. Wilschanski M, Sherman P, Pencharz P, Davis L, Corey M, Griffiths A. Supplementary enteral nutrition maintains remission in paediatric Crohn's disease. *Gut* 1996; **38:** 543–548.

33. King TS, Woolner JT, Hunter JO. The dietary management of Crohn's disease. *Aliment Pharmacol Ther* 1997; **11:** 17–31.

34. Aiges H, Markowitz J, Rosa J, Daum F. Home nocturnal supplemental nasogastric feedings in growth-retarded adolescents with Crohn's disease. *Gastroenterology* 1989; **97:** 905–910.

35. Larcher VF, Shepherd R, Francis DE, Harries JT. Protracted diarrhoea in infancy. Analysis of 82 cases with particular reference to diagnosis and management. *Arch Dis Child* 1977; **52:** 597–605.

36. Evans MA, Shronts EP. Intestinal fuels: glutamine, short-chain fatty acids, and dietary fiber. *J Am Diet Assoc* 1992; **92:** 1239–1246.

37. Harig JM, Soergel KH, Komorowski RA, Woods CM. Treatment of diversion colitis with short chain fatty acid irrigation. *N Engl J Med* 1989; **320:** 23–28.

38. Roberfroid MB. Health benefits of non-digestible oligosaccharides. *Adv Exp Med Biol* 1997; **427:** 211–219.

39. Khattak IU, Kimber C, Kiely EM, Spitz L. Percutaneous endoscopic gastrostomy in paediatric practice: complications and outcome. *J Pediatr Surg* 1998; **33:** 67–72.

40. Holden CE, MacDonald A, Ward M *et al.* Psychological preparation for nasogastric feeding in children. *Br J Nurs* 1997; **6:** 376–381 and 384–385.

41. Peters JM, Simpson P, Tolia V. Experience with gastro-jejunal feeding tubes in children. *Am J Gastroenterol* 1997; **92:** 476–480.

42. Melville CA, Bisset WM, Long S, Milla PJ. Counting the cost: hospital versus home central venous catheter survival. *J Hosp Infect* 1997; **53:** 197–205.

43. Milla PJ (ed) *Current perspectives on paediatric parenteral nutrition.* British Association for Parenteral and Enteral Nutrition, 2000.

44. Savidge C, Cullen M, Carmichael P, Long S, Hill S. Parents perceptions of caring for a child on home parenteral nutrition. *Proc Nutr Soc* 2000.

45. Suita S, Masumoto K, Yamanouchi T, Nagano M, Nakamura M. Complications in neonates with short bowel syndrome and long-term parenteral nutrition. *J Parenter Enteral Nutr* 1999; **23:** S106–S109.

46. Howard L, Ament M, Fleming C, Shike M, Steiger E. Current use of home parenteral and enteral nutrition therapies in the United States. *Gastroenterology* 1995; **109:** 355–365.

47. Andrew M, Marzinotto V, Pencharz P *et al.* A cross-sectional study of catheter-related thrombosis in children receiving total parenteral nutrition at home. *J Pediatr* 1995; **126:** 358–363.

48. Kucuk O, Gilman-Sachs A, Lis LJ, Westerman MP. Antiphospholipid antibody formation can be induced in mice by phospholipid. *Am J Hematol* 1993; **42:** 380–383.

49. Dollery C. Pulmonary embolism in parenteral nutrition. *Arch Dis Child* 1996; **74:** 95–98.

50. Sondheimer JM, Asturias E, Cadnapaphornchai M. Infection and cholestasis in neonates with intestinal resection and long-term parenteral nutrition. *J Pediatr Gastroenterol Nutr* 1998; **27:** 131–137.

51. Fell JME, Reynolds AP, Meadows N *et al.* Manganese toxicity in children receiving long-term parenteral nutrition. *Lancet* 1996; **347:** 1218–1221.

52. Committee on Clinical Practice Issues of the American Society for Clinical Nutrition. Guidelines for paediatric parenteral nutrition. *Am J Clin Nutr* 1988; **48:** 1324–1342.

53. Lockitch G, Taylor GP, Wong LT, Davidson AG, Dison PJ, Riddell D, Massing D. Cardiomyopathy associated with nonendemic selenium deficiency in a Caucasian adolescent. *Am J Clin Nutr* 1990; **52:** 572–577.

54. Hill S, Long S, Milla P. 14 years of home parenteral nutrition: long term outcome. *Arch Dis Child* 2000; **82:** A21.

55. Sondheimer JM, Cadnapaphornchai M, Sontag M, Zerbe GO. Predicting the duration of dependence on parenteral nutrition after neonatal intestinal resection. *J Pediatr* 1998; **132:** 80–84.

56. Kurkchubasche AG, Rowe MI, Smith SD. Adaptation in short-bowel syndrome: reassessing old limits. *J Pediatr Surg* 1993; **28:** 1069–1071.

57. Richards DM, Irving MH. Assessing the quality of life of patients with intestinal failure on home parenteral nutrition. *Gut* 1997; **40:** 218–222.

58. Royal College of Paediatrics and Child Health. *Witholding or withdrawing life saving treatment in children. A framework for practice.* RCPCH, London, 1997.

28

Quality of life assessment and cost-effectiveness

David M. Richards and Gordon L. Carlson

One of the key objectives of treating patients is to improve quality of life. Time in hospital, suffering, pain, disablement, emotional turmoil and disfigurement are quality of life issues which are very relevant to patients with intestinal failure. Data on these outcomes are not often collected, and consequently doctors themselves are frequently unaware of the extent to which treatment affects the quality of life of their patients.

Information on outcome can be used to inform patients and doctors about the effects of treatment and can also be used to compare different treatments for a particular condition. When the costs of treatment are also taken into account, then it is possible to describe the cost–effectiveness of interventions.

The introduction of the UK National Health Service reforms in 1990 led to a division between purchasers and providers of health care. Purchasers became required to provide reliable information concerning the services for which they were paying. In addition to morbidity and mortality statistics, detailed cost and quality of life (QoL) data are needed for contract negotiation.[1]

MEASUREMENT OF QoL

'When you can measure what you are speaking of and measure it in terms of numbers, you know something about it. When you cannot, your knowledge is of a meagre kind.'

Kelvin (1824–1907)

QoL assessment has to encompass many aspects of life and must be related to individual aims and goals.[2] It is generally accepted that a definition of the quality of life must include emotional state, social state, occupational state, physical state and psychological well-being.[3] Other domains such as self-esteem, body image and cognitive functioning might also be added.[1]

Objective quantification of subjective variables is difficult, mainly because of the wide variations in value that two people might attribute to a particular health state. Even if agreement is reached there is the equally difficult task of assigning a numerical value to that particular state. The measurement of health status has received much attention recently. It is now possible to use a variety of validated health status instruments to produce a meaningful, reproducible profile of health status.

PROBLEMS WITH MEASURING QoL

It is important to remember that health is a subjective state and perceptions of an acceptable health state will vary greatly from person to person. Some value life as more important than anything else and will seek life at any cost, no matter what the quality. This should be appreciated if doctors place an objective value on a patients' QoL. Wherever possible it is the patients' valuation of QoL that should be measured.

How a person values a new state of health depends on the original state of health. For example, a patient would view life on home parenteral nutrition differently depending on whether they were suffering from severe Crohn's disease or were completely well prior to a mesenteric infarction.

Using health status instruments to measure QoL outcomes is associated with several problems related to the nature of health care.[4] Outcomes are multidimensional, most are qualitative, and are affected by timing. Different disease subgroups will have different outcomes and these may not be attributable to specific treatments.

HEALTH STATUS INSTRUMENTS

There are many health status questionnaires available which can be divided into two main groups. The first are profile questionnaires which produce a broad description of the burden of illness on the patient. The second group are index assessments which yield a single figure relating to a quality of life scale. They can be further subdivided into general and disease-specific assessment tools.

An example of a general (profile) health status indicator is the Short Form 36, which can be used to describe the burden of illness on patients.[5] It measures subjective feelings and does not require clinicians or others to place their own values on QoL.

An example of a questionnaire which yields an index of QoL is the EuroQoL instrument (Fig. 28.1).[6] This type of instrument is valuable in economic appraisal. EuroQoL was developed in several European countries and can be used to make comparisons of health status between nations. This is of potential value in the field of intestinal failure research as there are now extensive links between European centres. EuroQoL examines six distinct domains with two or

EuroQoL

Patient number ....
Patient initials ....   Date

....

By placing a tick in one box in each group below, please indicate which statements best describe your own health state today.

Mobility

I have no problems in walking about ☐

I have some problems in walking about ☐

I am confined to bed ☐

Self-Care

I have no problems with self-care ☐

I have some problems washing or dressing myself ☐

I am unable to wash or dress myself ☐

Usual Activities (e.g. work, study, housework, family or leisure activities)

I have no problems with performing my usual activities ☐

I have some problems with performing my usual activities ☐

I am unable to perform my usual activities ☐

Pain/Discomfort

I have no pain or discomfort ☐

I have moderate pain or discomfort ☐

I have extreme pain or discomfort ☐

Anxiety/Depression

I am not anxious or depressed ☐

I am moderately anxious or depressed ☐

I am extremely anxious or depressed ☐

To help people say how good or bad a health state is, we have drawn a scale (rather like a thermometer) on which the best state you can imagine is marked by 100 and the worst state you can imagine is marked by 0.

We would like you to indicate on this scale how good or bad is your own health today, in your opinion. Please do this by drawing a line from the box below to whichever point on the scale indicates how good or bad your current health state is.

Best imaginable health state

100

Your own health state today

0

Worst imaginable health state

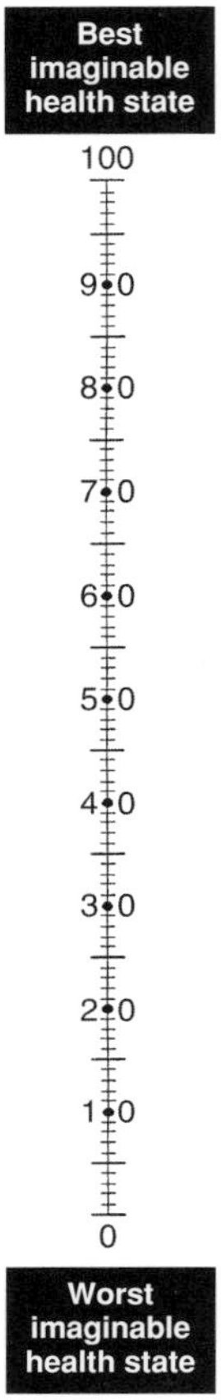

EUROQOL INSTRUMENT

Figure 28.1 – The EuroQol Questionnaire.[6]

three categories in each section. These are: mobility, self-care, main activity, social relationships, pain and mood. Each of the domains covers a wide range of severity. In essence this means that EuroQoL can be applied to a variety of subjects, from fairly healthy to severely ill. One problem of assessing patients with gastrointestinal disorders is the lack of disease–specific QoL instruments. Recent attempts to produce such instruments have failed, mainly because of lack of agreement over clinical definitions.[7]

ECONOMIC APPRAISAL

Economic appraisal is a rapidly growing area of medical research. The rise in popularity is due to increased (infinite) demands on scarce (finite) resources. By explicitly demonstrating the costs and outcomes associated with treatments it is possible to make better informed decisions on resource allocation. It also helps to decide the best 'mix' of

treatment programmes to achieve the maximum overall benefit from a healthcare system.

Knowledge of the opportunity cost is vital when considering expensive treatments for intestinal failure. Opportunity cost is the cost incurred by the allocation of resources to one programme which will deny resources to another healthcare need within a fixed budget.

There are three main types of economic appraisal:

1. Cost–Benefit Analysis (CBA): This involves the calculation of total cost and total benefit, and requires monetary valuation of outcomes. The methodology is problematic and they are rarely performed.

2. Cost-Effectiveness Analysis (CEA): This involves a comparison of outcome (e.g. lives saved) with cost. They are useful in the assessment of different treatments for the same condition, but they cannot

be compared to other treatments for different conditions.

3. Cost–Utility Analysis (CUA): This type of analysis differs from cost–effectiveness analysis in the way that outcomes are measured. The outcome in terms of survival is weighted by increases in QoL achieved. This is known as the quality-adjusted life year (QALY). This type of analysis can be used to compare a wide variety of healthcare interventions because the units of outcome measure are the same.

To answer questions on operational efficiency, CEA methodology is used. To answer questions regarding resource allocation, CUA is the preferred choice. As with all research proposals careful consideration of the research question and the answers required will determine which method to use.

With respect to intestinal failure there are two main areas where economic appraisal can be helpful. First, allocation efficiency: Why should resources be ear-marked for the treatment of intestinal failure rather than, for example, home haemodialysis? Second, operational efficiency: economic appraisal can be used to compare alternative treatments for intestinal failure (for example small bowel transplantation with home parenteral nutrition) or can be used to compare aspects of a treatment (for example the type of central venous access device used for the administration of parenteral nutrition).

Problems with economic appraisal

The methodology of cost–utility analysis is well described in the literature[8] and results are comparable providing all aspects of the methodology are followed. However, just because a study is published does not guarantee that it is relevant or of an acceptable standard. Therefore 'league tables' of cost-effective procedures must be interpreted with great caution because of the variation in the scientific rigour of the economic analysis. Criticisms exist because of differing methodologies used and failure to use marginal costs.[9] Marginal costs are defined as the cost of treating one additional patient which is more relevant in practice and is usually lower than the average cost.

Despite these criticisms, explicit presentation of costs and outcomes is an improvement on the less empirical decision-making processes of the past, when whoever 'shouted loudest' was allocated resources. Economic analysis should be thought of as an aid to decision-making rather than a precise tool. Resource allocation for healthcare programmes depends on many factors (e.g. political) in addition to the result of an economic analysis.

Patients with intestinal failure pose methodological problems for economic appraisal because of variations in practice, heterogeneity of the patients and uncertainty regarding outcomes. However, these are not reasons for abandoning attempts to combine costs with outcomes.

PREVIOUS QUALITY OF LIFE ASSESSMENTS OF HOME PARENTERAL NUTRITION (HPN)

HPN is complex and expensive and requires the patient to be dependent on a machine for nutritional support. The nature of the technology inevitably has an effect on QoL. Previous QoL studies are described in Table 28.1.

Anger, anxiety and depression result from the sense of loss sustained by the patient. The loss includes the inability to eat normally, loss of independence, loss of status and position in the social framework, lowered status at work and loss of control of bodily functions. These feelings vary in intensity according to the degree of severity of the underlying illness. The pre-morbid psychological and physical profile of the patient also have a bearing on the QoL achieved.[10]

Patients established on HPN can modify their lifestyles in order to minimize the impact of dependence on intravenous feeding. The usual practice is to infuse the nutrient solution overnight on a cyclical basis, allowing daytime 'freedom'. Patients are able to travel with the help of the HPN support groups that exist in the UK, Europe and the USA. Most are able to eat normally and can work, study and look after the home. Contact sports tend to be avoided but many patients swim, play golf and are involved in other leisure pursuits.

QoL scores for patients on HPN have been compared with estimated scores of patients receiving all their nutrition in hospital.[11] Moving patients from the hospital to the home setting has been demonstrated to result in a significant gain in QoL.

Life satisfaction scores of HPN recipients have been shown to be in the upper two-thirds of the index range; however, the scores were significantly lower

Table 28.1 – Results of quality of life assessments of patients on home parenteral nutrition

Study	Whose values?	Instrument used	Profile or index	Index scores	Best QoL	Worst QoL	Comments
Carlson DL, 1995[17]	Patient	Non-validated questionnaire	Index	0.64 0-1 scale †	-	-	QoL independent of variables tested. Younger patients keen on intestinal transplantation
Detsky AS, 1986[11]	Patient	Category scaling, time trade off	Index	0.73 0-1 scale †	Scores improve with time and peak at 4-5 years	Lowest scores seen in the first year of HPN	Scores were measured for 37 and estimated for 36. No subgroup analysis was performed
Duclaux IL, 1993[20]	Doctor	Non-validated questionnaire	Profile	-	-	-	QoL much improved at home. Development and psychological well-being were much improved.
Galandiuk S, 1990[21]	Both	QoL score, social activity score, psychological score	Index	Pre HPN = 7.1 On HPN = 5.3*	-	-	The instruments gave an index which showed that the better scores were obtained on HPN and that the pre HPN QoL was significantly worse ($P<0.01$). [All patients in this study had Crohn's disease]
Herfindal ET, 1989[12]	Patient	Multiple-validated instruments	Profile	-	Long duration (> 6 months)	Duration less than 6 months	HPN patients had lower (worse) scores than renal transplant recipients and the normal US population
King LA, 1993[34]	Doctor	Retrospective case note review	Profile	-	-	-	All patients had a gynaecological malignancy. Improvements were noted in pain, vomiting, fatigue, morale and social interactions ($P<0.05$) compared with the pre HPN status.
Ladefoged K, 1981[14]	Patient	Non-validated questionnaire	Profile	-	Acceptable in 213 of all cases	-	QoL parameters were independent of all variables. BUT not enough data to test
Messing B, 1989[22]	Doctor	Functional assessment	-	-	Age < 65. Benign	Age > 65. Malignancy Pseudo-obstruction	Simple 4-stage rehabilitation profile. Stage decided by physician, not the patient
O'Hanrahan T, 1992[13]	Doctor	Functional assessment	Profile	-	Crohn's disease	All other diagnostic groups	Data overlap with Messing (1989). Same 4-point scale used
Pironi L, 1993[35]	Doctor	Functional	Profile	-	-	-	Same 4-point scale as Messing + O'Hanrahan. Two-thirds of patients in the best outcome groups
Richards DM, 1995[18]	Patient	SF 36 and EuroQoL	Both	0.51 0-1 scale†	Age < 45	Age > 55. Narcotic addiction	No significant difference between disease subgroups, stomas, recent hospitalisation, and duration of HPN
Smith CE, 1993[36]	Patient	Multiple validated instruments	Profile	-	High self-esteem, good relationship	Long duration of HPN, poor income	Loss of friends, loss of employment and depression were noted in two-thirds of families

★ = Scale 3 to 9, 3 = best possible QoL, 9 = severe disablement. † = Scale 0 to 1, 0=death, 1 =best possible quality of life. QoL = quality of life.

than those obtained by patients with end-stage renal disease and the general population.[12]

The United Kingdom HPN Register classified patients into four groups according to their functional outcome,[13] these are shown in Figure 28.2. Patients with Crohn's disease tend to fall into groups 1 and 2, and increasing disease activity pushes patients into groups 3 and 4.[13–15]

Sexual functioning decreases in the majority of patients and only the occasional patient notices an improvement.[10] Sexual functioning among younger patients has been reported as normal[14] but it ceases completely in some patients over 55 years of age.

Some studies have shown that older patients experience the same QoL as young patients.[14,16] Older patients in the UK HPN Register did less well and tended to fall into groups 3 or 4.[13] A more recent study has reported that younger patients have a significantly better QoL than those over 55 years of age.[17] Younger patients are more interested in small bowel transplantation than older patients.[18] This may indicate an unwillingness to accept long-term HPN and to see a

transplant as a means of significantly improving their QoL. It is therefore interesting that patients with the highest quality of life scores expressed a desire for transplantation.

The ageing population of HPN patients will pose future management problems, particularly as they become less able to manage complex aseptic procedures. Older patients have a higher incidence of catheter infections[19] in addition to a lower QoL. The increased rate of catheter infections may contribute to the deterioration in QoL.

A sinister factor which affects a percentage of HPN patients is addiction to narcotic and sedative medication. In addition to the increase in morbidity and mortality, these drugs have a detrimental effect on QoL.[20]

Disease subgroups in HPN populations eventually report similar QoL scores,[17] but the early scores are different. Patients with severe Crohn's disease usually report low scores, then experience an improvement after starting HPN.[21] Patients who suffer a catastrophic loss of intestine following a mesenteric infarct experience an initial fall in their QoL, but this returns to the level of the general HPN population (Fig. 28.3).

The percentage of HPN recipients who are employed seems to be falling. A recent study has shown that only 5% of HPN patients are employed in full-time work or study.[18] This figure is much lower than previous reports on a similar cohort where 52% were fully employed.[22] The reasons for this are unclear but it may be due to illness-related financial benefits.

All QoL studies on intestinal failure report scores for patients with a benign pathology. The most obvious gap in the current literature is an appraisal of the QoL for patients with intestinal failure secondary to terminal malignant disease or AIDS. Approximately 90% of world-wide HPN programme growth is attributable to treating patients with malignant disease. It is vital that these patients receive treatments which improve their QoL. The need for urgent appraisal, supported by prospectively collected data, is therefore clear.

For many patients, HPN is lifesaving and therefore some reduction in the quality of life is acceptable. The aim should be to add the best possible quality to the years gained. When considering patients for HPN it is important to judge each case individually. Consideration should be given to the outcome that can be expected in older patients or those with other medical problems, but this should not be a limiting factor if other aspects are favourable.

HPN Patient Outcomes

UK HPN Register

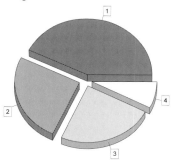

1	Full time work or looking after home and family unaided
2	Part time work or looking after the home with help
3	Unable to work but able to cope with HPN and go out occasionally
4	Housebound and needing major assistance with HPN

Figure 28.2 – Percentage of patients on the UK database in each functional category.[13]

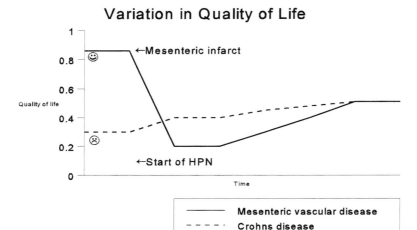

Variation in Quality of Life

←Mesenteric infarct

←Start of HPN

Mesenteric vascular disease
Crohns disease

(0 = death, 100 = best possible quality of life)

Figure 28.3 – Quality of life of HPN patient subgroups and variation with time.

PREVIOUS ECONOMIC APPRAISALS OF HPN

Economic analyses of HPN are scarce considering the cost of the technology. There have been seven studies examining the economics of HPN: two from the UK, four from the USA and one from Canada (Table 28.2). They examine the costs of HPN from the health service perspective and ignore patient costs.

Two studies examined costs and benefits as part of a cost–utility analysis. The marginal cost per QALY varied from $14 600 Canadian dollars in 1986 to UK £69 000 in 1995. This compares with a marginal cost per QALY of UK £190 000 for hospital TPN. A cost utility analysis of HPN in Toronto was based on utility scores measured in 37 patients and estimated for a further 36.[11] The net savings in healthcare costs were reported as Can. $19 232 per patient treated at home rather than repeated hospital admission. The cost per QALY was estimated to be Can. $27 375. The quality of life scores obtained were probably over estimated, which means that the true cost per QALY is higher than the figures reported in the study.[28]

The most recent estimate of costs to the UK National Health Service for HPN were UK £45 000 per annum for the first year and UK £36 000 per annum for subsequent years.[23] A significant reduction in costs (65–81% cheaper) can be achieved if care is transferred from the hospital to home.[23–26] The estimated savings for a patient receiving parenteral

nutrition for 4 years, treated at home rather than in hospital are UK £170 506.[23] For each patient on HPN, regular (6-monthly) assessment for compliance, appropriateness of formulation, infusion regimen, intestinal adaptation is required, so that optimally cost-effective care can be provided for each individual.[27]

The quality-adjusted survival for younger patients (< 44 years) is significantly better than for older (> 55) patients.[18] This reduces the marginal cost per QALY. Controversially this suggests that there is more to be gained by concentrating resources on younger patients.

In the USA and Italy, malignant disease is the commonest indication for HPN. If such patients were subjected to a cost–utility analysis, the poor survival figures associated with the expense of HPN treatment would produce very high cost per QALY ratios. This is the largest gap in the current economic literature on HPN.

It should be remembered that QALYs are not without their critics,[29,30] but measuring and valuing the QoL is an extremely difficult process. QALYs attempt to make this process as explicit as possible.[31] 'Marginal cost per QALY gained' league tables have been constructed in order to compare different healthcare interventions. When HPN treatment is compared with home haemodialysis it appears that HPN is much less cost-effective (UK £69 000 per QALY compared with UK £23 500). However, intestinal function recovers in approximately 75% of Crohn's patients and HPN becomes more competitive due to a fall in costs and an

Table 28.2 – Results of economic evaluations of HPN. Evidence of cost-effectiveness

Study	Year	Country	Perspective	Methodology	Findings (costs are given as reported and are not adjusted to current values)	Sensitivity analysis	% difference between hospital PN and HPN
Baptista RJ, 1984[27]	1984	USA	Health service	Cost analysis	Regular assessment of all aspects of patient care can result in significant fiscal savings	–	–
Bisset WM, 1992[37]	1992	UK	Health service	Cost analysis	HPN solutions, pump and consumables cost UK £23–30 000 per year	–	–
Dzierba SH, 1984[25]	1982–1983	USA	Health service	Cost analysis	Hospital PN more expensive than HPN. Can. $32 850 per year for HPN, Approx Can. $57 000 for hospital PN	–	72
Wateska LP, 1980[24]	1980	USA	Health service	Cost analysis	First year cost of HPN Can. $21 465, thereafter Can. $19 700 per year. Hospital PN costs Can. $73 720	–	73
Wesley JR, 1983[26]	1983	USA	Health service	Cost analysis	Can. $33–36 000 per year for HPN, Can. $182 000 for hospital PN	–	81
Richards DM, 1995[23]	1995	UK	Health service	Cost–utility analysis	First year cost of HPN = UK £44 288. The marginal cost per QALY was UK £69 000. One year of hospital PN costs UK £93 000	Sensitive to the age of the patient	65
Detsky AS, 1986[11]	1970–1982	Canada	Health service	Cost–utility analysis	Marginal cost per QALY Can. $14 600. Increase of 3.3 years of quality-adjusted survival compared with the alternative of intermittent hospital nutritional support. Cost–utility compares favourably with other healthcare programmes when used for benign diseases	Sensitive to the assumptions made regarding the costs of alternative treatments	–

increase in QALYS. In Oregon, USA, different treatments have been competing for scarce resources with regard to the marginal cost per QALY gained.[32] In the Oregon experiment, decisions on resource allocation were made if treatments could demonstrate good value for money in terms of cost per QALY. This might become a model for prioritization in resource allocation in the UK. It has, however, been argued that older HPN patients may lose out if decisions are made on this basis.

HPN is an expensive technology with a reasonable outcome for younger patients, while cost-effectiveness of HPN is lower for older patients. However, HPN is approximately 75% more cost-effective than keeping patients in hospital. The expense of the treatment is offset by the lifesaving nature of the technology and the possibility of future recovery of intestinal function.

REFERENCES

1. Morris J, Watt A. Assessing quality of life. In: Drummond MF, Maynard A (eds) *Purchasing and Providing Cost-effective Health Care*. Churchill Livingstone: Edinburgh, 1993.

2. Calman KC. Definition and dimension of quality of life. In: Aaronson NK. Beckmann J (eds) *The Quality of Life of Cancer Patients*. Raven Press: New York, 1987.

3. Aaronson NK. Quality of life. What is it, how should it be measured? *Oncology* 1988; **2**: 69–74.

4. Orchard C. Comparing health care outcomes. *Br Med J* 1994; **308**: 1493–1496.

5. Ware J. *SF 36 Health Survey, Manual and Interpretation Guide*. Medical Outcomes Trust: Boston, 1993.

6. EuroQoL Group. EuroQol – a new facility for the measurement of health related quality of life. *Health Policy* 1990; **16**: 199–208.

7. Kind P. Personal communication 1996.

8. Drummond MF. *Principles of Economic Appraisal in Health Care*. Oxford University Press: Oxford, 1990.

9. Mason JM, Drummond MF. Cost-effectiveness league tables and priority setting. In: Drummond MF, Maynard A (eds) *Purchasing and Providing Cost-effective Health Care*. Churchill Livingstone: Edinburgh, 1993.

10. Price BS, Levine EL. Permanent TPN, psychological and social responses to the early stages. *J Parenter Enteral Nutr* 1979; **3**: 49–52.

11. Detsky AS, McLaughlin JR, Abrams HB, L'Abbe KA, Whitwell J, Bombardier C, Jeejeebhoy KN. Quality of life of patients on long term total parenteral nutrition at home. *J Gen Intern Med* 1986; **1**: 26–33.

12. Herfindal ET, Bernstein LR, Kudzia K, Wong A. Survey of home nutritional support patients. *J Parenter Enteral Nutr* 1989; **13**: 255–261.

13. O'Hanrahan T, Irving MH. The role of HPN in the management of intestinal failure; report of 400 cases. *Clin Nutr* 1992; **11**: 331–336.

14. Ladefoged K. Quality of life in patients on home parenteral nutrition. *J Parenter Enteral Nutr* 1981; **5**: 132–137.

15. Robinovitch AE. HPN: a psycho-social viewpoint. *J Parenter Enteral Nutr* 1981; **5**: 522–525.

16. Burnes JU, Q'Keefe SJD, Fleming CR. Home parenteral nutrition: a 3-year analysis of clinical and laboratory monitoring. *J Parenter Enteral Nutr* 1992; **16**: 327–332.

17. Richards DM, Irving MH. Assessing the quality of life of patients with intestinal failure on home parenteral nutrition. *Gut* 1997; **40**(2): 218–222.

18. Carlson GL, Maguire G, Williams N, Bradley A, Shaffer J, Irving MH. Quality of life on home parenteral nutrition and attitudes towards intestinal transplantation. A single centre study of 37 patients. *Clin Nutr* 1995; **14**: 219–228.

19. Williams N, Carlson GL, Scott NA, Irving MH. Incidence and management of catheter related sepsis in patients receiving home parenteral nutrition. *Br J Surg* 1994; **81**: 392–394.

20. Richards DM, Scott NA, Shaffer JL, Irving MH. Narcotic addiction on home parenteral nutrition. *J Parenter Enteral Nutr* 1997 (in press).

21. Galandiuk S, O'Neill M, McDonald P, Fazio VW, Steiger E. A century of HPN for Crohn's disease. *Am J Surg* 1990; **159**: 540–545.

22. Messing B, Landais P, Goldfarb B, Irving MH. Home parenteral nutrition in adults: a multicentre survey in Europe. *Clin Nutr* 1989; **8**: 3–9.

23. Richards DM, Irving MH. A Cost–utility analysis of home parenteral nutrition. *Br J Surg* 1996; **83**: 1226–1229.

24. Wateska LP, Sattler LL, Steiger E. Cost of a HPN programme. *JAMA* 1980; **244**: 2303–2304.

25. Dzierba SH, Mirtallo JM, Grauer DW, Schnieder PJ, Latolais CJ, Fabri PJ. Fiscal and clinical evaluation of HPN. *Am J Hosp Pharm* 1984; **41**: 285–291.

26. Wesley JR. Home parenteral nutrition. Indications principles and cost-effectiveness. *Compr Ther* 1983; **9**: 29–36.

27. Baptista RJ, Lahey MA, Bistrian BR, Champagne CD, Miller DG, Kelley SE, Blackburn GL. Periodic reassessment for improved, cost-effective care in HPN: a case report. *J Parenter Enteral Nutr* 1984; **8**: 708–710.

28. Detsky A. Evaluating a mature technology, long-term HPN. *Gastroenterology* 1995; **108**: 129–131.

29. Harris J. OALYfying the value of life. *J Med Ethics* 1987; **13**: 117–123.

30. Rawles J. Castigating QALYS. *J Med Ethics* 1989; **15**: 143–147.

31. Mooney G. QALYS: are they enough? A health economists perspective. *J Med Ethics* 1989; **15**: 148–152.

32. Strosberg MA, Weiner JM, Baker R, Fein IA (eds). *Rationing Americas Healthcare: the Oregon plan and beyond.* Brookings Institute: Washington, DC, 1992.

33. Duclaux IL, DePotter S, Pharaon I, Olives JP, Hermier M. Qualite de vie des enfants en nutrition parenterale a domicile et de leurs parents. *Pediatrie* 1993; **718**: 555–560.

34. King LA, Carson LF, Konstantinides N, *et al.* Outcome assessment of HPN in patients with gynecologic malignancies: what have we learned in a decade of experience? *Gynecol Oncol* 1993; **51**: 377–382.

35. Pironi L, Miglioli M, Ruggeri E, *et al.* Home parenteral nutrition for the management of chronic intestinal failure; a 34 patient-year experience. *Ital J Gastroenterol* 1993; **25**: 411–418.

36. Smith C. Quality of life in long term total parenteral nutrition patients and their family caregivers. *J Parenter Enteral Nutr* 1993; **17**: 501–506.

37. Bisset WM, Stapieford P, Long S, Chamberlain A, Sokel B, Milia PJ. HPN in chronic intestinal failure. *Arch Dis Child* 1992; **67**: 101–114.

29

The patient's perspective

Carolyn Wheatley

*I*ncreasing numbers of patients are now living in their own homes whilst receiving artificial nutrition. For many this will be a welcome relief from long episodes of hospitalization, but for others it may mean a life of intense routine and isolation. Acceptance that life is dependent upon a specialized treatment, aseptic procedures, complex routines and mechanical equipment may be hard to comprehend. Once again the adult is dependent, like a child, and their confidence and trust must be placed in the hands of a highly specialized medical team whose skills will guide them back to a life that should integrate the therapy with their home and personal activities.

Patients are fully aware that home nutritional support will not cure their underlying condition, merely treat it. In the initial stages, and possibly for the duration of their therapy, patients may experience situations and emotions that are out of character. These changes can be hard to explain and are partly due to the psychological effects of both the nutritional support and the underlying illness.

Home parenteral nutrition (HPN) is a relatively new medical treatment, so many patients find themselves living in a society with no understanding of their problems or treatments. The public often regards anyone with a medical problem or receiving treatment as alien and someone to be avoided.

My personal plight to gain appropriate treatment for both my underlying condition and the subsequent disease-related undernutrition highlighted the lack of awareness and resources available within the British National Health Service. As a patient with diminishing strength, I was determined that all my efforts should be channelled into fighting for my life and appropriate care. My anger and frustration took control when I no longer felt in charge of my destiny and an inner strength willed me to carry on. When all attempts to resume a normal life appeared to fail, I felt a tremendous resentment about a world of which I felt no part and which seemed to be passing me by. Frequently I asked 'why can't anyone help me?'

This account relates both to my own experience and to reports I have had from fellow patients. It discusses, from a patient perspective, parenteral nutrition in the hospital and at home. The tables show results of questionnaires relating to both home parenteral and enteral nutrition and were completed by patients and/or carers.[1–3]

CARE IN HOSPITAL

Once the decision has been made, in the patient's best interest, to commence parenteral nutrition, the patient will experience apprehension and fears. They are fully aware that this treatment is only contemplated when all other avenues have been explored. As the patient may previously have had disappointments following treatments that failed, doubts again prevail. The patient will wonder 'can I afford to place my trust in yet another treatment which may not have a positive outcome?'

Weight loss will be a common factor; thus leaving the patient with poor body image in addition to the physical weaknesses this imposes. Watching one's body wasting away, despite all attempts to halt the deterioration, leaves the patient with a low self-esteem, feeling worthless and defeated. In certain circumstances the individual may lapse into a period of denial in the hope that it is not actually happening to them, and this state of mind will adversely influence and affect the outcome of their treatments.

Prior to insertion of venous access device/feeding tube

In order to boost the patient's confidence they need the opportunity to discuss any fears or concerns with the medical team in charge of their care. It is vital that the patient feels part of the decision processes, as the illness and treatments are happening to their body. Verbal communications need to be as normal as possible with no shouting or speaking slowly; while the patient may be undernourished they are not stupid. No two patients will live their lives in the same way, therefore the planning and preparation will vary from one to another. The hopeful end result for each patient must be that they control their treatment within sensible boundaries.

Prior to the insertion of the feeding line, each patient will need and benefit from variable amounts of support, understanding and time to express any concerns. Anxieties expressed should be discussed and systematically worked through to quell any fears. The patient will benefit from time spent familiarizing themself with the equipment that they will handle. This juncture is crucial to the acceptance of what will change their life forever, not only will they have a visual and constant reminder that they are now different, but their state of mind may be altered.

For many the process of inserting the feeding line will be a painless procedure. Depending upon the level of concern the patient is displaying, appropriate anaesthetics should be given to ensure calmness during the procedure. For those who have undergone many surgical procedures during the course of their illness, another procedure, no matter how minor in comparison to other experiences, may cause them distress with haunting memories.

After venous access device/feeding tube insertion

Patients report that shortly after nutritional support has commenced their bodies respond well to the much-needed nourishment. Slowly it becomes apparent that the patient is more attentive and shows a greater ability to concentrate. The patient will be bemused at the delight of those around them when normal responses are recognized, as they were probably unaware that they were lacking. After people had previously tried to tactfully say how terrible you looked, it is a satisfying experience to be told how well you now look. Improved appearance, increased weight and renewed energy enables the patient to actually believe that at last this could be the right treatment and that there is light at the end of the tunnel.

As the patient feels that they are starting to regain control of their life, confidence will return and they will be heartened by their improved appearance. A former dislike to weighing scales may vanish as they are now displaying signs that 'this treatment' is working. With a more positive attitude and a feeling of well-being, it can easily lead the patient into trying to rush the necessary training programme in order to achieve an early discharge from hospital.

A skilled medical team should be able to detect 'expected' emotions, which could easily be masking deep-rooted apprehension at the prospect of self-care in the community with a very highly technical treatment.

Training programme

It is essential that the patient understands the training programme which has been designed for them and appreciates the importance of taking each one step at a time. I had a close relationship with the nutrition nurse, who had a wealth of experience and was the appropriate person to determine my ability to learn the procedures. She became fully conversant with every aspect of my care. She spent much time sitting with me, getting to know me and became my advocate

when I found situations overwhelming or too emotional. I felt safe with her judgements and accepted that I would learn at a pace with which she knew I could cope.

Initially simple tasks, such as correct handling of medical items required to carry out the procedures, should be embarked on. For many, appreciating and understanding the need for good personal hygiene along with the complications that poor aseptic technique may bring, will be a major learning experience. As the patient's well-being improves, then the level of training can be increased until the trainer has complete confidence in their pupil. It may take several attempts, with mistakes along the way, to master the complex procedures, but the correct training is fundamental to the patient's future well-being.

The safe confines of the hospital provide the patient with instant access to advice and support 24 hours a day, which installs a sense of security. The security blanket will be called upon less frequently once confidence and well-being once again prevails.

LIFE AT HOME

When the day arrives for leaving the hospital, most patients have reached the position of being relatively self-sufficient. Going home brings a satisfying feeling, as it is comforting to be back home. Initial excitement can mask fears as previously the therapy has only been performed within the hospital environment. Once at home the realization that normal life must continue for family, relatives and friends may lead to long periods alone at home. The individual may experience loneliness and isolation, as they no longer have everyone's attention. Everyday issues that cause stress to a normal individual may be even harder for the patient to cope with. Many patients cope extremely well with the immense changes that have occurred to them. But these coping mechanisms, which partly depend upon the effects of their underlying condition and its treatment, are not automatic and they take time to develop.

When a patient has frequent admissions to hospital, it is difficult for the carers who in addition to the pressures of visiting are trying to maintain a job and home life.

Feeding

Being part of a normal household may bring unexpected pressures. Accommodating the feeding into other people's lifestyles may at first be a problem. Eating and drinking will be advised for each patient depending upon their situation. Where oral dietary restrictions are necessary, self-control must be steadfast. Eating and drinking are accepted social pastimes and exclusion from these can cause a state of deep depression. Food is everywhere, television commercials, magazines, advertising hoarding, it is also a key component in celebrating any major event.

The common belief that parenteral feeding at home is administered whilst the patient is asleep is not necessarily correct. Each patient will have their own sleeping patterns and may not wish to retire to bed at eight o'clock in the evening just because it is time to commence feeding. For some patients who feed for 12 hours, this may be too long to spend in bed. Their feeding pattern will not be constant and the time for connecting up will fluctuate. As part of the teaching process, the patient should be assured that it will be a natural occurrence for feeding times to vary from those that they have become used to in hospital. My training taught me to rule the treatment, not vice versa, and this philosophy has stayed with me ever since. The therapy should enable the individual, wherever possible, to live life to the full and to meet their personal goals.

Equipment

The patient will have to store the equipment and supplies in the home paying attention to their safety. Visitors to the home may find the ancillary equipment and feeding solutions interesting and wish to explore without realizing the dangers or consequences of misuse. The range of items required depends upon the procedure adopted by the patient's unit and needs to have been carefully planned, as inappropriate equipment will hamper progress.

The parenteral feeding solutions need to be kept within a safe cool temperature range, which necessitate the patient having a fridge. It may be a problem for many patients to find somewhere to keep a large fridge that can store 14–16 feeding bags; thus many fridges are kept in bedrooms, hallways or garages. Visitors to the home may assume that the fridge contains normally household food and drink and may open the door for long periods; however, this action may cause problems, as the temperature of the fridge must be maintained to guarantee the life and quality of the solutions and their contents.

The combined weight of a cumbersome dripstand, volumetric pump and feeding bag can present the individual with unexpected problems in trying to manoeuvre them around the home. For some this means being confined, when feeding, to one level removing the choice of total freedom whilst feeding. Normal households are not designed for hospital equipment to be used within them and various previously unrecognized obstacles will become apparent. The type of floor covering may restrict the movement of the equipment, for carpets do not allow the wheels of a dripstand to rotate freely. Thus the stand may become unstable and unbalanced causing sudden jerking or even tipping over of the equipment. This can cause the feeding-line to be pulled and thus become misplaced. In most homes, even bungalows or flats, there are likely to be some stairs, which can present a major task to negotiate without assistance. If the dripstand is tall, it may need to be angled in order to climb stairs, this may result in the feeding bag swinging freely leading to its attachment becoming weak and breaking. Patients tend to bump equipment down stairs and the vibrations from this may dislodge hooks, handles or loosen grips on pumps.

Any incident that causes concern to the patient will start to reduce their confidence. If the patient has a young family or leads an active lifestyle, incorporating the feeding into everyone else's life may take time.

Deliveries

It is essential that the patient has a reliable service that will minimize stress by delivering complete supplies at the time stated in accordance with the patient's needs. The initial stock items should be sufficient for 4–6 weeks. The chosen homecare provider will make regular deliveries and it is not uncommon for the delivery person to become a vital link for the patient. Having a good relationship with the homecare provider will be reassuring for the patient. However, the patient will have high expectations and these should be met and reviewed on a regular basis. Correct and appropriate stock levels will ensure that the home does not resemble a storeroom or warehouse. Certain items used will come in small boxes, others in larger ones – finding homes for them may mean using every inch of storage space. The equipment must be easily accessible in addition to being safe.

Hospital follow–up

If it is necessary for frequent admissions into hospital, the need to make arrangements for the family as well as trying to focus on the cause for the admission will result in additional stresses. If there are children, this can have a lasting effect on the patient, which will surface each time an admission is necessary.

For many patients a large proportion of their energy is channelled into maintaining an image of expected well-being. It becomes a natural part of being ill to put on a façade when beneath the surface the feelings are not so positive. The patient has quickly learnt the skills of each member of their team and adopts their roles at regular intervals. Self-diagnosis is common and they will endeavour to resolve a situation before accepting that it is time to bring in the professionals.

Continual support must be given to the patient and they must feel secure in the knowledge that advice is available 24 hours a day just as it was in the hospital. Contact numbers must be given, but more importantly they should be checked regularly or provide clear and precise instruction to gain access to a person able to provide support. The nurse is generally the team member that the patient turns to in a crisis, therefore their availability and accessibility is paramount to the patient's sense of security.

Unfortunately many of the problems faced by patients at home appear to occur late in the evening or at weekends. Most patients prefer to deal with their own team members who have knowledge and an understanding about the individual which eliminates the need to go over old ground before any help can be offered. Hopefully the unit supervising the care will have someone known to the patient on call all the time. Good training by the hospital team will have made the patient aware of all the hazards and complications that can occur. It is easy to know how to cope with them, but when it is for real, the patient is vulnerable and scared, being aware of the consequences if they make the wrong response.

Large units with specialized knowledge in intestinal failure care for many patients receiving home parenteral nutrition, this may pose problems as the distance between home and the hospital may be considerable. However, this does not deter many patients and they elect to stay under their care despite the distance involved. For some a shared care policy can add a reassuring back up for unexpected events.

Relationships

The introduction of parenteral nutrition into a family unit may have profound effects. Couples may experience added pressures that may weaken what was previously a solid relationship. Time and understanding can ease people through these hard times and it often helps to discuss these emotions with either the hospital team or other patients. Altered body image may inhibit both parties and only care and understanding will ease them through this period of insecurity. It is assumed that there are fewer psychosocial and sexual problems with an implanted intravenous access device rather than an external segment catheter;[4] however, this will vary from patient to patient.

An established relationship will learn how to cope with any obstacles. It is true that the real character and nature of the patient lies within, and is not just what the eye can see. Single patients often find it extremely difficult to be accepted socially. Forging friendships, which may lead to sexual contact, may bring extreme apprehension, but the patient learns where to place their trust and with whom. Self-confidence can be easily knocked when constant rejections are made, the treatment becomes the obvious obstacle, which can lead to diminished enthusiasm for trying again.

WORK AND HOLIDAYS

It can take several weeks if not months before life returns to normal. As time passes the patient may feel confident enough to venture into thinking about returning to work or taking a holiday. These two major events in anyone's life are even more of a feat when parenteral nutrition is included.

Work

Depending upon the circumstances and carer of the patient prior to treatment, it may be possible for them to return to work. For many it will be difficult enough coping with family life.

The prospect of finding a suitable job, which will cater for an individual requiring feeding, may be a daunting task. Hospital appointments along with the uncertainty of being well can greatly reduce anyone's chance of finding employment, and may also be restricted by a lack of non-feeding time to attend. The patient who has a portable feeding system (a rucksack-type bag containing the pump, battery and feed) may gain better opportunities. This system allows greater freedom, but the cost often means that it is not available to everyone.

Patients who have no work experience will find it difficult to acquire. Potential employers may be drawn to asking more questions than normal when there are

Table 29.1 – Results of a postal survey formulated and sent by LITRE to 320 members of PINNT in 1995. The questionnaire asked about venous access device/feeding tube, infusion pumps and stands, the home delivery service and holiday arrangements; 187 (58%) responded

Types of devices used for home nutritional support
Parenteral venous access device (*n* = 116 (24 children))

	%
Hickman–type line	84
Implanted port	13
Unknown	13

Enteral feeding tube (*n* = 71 (38 children))

	%
Nasogastric tube	38★
Gastrostomy	58
Jejunostomy	4

★ 40% passed a tube each night

Types and opinions about pumps	Parenteral (%)	Enteral (%)
Stationary pump	93	42
Ambulatory pump	7	58
Reliable	83	82
Easy to use	95	93
Good alarm system	94	73
Not regularly serviced	74	65
Repaired	51	30
Pump lights very bright	66	56

Transportation of equipment	Parenteral (%)	Enteral (%)
Easy to move		
Pump	29	59
Infusion stand	24	34

Kept awake at night by	Parenteral (%)	Enteral (%)
Pump lights	51	7
Pump noise	46	4
Pump lights and noise	15	–
Pump lights and/or noise	84	–

Delivery service	Parenteral (%)	Enteral (%)
Home delivery service	90	51
Supplies		
On time	90	81
Always complete	79	72
Clinical waste collection	39	21

Holidays	Parenteral (%)	Enteral (%)
One or more holidays	78	80
Travelled outside UK	30	21
Apprehensive about taking a holiday	66	68
Reason for apprehension		
Transportation of feed and equipment	31	45
Illness or dehydration	10	31

large gaps in employment records. Those determined to find employment have been successful, the knocks strengthen their desire and they usually achieve their goal.

Holidays

Planning a holiday requires close attention to detail and it is essential to try and foresee any problems and be prepared for them in advance. Selecting a safe destination, transporting the equipment and ancillaries can present obstacles that need to be overcome. Holiday accommodation has a large turnover and trying to ensure the use of a fridge that is clean, accessible and reliable can be a major task. It is advisable to consider the temperature of the resort for the duration of the stay, if very hot, dehydration can easily occur. Transporting the necessary equipment through the strict airport security can increase stress along with unforeseen delays. All equipment and feeds can safely pass through airport X-ray machines. Inadequate preparation can lead to company refusals, unexpected excessive baggage charges, difficulties in obtaining holiday insurance, or pumps that will not operate on a foreign voltage. Homecare providers can provide assistance with arranging holidays and should be consulted in advance. Their assistance can relieve some worries. It may be possible for them to deliver ancillary equipment and feeding bags to the holiday destination.

Caution is the key when travelling, never forgetting the basic principles that have been taught. Parenteral nutrition feeding bags have been transported all over the world.

SUPPORT GROUPS

A support group for patients on home artificial feeding, PINNT (Patients on Intravenous and Naso-gastric Nutrition Therapy), was established in the UK in 1987 to provide patients at home with a network of support and mutual understanding. Almost all problems experienced by a new patient have been encountered and resolved by a previous patient. It is reassuring to know that there are others in similar situations who can frequently offer support. Advice and assistance is tailored to the needs of patients, family and carers. There is a regular newsletter along with holiday guidelines and benefit advice. Their experiences have helped new patients to cope and adapt to a new life with renewed spirit. Many patients feel more able to discuss concerns with people outside of their family and close friends. All medical matters are referred back to the patient's medical team.

Another multidisciplinary group called LITRE (Looking Into The Requirements for Equipment) was established in UK in 1991 and it was from a postal questionnaire that Tables 29.1 and 29.2 are derived. They have highlighted some important problems, e.g. that pumps and infusion stands are generally heavy and difficult to move around, that the bright light displays and noise of parenteral pumps stop patients sleeping at night. Few patients have their pumps serviced regularly and few have a specific clinical waste collection.

CONCLUSIONS

Since the first patient survey in 1993[5] much work has been done to appreciate and recognize the needs of those people who require HPN. The voice of those on the receiving end is listened to in forums such as the British Association for Parenteral and Enteral Nutrition (BAPEN) where patient opinion is helping to shape future practice. The clear guidelines for the provision of nutrient fluids and equipment[6] were written after patient consultation.

HPN has provided the opportunity for people to live in their own homes where they are surrounded by familiar faces and objects. For most, it has brought the individual back from the depths of illness, but not provided a cure. All age groups, who receive parenteral nutrition at home, have achieved much. We all develop an inner strength that enables us to conquer each hurdle as it approaches. Life presents its ups and downs and we continually endeavour to overcome each of them in our own unique way.

Patients constantly face the problem of projecting a positive and healthy exterior with no visible signs of the pain and suffering they may be experiencing from their underlying condition. HPN has enabled patients to manage this, along with their lives to an acceptable standard. The permanent links with hospitals and healthcare professionals are accepted as part of their normal life and the patient becomes an active member of any healthcare team. Their continued support in addition to that of the homecare provider, partners, friends and family is essential to maintain the status quo and it is important for them to remember that each patient is an individual who must be treated accordingly. HPN does provide the desired outcome and provides patients with the opportunity to achieve their goals, enjoy a fulfilled life and feel a worthwhile member of society.

Table 29.2 – Information about gastrostomy tubes derived from a questionnaire of 65 questions that was distributed by dietitians and PINNT to 153 patients at home. There was a 59% response rate. The age of the patients varied from less than 2 to over 85 years old

Diagnosis	(%)
Cancer	22
Stroke	19
Multiple sclerosis	16
Motor neurone disease	14
Cystic fibrosis	14
Head injury	10
Other	5
Type of gastrostomy	**(%)**
PEG	69
Button	17
Foley catheter	14
Times of feeding	**(%)**
Daytime	35
Overnight	27
Day and night	17
Bolus during the day, drip at night	21
Information about patient use of gastrostomy tubes	**(%)**
Preferred it to naso-gastric feeding	93
Tube is comfortable	88
Fed for more than a year	24
Exit site bleeds a lot	20
Currently sore and painful	38
Treated with antibiotics for exit site infection	41
Problems with leakage	18
Loose stools	26
Felt left out at family meal times	51

REFERENCES

1. Carter D, Wheatley C, Martin R, *et al*. Nights of bright lights and noisy pumps – home parenteral feeding. *Proc Nutr Soc* 1996; **55**: 149A.

2. Porrett C, Carter D, Wheatley C, *et al*. Pumps and stands limit mobility, but sleep is uninterrupted – home enteral feeding. *Proc Nutr Soc* 1996; **55**: 189A.

3. Micklewright A, Carter D, McHattie G, *et al*. Gastrostomy feeding – a consumer survey by the LITRE working party. *Proc Nutr Soc* 1996; **55**: 203A.

4. Magnay S, Wheatley C, Wood S, Forbes A. Comparison of implanted ports with Broviac/Hickman-style tunnelled catheters for long-term home parenteral nutrition: the patient's view. *Proc Nutr Soc* 1995; **54**: 103A.

5. Carter DM, Wheatley C, Payne-James JJ, Pick A. Home nutrition survey in the UK: the patient's perspective. *Clin Nutr* 1993; **12**: 208–212.

6. Wood S (ed), Shaffer J, Wheatley C. *Home Parenteral Nutrition: Quality Criteria for Clinical Services and the Supply of Nutrient Fluids and Equipment*. BAPEN: London, 1995.

30

An intestinal failure unit

Miles Irving

The recognition of intestinal failure as a separate clinical entity has been slow to emerge compared with other organ/system failures. Nevertheless, it is now widely accepted as a distinct clinical entity and criteria for quality treatment are established and continuing to develop. As with other organ/system failures, single, early, uncomplicated intestinal failure can adequately be treated at district hospital (DGH) level, whereas severe and complicated cases associated with other organ/system failures are best referred to specialized units. Ideally there should be some degree of concentration and management of intestinal failure at DGH level.

Using the broad definition and classification of intestinal failure proposed in this book or the classical definition for relatively severe intestinal failure proposed by Fleming and Remington ('the reduction of functioning gut mass below the level necessary for digestion and absorption of nutrients')[1] (see Introduction), a logical way forward to provide the services for intestinal failure can be planned. It is apparent that intestinal failure can be total or partial and temporary (acute) or permanent (chronic). Management of partial and/or acute intestinal failure would be the category normally regarded as being within the scope of a DGH, whereas management of chronic/permanent intestinal failure would normally be the province of a specialized unit.

Thus acute intestinal failure, caused by postoperative ileus or obstruction, even when prolonged, can normally be successfully managed by either peripheral or central parenteral nutrition in the general wards of a DGH in the confident expectation that spontaneous resolution will occur in a matter of days up to a few weeks. Similarly DGH medical and surgical gastroenterologists with experienced nursing support can effectively handle intestinal failure caused by resection of up to two-thirds of the small intestine until adaptation occurs. However, the skills to cope with the much rarer problems of multiple fistulae, total small bowel resection, chronic intestinal obstruction, visceral myopathy, extensive radiation enteritis and total or near-total small bowel resection are likely only to be found in a specialized unit.

PRINCIPLES OF MANAGEMENT OF INTESTINAL FAILURE

The principles of management of intestinal failure are as follows:

- Recognize the presence of intestinal failure
- Establish appropriate fluid/nutritional support
- Investigate and identify the cause and nature of the underlying problem
- Eliminate compounding conditions such as sepsis
- Identify a long-term management plan
- Maintain treatment until the condition resolves or reveals itself as chronic.

These principles apply whether one is managing the intestinal failure patient in a DGH or in a specialized unit.

MANAGEMENT IN A DISTRICT GENERAL HOSPITAL

Whilst most gastrointestinal surgeons and physicians are familiar with the principles of management of intestinal failure, difficulties can arise from the associated technicalities, particularly the parenteral feeding lines. Although the rules for maintaining infection-free lines are well described, they are often broken unless they are under the control of nurses trained in their application. For this reason every DGH should have a multi-disciplinary nutrition team that will manage the nutritional support process wherever it is required in the hospital. Better still, however, is to have a high-dependency area where these patients can be concentrated so that nursing staff may become experienced in the control and management of the lines.

Keeping these patients on intensive care units is inappropriate unless their intestinal failure is accompanied by other organ system failure, and it is deleterious to patient morale and general management. Intensive care units are associated with high levels of infection and do not easily adjust to the regimen of nocturnal feeding that best suits these patients by allowing freedom for movement and exercise during daylight hours.

MANAGEMENT OF A SPECIALIZED UNIT

Specialized units have proved themselves clinically effective but have yet to prove themselves cost-effective. Their clinical effectiveness results from the concentration of experience of these difficult cases in the hands of expert medical practitioners, nurses and other specialities supplementary to medicine.

Running of the unit

As in all surgery-based specialities, the successful management of these patients requires strict discipline and attention to protocols. These features should be combined with a degree of informality and familiarity appropriate to those who have often had a confidence shattering experience prior to referral and who need restoration of both confidence and a degree of control over their treatment.

Successful management depends upon a multi-disciplinary approach. There should be a director of the unit responsible for ensuring unit policies are adhered to and that the administration of the unit is sound and effective. A business manager and a data manager should support the director, as patients generate a vast amount of financial and clinical information over the several months that is often necessary to treat them. There should be a clinical director who would normally be a gastrointestinal surgeon or physician depending upon the emphasis of the unit's work. The intestinal failure unit at Hope Hospital deals primarily with patients who have intestinal fistulae secondary to surgical complications and thus the nutritional and surgical management is directed by a surgeon, with a medical gastroenterologist in support.

As the main management of these difficult cases involves highly skilled multidimensional total nursing the nursing director of the unit should be a nurse practitioner with leadership skills able to establish and implement nursing protocols relevant to the unit's practise and based upon published guidelines.

Nurse/patient ratios will depend upon the unit's profile but will normally be 2:1. Additional staff required are a pharmacist, dietician, biochemist and physiotherapist. Secretarial support is essential to cope with the extensive documentation required for effective management of these patients. Although it may be thought that specialist psychological/counselling support would be required this has not been found to be necessary other than on very rare occasions. The reason for this is that intestinal failure patients are rare and few psychiatrists, psychologists or counsellors will have experience of the problem or understand its management. On the other hand nurses and doctors dealing with this condition on a daily basis soon acquire an understanding of the problems and become expert in giving support at the unusual times of the day or night that it is needed, particularly when the patient has gone home. A patient who has experienced the condition or is currently on treatment will often help a new patient cope with the problems of intestinal failure.

An intestinal failure ward should be bright and cheerful, with a special room equipped for training patients in the administration of intravenous feeding at home. Because patients with intestinal failure often have this single problem in an otherwise healthy body they should be encouraged to get dressed and go out and to take exercise on exercise machines in the ward.

TRAINING PATIENTS FOR HOME PARENTERAL NUTRITION

An intestinal failure unit can commence or take on the whole task of training patients for home enteral or parenteral nutrition. The latter will probably be required when the patient has multiple problems associated with their intestinal failure, which have to be dealt with simultaneously. The training process for home parenteral nutrition (HPN) is commenced as soon as the patient is well enough to concentrate on the techniques involved and can be continued at home, especially when there are commercial company financed nutritional support nurses in the community.

Continuing support for patients at home should be provided by a 24-hour telephone service available from the intestinal failure ward. Similar support should be available for medical practitioners wishing to consult their specialist colleagues on matters of intestinal failure and seek advice and refer patients. Equally, nursing staff in other hospitals faced with complex nursing problems associated with intestinal failure should have a similar degree of telephone advice available to them from their more experienced colleagues in the unit.

OUT-PATIENT SERVICES

The whole team involved in the patient's care should provide out-patient support for this complicated group of patients. This ensures continuity and means that patients do not have to gain familiarity and confidence in a new set of therapists every time they attend for follow-up.

WHEN TO REFER TO A SPECIALIZED UNIT

The threshold for referring a patient to a specialized unit will vary from hospital to hospital. Those with good nutrition teams will probably be able to cope with these patients for longer than those without such teams and appropriate experience. In general, the following cases should be referred to a specialized centre:

1. Persistence of intestinal, failure beyond six weeks without any evidence of resolution and complicated by venous access problems.

2. Multiple intestinal fistulation in a totally dehisced abdominal wound.

3. A third time recurrent intestinal fistula after two unsuccessful attempts to close it surgically.

4. Total or near-total small bowel enterectomy (less than 30 cm of residual small bowel).

5. Recurrent venous access problems in patients needing sustained parenteral nutrition. This definition includes recurrent severe infections and recurrent venous thrombosis where all upper limb and cervical venous access routes have become obliterated.

6. Persistent intra-abdominal sepsis, complicated by severe metabolic problems, characterized by hypo-albuminaemia, not responding to radiological and surgical drainage of sepsis and provision of nutritional support.

7. Metabolic complications relating to high output fistulae and stomas, and to prolonged intravenous feeding, not responsive to medication and adjustment of the feeding regimen. Disorders of hepatic and renal function associated with intravenous nutrition that are resistant to metabolic and nutritional manipulation.

8. End-stage visceral myopathy, not responding to medication, and resulting in continued hospitalization of the patient, and total failure of enteral nutrition.

REFERENCE

1. Fleming CR, Remington M. Intestinal failure. In: Hill GI (ed) *Nutrition and the Surgical Patient. Clinical Surgery International* (2). Churchill Livingstone: Edinburgh, 1981, pp. 219–235.

Section 7

Problems of treatment

31

Enteral nutrition

Hamish D. Duncan and David B. A. Silk

*P*atients who are undernourished[1] or at risk of undernutrition are common within hospitals. The treatment of undernutrition can cause complications, which partly depends on the route of access. While increasing oral energy intake with careful food selection and nutrient drink supplements is simplest, it is not always possible and enteral nutrition (EN) through an enteral tube inserted into the stomach or small bowel may be needed. Access to the gastro-intestinal tract may be either via a nasogastric or naso-enteric tube or by an enterostomy tube. Most short-term tube EN is given via a nasogastric tube.[2] The problems of enteral tube feeding can be divided into: mechanical, metabolic/biochemical and gastro-intestinal (Table 31.1).

Table 31.1 – Complications of enteral tube feeding

Mechanical
Unable to pass a tube
Misplacement
Blockage
Accidental and non-accidental removal
Nasopharyngeal pain, erosions, sinusitis, otitis media
Intracranial insertion
Hoarseness, laryngeal ulceration
Oesophageal erosions, oesophagitis and strictures
Tracheo-oesophageal fistula
Variceal rupture
Duodenal perforation
Pulmonary aspiration

Metabolic/Biochemical
Refeeding syndrome
Deficiency or excess
    Electrolytes
    Glucose
    Vitamins
    Trace elements
    Essential fatty acids
Abnormal liver function tests

Gastrointestinal
Nausea
Bloating
Reflux
Abdominal distention
Constipation
Diarrhoea

MECHANICAL PROBLEMS

Naso-enteric feeding tubes

The complications of naso-enteral feeding tubes are less common since the introduction of fine-bore naso-enteral feeding tubes in the 1970s.[4–6] Fine-bore tubes with a wire stiffener are easier to pass, being more flexible and smaller than Ryles tubes, and are less likely to cause nasopharyngeal or oesophageal erosions, oesophagitis or strictures. Tube blockage, physical complications (e.g. misplacement) and unwanted removal can cause problems.

Tube blockage

Tube blockage may occur if crushed medication is inserted into fine-bore tubes, if the tube is not flushed adequately or if there is precipitation of protein in the enteral feed.[7] It is best to avoid giving crushed medicines through a tube, liquid medicines are preferable and the tube should be flushed before and after giving the medication. Precipitation of enteral feed occurs because the iso-electric point of protein is between pH 4.5 and 5.3, and at this pH, protein precipitates causing tube blockage.[7] Many elixir medications have a pH of 5 or less[8] and thus may cause protein precipitation and tube blockage.

To prevent tube blockage a feeding tube should be flushed with sterile or boiled water at least before and after a feed or medication. A newly designed naso-gastric tube with a modified tapered outflow port reduces incidence of tube blockage compared to standard open-ended feeding tubes.[9] Obstructed tubes may be unblocked with water, a variety of solutions including fizzy drinks, pineapple or cranberry juice, alcohol or powdered pancreatic enzymes (Table 31.2). If enteric-coated pancreatic enzymes are used they need to be dissolved in a sodium bicarbonate solution before being administered (e.g. the contents of one Creon® capsule can be dissolved in 10 ml of 8.4% sodium bicarbonate).

Table 31.2 – Methods used to unblock an enteral feeding tube

Flush with 5 ml syringe of sterile or boiled water
Fizzy drinks or sodium bicarbonate solution
Pineapple or cranberry juice
Alcohol
Powdered pancreatic enzymes
Milking the tube like a drainage tube
Guidewire insertion★

To put solutions into the tube requires a push/pull technique
★ Not to be used with naso-enteric tubes due to risk of causing a perforation.

Physical complications

Physical complications of naso-enteric tubes may be due to the size, material and pliability of the tube used. Polyurethane naso-enteric feeding tubes are preferable to polyvinylchloride naso-enteric feeding tubes, as they are softer, less traumatic and easier to aspirate the gastric contents.[5,6] Intubation with a naso-enteric tube can cause discomfort for patients, and depends to some extent on the type and size of tube used. In general the larger the tube the greater the discomfort. We have observed that a nasogastric tube with a smooth tip causes less discomfort and is easier to insert than a standard tube.[9]

Although many problems are less common with the softer, more flexible fine-bore tubes, complications due to the physical presence of the feeding tube can occur. Nasopharyngeal discomfort persisting after intubation may be due to a reduced saliva production, due to mouth breathing and absence of chewing. Patients can develop a sore mouth, difficulty with swallowing, a sensation of thirst and dry mucous membranes. Simple measures such as mouthwashes, sucking ice cubes or using artificial saliva may help alleviate discomfort. Nasal erosions and occasionally an abscess can occur from pressure of the naso-enteric tube on the nasal alae. If the sinus tracts or Eustachian tubes are blocked by the naso-enteric tube, acute sinusitis or secondary otitis media infection respectively may occur. Both of these are less likely if a fine-bore tube is used.[5] The mucous membranes of the larynx can be irritated causing hoarseness. Accidental intracranial insertion of a feeding tube has been reported,[10] and may be less likely if a soft pliable tube is carefully inserted. Most modern fine-bore tubes are stiffened with a wire to aid passage of the tube, and it is important to be aware of this potentially fatal complication.

Gastro-oesophageal reflux occurs more frequently when a naso-enteric tube is used, particularly when the patient is in the supine position.[11] Nagler and Spiro[11] proposed that this is partly due to the patient lying flat, so losing the benefit of gravity in maintaining the gastric contents and partly due to the presence of a naso-enteric feeding tube which may impede the effectiveness of the gastro-oesophageal sphincter. Impedance of the gastro-oesophageal sphincter is likely to be less with small fine-bore feeding tubes. Nonetheless, it is still preferable not to feed patients lying flat, and the head of the bed should be raised to over 30°. If oesophagitis remains a problem despite using a fine-bore feeding tube, then treatment with H₂-receptor antagonists, proton pump inhibitors, cisapride or sucralfate may be used.

Excessive pressure against the oesophageal wall may cause ulceration with subsequent stenosis. The risk of oesophageal ulceration is increased in the presence of severe gastro-oesophageal reflux and oesophagitis. Modern fine-bore feeding tubes are less rigid and likely to exert less pressure against the oesophageal wall, and coupled with a reduced risk of gastro-oesophageal reflux, should make this unlikely to happen. Tracheo-oesophageal fistula may develop when large-bore naso-enteric tubes are used and a nasotracheal or tracheostomy tube is already in place. The fistula develops from pressure necrosis of the oesophagus and trachea. Excessive pressure from stiff, large-bore naso-enteric tubes can result in oesophageal variceal rupture, and although this risk is likely to be reduced with fine-bore tubes,[12] it may still be a complication, when inserting a feeding tube with a wire stiffener. Intestinal perforation with polyvinyl and polypropylene naso-enteric tubes has been reported.[13]

Fine-bore feeding tubes rarely cause any of the physical complications outlined, and in a study of over 800 intubations, these problems were not encountered.[5] Re-insertion of the guidewire with the feeding tube in situ should not be undertaken, as there is a risk of the guidewire inadvertently passing through an outflow port and causing a perforation.

Tube misplacement

Misplacement of the naso-enteric feeding tube into the lungs, with subsequent intrapulmonary infusion of an enteral diet can be fatal if not recognized. Other complications arising from tube misplacement include pneumothorax,[14] intrapleural infusion of enteral diet[15] and oesophageal perforation.[16]

Patients most at risk from tube misplacement include those on ventilators, with a reduced level of consciousness or with neuromuscular abnormalities such as impaired gag, swallow or cough reflexes.[17] If there is doubt regarding tube position in this group of patients, radiological confirmation of tube position should be undertaken before starting enteral feeding. In patients who are alert, verification of tube position can be safely made by aspirating gastric contents and checking for an acidic pH with litmus paper. This test does not work if the patient is taking a proton pump inhibitor. It is not always possible to aspirate gastric contents with fine-bore tubes, and to aid aspiration, the outflow port of some feeding tubes have been modified to improve the success rate of gastric aspiration.[5,6,9] The tube position can additionally be checked by auscultation over the epigastrium during air insufflation, although air insufflation into the pleural space or lung can produce similar sounds. If there is any doubt regarding the position of the feeding tube, a chest or abdominal radiograph should be taken.

Enterostomy tubes

There are alternative methods of feeding into the gastrointestinal tract apart from the nasogastric or nasoduodenal route. Tube enterostomies can be placed by surgical, endoscopic or radiological/ultrasound methods into the gastrointestinal tract. Tube enterostomies can be either temporary or permanent, and are usually placed if it is anticipated that long-term feeding (more than 4 weeks) will be required, or if naso-enteric access is compromised. The problems of tube blockage are treated in the same way as a nasogastric tube though occasionally, before a tube is removed, a guidewire may carefully be passed through a gastrostomy tube and often this will unblock it. A gastrostomy tube can become occluded by the gastric epithelium growing over the tube, this necessitates another tube being inserted and the remaining tube either cut short and left in situ or if infected being surgically removed. If a gastrostomy tube is gently rotated each week, this problem should be avoided.

Physical complications

Surgical enterostomy Adjunctive tube enterostomy is usually placed at the time of surgery, when it is expected that postoperative nutrient intake will be delayed. Primary surgical tube enterostomy is indicated for patients requiring long-term nutritional support.

Pharyngostomy Pharyngostomy involves inserting a tube into the oropharynx, and can be used in patients with congenital anomalies or trauma of the maxillofacial area, oro-pharyngeal tumours and following cervical or maxillofacial surgery or radiotherapy for partially obstructing oesophageal tumours. Contraindications include complete oesophageal obstruction, gastric, duodenal or jejunal obstruction or extensive neck tumours. Complications include cellulitis, wound infections, haemorrhage and aspiration pneumonia,[18] as well as mechanical complications including injury and stricture of the oesophagus, irritation of skin and soft tissue, tubal obstruction and accidental removal of the feeding tube.[19]

Surgical gastrostomy Surgical gastrostomy is indicated for patients in whom percutaneous endoscopic gastrostomy cannot be performed, or as adjunctive procedure when the patient is undergoing another surgical operation. Indications include oesophageal atresia, stricture and cancer, dysphagia due to neuromuscular disorders or following trauma. Relative contraindications include primary disease of the stomach, abnormal gastric and duodenal emptying, and significant oesophageal reflux, especially in patients with a poor gag reflex. Complications include local irritation, haemorrhage, skin excoriation from leakage of gastric contents, wound infection, accidental tube removal, tube blockage, aspiration, gastric outlet obstruction (from tube migration), intraperitoneal leakage of gastric contents, wound dehiscence, bleeding, hernia, delayed closure of the stoma, peritonitis and death.[20,21] The morbidity and mortality rate varies from 3 to 61%[21] and up to 37%[23] respectively. This variability in morbidity and mortality is likely to relate in part to the medical and surgical condition of the patient in whom a surgical gastrostomy is being performed. Such patients are often elderly, undernourished and suffering from strokes, cancers or head injury, and many surgical gastrostomies are performed under general anaesthesia, which may add to the potential morbidity.

Surgical jejunostomy Surgical jejunostomies and needle-catheter jejunostomies can be useful procedures when feeding into the stomach is contraindicated, for example following oesophageal, gastric, pancreatic or hepatobiliary surgery. Relative contraindications to their insertion include local Crohn's disease, ascites and coagulopathies. Following the procedure complications include accidental removal of the feeding tube, intraperitoneal leakage, tube blockage and displacement, bowel obstruction and volvulus.[22]

Endoscopic enterostomy

Percutaneous endoscopic gastrostomy (PEG) PEG tube insertion has become increasingly widely accepted.[24] PEGs are relatively simple and easy to insert, have a low morbidity and mortality,[25] avoid the need for a general anaesthetic and are cheaper than surgical gastrostomies.[24] The indication for a PEG is medium- to long-term feeding in a patient who cannot eat or swallow adequately or safely. Such patients include those with neuromuscular diseases (e.g. strokes, motor neurone disease), head and neck cancer or surgery, or oesophageal cancer. Relative contraindications include completely occluding pharyngeal or oesophageal tumour, ascites, peritoneal dialysis and disorders of coagulopathy.[24]

Complications of PEG tubes include peristomal infection, leakage, accidental tube removal, tube blockage, tube fracture, tube displacement and peritonitis, aspiration pneumonia, bleeding, gastric mucosa overgrowth and death.[24–26] If a peristomal abscess is suspected, an ultrasound examination should help confirm the diagnosis. Tube blockage and intraperitoneal leakage can be checked for by a tubogram with sterile water-soluble contrast. Complications such as infection and leakage arising from PEGs can be reduced by using smaller PEG tubes, without any increase risk of tube blockage.[25]

Percutaneous endoscopic gastrojejunostomy (PEGJ) and jejunostomy (PEJ) For patients at risk of oesophageal reflux, the PEG can be converted into a jejunostomy, using one of the commercially available kits, although the risk of aspiration is not completely eliminated.[27] Percutaneous jejunostomies can be placed using a long endoscope in the same way as a PEG, though this may need radiological guidance. Leakage at the entry site is a common problem with these as bile (acting as a soap) makes the tube and its skin fixative likely to become loose.

Radiological/ultrasound placed enterostomy

Tubes can be placed in the stomach or small bowel using a combination of radiological screening and ultrasound. It is helpful, though not essential, to pass a fine-bore tube into the stomach at the start of the insertion procedure to fill the stomach up with air. As the tubes inserted are often pig-tail catheters, leakage is common, or if a balloon-type catheter is used, balloon bursting and displacement may occur.

ASPIRATION

Reflux of feed can occur, particularly with larger bore nasogastric tubes, probably by affecting the integrity of the gastro-oesophageal junction. The development of aspiration pneumonia is a potential complication in all patients being tube fed into the stomach or small bowel. Aspiration of feed can occur without obvious evidence of vomiting, particularly in those patients with poor mental status and absent swallowing reflex. Such regurgitation is often a clinically silent event until signs of pneumonia develop. The incidence of clinically

significant aspiration occurs in up to 30% of patients with tracheotomies or translaryngeal intubation,[28] and 6.5–12.5% in neurological patients.[17] Those at particular risk are the aged, debilitated, demented or those with impaired consciousness and a poor gag reflex. If a large quantity of enteral diet is aspirated, the sudden onset of dyspnoea, cyanosis, tachycardia and hypotension and diffuse shadowing in the lung should not make a diagnosis of aspiration difficult. Small volumes of enteral diet may be aspirated and result in either no symptoms or the patient may develop features of pneumonia. Treatment includes stopping the feed, trying to aspirate as much feed as possible by endotracheal suction and/or bronchoscopy and institution of antibiotics if the patient is febrile.

Reducing the risk of pulmonary aspiration

Continuous pump controlled tube feeding is useful in delivering large volumes of feed reliably and was thought to reduce the likelihood of gastric pooling of feed, with a consequent possible reduction in risk of aspiration. Whether the patient is being fed continuously or by a bolus technique, the risk of aspiration may be reduced by elevating the head of the bed to 30° or more, to help aboral progression of feed by gravity. High osmolality feeds of 560 milli-osmoles or greater can significantly delay gastric emptying,[29] and so it is probably preferable to use iso-osmotic feeds in patients at risk from aspiration. Postpyloric feeding does not necessarily reduce risk of aspiration as nasoduodenal tubes can reflux back into the stomach[30] and may therefore give staff a false sense of security that aspiration will not occur. Pro-motility drugs (e.g. cisapride, metoclopramide or erythromycin) can be tried to reduce the chances of aspiration in those patients most at risk.

The risk of aspiration is greater when feed is administered overnight and since continuous feeding often means feeding over a 20- to 24-hour period, the risk may be greater in continuously fed patients.[31] Thus, the risk of aspiration may be reduced by reducing the amount of time that the feed runs at night. Pulmonary infections may occur subsequent to aspiration of gastric contents or from ascending contamination of the oropharynx.[32,33] This risk may be increased with continuous enteral tube feeding, as such a method of feeding results in a raised pH of gastric contents,[31,32,34,35] which may prevent the bactericidal effect of a low pH. This problem could be exacerbated by the high rate of bacterial colonization of enteral feed when fed continuously.[32] The incidence of pneumonic complications associated with continuous enteral feeding is reduced by changing to an intermittent regimen.[36]

METABOLIC/BIOCHEMICAL PROBLEMS

Metabolic problems include a deficiency or excess of variety of electrolytes, vitamins, trace elements and water,[37,38] which can usually be avoided by careful monitoring. Basic haematological and biochemical parameters are measured before starting nutritional support. Urea, creatinine, sodium, liver function, magnesium, calcium, potassium, phosphate and glucose are initially monitored frequently as fluctuations are common.[39] Patients on long-term EN may require vitamin and trace element analysis if clinically indicated.

Refeeding syndrome

Patients receiving artificial nutrition support should be monitored closely because of the risk of developing refeeding syndrome.[2]

Refeeding undernourished patients increases basal metabolic rate, with glucose being the predominant energy source.[39] This anabolic response causes intracellular movement of minerals, and serum levels may fall significantly. These rapid changes in metabolism and electrolyte movement may lead to severe cardiorespiratory and neurological problems resulting in cardiac and respiratory failure, oedema, lethargy, confusion, coma, convulsions and death.[39] These symptoms of the refeeding syndrome are thought to be due predominantly to hypophosphataemia, but hypokalaemia, hypomagnesaemia, hypocalcaemia, hypoglycaemia and thiamine deficiency can also contribute.[39] Intracellular fluid increases, and extracellular fluid may decrease or increase depending on the refeeding regimen and previous fluid intake.[39] Refeeding may cause extracellular fluid retention, due to refeeding with carbohydrates, resulting in marked sodium and water retention.[40] Thiamine deficiency may contribute to refeeding syndrome, with Wernicke's encephalopathy being precipitated by carbohydrate administration. Patients at high risk from the refeeding syndrome include those with chronic undernutrition, chronic alcoholics, prolonged fasting and those only given intravenous hydration.

To try and prevent the development of the refeeding syndrome, our policy on initiating feeding is to

measure urea and electrolytes daily with frequent monitoring of glucose (BM stix). Phosphate, magnesium, calcium and liver function tests are performed twice weekly, haematology weekly. Daily weight and fluid charts are recorded. The frequency of biochemical monitoring is adjusted according to the patients' clinical and metabolic status.

Hydration/hyper/hyponatraemia

Over-hydration may develop in up to 25% of tube fed patients,[38] with hypertonic dehydration being a complication in 5–10% of patients.[38,41] Hypertonic dehydration can occur secondary to the use of high osmolarity feeds, or high protein feeds, when the patient does not have access to, or is unable to ingest water.[41]

Hyponatraemia is usually due to a dilutional state from excessive use of intravenous dextrose.[38] Hypernatraemia may be due to water loss, and in neurosurgical patients from an inability to conserve water secondary to transient diabetes insipidus.[38]

Sodium loss is a major problem for patients with a short bowel and no colon. As jejunal mucosa is 'leaky' and unable to concentrate its contents, sodium absorption in the upper jejunum can only take place when the luminal sodium content is more than 90 mmol/L. If the concentration is less than this secretion rather than absorption of sodium will occur.[42] Maximal sodium absorption occurs at a sodium concentration of around 120 mmol/L, and is enhanced in the presence of glucose or amino acids.[42] Patients with a jejunostomy or high output fistula need sodium chloride added to their feeds.

Hyper- and hypoglycaemia

Rebound hypoglycaemia may rarely develop if nutrition is stopped abruptly following a high glucose load due to a relative excess of insulin, and may result in confusion, coma, convulsions and death. Rapid infusion of high carbohydrate enteral formulas can cause hyperglycaemia, particularly if the patient develops an intercurrent illness, which may cause a relative insulin resistance.[37] If hyperglycaemia remains uncontrolled, dehydration, coma, acidosis and death may result.

Potassium

Glucose uptake by muscle and fat induced by insulin facilitates the intracellular movement of potassium. Hypokalaemia may develop if anabolic requirements exceed potassium supplied.[40] Hypokalaemia occurs in up to 10% of malnourished patients, and may develop secondary to diuretics or insulin,[38] but is not usually a particular problem in patients with a short bowel.[42] Hypokalaemia can result in muscle weakness, confusion, coma, convulsions, lethargy and cardiac arrhythmias. If potassium fails to rise in patients with a short bowel and no colon, it is likely that the patient is either sodium-depleted with secondary hyperaldosteronism or magnesium-depleted.[43] These need to be treated before the potassium level can rise.

Hyperkalaemia is an uncommon complication of refeeding but may occur secondary to metabolic acidosis or renal disease[38,40] and can result in cardiac arrest.

Phosphate

Insulin-induced uptake of phosphate by cells in the presence of glucose during refeeding can cause hypophosphataemia.[40] Chronic alcoholics are often phosphate depleted and are at risk of developing refeeding hypophosphataemia. Although the risk of hypophosphataemia is greater with parenteral rather than enteral feeding, regular monitoring particularly during the early stages of enteral refeeding is still required. Hypophosphataemia can cause muscle weakness, confusion, paraesthesia, coma, convulsions, haemolytic anaemia, cardiac arrhythmias, rhabdomyolysis and respiratory depression.[40] Treatment is provided in the form of effervescent phosphate tablets (each containing 16.1 mmol), or initially intravenously if oral supplements are inadequate.

Magnesium

Patients at risk of hypomagnesaemia include those with severe undernutrition, on diuretics or with a short bowel. Magnesium deficiency is common in patients with a short bowel and a jejunostomy, and less common if the colon remains.[42] Hypomagnesaemia is often accompanied by hypocalcaemia and hypokalaemia.[43] Symptoms of hypomagnesaemia include anorexia, nausea, depression, irritability, tremors and paraesthesia; signs include hyper-reflexia and rarely tetany.[40] Treatment can be provided in the form of two to six magnesium oxide capsules (each containing 4 mmol), or intravenously initially if oral supplements are inadequate.

Calcium

Hypocalcaemia can develop secondary to magnesium deficiency.[43] Magnesium may need to be corrected before the hypocalcaemia improves. Hypocalcaemia can cause tetany and convulsions. Vitamin D is reasonably well absorbed even in short bowel, but if required vitamin D_2 (400–900 IU daily) can be administered.[42]

Liver function tests

Abnormalities of liver function tests, which are thought to be due to activation of hepatic enzymes by the influx of nutrients, may develop.[44] However, this may also result from the excessive storage of fat and glycogen in the liver as a result of persistently elevated insulin levels arising from continuous enteral tube feeding.[45,46] It is not always necessary to stop feeding, and unless severely abnormal we continue to feed with several hours break each day, which usually resolves the problem.

Vitamins and trace elements

Commercially produced polymeric enteral feeds contain adequate amounts of vitamins and trace elements. Supplementation may be required for some patients with severe malabsorption or specific deficiencies. Supplements of water-soluble vitamins including vitamin C and B complex are not usually required even in short bowel patients.[42] Parenteral vitamin B_{12} injections will be required in patients who have had a terminal ileal resection. Deficiency of fat-soluble vitamins A and E are uncommon, and seen only after several years of malabsorption.[42] Some enteral diets contain large amounts of vitamin K, which may reduce the effect of warfarin anticoagulation, thus the International Normalized Ratio (INR) may need to be checked more frequently. If clinically indicated, levels of zinc, copper, selenium, manganese, chromium and molybdenum can be quantified. Zinc sulphate capsules can be prescribed if zinc deficiency develops.

Gastrointestinal problems

The most common complications of enteral tube feeding are those related directly to the gastrointestinal tract.[37,47–49] Nausea can occur in 10–20% of patients,[47,50] with the pathogenesis thought to be multifactorial including smell,[51] diet osmolality,[29,52] altered gastric emptying,[29,52] too rapid infusion of feed[52] and psychological factors.[51]

There is little evidence that rapid bolus intragastric tube feeding causes significant gastrointestinal symptoms such as nausea, bloating or abdominal cramps.[52,53] Abdominal bloating and cramps may be due to delayed gastric emptying[29,52] and lactose intolerance,[54] although most modern commercial enteral tube feeds are now clinically lactose free.

Constipation, with resulting overflow diarrhoea, can be a problem with enteral feeding,[55] and it has been suggested that this is due to a lack of dietary fibre in many enteral feeds. There is currently, however, little conclusive evidence that using fibre-enriched enteral feeds increase stool frequency and weight.[55–58] The lack of improvement in constipation by adding fibre to enteral diets may be partly due to the manufacturing process which alters the physicochemical properties of the added fibre.[59] The viscosity of the feed is kept low by using fine rather than coarse fibre, however this reduces the water holding and bulking properties of the feed.[60] Furthermore, due to the requirement of having a small particle size renders the fibre highly fermentable, reducing the amount of fibre available to bulk faeces.[61]

Enteral tube feeding–associated diarrhoea

The commonest reported complication of enteral tube feeding is diarrhoea, which occurs in up to 30% of patients on general medical and surgical wards[47,50,62] and up to 68% of patients on intensive care units.[50,63–65] There is considerable variability in the reported incidence of enteral tube feeding-related diarrhoea, which is due in part to differences in definition of diarrhoea used by different investigators (Table 31.3). Some of these definitions rely on the ability to collect and measure every stool sample, which is often not a feasible proposition in patients who are bed-bound, faecally incontinent or uncooperative, and in females separating urine from the faecal collection can be difficult. As a result of the practical difficulties encountered in trying to collect and measure stool samples accurately, different investigators have tended to use their own definitions of diarrhoea (Table 31.3). This may explain in part the large differences of

Table 31.3 – Definitions of diarrhoea

Definition	Reference
Frequency	
Increased frequency (number of stools unspecified)	Walike and Walike, 1977[54]
> 3 stools/day	Pesola et al., 1989[75]
	Guenter et al., 1991[79]
	Bliss et al., 1992[48]
> 4 stools/day	Gottschlich et al., 1988[86]
Frequency and consistency	
> 2 liquid stools/day	Viall et al., 1990[144]
> 3 liquid stools/day	Kelly et al., 1983[63]
	Cataldi-Betcher et al., 1983[66]
> 4 liquid stools/day	Anderson et al., 1984[106]
Several liquid stools/day	Heymsfield et al., 1988[55]
Consistency	
Subjective assessment	
	Keohane et al., 1984[50]
	Meier et al., 1993[57]
	Jones et al., 1983[47]
	Lampe et al., 1992[58]
Stool weight	
> 300 g/day for 2 days	Brinson and Kolts, 1987[82]
> 250 g/day	Benya et al., 1991[64]
> 200 g/day	Turnberg, 1986[67]
Stool weight and consistency	
> 200 g liquid stool/day	Gottschlich et al., 1988[86]
Stool volume and consistency	
> 500 ml liquid or soft stool/day for 2 days	Edes et al., 1990[65]

reported incidence of diarrhoea ranging from 2.3%[66] to 68%.[63] Diarrhoea has been defined empirically as an increase in the frequency and/or volume of stool,[63] or a decrease in the consistency of stool[50] and quantitatively as an increase in stool weight of more than 200 g per 24 hours,[67] or as an increase in stool water of more than 500 ml per 24 hours,[65] or is simply not defined at all, when its presence is a function of the investigator or patients' subjective assessment.[47,66] These definitions are further confounded, because they do not take into account the patient's usual bowel habit and stool consistency. Diarrhoea usually occurs when the capacity of the colon to absorb fluid is exceeded or altered for whatever reason.

Clinical judgement is notoriously difficult to use to define diarrhoea. Benya et al.[64] reported that when stools were weighed from patients reported by nursing staff and by patients self-reporting diarrhoea, no stool weights were greater than 250 g per day. Thus no patient had diarrhoea when weight definition was used. Nonetheless, it is likely that some of the patients were passing liquid stool of a different consistency than normal and it would seem unreasonable to refute the patients' and nurses' assertions that diarrhoea had developed, or at least was a problem.

Diarrhoea is distressing for patients and their relatives, time-consuming for nursing staff and can add to potential problems such as infected pressure sores and altered fluid and electrolyte balance.[63] Diarrhoea, defined as an increase in bowel frequency and/or fluid content of the stool, can result in nutrient and electrolyte loss in patients being enterally tube fed. The complication of diarrhoea may also delay patient discharge and increase hospital costs. If diarrhoea is severe, it may be necessary to stop enteral feeding and institute parenteral nutrition with its attendant risks and costs.

Diarrhoea may result from a variety of causes including bacterial or viral infection, use of hyper-osmolar formula, lactose intolerance, antibiotic treatment, magnesium containing antacids, drug side-effects (e.g. digoxin and propanolol) and so called inert fillers of drugs which can include magnesium stearate, docusate sodium[68] and sorbitol. Some of these causes are discussed in more detail below.

In patients with short bowel and no colon additional factors that contribute to the development of diarrhoea including loss of the daily intestinal secretions produced in response to food, and rapid gastric emptying and small bowel transit.[41] A lack of peptide YY, which is known to delay gastric emptying

and small intestinal motility and which is found in the highest concentration in the colon[69] may be responsible for this.

Aetiology of enteral tube feeding-related diarrhoea

Several mechanisms have been proposed as contributing towards the development of enteral tube feeding-associated diarrhoea (Table 31.4), which are discussed below.

Table 31.4 – Proposed causes of enteral feeding-associated diarrhoea

Temperature of feed (cold)
Osmolality of feed (> 300 mOsmol)
Lactose intolerant
Fat malabsorption
Hypoalbuminaemia
Drugs (antibiotics★ or sorbitol containing)
Infected feed (includes gastroenteritis and *Clostridium difficile*)
Lack of fibre
Bolus tube feeding
Continuous tube feeding (rapid rate)
Constipation with overflow
Gastric feeding more commonly than jejunal feeding

★ Most common reason.

Temperature of liquid enteral diet

It has been suggested that the temperature of the enteral diet may play a role in the development of diarrhoea.[70] There is, however, little conclusive evidence that either refrigeration or warming of the liquid feed have clinically important effects on gastrointestinal complications including diarrhoea or abdominal cramps.[71,72]

Enteral diet osmolality

Enteral tube feed was often given using 'starter regimes', whereby the feed is diluted and/or infused at a slow rate, both of which are gradually increased over a period of time until the required strength and rate of feeding is reached. The rationale underlying this practice was that infusing a hypertonic feed was thought to cause diarrhoea[73,74] and consequently 'starter regimens' were and still are sometimes used. Starter regimes and hypotonic diets when feeding intragastrically do not reduce the incidence of gastrointestinal complications when antibiotic usage is accounted for, and serve only to delay reaching the patient's nutritional requirements.[50,75]

There appears currently, therefore, to be little conclusive evidence that diet osmolality plays any significant role in enteral feeding-related diarrhoea, when the diet is instilled directly into the stomach.

Lactase

Lactase deficiency is the most common disaccharidase deficiency, which can be subdivided into primary, secondary and relative deficiency (Table 31.5). Primary lactase deficiency is particularly common in Afro-Caribbeans, Orientals, Indians and Jews to varying degrees. Symptoms of carbohydrate malabsorption include abdominal cramps, flatulence, bloated sensation, nausea and watery diarrhoea, thought to be caused by bacterial fermentation of unabsorbed carbohydrate.[76]

Table 31.5 – Lactase-deficient states

Lactase deficiency
Primary
Secondary
Gastroenteritis
Drugs
Coeliac disease
Tropical sprue
Malnutrition
Relative
Short bowel
Rapid gastric emptying post surgery

Walike and Walike[54] were the first to suggest that lactose content of enteral feed could be a contributory factor in enteral feeding-associated diarrhoea. They reported that approximately 87% of patients fed a typical blenderized feed which contained lactose, developed diarrhoea. However, only 14% of these patients were lactase-deficient as indicated by a lactose tolerance test. Patients who can tolerate a small lactose load in their diet may become symptomatic if fed a milk-based diet, which can provide 80–210 g of lactose per 24 hours compared to an average normal lactose intake of 12 g per 24 hours.[54] Whether the patient has a true lactase deficiency or relative lactase deficiency in the presence of an excessive load of lactose, the resulting gastrointestinal complications are similar.

Relative lactase deficiency may develop due to reduced absorptive area and/or to reduced transit time. In this situation, lactose concentrations may be normal but total absorptive surface area is reduced as in patients with a short bowel, or the time available for enzyme action is diminished as with rapid gastric emptying, which may saturate the enzymes' ability to cope with the lactose load (concentration × rate of infusion), resulting in diarrhoea.[77]

Most commercially prepared enteral diets are now clinically lactose-free, and this potential causative problem has been removed. However, if a patient with diarrhoea is taking some oral food, it is important to check that they are not consuming much milk.

Fat malabsorption

Problems with fat absorption can cause diarrhoea in tube fed patients. Patients with severe pancreatic disease may have a deficiency of lipase necessary to hydrolyse triglycerides, and gastric surgery may prevent adequate mixing of lipase with luminal contents. Patients with biliary obstruction, ileectomy or ileitis may have insufficient bile salts for adequate fat absorption, resulting in diarrhoea and abdominal discomfort. Medium-chain triglycerides can also cause diarrhoea, flatulence and abdominal pain in patients intolerant to them.[78] Patients with a jejunostomy do not need to reduce their fat intake, but if the colon remains in continuity with the shortened small bowel, then steatorrhoea may develop. Using a feed containing a lower fat content (and thus lower energy density) may alleviate diarrhoea due to fat malabsorption in patients with a short bowel and retained colon.

Hypoalbuminaemia

There is a dichotomy of opinion as to the importance of serum albumin and its relevance in the development of diarrhoea. Several studies have suggested an association between hypoalbuminaemia and enteral feeding-related diarrhoea,[79–83] possibly by reducing intestinal water and solute absorption as a result of intestinal oedema and disruption of the intravascular osmotic force that contributes to the absorption of water and substrates across the intestinal cells.[84,85] However, patients who developed diarrhoea in the presence of hypoalbuminaemia were also on antibiotics, and it is likely that antibiotic use contributed towards development of diarrhoea.[79,81] Furthermore, patients with hypoalbuminaemia due to nephrotic syndrome or cirrhosis, or intestinal oedema from right heart failure often do not have diarrhoea. The majority of studies which have examined albumin levels, could find no definite association between hypo-albuminaemia and enteral tube feeding-associated diarrhoea.[48,75,86–89] Further evidence that hypo-albuminaemia may not be a major factor in enteral tube feeding associated diarrhoea, is provided by Foley et al.,[90] in which hypoalbuminaemic patients were given albumin supplementation with no clinical benefit on diarrhoea. Lack of a role for intravenous albumin in hypoalbuminaemic patients in preventing enteral feeding-associated diarrhoea has also been made by other investigators.[91,92]

Other researchers have also suggested there is little correlation between serum albumin and development of diarrhoea, and that drugs that can cause diarrhoea should be excluded first.[93] During a study of enteral feeding-related diarrhoea, seven patients developed diarrhoea, of which five were on broad-spectrum antibiotics, one was on lactulose and mylanta II and the remaining patient was also on mylanta II. Mylanta II contains magnesium and sorbitol, both of which have a laxative effect.[94]

Platt et al.[95] demonstrated the importance of providing adequate protein in the diet. Pigs fed low protein diets develop gastrointestinal mucosal atrophy, with development of diarrhoea. Starvation (or parenteral nutrition alone) results in flattening of microvilli, reduction in crypt depth and loss of intestinal villous brush border enzymes.[96,97] This atrophy of gut mucosa will result in a reduced ability of the gastrointestinal tract to digest and absorb an enteral feed, particularly if the 'load' (concentration × rate) of the feed is too great.

The role that hypoalbuminaemia per se may play in causing enteral feeding related diarrhoea is thus so far inconclusive. Hypoalbuminaemia is more likely to be a marker of disease severity and degree of under-nutrition rather than a direct cause of enteral feeding-associated diarrhoea, with the changes in bowel structure and function due to starvation, contributing to the risk of developing enteral tube feeding-associated diarrhoea.

Drugs and antibiotics

Diarrhoea is a recognized common complication associated with drugs and antibiotics.[47,50,79,81,86,87] Many drugs contain so called 'inert carriers' for the active compound, however they are osmotically active and the inert carrier may cause diarrhoea. For example, some drugs such as cimetidine, theophylline and acetaminophen (paracetamol) contain sorbitol,[65,94] and

others such as antacids and co-trimoxazole contain magnesium[68,94] or docusate sodium.[68] Sorbitol, magnesium and docusate sodium can all cause diarrhoea in their own right. Other drugs may cause diarrhoea as a result of recognized side-effects, such as H_2 blockers, anti-arrhythmics, anti-hypertensives, non-steroidal drugs or because they are designed to encourage bowel movements such as laxatives.

The incidence of diarrhoea associated with clindamycin is 7–26% and 5–10% for ampicillin, although the extent of the problem depends on the definition of diarrhoea used. Diarrhoea can result from primary structural (e.g. neomycin)[98] or functional (e.g. clindamycin)[99] damage to the small or large intestine. However, if this was the only reason, then the incidence of diarrhoea in enterally tube fed patients on antibiotics should be similar to that of patients on antibiotics who are eating normally, which is not the case. Thus there appears to be a synergistic effect of enteral tube feeding and anti-biotic usage, resulting in the high incidence of diarrhoea in tube fed patients.[77]

The reasons why antibiotics may cause diarrhoea are not entirely fully elucidated, although a proposed mechanism is that antibiotics alter the normal intestinal flora, allowing bacterial overgrowth of pathogenic bacteria (e.g. Klebsiella, Proteus, Escherichia coli).[100] Antibiotic usage is associated with isolation of Clostridium difficile and its toxin in some patients with diarrhoea.[65,79] C. difficile has been isolated in 20–50% of patients with antibiotic-related diarrhoea[79] and in 95% of cases of pseudomembranous colitis, although it is a normal commensal in approximately 4% of healthy adults.[101] The presence of C. difficile does not neces-sarily confirm that this organism is the cause of diarrhoea. Up to 25% of patients receiving antibiotics have positive C. difficile toxin but no diarrhoea.[101] C. difficile is thus likely to contribute to some cases of enteral feeding-related diarrhoea, but certainly not all.

Poorly metabolized carbohydrate or fibre enters the colon, where it is fermented by bacterial poly-saccharidases with the generation of short-chain fatty acids.[102] Short-chain fatty acids promote colonic absorption of water and electrolytes.[102,103] Antibiotics inhibit colonic bacterial polysaccharidase activity and markedly reduce short-chain fatty acid production.[61,104] Antibiotics can also reduce short-chain fatty acid production by reducing the population of endogenous bacteria such as Lactobacilli and Bifidobacteria[100] and thus limiting fibre fermentation still further. Therefore, antibiotics could increase the likelihood of diarrhoea developing, by reducing colonic short-chain fatty acid production, and increasing risk of overgrowth of potentially pathogenic bacteria.

When investigating the cause of enteral feeding-associated diarrhoea in the clinical situation, examination of the patients drug chart is essential before concluding that the enteral feed may be a contributory factor.

Contaminated feeds and feeding equipment

Enteral feed provides an excellent growth medium for bacteria, and once contaminated bacteria will rapidly multiply. A variety of micro-organisms have been cultured from enteral feeds including *Enterobacter* spp, *E. coli*, *Klebsiella* spp, *Proteus mirabilis*, *Salmonella enteriditis*, *Pseudomonas* spp, *Staphylococcus aureus* and *epidermidis*, *Streptococcus faecalis*, *Acinobacter* spp, *Citrobacter* spp and yeasts.[32]

Although enteral feeds are sterilized, as soon as the bottles or cans are opened, there is a risk of bacterial colonization of the feed, through a variety of routes, which is exacerbated by handling, type of delivery system, prolonged hanging time[105,106] and ascending spread of bacteria up the giving set.[32] Contaminated feeds reportedly cause not only diarrhoea, but also sepsis, pneumonia and urinary tract infections.[107–109]

Bacterial contamination of enteral feed can be a major problem, with up to 36% of enteral diet fed by a continuous drip method being contaminated.[110] Although the source of infecting organisms is often endogenous,[32] feed contamination can originate from a wide variety of exogenous sources. Retrograde spread of organisms from patient to a sterile feed chamber can occur and a drip chamber may prevent this problem from happening by interrupting continuity in the column of feed.[32] Continuous infusion of enteral feed raises gastric pH,[31,32,35] as does H_2 antagonists or other antisecretory drugs. Inhibiting gastric acid secretion allows bacterial overgrowth in the stomach,[109] whereas if the stomach is functioning normally and is acidic, most bacteria should be killed. A lower pH inhibits growth of bacteria within enteral feed, and thus a normal acidic stomach may help prevent ascending colonization of enteral feed. Allowing breaks in feeding may allow the pH of the stomach to fall between feeds with its subsequent bactericidal action.[33]

As bacterial colonization of the bowel and in particular small bowel bacterial overgrowth may cause diarrhoea, it is important to minimize the risk of gastrointestinal colonization by pathogenic bacteria. Continuous enteral tube feeding has been shown to be associated with a high incidence of bacterial contamination of the enteral bag and feeding system,[32] which combined with the resulting rise in gastric pH,[34] may increase the chances of small and large bowel colonization with pathogenic bacteria and contribute towards enteral feeding-associated diarrhoea. It has been recommended that feed containers and giving sets should be changed every 24 hours, to reduce the risk of bacterial contamination still further,[32,106] and there should probably be a break between feeds to allow gastric pH to fall.

Fibre in enteral tube feeds

Many commercially produced liquid enteral tube feeds are low in fibre (poorly metabolized carbohydrate). The earliest low residue diets were designed not only to provide a balanced diet to astronauts in space, but also to reduce the stool weight and frequency. It was subsequently realized, that one of the clinical advantages of the low residue diet was its low viscosity, enabling administration through fine-bore nasogastric feeding tubes. The ingestion of fibre has been found to increase slow intestinal transit time and delay rapid intestinal transit,[111,112] leading to the suggestion that the ingestion of fibre may produce a more regular bowel habit.[113] It has thus been suggested that supplementing commercially prepared enteral diets with fibre may be beneficial.[61]

In humans, the presence of fermentable polysaccharides in the diet has been shown to stimulate colonic microbial growth.[114] The increased bacterial mass is one of the mechanisms in which the presence of non-starch polysaccharides in the diet results in an increase in faecal output,[114] as it is not just the water-holding properties of fibre that increases stool weight. It has been estimated that between 40 and 55% of stool mass is due to the bacteria present within the stool.[115] Many of the microbial polysaccharidases are inducible, and so continuous fibre supplementation should increase short-chain fatty acid production.[116] During fermentation of fibre, not only to short-chain fatty acids, gas and energy produced but also to hydrogen ions.

Short-chain fatty acid absorption stimulates colonic sodium and water absorption,[103] but their presence in the colon, together with the generation of hydrogen ions from fibre fermentation, affects the pH of the colonic lumen. The lower pH inhibits growth of potentially pathogenic bacteria.[102,117]

The presence of either the highly soluble fibre pectin or the insoluble soy polysaccharide in enteral feed, significantly increases water absorption compared to a fibre-free diet.[118] The metabolism of short-chain fatty acids in epithelial cells may provide an energy source for active sodium transport.[119] Transport of non-ionized short-chain fatty acids into the cell may also drive the Na^+/H^+ exchange and so stimulate sodium absorption.[102] The administration of antibiotics active against colonic anaerobes can significantly reduce the production of short-chain fatty acids,[104] with potentially adverse consequences.

Short-chain fatty acids promote intestinal mucosal growth,[120] reduce colonic inflammation,[121] and help maintain intestinal mucosal barrier function,[122] whereas fibre free enteral diets can result in colonic mucosal atrophy.[123]

It has been demonstrated that continuous enteral feeding of a standard fibre-free polymeric feed via a nasogastric tube results in secretion of water and electrolytes into the colon and that this secretion can be reversed by the infusion of short-chain fatty acids into the caecum.[124] Thus short-chain fatty acids may play an important function in helping to maintain water and electrolyte homeostasis in the colon.

Diarrhoea is a common problem occurring in up to 60% of critically ill patients.[63] Possible causes of diarrhoea in these patients include altered colonic bacterial microflora due to the administration of broad-spectrum antibiotics and fibre-deficient diets. The reduced bacterial load together with reduced fibre intake, will lead to a decrease in short-chain fatty acid production, which may result in a reduction of water and sodium absorption.

However, the addition of fibre to enteral diets has not been uniformly successful in preventing development of enteral tube feeding-related diarrhoea. Dobb and Towler[125] found the incidence of diarrhoea to be similar whether patients were on a fibre-supplemented or fibre-free diet. Patil et al.[56] reported that an enteral feed supplemented with mixed fibre had no beneficial effect on stool wet weight and frequency of bowel action, compared to fibre-free enteral diet. We have also recently demonstrated that drinking fibre-free or fibre-supplemented enteral diet does not cause diarrhoea and has no significant effect on colonic motor activity.[126–128] We have shown that the addition of a mixed fibre source to an enteral diet does not affect stool weight nor bowel frequency, but does normalize or prolong gut transit time.[57,59,126]

The reason for this apparent lack of an effect by fibre on bowel function may lie in the small particle size of soy polysaccharide in enteral feeds, which is to help reduce viscosity of the feed. Reducing particle size increases the surface area available for fermentation,[60,61] which together with inducibility of the colonic bacterial polysaccharidase enzymes by fibre substrate will increase fermentation over time,[61,114] reducing the amount of undigested fibre available to hold water. In addition, the manufacturing process of enteral feeds may alter the physiological properties of the added fibre,[59] with a potential effect on fibre fermentability. Fine bran, which is better digested due to its reduced particle size and increased available surface area, has less effect on large bowel function than coarse bran which is less well fermented,[60] and thus has a greater water holding property than fine bran.[60] We have recently confirmed that the addition of fibre does not prevent the development of diarrhoea when fed by nasogastric tube,[128] which may be due to a combination of failure to stimulate a cephalic response and suppression of distal colonic motor activity with tube feeding.[127]

There is thus currently little evidence to suggest that the addition of fibre to enteral diets can overcome the diarrhoea associated with enteral tube feeding.

However, absorbed short-chain fatty acids can provide up to 500 kcal of energy in patients with an intact colon and shortened small bowel. If excessive carbohydrate enters the colon and remains un-fermented, however, an osmotic diarrhoea may result.[42]

There is currently much research taking place about the use of prebiotics (substrates used for bacterial growth, e.g fructo-oligosaccharide) and probiotics which are the bacteria (e.g. lactobacillus) that will act upon the substrate.

Nasogastric versus post-pyloric feeding

It has been suggested that continuous post-pyloric feeding may be more physiological than continuous intragastric tube feeding and cause diarrhoea less often than intragastric tube feeding.[129–132] However, this is not necessarily correct, as continuous intraduodenal feeding does not produce normal colonic responses.[132–134] There are logistical and practical problems to be overcome in trying to feed patients by the post-pyloric route, and currently it is not a practical method of feeding most patients.

Bolus versus continuous modes of enteral tube feeding

The method of 'bolus feeding' is frequently reported to be associated with a high incidence of complications such as nausea, bloating and diarrhoea,[135–137] although there has previously been little scientific substantiation of this statement.

It has been suggested that continuous intragastric feeding is generally better tolerated than intermittent feedings[138] although this has been disputed.[139] Several investigators have reported that bolus nasogastric tube feeding does not cause nausea, vomiting, bloated sensation,[52,140–142] or diarrhoea.[143] Kocan et al.[139] reported no significant differences in stool consistency, number of stools per day, or caloric intake between continuous and intermittent methods of enteral tube feeding.

We have recently shown that there is little evidence that bolus feeding causes diarrhoea more frequently than continuous nasogastric tube feeding.[53,131] Continuous nasogastric enteral tube feeding may cause diarrhoea.[131] Continuous nasogastric tube feeding fails to provoke a normal postprandial response, suppresses distal colonic segmenting motor activity,[131] and causes an abnormal secretory response in the ascending colon.[132] Bolus intragastric tube feeding high or low loads (load = rate × concentration) however, promotes a pro-absorptive response in the ascending colon (unpublished observation). Low loads of enteral diet bolus tube fed intragastrically does not cause diarrhoea,[53] but high loads of enteral diet bolus tube fed intragastrically causes suppression of distal colonic motor activity associated with diarrhoea. We have recently shown that enteral diet itself does not cause enteral tube feeding-related diarrhoea, but that the lack of a cephalic response with nasogastric tube feeding is likely to be significant in the pathogenesis of enteral tube feeding-related diarrhoea.[142]

If diarrhoea is a problem despite attention to possible causes as discussed, then loperamide (or codeine phosphate) can be instituted to control symptoms and there are anecdotal reports of live yogurt being helpful.

SUMMARY

Enteral tube feeding can cause a number of complications which can be mechanical, metabolic/biochemical or gastrointestinal. The type of complications may be dictated by the underlying disease, the route of enteral access, type of enteral diet used and concomitant use of drugs. A number of these problems can be anticipated and prevented or treated, provided that the physician or surgeon is aware of the possibility that enteral tube feeding-related complications can develop, particularly in patients with a short bowel. Regular clinical and biochemical monitoring and early involvement of nutrition teams should result in early recognition of developing complications, and thus be prevented from progressing further. The common complication of enteral tube feeding-related diarrhoea is unlikely to be due to the enteral diet itself, and other reasons must be sought (especially concomitant use of antibiotics and other drugs).

REFERENCES

1. McWhirter JP, Pennington CR. Incidence and recognition of malnutrition in hospital. *Br Med J* 1994; **308**: 945–948.

2. Pennington CR, Powell-Tuck J, Shaffer J. Review article: Artificial nutritional support for improved patient care. *Aliment Pharmacol Ther* 1995; **9**: 471–481.

3. Rana SK, Bray J, Menzies-Gow N, Jameson J, Payne-James JJ, Frost P, Silk DBA. Short term benefits of post-operative oral dietary supplements in surgical patients. *Clin Nutr* 1992; **11**: 337–344.

4. Keohane PP, Attrill H, Jones BJM, Silk DBA. Limitations and drawbacks of 'fine-bore' nasogastric feeding tubes. *Clin Nutr* 1983; **2**: 85–86.

5. Silk DB, Rees RG, Keohane PP, Attrill H. Clinical efficacy and design changes of 'fine-bore' nasogastric feeding tubes: a seven-year experience involving 809 intubations in 403 patients. *J Parenter Enteral Nutr* 1987; **11**: 378–383.

6. Rees RG, Attrill H, Quinn D, Silk DBA. Improved design of nasogastric feeding tubes. *Clin Nutr* 1986; **5**: 203–207.

7. Marcaud SP, Perkins AM. Clogging of feeding tubes. *J Parenter Enteral Nutr* 1988; **12**: 403–405.

8. Altman E, Cutie A. Compatability of enteral products with commonly employed drug additives. *Nutr Support Serv* 1984; **4**: 8–17.

9. Silk DBA, Bray MJ, Keele AM, Walters ER, Duncan HD. Clinical evaluation of a newly designed nasogastric enteral feeding tube. *Clin Nutr* 1996; **15**: 285–290.

10. Wyler AR, Reynolds AF. An intracranial complication of nasogastric intubation. *J Neurosurg* 1977; **47**: 297–298.

11. Nagler R, Spiro SM. Persistent gastro-oesophageal reflux induced during prolonged gastric intubation. *N Engl J Med* 1963; **269**: 495–500.

12. Keohane PP, Attrill H, Grimble GK, Spiller R, Frost P, Silk DB. Enteral nutrition in malnourished patients with hepatic cirrhosis and acute encephalopathy. *J Parenter Enteral Nutr* 1983; **7**: 346–350.

13. Siegle RL, Rabinowitz JG, Sarasohn C. Intestinal perforation secondary to nasojejunal feeding tubes. *Am J Roentgenol* 1976; **126**: 1229–1232.

14. Eldar S, Meguid MM. Pneumothorax following attempted nasogastric intubation for nutritional support. *J Parenter Enteral Nutr* 1984; **8**: 450–452.

15. James RH. An unusual complication of passing a narrow-bore nasogastric tube. *Anaesthesia* 1978; **33**: 716–718.

16. Iyer V, Reichel J. Perforation of the oesophagus by a fine-bore feeding tube. *NY State J Med* 1981; 63–64.

17. Olivares L, Segovia A, Revuelta R. Tube feeding and lethal aspiration in neurological patients: a review of 720 autopsy cases. *Stroke* 1974; **5**: 654–657.

18. Meehan SE, Wood RAB, Cushier A. Percutaneous cervical pharyngostomy. A comfortable and convenient alternative to protracted nasogastric intubation. *Am J Surg* 1984; **148**: 325–330.

19. Balkany TJ, Jafek BW, Wong ML. Complications of feeding esophagotomy. Advantages of a new esophagotomy tube. *Arch Otolarnygol* 1980; **106**: 122–123.

20. Engel S. Gastrostomy. *Surg Clin North Am* 1969; **49**: 1289–1295.

21. Torosian M, Rombeau JL. Feeding by tube enterostomy. *Surg Gynecol Obstet* 1980; **150**: 918–927.

22. Blebea J, King TA. Intraperitoneal infusion as a complication of needle cather jejunostomy. *J Parenter Enteral Nutr* 1985; **9**: 758–759.

23. Jarnagin WR, Duh QY, Mulvihill SJ, Ridge JA, Schrock TR, Way LW. The efficacy and limitations of percutaneous endoscopic gastrostomy. *Arch Surg* 1992; **127**: 261–264.

24. Moran BJ, Taylor MB, Johnson CD. Percutaneous endoscopic gastrostomy. *Br J Surg* 1990; **77**: 858–862.

25. Duncan HD, Bray MJ, Kapadia SA, *et al*. Prospective randomized comparison of two different sized percutaneous endoscopically placed gastrostomy tubes. *Clin Nutr* 1996; **15**: 317–320.

26. Hull MA, Rawlings J, Murray FE, *et al*. Audit of outcome of long term enteral nutrition by percutaneous endoscopic gastrostomy. *Lancet* 1993; **341**: 869–872.

27. DiSario JA, Foutch PG, Sanowski RA. Poor results with percutaneous endoscopic jejunostomy. *Gastrointest Endosc* 1990; **36**: 257–260.

28. Winterbauer RH, Duming RB, Barron E, McFadden MC. Aspirated nasogastric feeding solution detected by glucose strips. *Ann Intern Med* 1981; **95**: 67–68.

29. Bury KD, Jambunathan G. Effects of elemental diets on gastric emptying and gastric secretion in man. *Am J Surg* 1974; **127**: 59–66.

30. Rees RG, Payne-James JJ, King C, Silk DB. Spontaneous transpyloric passage and performance of 'fine bore' polyurethane feeding tubes: a controlled clinical trial. *J Parenter Enteral Nutr* 1988; **12**(5): 469–472.

31. Jacobs S, Chang RWS, Lee B, Bartlett FW. Continuous enteral feeding: A major cause of pneumonia among ventilated intensive care unit patients. *J Parenter Enteral Nutr* 1990; **14**: 353–356.

32. Payne-James JJ, Rana SK, Bray MJ, McSwiggan DA, Silk DB. Retrograde (ascending) bacterial contamination of enteral diet administration systems. *J Parenter Enteral Nutr* 1992; **16**: 369–373.

33. Atkinson S, Bihari D. The benefits of enteral feeding in the critically ill patient. *Curr Opinion Anaesth* 1994; **7**: 131–135.

34. Hopert R, Liehr RM, Riecken EO. Reduction of 24-hour gastric acidity by different dietary regimens: A randomised controlled study in healthy volunteers. *J Parenter Enteral Nutr* 1989; **13**: 292–295.

35. Armstrong D, Castiglione F, Emde C, *et al*. The effect of continuous enteral nutrition on gastric acidity in humans. *Gastroenterology* 1992; **102**: 1506–1515.

36. Lee B, Chang RWS, Jacobs S. Intermittent nasogastric feeding: a simple and effective method to reduce pneumonia among ventilated ICU patients. *Clin Intens Care* 1990; **1**: 100–102.

37. Woolfson AMJ, Ricketts CR, Hardy SM, Saour JN, Pollard BJ, Allison SP. Prolonged nasogastric tube feeding in critically ill and surgical patients. *Postgrad Med J* 1976; **52**: 678–682.

38. Vanlandingham S, Simpson S, Daniel P, Newmark SR. Metabolic abnormalities in patients supported with enteral tube feeding. *J Parenter Enteral Nutr* 1981; **5**: 322–324.

39. Solomon S, Kirby DF. The refeeding syndrome: a review. *J Parenter Enteral Nutr* 1990; **14**: 90–97.

40. Havala T, Shronts E. Managing the complications associated with refeeding. *Nutr Clin Prac* 1990; **5**: 23–29.

41. Gault MH, Dixon ME, Doyle M, Cohen WM. Hypernatraemia, azotaemia and dehydration due to high protein tube feeding. *Ann Intern Med* 1968; **68**: 778–791.

42. Lennard-Jones JE. Review article: practical management of the short bowel. *Aliment Pharmacol Ther* 1994; **8**: 563–577.

43. Elia M, Crozier C, Neale G. Mineral metabolism during short-term starvation in man. *Clin Chim Acta* 1984; 13937–13945.

44. Grant J, Cox CE, Kleiman LM, *et al*. Serum hepatic enzyme and bilirubin elevations during parenteral nutrition. *Surg Gynecol Obstet* 1977; **145**: 573–580.

45. Blackburn GL, Bristian BR. Nutritional care of the injured and/or septic patient. *Surg Clin North Am* 1976; **56**: 1195–1224.

46. Flatt JP, Blackburn GL. The metabolic fuel regulatory system: implications for protein-sparing therapies during caloric deprivation and disease. *Am J Clin Nutr* 1974; **27**: 175–187.

47. Jones BJM, Lees R, Andrews J, Frost P, Silk DB. Comparison of an elemental and polymeric enteral diet in patients with normal gastrointestinal function. *Gut* 1983; **24**: 78–84.

48. Bliss DZ, Guenter PA, Settle RG. Defining and reporting diarrhoea in tube-fed patients – what a mess! *Am J Clin Nutr* 1992; **55**: 753–759.

49. Silk DBA, Grimble GK, Payne-James JJ. Enteral nutrition. *Curr Opin Gastroenterol* 1992; **8**: 290–295.

50. Keohane PP, Attrill H, Love M, Frost P, Silk DBA. Relation between osmolality of diet and gastrointestinal side effects in enteral nutrition. *Br Med J* 1984; **288**: 678–680.

51. Haynes-Johnson V. Tube feeding complications: causes, prevention, therapy. *Nutr Support Serv* 1986; **6**: 17–21.

52. Heitkemper MM, Martin MN, Hansen BC, Hanson R, Vanderburg V. Rate and volume of intermittent feeding. *J Parenter Enteral Nutr* 1981; **5**: 125–129.

53. Duncan HD, Cole SJ, Bowling TE, Silk DBA. The effect of bolus enteral feeding on human colonic motor activity. *Gastroenterology* 1996; **110**: A659.

54. Walike BC, Walike JW. Relative lactose intolerance: a clinical study of tube fed patients. *JAMA* 1977; **238**: 948–951.

55. Heymsfield SB, Roongspisuthipong C, Evert M, Casper K, Heller P, Akrabawi SS. Fiber supplementation of enteral formulas: effects on the biovailability of major nutrients and gastrointestinal tolerance. *J Parenter Enteral Nutr* 1988; **12**: 265–273.

56. Patil DH, Grimble GK, Keohane P, Attrill H, Love M, Silk DBA. Do fibre containing enteral diets have an advantage over existing low residue diets? *Clin Nutr* 1985; **4**: 67–71.

57. Meier R, Beglinger C, Schneider H, Rowedder A, Gyr K. Effect of a liquid diet with and without soluble fibre supplementation on intestinal transit and cholecystokinin release in volunteers. *J Parenter Enteral Nutr* 1993; **17**: 231–235.

58. Lampe JW, Effertz ME, Larson JL, Slavin JL. Gastrointestinal effects of modified guar gum and soy polysaccharide as part of an enteral formula diet. *J Parenter Enteral Nutr* 1992; **16**: 538–544.

59. Kapadia SA, Raimundo A, Silk DBA. The effect of a fibre free and fibre supplemented polymeric enteral diet on normal human bowel function. *Clin Nutr* 1993; **12**: 272–276.

60. Heller SN, Hackler LR, Rivers JM, Van Soest PJ, Roe DA, Lewis BA, Robertson J. Dietary fibre: the effect of particle size of wheat bran on colonic function in young adult men. *Am J Clin Nutr* 1980; **33**: 1734–1744.

61. Silk DBA. Fibre and enteral nutrition. *Gut* 1989; **30**: 246–264.

62. Rees RG, Keohane PP, Grimble GK, Frost PG, Attrill H, Silk DB. Elemental diet administered nasogastrically without starter regimens to patients with inflammatory bowel disease. *J Parenter Enteral Nutr* 1986; **10**: 258–262.

63. Kelly TWJ, Patrick MR, Hillman KM. Study of diarrhea in critically ill patients. *Crit Care Med* 1983; **11**: 7–9.

64. Benya R, Layden TJ, Morbarhan S. Diarrhea associated with tube feeding: the importance of using objective criteria. *J Clin Gastroenterol* 1991; **13**: 167–172.

65. Edes TE, Walk BE, Austin JL. Diarrhea in tube-fed patients: feeding formulas not necessarily the cause. *Am J Med* 1990; **88**: 91–93.

66. Cataldi-Betcher EL, Seltzer MH, Slocum BA, Jones KW. Complications occurring during enteral nutrition support: a prospective study. *J Parenter Enteral Nutr* 1983; **7**: 546–552.

67. Turnberg LA. Mechanisms of diarrhoea. *Curr Concepts Gastroenterol* 1986; (Spring): 3–9.

68. Guidotti JL. Laxative components of a generic drug. *Lancet* 1996; **347**: 621.

69. Adrian TE, Ferri GL, Bacarese-Hamilton AJ, Fuessel HS, Polak JM, Bloom SR. Human distribution and release of a putative new gut hormone, peptide YY. *Gastroenterology* 1985; **89**: 1070–1077.

70. Gershon-Cohen J, Shay H, Feks SS. The relation of meal temperature to gastric motility and secretion. *Am J Roentgenol Radium Ther Nucl Med* 1940; **43**: 237–242.

71. Hanson RL. A study to determine the differences in effects of administering cold and warmed tube feedings. *Commun Nurs Res* 1974; **6**: 136–140.

72. Kawaga-Busby KS, Heitkemper MM, Hansen BC, Hanson RL, Vanderburg VV. Effects of diet temperature on tolerance of enteral feedings. *Nutr Res* 1980; **29**: 276–280.

73. Masterton JP, Dudley H, Macrae S. Design of tube feeds for surgical patients. *Br Med J* 1963; **2**: 909–913.

74. Lee H. Why enteral nutrition. *Res Clin Forums* 1979; **1**: 15–25.

75. Pesola GE, Hogg JE, Yonnios T, McConnell RE, Carlton GC. Isotonic nasogastric feedings: do they cause diarrhoea? *Crit Care Med* 1989; **17**: 1151–1155.

76. Olsen WA. Carbohydrate digestion and absorption. *Postgrad Med* 1972; **51**: 149–152.

77. Silk DBA. Towards the optimization of enteral nutrition. *Clin Nutr* 1987; **6**: 61–74.

78. Chernoff R. Enteral feedings. *Am J Hosp Pharm* 1980; **37**: 65–74.

79. Guenter PA, Settle RG, Perlmutter S, Marino PL, DeSimone GA, Rolandelli RH. Tube feeding-related diarrhoea in acutely ill patients. *J Parenter Enteral Nutr* 1991; **15**: 277–280.

80. Hwang TL, Lue MC, Nee NJ, Jan YY, Chen MF. The incidence of diarrhoea in patients with hypoalbuminaemia due to acute or chronic malnutrition during enteral feeding. *Am J Gastroenterol* 1994; **89**: 376–378.

81. Heimburger DC, Sockwell DG, Geels WJ. Diarrhoea with enteral feeding: prospective reappraisal of putative causes. *Nutrition* 1994; **10**: 392–396.

82. Brinson RR, Kolts BE. Hypoalbuminaemia as an indicator of diarrhoeal incidence in critically ill patients. *Crit Care Med* 1987; **15**: 506–509.

83. Ford EG, Jennings M, Andrassy RJ. Serum albumin (oncotic pressure) correlates with enteral feeding tolerance in the pediatric surgical patient. *J Pediatr Surg* 1987; **22**: 597–599.

84. Moss G. Post-operative metabolism: The role of plasma albumin in the enteral absorption of water and electrolytes. *Pac Med Surg* 1967; **75**: 355–358.

85. Moss G. Editorial comment: The role of albumin in nutritional support. *J Am Coll Nutr* 1988; **7**: 441–442.

86. Gottschlich MM, Warden GD, Michel M, Havens P, Kopcha R, Jenkins M, Alexander JW. Diarrhoea in tube-fed burn patients: incidence, etiology, nutritional impact, and prevention. *J Parenter Enteral Nutr* 1988; **12**: 338–345.

87. Byers PH, Wiggins CL, Morelli CC. Effect of enteral alimentation and antibiotic usage on diarrhoea. *Nutr Support Serv* 1988; **8**: 14–15.

88. Patterson ML, Dominguez JM, Lyman B, Cuddy PG, Pemberton LB. Enteral feeding in the hypoalbuminaemic patient. *J Parenter Enteral Nutr* 1990; **14**: 362–365.

89. Levinson M, Bryce A. Enteral feeding, gastric colonization and diarrhoea in the critically ill patient: Is there a relationship? *Anaesth Intens Care* 1993; **21**: 85–88.

90. Foley EF, Borlase BC, Dzik WH, Bistrian BR, Benotti PN. Albumin supplementation in the critically ill. A prospective randomised trial. *Arch Surg* 1990; **125**: 739–742.

91. D'Angio RG. Is there a role for albumin administration in nutrition support. *Ann Pharmacother* 1994; **28**: 478–482.

92. Koretz RL. Intravenous albumin and nutrition support: going for the quick fix. *J Parenter Enteral Nutr* 1995; **19**: 166–171.

93. Forlaw L, Chernoff R, Rombeau JL, Caldwell MD (eds) *Clinical Nutrition: Enteral and Tube Feeding*, 1st edn. WB Saunders: Philadelphia, 1984, p. 231.

94. Harvey SC, Goodman LS, Gilman A (eds) *The Pharmacological Basis of Therapeutics*, 5th edn. Macmillan: New York, 1975, pp. 960–973.

95. Platt BS, Heard CRC, Stewart RJC. Munro HN (eds) *The Role of the Gastrointestinal Tract in Protein Metabolism*. FA Davis: Philadelphia, 1964, pp. 227–238.

96. Levine GM, Deren JJ, Steiger E, Zinno R. Role of oral intake in maintenance of gut mass and disaccharidase activity. *Gastroenterology* 1974; **67**: 975–982.

97. Raul F, Noriega R, Doffoel M, Grenier JF, Haffen K. Modifications of brush border enzyme activities during starvation in the jejunum and ileum of adult rats. *Enzyme* 1982; **28**: 328–335.

98. Dobbins WO, Herrero BA, Mansback CM. Morphological alteration associated with neomycin-induced malabsorption. *Am J Med Sci* 1968; **255**: 63–77.

99. Spiller RC, Higgins BE, Frost PG, Silk DBA. Inhibition of jejunal water and electrolyte absorption by therapeutic doses of clindamycin in man. *Clin Sci* 1984; **67**: 117–120.

100. Wang X, Gibson GR. Effects of the in vitro fermentation of oligofructose and inulin by bacteria growing in the human large intestine. *J Appl Bacteriol* 1993; **75**: 373–380.

101. George WL, Rolfe RD, Finegold SM. *Clostridium difficile* and its cytotoxin in faeces of patients with antimicrobial agent-associated diarrhoea and miscellaneous conditions. *J Clin Microbiol* 1982; **15**: 1049–1053.

102. Cummings JH. Short-chain fatty acids in the human colon. *Gut* 1981; **22**: 763–779.

103. Ruppin H, Bar-Meir S, Soergal KH, Wood CM, Schmitt MG. Absorption of short-chain fatty acids by the colon. *Gastroenterology* 1980; **78**: 1500–1507.

104. Raimundo AH, Wilden S, Rogers J, Filden P, Silk DBA. Influence of metronidazole on volatile fatty acid (VFA) production from soy polysaccharide – relevance to enteral feeding related diarrhoea. *Gastroenterology* 1990; **98**: A197.

105. Kohn CL. The relationship between enteral formula contamination and length of enteral delivery set usage. *J Parenter Enteral Nutr* 1991; **15**: 567–571.

106. Anderson K, Norris D, Godfrey L, Avent C, Butterworth C. Bacterial contamination of tube-feeding formulas. *J Parenter Enteral Nutr* 1984; **8**: 673–678.

107. Levy J, Van Laethem Y, Verhaegen G. Contaminated enteral nutrition solutions as a cause of nosocomial bloodstream infection: a study using plasmid finger-printing. *J Parenter Enteral Nutr* 1989; **13**: 228–234.

108. Thurn J, Crossley K, Gerdts A, Maki M, Johnson J. Enteral hyperalimentation as a source of nosocomial infection. *J Hosp Infect* 1990; **15**: 203–217.

109. Driks MR, Craven DE, Celli BR, *et al.* Nosocomial pneumonia in intubated patients given sucralfate as compared with antacids or histamine type 2 blockers. The role of gastric colonization. *N Engl J Med* 1987; **317**: 1376–1382.

110. Schreiner RL, Eitzen H, Gfell MA, Kress S, Gresham EL, French M, Moye L. Environmental contamination of continuous drip feedings. *Pediatrics* 1979; **63**: 232–237.

111. Harvey RF, Pomare EN, Heaton KW. Effects of increased dietary fibre on intestinal transit. *Lancet* 1973; **1**: 1278–1280.

112. Paylor DK, Pomare EW, Heaton KW, Harvey RF. The effect of wheat bran on intestinal transit. *Gut* 1975; **16**: 209–213.

113. Eastwood MA, Brydon WG, Tadasse K, Spiller GA, Kay RM (eds) *Medical Aspects of Dietary Fibre*. Plenum Press: New York, 1980, p. 1.

114. Stephen AM, Cummings JH. Mechanisms of action of dietary fibre in the human colon. *Nature* 1980; **284**: 283–284.

115. Stephen AM, Cummings JH. The microbial contribution to human faecal mass. *J Med Microbiol* 1980; **13**: 45–46.

116. Salyers AA, Palmer JK, Wilkins TD. Degradation of polysaccharides by intestinal bacterial enzymes. *Am J Clin Nutr* 1978; **31**(Suppl.10): 5128–5130.

117. Duncan HD, Walters E, Silk DBA. Inulin and oligofructose: an overview. *Essentials* 1996; **12**: 6–8.

118. Levine GM, Rosenthal J. Effects of fibre-containing liquid diets on colonic structure and function in the rat. *J Parenter Enteral Nutr* 1991; **15**: 526–529.

119. Engelhardt W, Rechkemmer G. The physiological effects of short-chain fatty acids in the hind gut. *Bull R Soc NZ* 1983; **20**: 149–155.

120. Kripke SA, Fox AD, Berman JM, Settle RG, Rombeau JL. Stimulation of intestinal growth with intracolonic infusion of short-chain fatty acids. *J Parenter Enteral Nutr* 1989; **13**: 109–116.

121. Harig JM, Soergal KH. Treatment of diversion colitis with short-chain fatty acids (SCFA) irrigation. *N Engl J Med* 1989; **320**: 23–28.

122. Alverdy J, Aoys E, Moss G. Effects of commercially available chemically defined liquid diets on the intestinal microflora and bacterial translocation from the gut. *J Parenter Enteral Nutr* 1990; **14**: 1–6.

123. Janne P, Carpenter Y, Williams G. Colonic mucosal atrophy induced by a liquid elemental diet in rats. *Dig Dis Sci* 1977; **22**: 808.

124. Bowling TE, Raimundo AH, Grimble GK, Silk DBA. Reversal by short-chain fatty acids of colonic fluid secretion induced by enteral feeding. *Lancet* 1993; **342**(8882): 1266–1268.

125. Dobb GJ, Towler SC. Diarrhoea during enteral feeding in the critically ill: a comparison of feeds with and without fibre. *Intens Care Med* 1990; **16**: 252–255.

126. Walters ER, Duncan HD, Green CJ, *et al.* Effect of new mixed fibre-supplemented enteral formula on healthy volunteers bowel function. *Proc Nutr Soc* 1997; **56**: 274A.

127. Duncan H, Cole S, Bowling T, Silk D. Is mode of feeding important in enteral feeding-related diarrhoea? *Gastroenterology* 1997; **112**: A725.

128. Duncan H, Cole S, Bowling T, Green C, Silk D. An investigation of the effects of a novel mixed fibre enteral feed on colonic motility. *Gastroenterology* 1997; **112**: A725.

129. Raimundo AH, Rogers J, Spiller RC, Grimble GK, Silk DBA. Effect of continuous intraduodenal enteral feeding on human colonic inflow volumes and small bowel motility. *Gastroenterology* 1989; **96**: A404.

130. Raimundo AH, Rogers J, Silk DBA. Is enteral feeding related diarrhoea initiated by an abnormal colonic response to intragastric diet infusion? *Gut* 1990; **31**: A1195.

131. Bowling TE, Raimundo AH, Jameson JS, Rogers J, Silk DBA. The effect of enteral feeding on colonic motility in man. *Gut* 1993; **34**: S64.

132. Bowling TE, Raimundo AH, Grimble GK, Silk DBA. Colonic secretory effect in response to enteral feeding in humans. *Gut* 1994; **35**: 1734–1741.

133. Raimundo AH, Jameson JS, Rogers J, Silk DBA. The effect of enteral nutrition on distal colonic motility. *Gastroenterology* 1992; **102**: A573.

134. Raimundo AH, Jameson JS, Rogers J, Silk DBA. Colonic motility during enteral nutrition. *Gastroenterology* 1992; **33**(Suppl): S17.

135. Allison S, Walford S, Todorovic V, Elliot E. Practical aspects of nutritional support. *Res Clin Forum* 1979; **1**: 49–57.

136. Allison S. Enteral and parenteral feeding. *Prescribers J* 1984; **24**: 1–11.

137. Powell-Tuck J, Goode AW. Principles of enteral and parenteral nutrition. *Br J Anaesth* 1981; **53**: 169–181.

138. Heibert JM, Brown A, Anderson RG, Halfacre S, Rodeheaver GT, Edlich RF. Comparison of continuous versus intermittent tube feeding in adult burn patients. *J Parenter Enteral Nutr* 1981; **5**: 526–527.

139. Kocan MJ, Hickisch SM. A comparison of continuous and intermittent enteral nutrition in NICU patients. *J Neuroscience Nurs* 1986; **18**: 333–337.

140. Heitkemper MM, Hansen BC, Hanson RL, Vanderburg VV. Effects of rate and volume of tube feeding on gastric motility and feeding tolerance. *J Parenter Enteral Nutr* 1977; **1**: 1A.

141. Heitkemper MM, Hanson RL, Hansen BC. Effects of rate and volume of tube feeding in normal human subjects. *Commun Nurs Res* 1978; **10**: 71–89.

142. Duncan HD, Cole SJ, Bowling TE, *et al*. Does the mode of feeding play a role in the pathogenesis of enteral feeding-related diarrhoea? *Proc Nutr Soc* 1997; **56**: (2) 216A.

143. Walike BC, Padilla G, Bergstrom N, Hanson RL, Kubo W, Grant M, Wong HL. Patient problems related to tube feeding. *Commun Nurs Res* 1975; **7**: 89–112.

144. Viall C, Porcelli K, Teran C, Varma N, Steffee WP. A double-blind clinical trial comparing the gastro-intestinal side-effects of two enteral feeding formulas. *J Parenter Enteral Nutr* 1990; **14**: 265–269.

32

Parenteral nutrition

C. R. Pennington

Soon after the introduction of parenteral nutrition (PN) it became apparent that this treatment may cause significant morbidity and mortality, principally through catheter-related complications. Now with increased experience and knowledge, and expert management, it has become a safe and highly effective therapeutic modality which can save the lives of patients who suffer from intestinal failure. For the majority of such patients the morbidity associated with PN is very much less than that which accompanies intestinal transplantation

This chapter will describe the clinical recognition, management and prevention of PN-related complications (Table 32.1). These can conveniently be considered in three groups: catheter-related problems, metabolic and nutritional disorders, and the effect of PN on other organ function. Catheter-related complications are relatively common.

Table 32.1 – Problems of parenteral nutrition

Catheter-related complications
Nutritional and metabolic problems
Effect of parenteral nutrition on organ function

CATHETER-RELATED COMPLICATIONS

Patients with intestinal failure usually require central venous access, most emphasis will be given to central catheter complications (Table 32.2). Catheter complications include infection, venous thrombosis, catheter occlusion and catheter fracture. Catheter infection is still a particular problem in some units and in some patients.

Table 32.2 – Catheter-related complications

Catheter-related infection
Central vein thrombosis
Catheter occlusion
Mechanical complications

Catheter infection

Catheters can become infected on the luminal surface, or the external surface.

External catheter infection

The exit site was originally thought to be the most common source of catheter-associated septicaemia. After the first 2 weeks most episodes of catheter-related septicaemia originate from the hub.[1] Exit site infections can be minimized with the use of appropriate dressing such as 'IV 3000' which is permeable to moisture from the skin surface but prevents external water penetration. These infections are recognized by redness and discharge at the catheter exit. Most can be treated with frequent dressings, the use of systemic antibiotics active against the most common pathogens, *Staphylococcus epidermidis* or *Staph. aureus*, should also be considered. Treatment will not succeed when the catheter cuff is located at the exit site, rather than in the mid point of the tunnel. Decontamination of the cuff is unlikely to be achieved, and under these circumstances the catheter will need to be removed. Delay in management will lead to the spread of infection proximal in the skin tunnel.

Tunnel infection leads to a discharge from the exit site, and pain on palpation over the tunnel. Such infections usually occur from retrograde spread from the exit site, rarely infection may spread distally in the tunnel from infected thrombophlebitis in the superior vena cava. Recurrent tunnel infection with the same organism should suggest this possibility. The recognition of a tunnel infection is an indication for the removal of the catheter.

Both exit site and tunnel infections may be accompanied by systemic sepsis. Under these circumstances clinical inspection of the exit site and the tunnel will usually indicate the source of infection.

The intravascular external surface of catheter can also be contaminated during episodes of septicaemia from any source. Management is determined by the underlying condition. When bloodstream infection with aggressive pathogens occurs difficult management decisions are required (see below). Some authorities recommend the prophylactic antibiotic therapy for procedures that may lead to bacteraemia, such as dental treatment, although there is no evidence to support this practice.

Luminal catheter infection

Infection of the internal luminal catheter surface is normally heralded by the sepsis syndrome. Patients become ill with fever and tachycardia, often during the nutrient infusion. Infections gain access from the nutrient infusions or the catheter junctions. With the rare exception of errors during compounding, prospective microbiological studies demonstrate that contamination is usually via the catheter junctions.[1]

Infections are caused by poor techniques for catheter care. The observance of appropriate protocols[2] will almost eliminate the problem in the stable patient; the use of catheter hubs impregnated with iodine and ethanol[3] is no substitute for proper techniques. The introduction of the team approach in the hospital setting has greatly reduced catheter infection.[4] Catheter infection rates in patients who receive home parenteral nutrition (HPN) are currently less than 0.25 per patient year of treatment.[5,6] Undoubtedly some patients are especially prone to infection. These include patients who require opiates for the control of pain.[7] The location of the catheter also influences the risk of infection, the incidence of infection is greater in catheters placed in the inferior vena cava which exit on the thigh.[8]

Catheter-related infection is probable in the previously well patient who suddenly develops features of infection while undergoing PN. Diagnosis can be more difficult in the hospital patients in whom many other possible reasons for infection or illness exist. Fever may reflect other infections such as pneumonia or intra-abdominal infection, or venous thrombosis. All patients with the sepsis syndrome in whom catheter infection is suspected should have blood cultures from peripheral veins and from blood drawn back through the central catheter.[9] The use of quantitative cultures of blood obtained through the central catheter, with a colony count fivefold greater than from peripheral blood, may improve diagnostic precision.[10] Recently an endoluminal brush has been advocated for more accurate diagnosis.[11] However, the brushes that are currently available are only suitable for large diameter Hickman catheters, they will not fit the catheters commonly used for long-term PN.

When patients present with features of catheter infection, parenteral feeding should be discontinued, cultures obtained and a decision made on the continuing need for central parenteral feeding. The practice of immediate catheter removal when symptoms of infection occur is to be discouraged in patients who continue to require central venous access. Other sources of infection are found in up to 80% of these patients.[11,12] The catheter is locked and the patients given antimicrobial therapy pending the results of the blood

cultures. The choice of drug will reflect local policy and the anticipated micro-organism. *Staph. epidermidis* is a common catheter pathogen, a minority of catheters may be infected with *Candidia* spp. Catheters which exit on the thigh may be infected with *Klebsiella* spp.[8] The short-term use of vancomicin and gentamicin will cover most common pathogens until the relevant information is available. If the culture results support the suspected diagnosis of catheter infection management is re-assessed. Removal of the feeding catheter should occur when a central catheter is no longer essential, there is a subcutaneous port, and when there is infection with especially pathogenic micro-organisms.

Clearance of infection can be achieved in many external catheters by the infusion of antibiotic through the catheter.[13] Anecdotal experience suggests that the clearance of infection from a subcutaneous port is unlikely to be successful. A urokinase lock may facilitate antibiotic penetration by dispersing fibrin around the catheter tip.[14] Antibiotic locks may reduce the period necessary to achieve clearance. Some authorities use antibiotic locks for 2 weeks, do not advocate the routine use of systemic antibiotic treatment, and recommence parenteral feeding through the catheter after only 2 days.[13,15] We use systemic antibiotics, and antibiotic alternating with urokinase locks for 2 weeks. Nutrient solutions are not infused through the catheter until after this period, and then only after negative catheter drawback blood cultures have been obtained. Catheter clearance may be successful with organisms such as *Staph. epidermidis*, or *Escherichia coli*, many would argue that there should be no attempt to clear other pathogens such as *Staph. aureus* and particularly fungal infections such as *Candida* spp. The risk of metastatic infection with endocarditis and osteomyelitis is significant.[16] In one study 25% of affected patients developed ocular infection following fungal line sepsis, the author drew attention to the teeth as the source in some of these patients.[17] The need for echocardiography should be considered, especially when presentation has been delayed.

Rare patients are prone to recurrent infections.[17a] Attempts at prophylaxis have been attempted by compounding substances in the nutrition bag which have antimicrobial properties, yet which are safe. One such example is Taurolin, a preparation which contains Taurolidine and povidone. When compounded with the nutrient solutions it has an extensive antimicrobial spectrum including the common pathogens which cause catheter infection.[6] Taurolidine has also been used as a catheter lock after the feed solution is flushed, this was also effective for the prevention of recurrent catheter infection.[18]

In summary, endoluminal infection can be prevented by the careful application of suitable catheter care protocols, when an infection occurs the line should be removed if it is not required, bacterial clearance can be attempted in patients who need prolonged venous access providing there is no evidence of fungal infection and they do not have a subcutaneous port.

Central vein thrombosis

The development of central vein thrombosis during treatment with central PN is a serious complication which may lead to the loss of venous access, a prolonged illness, and even the death of the patient.[19] The incidence of thrombosis during prolonged PN may be assessed by reference to HPN registers. In the UK and Europe it varied from 6% to 9% with 0.06 episodes per annum.[20–22] Whereas the American data suggested the problem was less common, the fact that large numbers of these patients suffered from terminal cancer or AIDS with a short lifespan may have influenced the reported incidence.[23] Furthermore, during central PN thrombosis occurs relatively early with a mean time of 12 or 35 days.[24,25] Thus many episodes will occur during the hospital course and will not be recorded in the registers. Evidence that thrombosis occurs more frequently than previously thought was provided in a study of 255 silicon catheters inserted into 233 patients for nearly 100 catheter-years. There were 35 cases of venous thrombosis, 1 episode for 1033 catheter days.[26]

Following catheter insertion, plasma proteins, preferentially fibrinogen, are adsorbed onto the catheter surface. They attract platelets and activate the intrinsic coagulation pathway. Subsequent conformational change results in the proteins becoming less reactive.[27] A fibrin sleeve encases the catheter. Thrombus may form on the wall of the vessel. These events do not usually lead to clinically significant sequelae in the majority of patients. Risk factors for significant thrombus can be considered in three groups: those relating to the patient, the catheter and the nutrient solution. Sepsis may also be a precipitating factor. Patients with thrombotic tendency due to antithrombin III, protein S or C deficiency or activated protein C resistance (factor V Leiden), are at great risk of central vein thrombosis. There is also evidence of enhanced coagulation in patients with inflammatory bowel disease.[28] Early studies attested to the thrombogenicity of PVC catheters which are no

longer used. Thrombosis is more likely to occur with the catheter tip in the proximal superior vena cava compared to the placement at the distal cava or the junction of the vein and the atrium.[29] This may be due to the closer proximity of potentially thrombogenic nutrient solutions to the vessel wall with proximal placement. Highly concentrated solutions of glucose and amino acids are especially thrombogenic, standard lipid containing mixes of similar energy density rarely cause thrombosis.[25] This clinical observation is supported by *in vitro* and *in vivo* evidence of increased thrombogenicity of glucose amino acid mixes, compared with glucose amino acid lipid mixes.[30,31]

Central vein thrombosis may be recognized clinically by symptoms such as pain in the chest, shoulder, or intrascapular area;[31] or signs of venous occlusion with swelling of ipsilateral arm, or the superior vena cava syndrome (Fig. 32.1). Some patients present with pyrexia that may be mistaken for catheter infection. Thrombus may rarely occlude the catheter, or even encase it so that the infusion fluid tracks back through the exit site. Pulmonary embolism[32] and intracardiac thrombus[33,34] have been described. Infected thrombophlebitis poses a major problem, it may be difficult to establish if the infection or the thrombus occurred first.

The diagnosis of central vein thrombosis is confirmed by bilateral upper limb phlebography, the clot may be proximal to the catheter tip when it is missed with a catheter venography. Doppler ultrasound is a useful alternative method for identifying thrombosed veins, or veins with small lumens prior to catheter insertion.[34a]

Prevention of thrombotic complications involves attention to the catheter tip position, the choice of nutrient infusion and the use of prophylactic anticoagulation. Low dose warfarin in a dose of 1 or 2 mg per day, which does not significantly affect the prothrombin time, may be effective.[35] The commonly used regimen of heparin in a dose of 1 unit per ml of feed solution may not be adequate.[24] Heparin in a dose of 3 units per ml will prevent thrombosis,[36] but there are concerns about lipid stability when mixed with heparin in the feed solution, and in the long-term heparin could promote osteoporosis.

Established thrombosis can be treated with fibrinolysis, streptokinase or TPA, for 48 hours followed by heparin anticoagulation.[25,37] Although data are lacking to guide policy, we leave the central catheter in situ, assuming there is no infection. This is because there is a theoretical risk of dislodging thrombus, central access

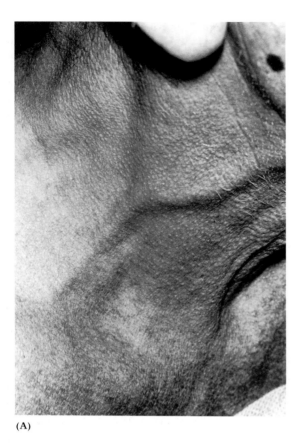

(A)

(B)

Figure 32.1 – (**A**) A patient with central vein thrombosis showing engorged jugular vein. (**B**) Upper limb venography demonstrating central vein thrombosis.

may be required if there is a large pulmonary embolus, and following thrombosis there may be difficulty in regaining central access. Refractory obstruction that threatens venous access or leaves the patient with the superior vena cava syndrome has been treated with expandable metal stents.[38]

Catheter occlusion

Catheter occlusion occurs on account of fibrin, lipid, or amorphous debris. The diagnosis of the cause of occlusion is difficult. When lipid-containing bags are employed the occlusion is more likely to be lipid, with the conventional bags which do not contain lipid, or following blood 'flash back', fibrin may be responsible. Rarely the catheter is intermittently compressed between the first rib and the clavicle. This occurs shortly after placement and is related to posture.[39]

The fibrin sleeve which grows around the catheter may initially form a flap which can act as a valve,[40] thus preventing the aspiration of blood through the catheter when cultures are needed. Occasionally the fibrin may engulf the catheter; this can cause occlusion or the infused fluid may track back around the catheter in the fibrin sack to emerge at the exit site.[41] Blood which gains access to the catheter may cause a thrombotic occlusion. Treatment is with a urokinase lock, 1000 units per ml.[40] When there is a complete block so that urokinase cannot be instilled into the catheter, a syringe containing 1000 units per ml of urokinase is left attached to the end of the catheter for up to 24 hours, following which catheter patency is sometimes restored.[41] The urokinase probably diffuses down the solution in the catheter to reach the fibrin at the tip. Urokinase is preferred to streptokinase which is reserved for major thrombotic episodes.

The use of lipid containing '3 in 1' mixes has caused the deposition of waxy lipid material in the catheter lumen.[42] Resistance in the catheter increases over 2–3 days before there is complete occlusion (Fig. 32.2). The use of a 70% ethanol lock can free such partial occlusions, presumably by the dissolution of the lipid material.[43a] The flushing of this material into the patient did not appear harmful in this report, but it is not desirable. Replacing saline with a flush of 10 ml of 20% ethanol solution, before the application of a heparin lock, appears to prevent this problem.[43]

There have also been reports of catheters becoming occluded with amorphous debris which responds to hydrochloric acid.[44]

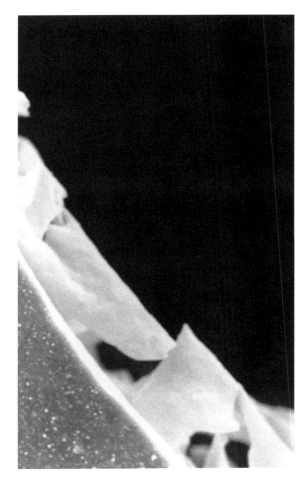

Figure 32.2 – Lipid material deposited on the luminal wall of the catheter which can eventually lead to occlusion. The catheter had been electively removed at the end of a 3-month course of treatment.

Catheter damage

Catheter fracture is hazardous but fortunately rare. With the external catheter there is a risk of air embolism, infection and haemorrhage. Damage to the port will lead to leakage of nutrient solution and pain during infusion. Both external catheters and subcutaneous ports when damaged may lead to catheter embolism.

Fracture of the external catheter usually occurs close to the hub where it has been clamped. Previously the use of an extension tube between the catheter and the giving set was used for clamping and changed at regular intervals. The use of sealed connection devices such as the 'Interlink'®, or polyurethane catheter with terminal switches offer an alternative approach.

Patients with external catheters on HPN are supplied with clamps for use in an emergency should the catheter fracture. They should clamp between the site of damage and the exit site and report to the base hospital where repair kits are available. Failure to clamp a fractured external catheter risks the development of air embolism which may be heralded by central chest pain and hypotension. When the diagnosis is suspected the patients should be placed in a steep Trendelenburg position (head down) in the left lateral decubitus.

The subcutaneous port will eventually leak. Port failure may be recognized by pain during nutrient infusion. When this happens a new port can be connected to an existing catheter. The life of the port can be prolonged by encouraging the patient to access different points on each occasion (Fig. 32.3).

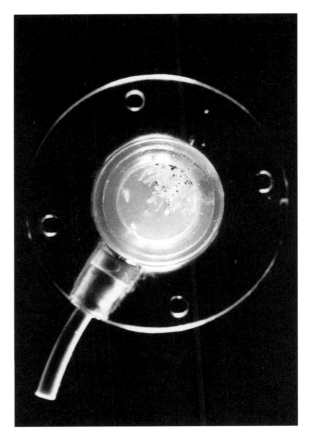

Figure 32.3 – A subcutaneous port; the patient had repeatedly accessed the port in one half of the membrane, this may have led to the premature failure.

Peripheral venous catheters

PN may be delivered by peripheral veins while awaiting central catheter placement, or evaluation of the residual intestinal capacity. Fine-bore peripheral catheters are inserted in a cubital vein and managed with the same care as a central catheter.[45] The main problem is thromboplebitis and infection, some authorities advocate the use of glyceryl trinitrate patches over the vein and hydrocortisone and heparin in the nutrient bag to minimize this complication.[46] The catheter should be removed if redness or tenderness is evident along the vein. The tendency for these very fine catheters to occlude makes cyclical feeding problematic. Cyclical feeding can be delivered through peripheral veins through standard teflon cannulae which are removed after each infusion.[47] PICC lines are unlikely to gain favour in the context of intestinal failure. They are associated with a high incidence of central vein thrombosis, especially when the tip lies proximal to the superior vena cava.[48]

NUTRITIONAL AND METABOLIC PROBLEMS

The administration of excess or insufficient amounts of macronutrients and micronutrients can lead to morbidity, which is avoided by careful prescribing and monitoring.

Macronutrients

Glucose

Hyperglycaemia may develop in the diabetic patient, and when patients are septic. The majority of adult patients are maintained in the range of 25–35 non-protein Kcal/kg body weight. These energy needs are reduced during periods of weaning from parenteral to enteral nutrition and when PN is used as an adjunct to enteral feeding. Energy should be supplied below the estimated needs when initiating PN in the severely depleted or critically ill patient. An upper limit of 40 Kcal/kg should not be exceeded in the adult. The administration of excess glucose leads to lipogenesis and is associated with hyperglycaemia, and increased respiratory demands leading to tachypnoea. Glucose administration should be limited to 4 mg/kg/min in the stressed patient to avoid hyperglycaemia.[49] Hypoglycaemia can accompany the sudden cessation

of parenteral feeding due to the effect of endogenous insulin. The problem can be avoided by the tapering of glucose infusions before the end of the feed.

Lipid

Energy should be provided by a combination of glucose and lipid. This will supply essential fatty acids. The continuous infusion of concentrated glucose solutions leads to hyperinsulinaemia which prevents the mobilization of endogenous lipid. The simultaneous infusion of fat, supplying 30–50% of the energy, with other nutrients in compounded bags, has other metabolic advantages. There is reduced water and electrolyte retention and a reduced propensity to reactive hypoglycaemia after the infusion has been discontinued. The provision of a high fat regimen may have theoretical advantages in the patient with portal systemic encephalopathy by increasing the serum concentration of branched-chain amino acids.

The disadvantages of using fat emulsions include: cost, concern about possible immunosuppressive effects, the risk of catheter occlusion with compounded solutions (in patients who need prolonged PN) and pharmaceutical limitations on stability and shelf-life. Immunosuppressive effects and other potential deleterious consequences of fat emulsions such as pulmonary complications have not been shown to be clinically significant if fat emulsions are infused at appropriate rates.[50] This is ensured if fat emulsions are administered as compounded solutions with amino acids and glucose. Provided that the rate of lipid infusion does not exceed 50 mg/kg/h there is no adverse effect on respiratory function.[51] Hypoxaemia was previously demonstrated with the infusion of 250 ml of 20% lipid over 4 hours, and was attributed to alterations in the production of arachidonic acid metabolites reversing arteriolar constriction found in unventilated pulmonary segments. Similarly, these recommended rates of infusion are not associated with significant effects on immune function.

Micronutrients

Trace elements

Trace elements are provided in most patients in the UK by the prescription of Additrace, 10 ml/day. Measurement of trace element status is recommended in the severely depleted patient and the patient who needs long-term treatment.

The requirements for parenteral trace elements are estimates based on the proportion of trace elements in the diet which are absorbed. This may vary from 1% for chromium to 75% in the case of selenium.[52]

Too little Deficiency syndromes due to the inadequate provision of trace elements have been described especially in patients on long–term PN. Examples include cardiomyopathy due to selenium depletion, diabetes in patients who were not given adequate chromium, and pancytopenia in patients who become deficient in copper.[52,53]

PN has been associated with impairment of the normal renal homeostatic mechanisms for selenium conservation, and increased supplementation may be needed.[54] Additional amounts of some elements such as selenium will be needed in the severely depleted patient. Most commercial trace element solutions provide sufficient nutrient to meet estimated daily needs with no excess provision for the restoration of body stores. Thus patients who are treated by HPN and require less than seven PN bags a week are at risk of selenium deficiency without additional supplementation.[55]

The requirements for trace elements in the critically ill and stressed patient remain uncertain and difficult to estimate. Initiation of the cytokine cascade results in alterations of certain trace elements. For example, a reduction in serum iron and zinc and a rise in serum copper may be seen in the septic state.

Too much Compensatory excretion of trace elements administered in excessive doses may not be achieved. Furthermore copper and manganese are excreted via the biliary tract and the development of cholestatic syndromes will impair excretory capacity necessitating adjustment of prescribed amounts. This has led to the accumulation of manganese, a problem compounded by errors in the estimation of manganese absorption which lead to excessive administration of manganese in PN solutions. Some patients developed neurological toxicity with psychological symptoms and Parkinsonian–like features[56] (Fig. 32.4). However, there are concerns that even with the reduced mangenese content of current trace element solutions such as Additrace®, excessive accumulation has been described in the absence of cholestasis (Fig. 32.4).[57]

Vitamins

The degradation of vitamins in the nutrient solution reduces substantially the amount which is delivered to the patient. Sunlight will degrade vitamin A with the

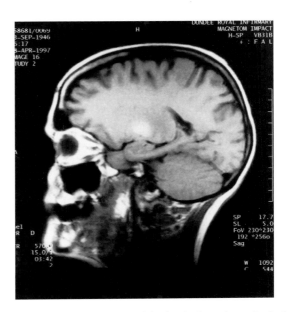

Figure 32.4 – An MRI scan of the head of a patient who had received home parenteral nutrition for 5 years with standard nutrient and trace element solutions (Kabimix and Additrace). He had very high serum concentrations of manganese. The scan shows an increased signal in the basal ganglia compatible with manganese deposition.

loss of 40–98% during a 24–hour infusion.[58] Protection from sunlight will prevent this problem, and the use of multi–layer bags greatly reduces the loss of vitamin C which is susceptible to oxidation.[59] There may be loss of up to 90% of thiamine and 35% of vitamin E when they are compounded with some amino acid solutions which contain sulphite as an anti–oxidant.

The possible need for the administration of thiamine before the initiation of PN in severely under–nourished patients, especially those with a history of alcohol abuse should be considered as requirements increase when the patient becomes anabolic and utilizes carbohydrate.

Water and electrolytes

Whereas patients with high jejunostomies and high output fistulae will need additional water and electrolytes, sodium and water retention can be a problem when malnourished patients are provided regimens in which all the non–protein energy is supplied as carbohydrate. This is a consequence of the anti–natriuretic effect of insulin on the proximal renal tubule. There is evidence that preoperative PN with conventional solutions may lead to water and sodium retention and depression of the serum albumin concentration, it has been suggested that these events could contribute to postoperative respiratory problems.[60] Furthermore the major intracellular electrolytes, potassium, magnesium and phosphorus, are required for protein synthesis. Serum concentrations of these electrolytes may fall rapidly once adequate energy and nitrogen have been provided.[61] Magnesium deficiency is common in undernourished alcoholic patients and in those with excessive gastrointestinal losses such as may occur in Crohn's disease or patients with a jejunostomy. It may be associated with significant hypokalaemia and hypocalcaemia which are resistant to respective supplements. Hypophosphataemia is relatively common and potentially dangerous; it may present with thrombocytopenia, confusion, cardiac dysrythmia and lead to death.[61] The administration of glucose stimulates insulin secretion which increases the transport of glucose and phosphate into the cell; this may result in profound hypophosphataemia in the previously malnourished patient. Such patients should receive phosphate replacement before commencing PN.

The rapid intracellular shifts of magnesium, potassium, phosphate and the increased need for thiamine and folate, which occurs when the severely depleted patient becomes anabolic is described as the 'refeeding syndrome'. This may reflect the switch in fuel from endogenous lipid to exogenous carbohydrate. The need for electrolytes may exceed the capacity of the bag because of stability considerations. Under these circumstances separate infusions will be necessary.

THE EFFECTS OF PN ON ORGAN FUNCTION

Patients who receive PN can develop disorders of organ function which has a direct or indirect relationship to the technique of parenteral feeding (Table 32.3). For example, cardiac problems may arise from atrial thrombus formation, endocarditis and cardiomyopathy due to selenium depletion. The recognition of new cardiac murmurs or unexplained pulmonary emboli should lead to transoesophageal echocardiography. There is impairment of aspects of immune function with lipid formulations, and the failure to stimulate the gut-associated lymphoid tissue; in most patients this is of no obvious clinical significance, and is irrelevant in relation to the problems that arise with starvation. Changes in intestinal function have been described, with increased permeability and microbial

Table 32.3 – The direct and indirect effect of parenteral nutrition on organ function

Organ or system	Effect
Liver	Steatosis Cholestasis Cirrhosis
Gallbladder	Biliary sludge Gallstones
Intestine	Bacterial overgrowth Increased permeability Microbial translocation
Immune system	Immunosuppression
Kidney	Renal impairment
Skeletal	Osteoporosis

translocation. This has mainly been demonstrated in the animal model.[62] The overgrowth of intestinal bacteria, microbial bile acid metabolism, the impairment of the intestinal barrier function which may in part be attributable to the loss of luminal nutrition and absence of glutamine from most conventional PN formulations,[63] could collectively contribute to impaired intestinal and hepatobiliary function. For these reasons, and in particular the need to encourage intestinal adaptation, patients with intestinal failure should be encouraged to take some oral nutrition. Deterioration in renal function in patients on long-term PN has been described.[54] The reason for this observation was not known.

Particular interest has focused on hepatobiliary disease and skeletal abnormalities in patients who need prolonged PN.

Hepatobiliary complications

There are many reasons why patients who need to be fed by the parenteral route may have disease of the liver or biliary tree. Some forms of hepatobiliary disease occur in association with the intestinal disease which is the cause of intestinal failure and the reason for PN. Examples include sclerosing cholangitis and cholelithiasis in Crohn's disease. Hepatobiliary disease can occur as a consequence of the failure to take an oral diet which can promote the increased absorption and translocation of toxins and micro-organisms,[65] and leads to biliary stasis and the formation of biliary sludge.

Liver disorders in patients who receive PN may reflect nutrient deficiency or excess. The lack of glutamine in conventional PN solutions may be a factor in the mucosal barrier dysfunction. The lack of taurine could also be relevant, this amino acid protects against bile acid induced hepatic damage in animals, and stimulates bile flow in infants.[64] Rarely micronutrient deficiencies have been incriminated in the genesis of liver disease; molybdenum deficiency has been associated with cholestasis.[65]

The excess administration of glucose which increases insulin secretion and stimulates acetyl CoA carboxylase, the rate-limiting enzyme for lipid synthesis, will cause hepatic steatosis.[66] The excessive administration of amino acids can cause cholestasis in infants.[67]

Hepatobiliary disease which occurs in the context of PN is multifactoral in origin. Biliary sludge is common in both adults and children, cholestasis predominates in children and steatosis in adults.[68] The recognition of abnormal hepatic function should prompt an assessment of the probable cause in the patient. The introduction of an oral or enteral diet to promote bile flow and improve the gut barrier function, the adjustment of the nutrient prescription, the exclusion of mechanical bile duct obstruction, and the trial of oral antibiotics such as metronidazole are examples of management approaches to the development of liver disease in these patients.

Bone disease

A spectrum of bone disease, osteomalacia, osteoporosis and hyperparathyroid disease, may be present at the onset of treatment due to effects of intestinal disease and corticosteroid treatment. Severe metabolic bone disease was reported with the use of caesein hydrolysates and attributed to the aluminium content of these solutions.[69] In some patients there is an excessive excretion of calcium and phosphorus, this may reflect acidosis associated with rapid nutrient infusion. There have been reports of improvement in the calcium balance by increasing the delivery of phosphorus, and thereby increasing renal tubular absorption of calcium.[70] Osteoporosis has improved after the withdrawal of vitamin D. The effect of vitamin D on the intestinal absorption of calcium is not likely to be relevant when patients are dependent on parenteral feeding while the resorptive effect on bone is a disadvantage.[71] Studies in patients receiving HPN indicate increased bone resorption during the early phase of treatment. Resorption had returned to normal by 6 months.[72]

The recognition of osteoporosis should prompt assessment of calcium and phosphorus provision, consideration of the withdrawal of heparin, the encouragement of exercise and consideration of the use of oestrogen in the female patients with ovarian failure. Use of the latter has to be balanced against the risk of catheter associated central vein thrombosis.

MINIMISING THE PROBLEMS OF PN

Monitoring

Patients require careful monitoring of clinical, laboratory and nutritional indices. Before treatment is commenced the weight and height of the patient should be obtained together with baseline measurements of temperature, pulse and respiratory rate. Baseline laboratory measurements consist of a full blood count, urea and electrolytes which should include calcium, magnesium, and phosphate, as well as liver function tests. The need for a micronutrient screen should be considered in the severely depleted patient, and when prolonged treatment is envisaged. This involves the analysis of vitamins and trace elements, blood has to be obtained using specific equipment to avoid contamination. Trace element kits can be obtained from supra-regional centres where the analysis is performed.

When central lines are used a post insertion chest X-ray must be viewed to confirm that the catheter is in a satisfactory position and to exclude such immediate complications as pneumothorax. No patient should receive PN through any central catheter until the position has been confirmed in this way, regardless of the use of image intensification during insertion.

Charts of temperature, pulse and respiration should be completed to ensure early recognition of septic or metabolic complications. Daily fluctuations in weight of more than 1 kilogram reflect changes in fluid balance. Blood glucose is usually measured 12 hourly for the first 2 days. Persistent hyperglycaemia may require supplemental insulin. Blood is checked for lipaemia after the first day. It is essential that an accurate fluid balance chart is kept and that fluid losses through vomiting or enterocutaneous fistulae are recorded. Additional intravenous fluids may be needed in a few patients with high output fistulae. The exit-site dressing should be changed according to local protocol.

Patients who require long-term treatment will also need monitoring with reference to the underlying disease process, and the possibility of transfer from parenteral to enteral feeding following intestinal adaptation should always be considered. Psychological and social aspects should be considered especially in patients who require prolonged PN.

The frequency with which laboratory measurements are obtained will be governed by the condition of the patient. Unstable patients, and patients who are severely malnourished will require more frequent monitoring often on a daily or less commonly, a twice daily basis. In general, urea and electrolytes should be measured every other day, and liver function and haematological tests twice weekly. Initially, magnesium and phosphate should be included with the electrolyte request, this is especially important in malnourished patients. Twice-weekly 24-hour urine collections for measurement of urea and electrolytes should be obtained. Urinary urea excretion may be used to estimate nitrogen balance. The measurement of the electrolyte content of fistula fluid may also be required. When patients are severely depleted, or when prolonged treatment is necessary trace element status is measured at the outset and thereafter every 6–12 weeks.

Nutritional repletion restores function before structure. At present there are no satisfactory non-invasive bedside tests of function, however, some authorities recommend hand grip dynamometry and measurement of respiratory function tests. Structural measurements include mid-arm circumference and triceps skin fold thickness when prolonged PN is given. Continued weight loss over a long period should alert the clinician to the possibility that PN is inadequate although it must be recognized that this can occur with optimal PN, for instance, in patients with sepsis.

Resources for PN

The management of PN is facilitated by the presence of a nutrition support team.[2] Not only do these teams result in a reduction in PN-related morbidity they also significantly reduce the material costs of PN by rationalizing its use in the hospital and home environment. The nutritional support team may vary in composition and role between different hospitals. Most successful teams will include a nurse specialist in nutrition, a pharmacist, dietitian, biochemist and a clinician. There may, in larger institutions, be more than one team each representing specific areas within the hospital. For example, intensive care, neonatology,

medical gastroenterology and surgery may all have their own groups. Nutrition teams should ideally have an interventional role in patient management and be able to implement previously agreed treatment protocols. There should be a programme for staff education and training. Audit of nutritional practice should be supervised by the nutrition team.

PN can be undertaken on most wards in adequately equipped hospitals. There is, however, an advantage in confining central PN to parts of the hospital with sufficient experience of this treatment to maintain an adequate standard of expertise and practice. Furthermore both the British Society of Gastroenterology, and the British Association for Parenteral and Enteral Nutrition recommend that patients who need HPN are looked after in regional centres which offer appropriate resources.[73]

REFERENCES

1. Linares J, Sitges-Serra A, Garaas J, et al. Pathogenesis of catheter sepsis: a prospective study with quantitative and semi quantitative culture of hub and segments. J Clin Microbiol 1985; 21: 357–360.

2. Sizer T. Standards and Guidelines for Nutritional Support of Patients in Hospitals. A report by a Working Party of the British Association for Parenteral and Enteral Nutrition. 1996.

3. Segura M, Alvarez-Lerma F, Ma Tellado J, et al. A clinical trial on the prevention of catheter-related sepsis using a new hub model. Ann Surg 1996; 223: 363–369.

4. Keohane PP, Jones BJ, Attrill H, Cribb A, et al. Effect of catheter tunnelling and a nutrition nurse on catheter sepsis during parenteral nutrition. A controlled trial. Lancet 1983; 2(8634): 1388–1389.

5. Mughall MM. Complications of intravenous feeding catheters. Br J Surg 1989; 76: 15–21.

6. Johnston DA, Richards K, Pennington CR. Auditing the effect of experience and change on home parenteral nutrition related complications. Clin Nutr 1994; 13: 341–344.

7. Richards DM, Scott NA, Shaffer JL, Irving M. Opiate and sedative dependence predicts a poor outcome for patients receiving home parenteral nutrition. J Parenter Enteral Nutr 1997; 21: 336–338.

8. Rannem T, Ladefoged K, Hegnhoj J, Hylander Moller E, Bruun B, Jarnum S. Catheter-related sepsis in long-term parenteral nutrition with broviac catheters. An evaluation of different disinfectants. Clin Nutr 1990; 9: 131–136.

9. Bozzetti F, Terne G, Bonfanti G. Blood culture as a guide for the diagnosis of central venous catheter sepsis. J Parenter Enteral Nutr 1984; 8: 396–398.

10. Mosca R, Curtas S, Forbes B, Meguid MM. The benefits of isolator cultures in the management of suspected catheter sepsis. *Surgery* 1987; **102**: 718–723.

11. Tighe M, Kite P, Thomas D, Fawley W, McMahon M. Rapid diagnosis of catheter-related sepsis using the acridine orange leukocyte cytospin test and an endoluminal brush. *J Parenter Enteral Nutr* 1996; **20**: 215–218.

12. Pettigrew RA, Lang SDR, Haydock DA, *et al.* Catheter related sepsis on intravenous nutrition: a prospective study of quantitative cultures and guidewire changes for suspected sepsis. *Br J Surg* 1985; **72**: 52–55.

13. Messing B, Man F, Colimon R, *et al.* Antibiotic-Lock technique is an effective treatment of bacterial catheter-related sepsis during parenteral nutrition. *Clin Nutr* 1990; **9**: 220–225.

14. Glynn MFX, Langer B, Jeejeebhoy KN. Therapy for thrombotic occlusion of long-term intravenous alimentation catheters. *J Parenter Enteral Nutr* 1980; **4**: 387–390.

15. Messing B. Catheter sepsis during home parenteral nutrition: use of the antibiotic lock technique. *Nutrition* 1998; **14**: 466–476.

16. Corso FA, Shaul DB, Wolfe BM. Spinal osteomyelitis after TPN catheter-induced septicaemia. *J Parenter Enteral Nutr* 1995; **19**(4): 291–295.

17. Nightingale JMD, Simpson AJ, Towler HMA, Lennard-Jones JE. Fungal feeding-line infections: beware the eyes and teeth. *J R Soc Med* 1995; **88**: 258–263.

17a. O'Keefe SJD, Burnes JU, Thompson RL. Recurrent sepsis in home parenteral nutrition patients: an analysis of risk factors. *J Parenter Enteral Nutr* 1994; **18**(3): 256–263.

18. Jurewitsch B, Lee T, Park J, Jeejeebhoy K. Taurodiline 2% as an antimicrobial lock solution for prevention of recurrent catheter-related bloodstream infections. *J Parenter Enteral Nutr* 1998; **22**(4): 242–244.

19. Pennington CR. Central vein thrombosis during home parenteral nutrition. *Clin Nutr* 1995; **14** (Suppl 1): 52–55.

20. Messing B, Landais P, Goldfarb B, Irving M. Home parenteral nutrition in adults: a multicentre survey in Europe. *Clin Nutr* 1989; **8**: 3–9.

21. O'Hanrahan T, Irving MH. The role of home parenteral nutrition in the management of intestinal failure – report of 400 cases. *Clin Nutr* 1992; **11**: 331–336.

22. Schmidt-Somerfield E, Snyder G, Rossi TM, Lebenthal E. Catheter-related complications in 35 children and adolescents with gastrointestinal disease receiving home parenteral nutrition. *J Parenter Enteral Nutr* 1990; **14**: 148–151.

23. Oley Foundation. North American home parenteral and enteral patient registry: annual report with patient profiles, 1985–1990. 1992.

24. Bozzetti F, Scarpa D, Terno G, *et al.* Subclavian vein thrombosis due to indwelling catheters: A prospective study on 52 patients. *J Parenter Enteral Nutr* 1983; **7**: 560–562.

25. Pithie AD, Pennington CR. The incidence, aetiology and management of central vein thrombosis during parenteral nutrition. *Clin Nutr* 1987; **6**: 151–153.

26. Gould JR, Carloss HW, Skinner WL. Groshong catheter-associated subclavian venous thrombosis. *Am J Med* 1993; **95**: 419–423.

27. Forbes CD, Courtney JM. Thrombosis and artificial surfaces. In: Bloom L, Thomas D (eds) *Haemostasis and Thrombosis.* Churchill Livingstone: Edinburgh, 1987, pp. 902–921.

28. Williams N, Wales S, Scott N A, Irving MH. Incidence and management of catheter occlusion in patients on home parenteral nutrition. *Clin Nutr* 1993; **12**: 344–349.

29. Pithie A, Soutar S, Pennington CR. Catheter tip position in central venous thrombosis. *J Parenter Enteral Nutr* 1988; **12**: 613–614.

30. Wakefield A, Cohen Z, Craig M, *et al.* Thrombogenicity of total parenteral nutrition solutions: I. Effect on induction of monocyte/macrophage procoagulant activity. *Gastroenterology* 1989; **97**: 1210–1219.

31. Wakefield A, Cohen Z, Rosenthal A, *et al.* Thrombogenicity of total parenteral nutrition solutions: II. Effect on induction of endothelial cell procoagulant activity. *Gastroenterology* 1989; **97**: 1220–1228.

31a. Passaro ME, Steiger E, Curtas S, Seidner DL. Long-term silastic catheters and chest pain. *J Parenter Enteral Nutr* 1994; **18**(3): 240–242.

32. Leiby JM, Purcell H, De Maria JJ, *et al.* Pulmonary embolism as a result of Hichman Catheter related thrombosis. *Am J Med* 1989; **86**: 228–231.

33. Champsi-Pasha H, Irving MH. Right atrial thrombus, a complication of total parenteral nutrition in an adult. *Br Med J* 1987; **295**: 308.

34. McCulloch I, Pennington CR. Intracardiac thrombus complicating prolonged parenteral nutrition in an adult. *J Parenter Enteral Nutr* 1989; **13**: 557–559.

34a. McIntyre AS, Gertner DJ, Levison RA, Wood S, Phillips RHS, Lennard-Jones JE. Central venous thrombosis and intravenous nutrition: problems of venous access and assessment by Doppler ultrasound. *Gut* 1990; **31**: A590–591.

35. Bern MM, Lockich J, Wallach SR, *et al.* Very low doses of warfarin can prevent thrombosis in central venous catheters. *Ann Int Med* 1990; **112**: 423–428.

36. Fabri PJ, Mirtallo JM, Ruberg RL, et al. Incidence and prevention of thrombosis of subclavian vein. Surg Gynaecol Obstet 1982; **155**: 238–240.

37. Barclay GR, Pennington CR. Tissue plasminogen activator in the management of superior vena cava thrombosis associated with parenteral nutrition. Postgrad Med J 1990; **66**: 398–400.

38. Hemphill DJ, Sniderman KW, Allard JP. Case report: Management of total parenteral nutrition-related superior vena cava obstruction with expandable metal stents. J Parenter Enteral Nutr 1996; **20**(3): 222–227.

39. Andris DA, Krzywda EA, Schulte W, Ausman R, Quebbeman EJ. Pinch-off syndrome: A rare aetiology for central venous catheter occlusion. J Parenter Enteral Nutr 1994; **18**(6): 531–533.

40. Schneider TC, Krywda E, Andris D, Quebbman EJ. The malfunctioning silastic catheter: radiological assessment and treatment. J Parenter Enteral Nutr 1986; **10**: 70–73.

41. Rich AJ. The surgical management of venous access. In: Donnelly TK, Watkin E (eds) Access 88 Symposium Proceedings. Quest Design Studios: Hertford, 1990.

42. Erdman SH, McElwee RN, Kramer Jan M, Zuppan CW, White JJ, Grill BB. Central line occlusion with three-in-one nutrition admixtures administered at home. J Parenter Enteral Nutr 1994; **18**(2): 177–181.

43. Johnston DA, Walker K, Richards J, Pennington CR. Ethanol flush for the prevention of catheter occlusion. Clin Nutr 1992; **11**: 97–100.

43a. Pennington CR, Pithie AD. Ethanol lock in the management of catheter occlusion. J Parenter Enteral Nutr 1987; **8**: 507–508.

44. Werlin S, Lausten T, Jessen S, et al. Treatment of central venous catheter occlusions with ethanol and hydrochloric acid. J Parenter Enteral Nutr 1995; **19**: 416–418.

45. Payne-James J, Kwaja HT. First choice for total parenteral nutrition: the peripheral route. J Parenter Enteral Nutr 1993; **17**: 468–471.

46. Tighe MJ, Wong C, Martin IG, McMahon MJ. Do heparin, hydrocortisone, and glyceryl trinitrate influece thrombophlebitis during full intravenous nutrition via a peripheral vein? J Parenter Enteral Nutr 1995; **19**(6): 507–509.

47. May J, Murchan P, MacFie J, Sedman P, Donat R, Palmer D, Mitchell CJ. Prospective study of the aetiology of infusion phlebitis and line failure during peripheral parenteral nutrition. Br J Surg 1996; **83**: 1091–1094.

48. Kearns PJ, Coleman S, Wehner JH. Complications of long arm-catheters: a randomised trial of central vs peripheral tip location. J Parenter Enteral Nutr 1996; **20**: 20–24.

49. Rosmarin D, Wardlaw G, Mirtallo J. Hyperglycaemia associated with high, continuous infusion rates of total parenteral nutrition dextrose. Nutr Clin Pract 1996; **11**: 151–156.

50. Ota DM, et al. Immune function during intravenous administration of a soybean oil emulsion. J Parenter Enteral Nutr 1985; **9**(1): 23–27.

51. Askanazi J, et al. Nutrition for the patient with respiratory failure: Glucose vs fat. Anaesthesiology 1981; **54**: 373–377.

52. Elia M. Changing concepts of nutrient requirements in disease: Implications for artificial nutritional support. Lancet 1995; **1**: 279–1284.

53. Wasa M, Stani M, Tanano H, Nezu R, Takagi Y, Okada A. Copper deficiency with pancytopenia during total parenteral nutrition. J Parenter Enteral Nutr 1994; **18**: 190–192.

54. Buchman AL, Moukarzel A, Ament ME. Selenium renal homeostasis is impaired in patients receiving long-term total parenteral nutrition. J Parenter Enteral Nutr 1994; **18**(3): 231–233.

55. Malone M, Shenkin A, Fell GS, Irving MH. Evaluation of a trace element preparation in patients receiving home intravenous nutrition. Clin Nutr 1989; **8**: 307–312.

56. Mirowitz SA, Westrich TJ, Hirsh JD. Hyperintense basal ganglia on TI weighed images in patients receiving parenteral nutrition. Radiology 1991; **181**: 117–120.

57. Reynolds N, Blumsohn A, Baxter J, Houston G, Pennington CR. Manganese requirement and toxicity in patients on home parenteral nutrition. Clin Nutr 1998; **17**: 227–230.

58. La France RJ, Miyagawa CI. Pharmaceutical considerations in total parenteral nutrition. In: Fischer JE (ed) Total Parenteral Nutrition, 2nd edn. Little Brown: Boston, 1991, pp. 57–92.

59. Allwood MC, Brown PW, Ghenddini C, Hardy G. The stability of ascorbic acid in TPN parenteral nutrition admixtures stored in a multilayered bag. Clin Nutr 1992; **11**: 284–290.

60. Gil MJ, Franch G, Guirao X, Oliva A, Sitges-Serra. Response of severely malnourished patients to pre-operative parenteral nutrition: a randomised clinical trial of water and sodium restriction. Nutrition 1997; **13**(1) 26–31.

61. Solomon SN, Kirby DS. The refeeding syndrome: a review. J Parenter Enteral Nutr 1990; **14**: 90–95.

62. Silk DBA, Grimble GK. Dietary nucleotide and gut mucosal defence. Gut 1994; (Suppl 1): S46–S51.

63. Bengmark S. Econutrition and health maintenance – a new concept to prevent GI inflammation, ulceration and sepsis. Clin Nutr 1996; **15**: 1–10.

64. Dorvil NP, Yousek M, Uchweber B. Taurine prevents cholestasis induced by lithocholic acid in guinea pigs. *Am J Clin Nutr* 1983; **37**: 221–230.

65. Fisher RL. Hepatobiliary disorders associated with total parenteral nutrition. *Gastroenterol Clin N Am* 1989; **18**: 645–667.

66. Kaminski DI, Dams A, Jellink M. The effect of hyperalimentation on hepatic liquid content and lipogenic enzyme activity in rats and man. *Surgery* 1980; **88**: 93–98.

67. Black DD, Suttle EA, Whittington PF. The effect of short-term parenteral nutrition on hepatic function in the human neonate. A prospective randomised study demonstrating alteration of hepatic canalicular function. *J Paediatrics* 1981; **99**: 445–454.

68. Quigley EMM, Marsh MN, Shaffer JL, Markin RS. Hepatobiliary complications of total parenteral nutrition. *Gastroenterology* 1993; **104**: 286–301.

69. Shike M, Harrison JE, Sturtridge WC, *et al.* Metabolic bone disease in patients receiving long-term total parenteral nutrition. *Ann Int Med* 1980; **92**: 343–350.

70. Wood RJ, Sitrin MD, Cusson CJ, Rosenberg IH. Reduction of total parenteral nutrition induced urinary calcium loss by increasing the phosphorus in the TPN prescription. *J Parenter Enteral Nutr* 1986; **10**: 188–190.

71. Verhage AH, Cheong WK, Allard JP, Jeejeebhoy KN. Increase in lumbar spine bone mineral content in patients on long term parenteral nutrition without vitamin D supplementation. *J Parenter Enteral Nutr* 1995; **19**: 431–436.

72. Pironi L, Maghetti A, Zolezzi C, *et al.* Bone turnover in patients on home parenteral nutrition: a longitudinal observation by biochemical markers. *Clin Nutr* 1996; **15**(4): 157–163.

73. Wood S, Shaffer J, Wheatley C. Home parenteral nutrition: Quality criteria for clinical services and the supply of nutrient fluids and equipment. *BAPEN* 1995;

Section 8

Surgical treatment of intestinal failure

33

Surgery for patients with a short bowel

Jon S. Thompson

*T*here are two important roles for surgical procedures in the management of patients with a short bowel. One is the management of complications related to the massive intestinal resection and the resulting pathophysiology. The other is to employ surgical procedures therapeutically to maximize the function of existing intestine.

SURGICAL MANAGEMENT OF COMPLICATIONS

Approximately 50% of patients with a short bowel will require re-operation after their initial time in hospital.[1] These procedures are most frequently required for intestinal problems, cholelithiasis and gastric hypersecretion. The important aspects of management are shown in Table 33.1.

Table 33.1 – Surgical management of complications

Intestinal problems
- Preserve intestinal remnant length

Cholelithiasis
- Early diagnosis
- Prophylactic cholecystectomy

Peptic ulcer disease
- Medical therapy
- Avoid resection if operation required

Intestinal problems

Two-thirds of re-operations in patients with a short bowel are for intestinal problems. Many are related to the underlying intestinal disease, requiring further resection or management of obstruction or fistula. During these procedures an important goal is to preserve as much of the intestinal remnant as possible. There are several strategies that can be used to preserve intestinal length when further intestinal disease occurs in patients with short intestinal remnants. These include employing intestinal tapering for dilated segments, stricturoplasty for strictures and serosal patches for strictures and perforations to avoid resection[2] (Fig. 33.1). If resection is necessary, minimal resection should be performed whenever possible. End-to-end anastomosis is preferred when maintaining length is the goal. Whereas normally a surgeon might discard a few inches of intestine to avoid another anastomosis, this should be given careful consideration in patients with a short bowel where each additional centimetre of bowel becomes significant.

Cholelithiasis

As discussed in Chapter 14, cholelithiasis occurs in approximately one-third of patients with a short bowel.[3–6] These patients have a significantly increased risk of developing cholelithiasis when the remnant length is less than 120 cm, total parenteral nutrition (TPN) is required and the terminal ileum is resected.[4] Furthermore, these patients have more complicated biliary tract disease and increased postoperative morbidity and mortality rates.[3,4] In one study, 40% of these procedures were performed as an emergency, with a complication rate of 54% and mortality of 11%.[3] Delay in diagnosis may contribute to this outcome, particularly because of the confounding effect of PN-induced liver disease. Thus, the diagnosis should be suspected and ultrasonography performed liberally to permit early diagnosis. The significant morbidity of symptomatic cholelithiasis in these patients has led to recommendation of prophylactic cholecystectomy, even before cholelithiasis develops.[3,4] This is particularly appropriate in patients with benign conditions and anticipated long-term survival. While cholecystectomy may not be advisable at the time of the initial massive resection, it should be considered at the time of other abdominal operations.

Gastric hypersecretion

Patients with a short bowel may develop hypergastrinaemia and gastric hypersecretion.[7] This problem is usually transient but lasts several months and may be associated with complications of peptic ulcer disease. While the majority of patients respond to medical management, we found that one-third of our patients with a short bowel who developed peptic ulcer disease required operation.[1] The most desirable procedure would be the one that is least disruptive to normal digestive function. Thus, a highly selective vagotomy is performed if possible.[8] However, we have found that resection is often required because of the severe nature of the peptic ulcer disease.

SURGICAL THERAPY FOR PATIENTS WITH A SHORT BOWEL

The goal of surgical therapy is to increase intestinal absorptive capacity by either improving absorption by existing intestine or by increasing the area of absorption (Table 33.2). Absorption can often be

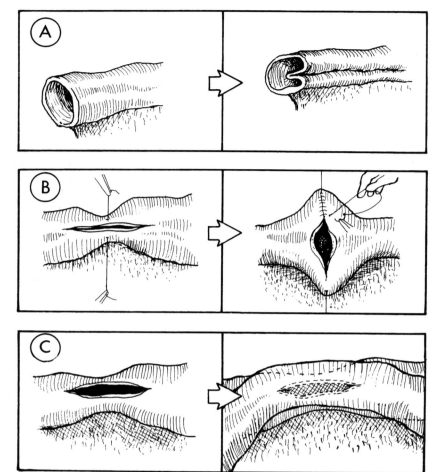

Figure 33.1 – Techniques for preserving intestinal length include tapering of dilated segments rather than resection (**A**), stricturoplasty for strictures (**B**), and serosal patches for strictures and perforated (**C**). Reproduced with permission from Thompson JS, Recent advances in the surgical treatment of the short bowel syndrome. *Surg Annu* 1990; **22**: 110.

Table 33.2 – Surgical therapy for patients with a short bowel

---

Optimize intestinal function
- Restore continuity
- Relieve obstruction
- Taper dilated bowel

Slow intestinal transit
- Reversed intestinal segment
- Artificial valve
- Colon interposition

Increase intestinal length
- Intestinal lengthening

---

improved by recruiting additional intestine into continuity, relieving obstruction, or slowing intestinal transit. Intestinal lengthening is feasible in selected patients but obviously the most significant increase in length is achieved by intestinal transplantation (Chapter 34).

Adjunctive procedures for surgical therapy of patients with a short bowel should not be performed at the time of initial resection.[9,10] They add potential morbidity in patients who are already quite ill. Furthermore, intestinal adaptation, in patients with retained ileum and/or colon, will often result in sufficient improvement in absorption to obviate the need for additional therapy. This is particularly true in children, where additional growth occurs. Adaptation avoided the need for PN in almost half of patients in our experience.[11] Moreover, there is evidence to suggest that performing such procedures, e.g. colon interposition and serosal patching, at the initial resection may diminish the degree of adaptation that occurs.[11,12] Thus, surgical therapy for patients with a short bowel should only be undertaken after the initial adaptive period and even then with specific objectives in mind.

The nature of nutritional support is the primary factor to be considered when surgical therapy for patients with a short bowel is contemplated. Patients supported by enteral nutrition (EN) alone should be considered for operation only if they demonstrate worsening malabsorption, are at risk for receiving PN or have other symptoms related to malabsorption. Patients who are stable on PN should undergo surgical therapy only if this would permit them to discontinue or markedly reduce PN. Patients who develop significant complications from PN will eventually require either combined liver–intestine or solitary intestine transplantation.

Optimising intestinal function

Recruiting any additional intestine into continuity with the gastrointestinal tract is an important objective in managing patients with a short bowel. Intestinal absorptive capacity can be increased and transit time prolonged. Recruiting downstream intestine may simply entail exchanging a more proximal jejunostomy for a more distal colostomy or actually closing a stoma. However, occasionally other intestinal segments are available as well. We have recently restored to continuity an ileal segment previously used as a urinary conduit in a patient with a short bowel; this ameliorated diarrhoea and steatorrhoea.[13]

Many patients have stomas created at the time of massive resection.[14] Whether or not intestinal continuity should be restored at a later time will depend on several factors, including length of intestinal remnant, status of the ileocaecal valve and colon and the overall condition of the patient. While some persons function well with very short intestinal remnants, generally at least a metre of small intestine is required to prevent severe diarrhoea and perianal complications.[14,15] We found that only 20% of the patients with an initial stoma had intestinal continuity restored at a later time.[14] Moreover, only one-third of the patients in whom continuity was maintained at initial resection had a satisfactory long-term outcome. In addition to improving absorption, maintaining intestinal continuity eliminates the inconvenience of the stoma. This has more than psychological advantages since patients with a stoma are more likely to have venous catheter infections.[16] Furthermore, malabsorbed carbohydrates that reach the colon are metabolized to short-chain fatty acids by colonic bacteria.[17] Short-chain fatty acids improve fluid and electrolyte absorption, are absorbed as additional energy and may be trophic to the intestinal remnant.[17,18]

There are a number of potential disadvantages to restoring intestinal continuity. Bile acids cause secretion of fluid in the colon and may exacerbate diarrhea. Thus, there may be more perianal complications and resultant dietary restrictions. In our experience 60% of patients had dietary restrictions with intestinal continuity compared to 33% with a stoma.[14] Also, calcium oxalate kidney stones occur more frequently because of absorption of unbound oxalate from the colon (Chapter 15). In one study no patients with a jejunostomy had nephrolithiasis compared to one-fourth of patients with a short bowel and an intact colon.[6]

Predicting the functional outcome after restoring intestinal continuity in individual patients with short remnants is difficult. In general, Carbonnel et al.[19] found that a jejuno-ileal anastomosis is equivalent to adding 80 cm of small bowel and a jejuno-colic anastomosis equivalent to 25 cm of small bowel in terms of improved absorptive function compared to a jejunostomy. Patients with a marked increase in stomal output in response to feeding will not do well unless a significant amount of small intestine is recruited distally. Assessing the effect of the distal bowel on absorption has been evaluated by using an external reinfusion apparatus.[20] This technique is somewhat cumbersome and requires access to the distal remnant. If distal reinfusion of stomal effluent into a mucous fistula results in a decreased stoma output, then restoring continuity is likely to be of benefit.

The proximal intestine may become markedly dilated secondary to chronic obstruction and/or structural adaptation in patients with a short bowel. In adults this is usually due to obstruction secondary to stenosis. A useful approach in these patients is simply to relieve the obstruction. We have found stricturoplasty to be efficacious.[11] Dilated bowel is less frequently due to obstruction in children and may be a variant of intestinal pseudo-obstruction. The resultant stasis and bacterial overgrowth further aggravates malabsorption. These large diameter segments of intestine have low contraction pressures that result in poor propulsion.[21] Therefore, tapering dilated segments should improve motility in these patients.

Intestinal tapering

Intestinal tapering has been reported in at least 27 children with a short bowel and dilated intestine.[11,21,22] Absorptive function, growth and development improved in all cases. All of our patients had bacterial overgrowth but only one-fourth had an associated mechanical obstruction.[11] In our experience all patients had transient functional improvement but two of 11 required further procedures for recurrent mal-absorption. Many patients experienced a prolonged postoperative ileus. Segments ranging from 15 to 35 cm in length were tapered on the antimesenteric border. Tapering can be accomplished by either resection or simply turning in the redundant tissue. Overlapping the redundant intestine results in more normal intestinal structure and function than tapering by longitudinal transection and is the preferred approach.[23]

Slowing intestinal transit

The earliest surgical attempts at therapy for patients with a short bowel involved techniques for retarding intestinal transit.[24] These have included antiperistaltic segments, artificial valves, colon interposition and other approaches (Fig. 33.2). These procedures are most appropriate in patients with sufficient intestinal surface area but rapid intestinal transit. Massive intestinal resection results in markedly shortened intestinal transit time, which contributes to mal-absorption and diarrhoea. Clinical experience with these procedures is summarized in Table 33.3.

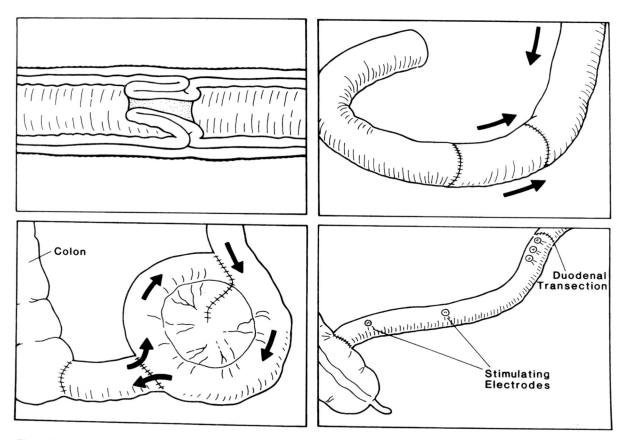

Figure 33.2 – Techniques for slowing intestinal transit: Intestinal valve (upper left), antiperistaltic segment (upper right), recirculating loop (lower left) and intestinal pacing (lower right). Reproduced with permission from Thompson JS, *et al.* Surgical alternatives for the short bowel syndrome. *Am J Gastroent* 1987; **82**: 97–106.

Table 33.3 – Non-transplant procedures to prolong transit for patients with a short bowel

Procedure	Number	References	Clinical improvement (%)	Children (%)
Reversed segment	40	Carbonnel et al., 1996[19] Dorney et al., 1985[35] Lopes-Perez et al., 1981[38] Careskey et al., 1981[39] Sawchuk et al., 1987[40]	80	15
Intestinal valve	6	Carbonnel et al., 1996[19] Kurz and Sauer, 1983[30] Pigot et al., 1990[31]	67	16
Colon interposition	10	Sidhu et al., 1985[49] Carner and Raju, 1981[50] Belin et al., 1972[51] Garcia et al., 1981[52] Glick et al., 1984[53]	60	90
Pouch or loop	4	Watkins et al., 1984[57] Camprodon et al., 1975[58] Poth, 1969[59]	25	25
Intestinal pacing	1	Devine and Kelly, 1989[65]	0	0

Antiperistaltic segments

Reversing segments of intestine to slow intestinal transit has been studied extensively. The antiperistaltic segment acts as a 'physiologic valve' by causing retrograde peristalsis and disrupting the motility of the proximal intestine. The disruption of the intrinsic nerve plexus slows distal myoelectrical activity.[25] Although retrograde peristalsis has been demonstrated radiologically, this finding does not always correlate with improved function.[26] Antiperistaltic segments slow intestinal transit, improve absorption, reduce weight loss and prolong survival after intestinal resection in some experimental studies but others report no beneficial effect.[15–29] These conflicting results may be partly explained by the different lengths of antiperistaltic segments used. While the ideal length of the antiperistaltic segment is not clear, lengthy segments may produce significant obstruction and short segments may be ineffective. In one study an intestinal valve was more effective than an antiperistaltic segment in prolonging transit time after resection, but neither procedure improved absorption.[29]

Antiperistaltic segments have been used clinically in more than 40 patients, the majority being adults.[11,27,30–32] Slowed intestinal transit and increased absorption with resultant clinical improvement have been reported in 80% of patients. However, transient obstructive symptoms and anastomotic leak are potential problems.[27,31] While the length of the segment has varied from 5 to 15 cm in these reports, the ideal length of the reversed segment seems to be approximately 10 cm in adults and 3 cm in children. In one study a reversed segment that initially increased absorption could not be demonstrated radiologically 6 months later.[33] Furthermore, initial manometric abnormalities in the proximal intestine may resolve with time which also raises questions about long-term function with this procedure.[34] A limitation of this procedure is that patients with shorter intestinal remnants may not be able to afford to sacrifice a 10-cm segment for reversal.

Intestinal valves and sphincters

The terminal ileum and ileocaecal valve may be important in retarding intestinal transit of nutrients and preventing reflux of colonic contents. The presence of colonic contents in the small intestine may alter motility and may contribute to bacterial colonization of the small intestine and further malabsorption. An intact ileocaecal valve permits survival in children with only 11 cm of small intestine remaining, whereas those who lost their ileocaecal valve required at least 25 cm of small intestine for survival without PN.[35]

Intestinal valves and sphincters have been created by a variety of different techniques. These include constricting the intestine externally, denervating segments of intestine and increasing intraluminal pressure by intussuscepting intestinal segments.[36-43] We have generally created a sphincter similar to that employed in the continent ileostomy procedure but only 2 cm in length.[11] The effect of valves and sphincters on intestinal motility is complex, involving several different mechanisms. They create a partial mechanical obstruction, prevent retrograde reflux of colonic contents and disrupt the normal motor pattern of the small intestine, converting jejunal motor activity to a pattern more similar to the ileum.[36,38,42] While intestinal valves and sphincters have been shown to lengthen transit time, increase absorptive capacity and prolong survival in several experimental studies, results have been inconsistent.[36-40] Effective valves usually cause some dilation of the proximal intestine and may result in obstructive symptoms. Necrosis of the valve, complete obstruction and intussusception are potential complications. Valves may lose the sphincter function with time.[38]

Clinical experience with intestinal valves and sphincters has been limited. Intussuscepted valves have been reported in six patients with a short bowel.[11,42,43] Four patients improved markedly, one remained unchanged and the other had an obstruction necessitating take down of the valve. However, in one long-term study ileocolic nipple valves were lost in one-third of patients followed for more than 5 years.[44] As described below, nipple valves have recently been utilized to cause dilation of the intestine to permit subsequent intestinal lengthening.[45]

Colon interposition

Isoperistaltic and antiperistaltic colon interposition will retard intestinal transit. Isoperistaltic transposition is performed proximally and functions by slowing down the rate at which nutrients are delivered to the distal small intestine.[12,46] The antiperistaltic colon interposition is placed distally, similar to the reversed small intestinal segment, but has the advantage that none of the small intestine remnant is used. In addition to the effect on transit time, interposed segments absorb water, electrolytes and nutrients.[47] Experimental studies demonstrate that isoperistaltic colon interposition, either proximal or distal to the small intestinal remnant, resulted in slower transit time, less weight loss and increased survival without producing intestinal obstruction.[46-48] While one investigator also demonstrated prolonged transit time with isoperistaltic colon interposition, no significant improvement in body

weight or intestinal absorption was found.[12] The length of colon interposed seems to be less critical than with reversed segments. However, results with antiperistaltic colon interposition have been less consistent.[49,50]

The use of colon interposition has been reported in ten patients. Isoperistaltic interposition was performed in nine of these patients, of whom eight were infants less than 1 year of age.[51-55] The length of colon interposed varied between 8 and 24 cm. All patients were dependent on PN and had intestinal remnants ranging from 15 to 63 cm in length. Four infants were weaned off PN within 4 months and survived. Diarrhoea improved in one infant who subsequently died of pneumonia. Three patients did not improve and subsequently died of sepsis or hepatic failure. An adult patient had transit time prolonged from 10 to 25 minutes and a 50% reduction in PN.[54] Thus, isoperistaltic colon interposition has shown some promise as a therapeutic alternative. In a single report of antiperistaltic colon interposition, an infant eventually died after initial increase in weight and slowing of intestinal transit time.[55]

Recirculating loops

Theoretically, intestinal pouches and recirculating loops would prolong transit time by permitting repeated or prolonged exposure of luminal nutrients to the intestinal absorptive surface. However, these procedures have been associated with high morbidity and mortality rates in experimental studies and do not clearly improve absorption or survival rates after massive resection.[56,57] The results of few anecdotal clinical reports using recirculating loops have not demonstrated clear benefit.[58-60] The three adults were followed for 7, 10 and 24 months. Two died and increased absorption was not clearly demonstrated. Cywes[61] previously created a proximal jejunal pouch with a distal 4-cm antiperistaltic segment in an infant. After 3 months transit time was prolonged, but improved absorption was not demonstrated.

Retrograde electrical pacing

Retrograde electrical pacing has also been investigated as a means of prolonging transit time.[62-64] This promotes peristalsis in a reverse direction and also alters the motility of non-paced intestine, presumably through a hormonal mechanism.[64] In experimental studies, postcibal retrograde pacing improved absorption of water and minerals after intestinal resection.[62,63] In addition, weight loss and faecal fat and nitrogen excretion were decreased.

Intestinal pacing has been used clinically in only one patient with a short bowel, but the pacemaker failed to stimulate the intestine.[65] In humans, the natural pacemaker potential frequency is similar throughout the length of the small intestine. Intestinal transection does not alter the pacemaker frequency of the distal intestine.[66] Because the pacemaker frequency cannot be increased above the natural rate in the intact intestine, it may not, in fact, be feasible to entrain the intestine to achieve retrograde pacing in humans.[67]

Increasing intestinal length

Intestinal tapering and lengthening, which has the attraction of not only tapering the dilated intestine but also using the redundant intestine for additional

length, was initially described by Bianchi.[68] Dissection is performed longitudinally between the blood vessels on the mesenteric border of the intestine, allocating vessels to either side of the intestinal wall (Fig. 33.3). A relatively avascular plane can be developed because these vessels enter the intestine from either side of midline. The intestine is then transected longitudinally with clamps or a stapler. The resultant parallel intestinal segments are then anastomosed end–to–end so that the initial dilated segment becomes a segment of one-half the diameter and twice the length. In the short-term this procedure disrupts motor activity and alters the hormonal response to resection.[69] However, long-term patency and function of divided segments has been demonstrated with resultant improved absorption.

Intestinal lengthening has been reported in more

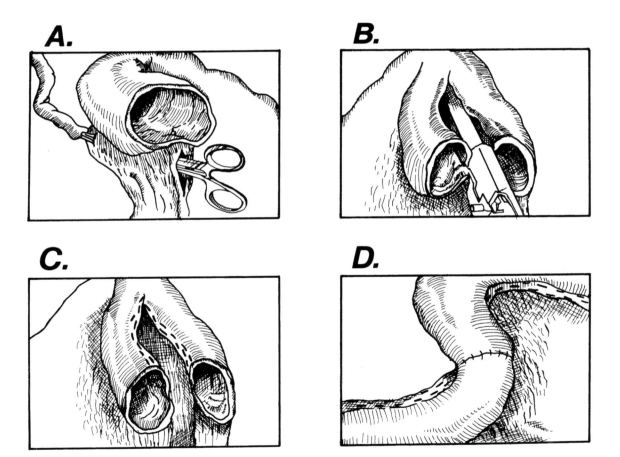

Figure 33.3 – Intestinal tapering and lengthening. Dissection longitudinally between the blood vessels on the mesenteric border (**A**) permits the stapler to be used to divide the bowel longitudinally (**B** and **C**). The two parallel segments are then anastomosed end-to-end (**D**). Reproduced with permission from Thompson JS, Recent advances in the surgical treatment of the short bowel syndrome. *Surg Annu* 1990; **22**: 110.

than 50 children ranging in age from 1 day to 19 years.[45,68,70,71] Bacterial overgrowth and complications of TPN were present frequently. Significant improvement in nutritional status occurred in approximately 90% of patients in these reports. Follow-up now extends 10 years in many patients. Segments as long as 55 cm have been tapered and lengthened. Complications have been reported in 20% of cases. In one of our patients in whom a 25-cm segment of proximal intestine was divided longitudinally, one-half of the divided segment became ischaemic and required resection. Intestinal motility is slow to return in these patients and gastrostomy tubes are frequently used. Two deaths have been reported, one as a result of sepsis related to an anastomotic leak and the other because of hepatic failure. The deaths have been reported in the youngest patients, 1 day and 3 months old. Thus, although intestinal lengthening is beneficial in selected patients with a short bowel, the procedure should be applied cautiously because there is the risk of jeopardizing the divided segments. The vascular anatomy must be favourable and the intestinal diameter of the segment to be tapered should be at least 4 cm.

At present intestinal lengthening can only be applied to a fairly select group of patients. They must have a short remnant and an intestinal diameter greater than 4 cm. Thus, there has been recent interest in sequential procedures, first employing a distal valve or sphincter to dilate the proximal bowel and then performing the lengthening procedure.[45] Alternative methods to increase blood supply to isolated segments (e.g. from liver or omentum) and thus, permit repeated lengthening have also been investigated.[72]

Another potential technique for expanding the intestinal surface area takes advantage of the regenerative capability of the intestine. Intestinal regeneration will occur in full thickness intestinal defects patched with a variety of surfaces, including adjacent serosal surfaces. Whether or not sufficient mucosa can be produced by intestinal patching to significantly increase intestinal absorption remains unclear.[10] Further experimental study is necessary to assess the safety and efficacy of this approach. Clinical experience with intestinal patching to increase absorptive surface in patients with a short bowel has not been reported. This remains a useful technique, however, for managing intestinal defects and strictures when it is desirable to avoid resection.

SUMMARY

The choice of surgical therapy for patients with a short bowel is influenced by intestinal length, intestinal function and the caliber of the intestinal remnant (Table 33.4). Procedures designed to optimize intestinal function by recruiting additional intestine, relieving obstruction, or tapering dilated bowel are usually appropriate when feasible. A reversed intestinal segment is the most frequently reported procedure for prolonging intestinal transit and appears to be efficacious in the short-term. There has been less clinical experience with colon interposition and intestinal valves but they might also have merit in selected patients. Intestinal lengthening has proven efficacy in patients with dilated intestinal segments. Unfortunately, only a small proportion of patients with

Table 33.4 – Surgical options for patients with a short bowel

Remnant length	Clinical condition	Surgical options
Remnant > 120 cm	Normal diameter Enteral nutrition	Optimize intestinal function
	Dilated bowel with bacterial overgrowth, stasis	Treat obstruction Intestinal tapering
Remnant > 90 cm	Rapid transit Need for PN	Recruit additional length Reversed intestinal segment Artificial valve Colon interposition
Remnant 60–90 cm	Normal diameter Dilated bowel Need for PN	Optimize intestinal function Intestinal lengthening
Remnant < 60 cm	Complications of PN	Intestinal transplantation

a short bowel are candidates for these non–transplant procedures. For most, intestinal transplantation holds the greatest future promise for the surgical treatment of patients with a short bowel.

REFERENCES

1. Thompson JS. Reoperation in patients with the short bowel syndrome. *Am J Surg* 1992; **164**: 453–457.

2. Thompson JS. Strategies for preserving intestinal length in the short bowel syndrome. *Dis Col Rectum* 1987; **30**: 208–213.

3. Roslyn JJ, Pitt HA, Mann LL, Fonkalsrud EW, Den Besten L. Parenteral nutrition-induced gallbladder disease: a reason for early cholecystectomy. *Am J Surg* 1984; **148**: 58–63.

4. Thompson JS. The role of prophylactic cholecystectomy in the short bowel syndrome. *Arch Surg* 1996; **131**: 556–560.

5. Manjo N, Bistrian BR, Mascioloi EA, Benotti PA, Blackburn GL. Gallstone disease in patients with severe short bowel syndrome dependent on parenteral nutrition. *J Parenter Enteral Nutr* 1989; **12**: 461–464.

6. Nightingale JMD, Lennard-Jones JE, Gertner DJ, Wood SR, Bartram CI. Colonic preservation reduces need of parenteral therapy, increases incidence of renal stones, but does not change high prevalence of gallstones in patients with a short bowel. *Gut* 1992; **33**: 1493–1497.

7. Tilson DM. Pathophysiology and treatment of short bowel syndrome. *Surg Clinic North Am* 1980; **60**: 1273–1284.

8. Wolf SA, Telander RL, Go VLW, Dozois RR. Effect of proximal gastric vagotomy and truncal vagotomy and pyloroplasty on gastric functions and growth in puppies after massive small bowel resection. *J Pediatr Surg* 1979; **14**: 441–445.

9. Burrington JD. Surgery after massive bowel resection. *Am J Surg* 1971; **121**: 213–214.

10. Thompson JS, Harty RJ, Saigh JA, Giger DK. Morphological and nutritional responses to intestinal patching following intestinal resection. *Surgery* 1988; **103**: 79–86.

11. Thompson JS, Langnas AN, Pinch LW, Kaufman S, Quigley EMM, Vanderhoof JA. Surgical approach to the short bowel syndrome: experience in a population of 160 patients. *Ann Surg* 1995; **222**: 600–607.

12. Lloyd PA. Colonic interposition between the jejunum and ileum after massive small bowel resection in rats. *Prog Pediatr Surg* 1978; **12**: 51–106.

13. Kaveggia FF, Thompson JS, Taylor RJ. Placement of an ileal loop urinary diversion back into continuity with the intestinal tract. *Surgery* 1991; **110**: 557–560.

14. Nguyen BT, Blatchford GJ, Thompson JS, Bragg LE. Should intestinal continuity be restored after massive intestinal resection. *Am J Surg* 1989; **158**: 577–580.

15. Gouttebel MC, Saint-Aubert B, Astre C, Joyeux H. Total parenteral nutrition needs in different types of short bowel syndromes. *Dig Dis Sci* 1986; **31**: 718–723.

16. O'Keefe SJD, Burnes JU, Thompson RL. Recurrent sepsis in home parenteral nutrition patients: an analysis of risk factors. *J Parenter Enteral Nutr* 1994; **18**: 256–263.

17. Rombeau JL, Kripke SA. Metabolic and intestinal effects of short chain fatty acids. *J Parenter Enteral Nutr* 1990; **14**: 181S–185S.

18. Koruda MJ, Rolandelli RH, Settle RG, Saul SH, Rombeau JL. The effect of a pectin-supplemented elemental diet on intestinal adaptation to massive small bowel resection. *J Parenter Enteral Nutr* 1986; **10**: 343–350.

19. Carbonnel F, Cosnes J, Chevret S, et al. The role of anatomic factors in nutritional autonomy after extensive small bowel resection. *J Parenter Enteral Nutr* 1996; **20**: 275–280.

20. Levy E, Frileux P, Sandrucci S, et al. Continuous enteral nutrition during the early adaptive stage of the short bowel syndrome. *Br J Surg* 1988; **75**: 549–553.

21. Weber TR, Vane DW, Grosfield JL. Tapering enteroplasty in infants with bowel atresia and short gut. *Arch Surg* 1982; **117**: 684–688.

22. Borgstein ES, Munro A, Youngson GG. Intestinal plication: an alternative to tapered jejunostomy in functional small bowel obstruction. *Br J Surg* 1991; **78**: 1075–1076.

23. Ramanujan TM. Functional capability of blind small loops after intestinal remodeling techniques. *Aust NZ J Surg* 1986; **54**: 145–150.

24. Mall F. Reversal of the intestine. *Johns Hopkins Hosp* 1896; **1**: 93–110.

25. Thompson JS, Quigley EMM, Adrian TE. Effect of reversed intestinal segments on intestinal structure and function. *J Surg Res* 1995; **58**: 19–27.

26. Persemlidis D, Kark AE. Antiperistaltic segments for the treatment of short bowel syndrome. *Am J Gastroent* 1974; **62**: 526–530.

27. Barros D'Sa AAB. An experimental evaluation of segmental reversal after massive small bowel resection. *Br J Surg* 1979; **66**: 493–500.

28. Delaney HM, Parker JG, Gliedman ML. Experimental massive intestinal resection: comparison of surgical measures and spontaneous adaptation. *Arch Surg* 1970; **101**: 599–604.

29. Williams NS, King RFG. The effect of reversed ileal segments and artificial valve on intestinal transit and absorption following colectomy and low ileorectal anastomosis in the dog. *Br J Surg* 1985; **72**: 169–174.

30. Kurz R, Sauer H. Treatment and metabolic finding in extreme short bowel syndrome with 11 cm jejunal remnant. *J Pediatr Surg* 1983; **18**: 257–263.

31. Pigot F, Messing B, Shaussade S, Pfeiffer A, Pouliguen Y, Jiau R. Severe short bowel syndrome with a surgically reversed small bowel segment. *Dig Dis Sci* 1990; **35**: 137–144.

32. Panis Y, Messing B, Rivet P, et al. Segment reversal of the small bowel as an alternative to intestinal transplantation in patients with short bowel syndrome. *Ann Surg* 1997; **225**: 401–407.

33. Wilmore DW, Johnson DJ. Metabolic effect of small bowel reversal in treatment of the short bowel syndrome. *Arch Surg* 1968; **97**: 784–791.

34. Richards WO, Golzarian J, Wasuder N, Sawyers JL. Reverse phasic contractions are present in antiperistaltic jejunal limbs up to 21 years postoperatively. *J Am Coll Surg* 1994; **178**: 557–563.

35. Dorney SF, Ament ME, Berquist WE. Improved survival in very short small bowel of infancy with use of long-term parenteral nutrition. *J Pediatr* 1985; **107**: 521–525.

36. Quigley EMM, Thompson JS. Effects of an artificial ileocolonic sphincter on motility in the intestinal remnant following subtotal small intestinal resection. *Dig Dis Sci* 1994; **39**: 1222–1229.

37. Stacchini A, DiDo LJ, Primo ML, Borelli V, Andretto R. Artificial sphincter as surgical treatment for experimental massive resection of small intestine. *Am J Surg* 1982; **143**: 721–726.

38. Lopes-Perez, GA, Martinez AJ, Machcua J, Lopez S, Unda A, Rodriguez M, Miguelez C. Experimental antireflux intestinal valve. *Am J Surg* 1981; **141**: 597–600.

39. Careskey J, Weber TR, Grosfield JL. Ileocecal valve replacement: its effect on transit time, survival and weight change after massive intestinal resection. *Arch Surg* 1981; **116**: 618–622.

40. Sawchuk A, Goto S, Yount J, Grosfield JA, Lohmuller J, Grosfield MD. Chemically induced bowel denervation improved survival in short bowel syndrome. *J Pediatr Surg* 1987; **22**: 492–496.

41. Chardovoyne R, Isenberg H, Tindel M, Stein T, Wise L. Efficacy of a surgically constructed nipple valve following massive small bowel resection. *Gastroenterology* 1983; **84**: 1122.

42. Ricotta J, Zuidema FD, Gadacz RT, Sadri D. Construction of an ileocecal valve and its role in massive resection of the small intestine. *Surg Gynecol Obstet* 1981; **152**: 310–314.

43. Waddell WR, Kern F, Halgrimson CF, Woodbury JJ. A simple jejunocolic valve for relief of rapid transit and the short bowel syndrome. *Arch Surg* 1970; **100**: 438–444.

44. Smedh K, Olaison G, Sjodahl R. Ileocolic nipple valve anastomosis for preventing recurrence of surgically treated Crohn's disease. *Dis Colon Rectum* 1990; **33**: 987–990.

45. Georgeson K, Halpin D, Figuera R, Vincente Y, Hardin W. Sequential intestinal lengthening procedures for refractory short bowel syndrome. *J Pediatr Surg* 1994; **29**: 316–321.

46. Hutcher NE, Mendez-Picon G, Salzberg AM. Prejejunal transposition of colon to prevent the development of the short bowel in puppies with 90% small intestine resection. *J Pediatr Surg* 1973; **8**: 771–777.

47. Sidhu GS, Narasimharao V, Rani V, Sarkar AK, Chakravarti RN, Mitra Sk. Morphological and functional changes in the gut after massive small bowel resection and colon interposition in Rhesus monkeys. *Digestion* 1984; **129**: 47–54.

48. Hutcher NE, Salzberg AM. Pre-ileal transposition of colon to prevent the development of the short bowel syndrome in puppies with 90% small intestinal resection. *Surgery* 1971; **70**: 189–197.

49. Sidhu GS, Narasimharao V, Rani V, Sarkar AK, Mitra SK. Absorptive studies after massive small bowel resection and antiperistaltic colon interposition in Rhesus monkeys. *Dig Dis Sci* 1985; **30**: 483–488.

50. Carner DV, Raju S. Failure of antiperistalsis colon interposition to ameliorate short bowel syndrome. *Am Surg* 1981; **47**: 538–540.

51. Belin RP, Richardson JD, Medley ES. Transit time and bacterial overgrowth as determinants of absorptive capacity. *J Surg Res* 1972; **3**: 185–192.

52. Garcia VF, Templeton JM, Eichelberger MR, Koop CE, Vinograd I. Colon interposition for the short syndrome. *J Pediatr Surg* 1981; **16**: 994–995.

53. Glick PL, de Lorimier AA, Adzick NS, Harrison MR. Colon interposition: an adjuvant operation for short gut syndrome. *J Pediatr Surg* 1984; **19**: 719–725.

54. Brolin RE. Colon interposition for extreme short bowel syndrome: a case report. *Surgery* 1986; **100**: 576–580.

55. Trinkle JK, Bryant LR. Reversed colon segment in an infant with massive small bowel resection. A case report. *J Ky Med Assoc* 1967; **65**: 1090–1091.

56. Budding J, Smith CG. Role of recirculating loops in the management of massive resection of the small intestine. *Surg Gynecol Ostet* 1967; **125**: 213–249.

57. Watkins RM, Dennson AR, Collin J. Do intestinal pouches have a role in the treatment of the short bowel syndrome? *Br J Surg* 1984; **71**: 384.

58. Camprodon R, Guerrero JA, Salva JA, Jronet J. Shortened small bowel syndrome: Mackby's operation. *Am J Surg* 1975; **129**: 585–586.

59. Poth EJ. Use of gastrointestinal reversal in surgical procedures. *Am J Surg* 1969; **118**: 893–899.

60. Mackby MJ, Richards V, Gilfillan RS, Floridia R. Methods of increasing the efficiency of residual small bowel segments. *Am J Surg* 1965; **109**: 32–38.

61. Cywes S. The surgical management of massive bowel resection. *J Pediatr Surg* 1968; **3**: 740–748.

62. Gladen HE, Kelly KA. Enhancing absorption in the canine short bowel syndrome by intestinal pacing. *Surgery* 1980; **88**: 281–286.

63. Layzell T, Collin J. Retrograde electrical pacing of the small intestine: a new treatment for the short bowel syndrome? *Br J Surg* 1981; **68**: 711–713.

64. Bjored WS, Phillips SF, Kelly KA. Mechanisms of enhanced intestinal absorption with electrical pacing. *Gastroenterology* 1984; **86**: 1029.

65. Devine RM, Kelly KA. Surgical therapy for the short bowel syndrome. *Gastroenterol Clin North Am* 1989; **18**: 603–617.

66. O'Connell PR, Kelly KA. Enteric transit and absorption after canine ileostomy: effect of pacing. *Arch Surg* 1987; **122**: 1011–1017.

67. Soper NJ, Sarr MG, Kelly KA. Human duodenal myoelectric activity after operation and with pacing. *Surgery* 1990; **107**: 63–68.

68. Bianchi A. Intestinal lengthening: An experimental and clinical review. *J R Soc Med* 1984; **77**: 35–41.

69. Thompson JS, Quigley EMM, Adrian TE. Effect of intestinal tapering and lengthening on intestinal structure and function. *Am J Surg* 1995; **169**: 111–119.

70. Thompson JS, Pinch LW, Murray N, Vanderhoof JA, Schultz LR. Initial experience with lengthening for the short bowel syndrome. *J Pediatr Surg* 1991; **26**: 721–724.

71. Pokorny WJ, Fowler CL, Isoperistaltic intestinal lengthening for short bowel syndrome. *Surg Gynecol Obstet* 1991; **173**: 39–43.

72. Kimura K, Soper RT. A new bowel elongation technique for the short bowel syndrome using the isolated bowel segment Iowa models. *J Pediatr Surg* 1993; **28**: 792–794.

34

Small intestinal transplantation

Richard F. M. Wood and A. Graham Pockley

Successful transplantation of the small intestine is still a major clinical challenge. Near perfect function of the transplanted bowel is required for the recipient to maintain adequate nutrition. In addition the intestine is more susceptible to rejection than other forms of organ graft and it also has the potential to induce graft-versus-host disease (GVHD) in the recipient. The aggressive immunosuppressive regimens required to control rejection have rendered patients at risk of sepsis and malignancy (Table 34.1). The causes of small bowel failure which give rise to a need for transplantation have been described in detail earlier in this book. There is a specific issue in relation to transplantation in children. Infants with intestinal failure who are started on total parenteral nutrition (TPN) within their first year of life frequently manifest signs of liver failure by the time they are 3 or 4 as the immature liver has difficulty in metabolizing the amino acids in the feed. These children may therefore require a combined liver and small bowel transplant.

The first part of this chapter considers how the problems of small intestinal transplantation have been addressed in experimental studies and the second part provides an overview of current clinical experience. There is a glossary of terms at the end of this chapter.

MECHANISMS OF REJECTION AND GVHD

Immunological factors

The normal small intestine contains a great deal of lymphoid tissue (especially in the ileum) (Chapter 2).

Table 34.1 – Cause of death in small intestinal transplant recipients (as at February 1999). Data were reprinted with permission from the Intestinal Transplant Registry (© 1999 Intestinal Transplant Registry

Cause of death	%
Sepsis	55
Non-transplant organ failure	14
Lymphoma	14
Thrombosis/ischaemia/bleeding	13
Graft rejection	12
Other	5

There is also a constant circulation of lymphocytes between the gut and peripheral lymphatic tissues such as the spleen, lymph nodes and other mucosal sites (e.g. lacrimal and salivary glands).[1] This cell traffic continues after small bowel transplantation.[2-6]

Migration of host immunological cells into the lymphoid areas of the grafted intestine stimulates direct lymphocyte sensitization and an aggressive, early rejection response if no immunosuppressive drugs are given. Graft lymphocytes also migrate to the recipient tissues. In the absence of immunosuppression the graft cells will be rapidly destroyed by the host immune system. However, when rejection has been suppressed by drug therapy the graft cells usually remain quiescent in the recipient although they have the potential to attack host tissue causing GVHD.

Rejection

The potent immunosuppressive drugs cyclosporin and tacrolimus are both capable of eliciting long-term graft survival in rodents. In these experimental studies the use of strain-specific monoclonal antibodies has allowed the migration pattern of host and graft lymphocytes to be tracked in detail. Even when immunosuppression is sufficient to prevent rejection there is still extensive infiltration of the graft by host lymphoid cells.[4,7] Cell migration is a prolonged response and by 1 month after transplantation in immunosuppressed animals the lymphoid population of the graft mesenteric lymph node has been completely replaced by recipient cells (Fig. 34.1). Concomitantly, significant numbers of graft lymphocytes can be detected in the host spleen.[4,5] This re-population of donor lymphoid compartments by host cells has also been observed in the clinical setting.[8] This is a feature unique to intestinal transplantation. In other organ grafts, for example the kidney, lymphocyte infiltration is the hallmark of rejection. Only if the infiltrating lymphocytes reach the intra-epithelial compartment can their presence be correlated with rejection.[7] Although the exchange migration of cells is slowed after treatment with immunosuppression, there is evidence to suggest that the presence of these cells is necessary for tolerance (i.e. non-rejection of the graft) to become established.[9-11] Extending this concept has been the controversial suggestion that micro-chimerism (see Glossary) is involved in the maintenance of tolerance to a number of organ allografts.[12] The clinical difficulty is maintaining the cells in a state of stable chimerism without immunological changes triggering either GVHD on the one hand, or rejection on the other.

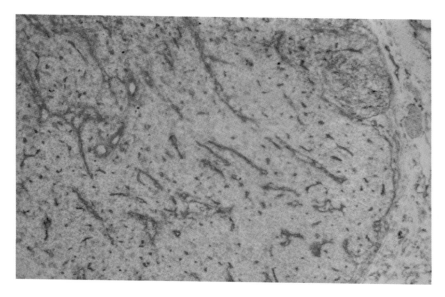

Figure 34.1 – Graft mesenteric lymph node from a cyclosporin treated (15 mg/kg/day) recipient 28 days after rat heterotopic small bowel transplantation. Tissue was snap-frozen in liquid nitrogen and cryostat sections stained by an indirect immunoperoxidase technique using monoclonal antibodies specific for the MHC class I expressed by graft cells. Donor lymphocytes have been almost totally replaced by infiltrating recipient cells.

T lymphocytes

Studies of basic immune mechanisms have shown that, in addition to recognition of antigenic peptides by the T-cell receptor complex, a number of adhesive and co-stimulatory events are required to cause T-cell activation. Adhesion of lymphocytes to the lining of vascular capillaries involves the interaction of lymphocyte function antigen-1 (LFA-1) on the surface of T-cells with its receptor – intercellular adhesion molecule-1 (ICAM-1) – on the vascular endothelium.[13–15] There is also an interaction between the CD28 antigen on T-cells with CD80 (B7–1) and CD86 (B7–2) molecules on antigen-presenting cells. If these antigen-presenting cells are absent or this interaction is blocked, then the T-cells are rendered unresponsive or anergic.[16,17] The role of adhesion molecules in the rejection of small bowel transplants and the possible value of their expression as a predictor of rejection has received little attention. Immunohistochemical analysis of rejecting rat small bowel transplants has demonstrated an up-regulation of ICAM-1 and LFA-1α expression, whereas LFA-1β and VLA-4 antigen expression remain unchanged.[18,19] Funayama *et al.* also reported that adhesion molecule upregulation was prevented by the administration of tacrolimus.[18] The expression of CD44 by villus intestinal epithelial cells also appears and progresses towards the villus tip as rejection proceeds.[20] These data are particularly interesting, as CD44 expression is apparent 2 days before histological evidence of rejection.[20] The factors and mechanisms leading to the induction of CD44 expression and the potential value of monitoring CD44 in the clinical situation remain to be elucidated.

Neutrophils

Neutrophils, which are noted for their activity against pathogenic microbes and tumours,[21,22] are now being recognized as having a role in rejection. They may be involved in both the induction and active stages of the immune response, predominantly through their ability to synthesize and secrete immunoregulatory cytokines such as γ-interferon (γ-IFN), interleukins (ILs) 1, 2, 6, 8 and tumour necrosis factor-α (TNF-α).[23,24] These cytokines act locally to activate cells and induce the expression of adhesion molecules and the molecules to which they bind (ligands) on vascular endothelial cells. Cytokine-mediated events promote the accumulation of neutrophils at inflammatory sites.[23] Neutrophils have been implicated in allograft rejection and the aetiology of chronic obliterative disease in lung transplant recipients,[25,26] although their relative importance in the creation of tissue damage remains elusive. The observation that peripheral blood neutrophils express high levels of the natural killer cell molecule NKR-P1 as early as 24 hours after allogenic rat small bowel transplantation,[27] suggests that this antigen may be an indicator of neutrophil activation and that these activated cells may participate in the rejection process. It is interesting that neutrophils disappear from the peripheral circulation on day 5, a time that coincides with the first histological signs of rejection in the PVG to DA strain combination used for these studies.[27]

The complex nature of the cell migratory responses after small bowel transplantation makes immune events within the graft difficult to assess. A number of groups have attempted to define the role of cytokines in small bowel allograft rejection, but with variable results. A wide array of cytokine genes is expressed in the graft during the rejection of rat small bowel transplants.[28-32] Quan *et al.* showed in a mouse model that IL-2, -4, -5 and -6 mRNA levels increased during the onset of rejection.[30] Using rat models, McDiarmid *et al.*[29] and Farmer *et al.*[28] have reported an early increase in γ-IFN, TNF-α and IL-6 correlating with the severity of rejection and suggesting that this may serve as a useful marker for developing rejection. A subsequent study has reported an early increase in some cytokine gene transcripts in the mesenteric lymph nodes and Peyer's patches of rejecting small bowel allografts.[32] Levels were elevated in the first 24 hours after transplantation and in the case of IL-2 and IL-10 peaked within 1–3 days. Toogood *et al.* proposed that this early increase in cytokine production may be difficult to control using immunosuppression administered at the time of operation and may, to some extent, explain why rejection in intestinal transplantation is such a problem.[32]

Another confounding issue in the induction and progression of the rejection response is the interplay between infiltrating recipient and resident graft cells. Although in the clinical situation and in the majority of fully allogeneic animal models, the appearance of overt GVHD is rare, it is possible that such responses are occurring within the graft. Flow cytometric morphological analysis has identified activated populations of donor cells in the graft mesenteric lymph nodes and Peyer's patches.[33] These localized graft-versus-host responses will influence the development of rejection as the cytokine production they induce will directly or indirectly promote the development of immunological responses against the intestinal graft.

EXPERIMENTAL TRANSPLANTATION

The emerging programs of clinical small intestinal transplantation have been based on extensive experimental work primarily in rats and pigs.

Ischaemia/reperfusion (I/R) injury

The small intestine is particularly sensitive to the effects of ischaemia and reperfusion. Deprivation of blood supply induces rapid changes in cell metabolism. Intracellular calcium concentrations rise quickly and the breakdown of adenosine triphosphate to adenine and hypoxanthine provides substrates for the development of oxygen free radicals (OFRs) when the tissue is reperfused with blood. Lipid peroxidation within the endothelial cell, triggered by OFRs, leads to up-regulation of molecules such as selectins on the cell membrane. Selectins and other adhesion molecules allow neutrophil and lymphocyte attachment to the cell membrane and their transportation to the sub-endothelial layer by diapedesis. There is evidence, from other forms of transplantation, that I/R injury promotes rejection and graft loss.[34] Long-term survival of small bowel transplants is hampered by chronic rejection[35-37] and it has been suggested that this is a consequence, at least in part, of preservation and I/R-induced tissue damage.[38] In small bowel transplantation, the presence of neutrophil activation and OFR production has been confirmed following I/R injury.[39] Methods to combat the problem include the addition of glutamine to perfusion systems and the use of agents such as mannitol and the lazaroid compounds which can prevent a build up of OFRs.[40] The use of reagents capable of blocking adhesion molecules may be helpful and recent research has suggested that soluble P-selectin glycoprotein ligand can effectively reduce neutrophil binding to the endothelium of the graft microcirculation in experimental renal transplantation.[41]

Mucosal barrier function

Damage to the integrity of the villi can result in bacterial translocation from the gut lumen into the portal circulation with the development of systemic sepsis. I/R injury and rejection predispose to villus damage and experimental studies have shown a clear correlation between the development of rejection and bacterial translocation.[42,43] Another factor that may affect translocation is the spectrum of bacterial flora within the gut. In early clinical transplants both ends of the gut were initially exteriorized in the belief that this would reduce the risks of sepsis. However, taking the gut out of continuity in this way induces villus atrophy from the loss of the trophic factors present in normal intestinal content. Atrophy is accompanied by a change in the gut flora towards organisms such as

Staphylococcus epidermidis which have a particular predilection to translocate.[44] Placing an intestinal graft back into continuity corrects the changes in intestinal microflora and stresses the importance and potential benefits of anastomosing the proximal end of the transplanted gut to the host gastrointestinal tract at the time of transplantation.[45] Attempts to flush the lumen of the donor intestine prior to transplant may also be unhelpful as this may remove the protective mucus layer from the surface of the villi.

In addition to the mechanical aspects of barrier function, secretory IgA (the predominant immuno-globulin produced in the small intestine) is central to an effective immunological defense against infectious agents within the gut lumen.[1] Heterotopic rat small bowel allografts do not produce antigen-specific IgA in response to newly presented antigen in the presence of cyclosporin.[46] However, additional studies will be required to establish the extent to which normal immune responses to orally ingested antigens are preserved in orthotopic (in-continuity) small bowel allografts.

Lymphatic and neurological disruption

It is inevitable that the lymphatics and the autonomic nerve supply of the donor intestine will have been divided at the time of organ harvesting. Experimental studies have shown that a network of fine lymphatic connections develops within a week to 10 days after transplantation.[47,48] In rodent experiments it has proved possible to achieve lymphatic duct drainage with a marked improvement in graft outcome.[49,50] Impaired lymphatic drainage is a potential clinical problem, particularly with respect to achieving good absorption of fat-soluble drugs such as cyclosporin.[48] Neuro-logical disruption leads to an initial hyper-secretion of water and chloride from the crypts that overwhelms the absorptive capacity of the villus tip and results in watery diarrhoea.[48,51] However, this problem usually settles within the first 2 weeks after clinical trans-plantation and has not proved to be a major long-term problem.

Portal versus systemic drainage

Practically it may be easier to drain the venous effluent from the graft to the systemic rather than the portal system. This is essential if the portal venous system is already thrombosed. Although satisfactory nutrition can be achieved with systemic drainage, there is experimental evidence that portal drainage confers immunological advantages.[52]

Immunosuppression

Experimental studies have demonstrated that cyclosporin and subsequently tacrolimus are effective in controlling the immune response after small bowel transplantation.[53] Studies with some of the newer agents have shown that sirolimus (Rapamycin®) may be an effective adjunct to current immunosuppressive regimens, however, mycophenylate mofetil (MMF), the pro-drug of mycophenolic acid, also shows considerable promise. Porcine studies have shown that combining tacrolimus with MMF results in excellent long-term survival with minimal infective complications when compared to a regimen using tacrolimus alone.[54]

Experimental studies have shown that monoclonal antibodies to adhesion molecules or to the CD4 antigen can prolong the survival of a number of allografts.[55] In addition, the injection of donor antigen into the recipient thymus concomitant with anti-lymphocyte serum to deplete T lymphocytes in the periphery of the recipient has been shown to induce tolerance to a subsequently transplanted kidney, liver or heart.[56–58] Despite these promising results, admini-stration of anti-CD4 monoclonal antibodies causes only a modest prolongation in small bowel allograft survival.[59,60] Results following intrathymic injection have been mixed, with Karim *et al.*[61] reporting a slight prolongation of graft survival and Goss *et al.*[62] a 2.5-fold longer survival.

Attempts to modify the rejection response by using anti-adhesion molecule monoclonal antibodies have also met with mixed success. Administration of anti-LFA-1 antibodies to DA rats that had received PVG strain small bowel heterotopic grafts induced only a modest prolongation of graft survival,[60] whereas monoclonal antibodies to ICAM-1 appear to prevent rejection in the Fischer to Lewis combination.[63] Tice *et al.* have shown that although an anti-VLA-4 mono-clonal antibody alone was ineffective significant prolongation of rat small bowel graft survival was achieved when the antibody was combined with sub-therapeutic doses of cyclosporin.[64]

The evidence to date confirms that the intestinal allograft presents a potent target for the rejection response and that approaches which may be effective in delaying/preventing graft rejection in other situations are likely to be less effective when applied to small bowel transplantation. From an immunological perspective much remains to be elucidated before it will be possible to specifically target the immunological events that lead to intestinal graft loss.

CLINICAL TRANSPLANTATION

Early attempts at small bowel transplantation before cyclosporin became available were uniformly unsuccessful, although one patient transplanted in New York survived for 75 days.[65] Most patients appear to have succumbed to overwhelming infection within a few days of transplantation. Cyclosporin, which is derived from the fungus *Tolypocladium inflatum Gams*, was used as the basis of immunosuppression in a series of four cases transplanted in Kiel (Germany) in the 1980s. One patient who received a live-related transplant from her half-sister with a favourable HLA match survived in the long-term.[66] From a series of seven paediatric transplants performed in Paris at about the same time, there remains one long-term survivor in whom a neo-natal intestine was used as the graft source. The neo-natal intestine is less immunogenic and this may partly account for the good outcome.[67]

Calne and colleagues had shown that the presence of a functioning liver transplant enhanced the survival of other transplanted organs (e.g. kidney) in pigs.[68] Grant and his colleagues in London, Ontario[69] made an important breakthrough by performing a combined liver and small bowel transplant and showing that the liver conveyed an immunological advantage. However, Grant's first combined case demonstrated that GVHD could be a problem, as the female recipient developed the typical skin rash of GVHD and lymphocytes from the male donor were detected in the recipient peripheral blood.[70]

The Pittsburgh series

Tacrolimus, an immunosuppressive drug discovered in a soil sample taken at the foot of Mount Tsukuba in Japan, had been demonstrated to improve the outcome after liver transplantation. It was made available to the Pittsburgh transplantation programme for a series of both isolated intestinal and combined liver and small bowel transplants. This series highlighted not only the potential benefits of small transplantation, but also the significant problems that remained.[70] A total of 71 transplant procedures were performed in 63 patients and at the time of the report in 1995, 32 patients (50%)

were surviving from 1 to 5 years after surgery. Twenty-eight patients had functioning primary grafts and the remaining four individuals had been returned to treatment with total parenteral nutrition. Analysing the 35 graft losses, ten were ascribed to technical and management errors, six to rejection and 19 to infection. Cytomegalovirus (CMV) enteritis was prone to occur in recipients that required repeated treatment with high dose immunosuppression, especially those receiving the OKT3 monoclonal antibody. A proportion of paediatric patients with CMV enteritis went on to develop Epstein-Barr virus-related post-transplant lymphoproliferative disease.[71]

Although the inclusion of the ileocaecal valve and some proximal ascending colon may improve gut function,[72] including the colon with a transplant causes some problems.[73] First, postoperative management can be complicated, as the colon may appear normal while rejection is occurring in the small bowel. Second, studies in pigs have shown that the addition of the colon can increase the risk of GVHD.[74]

How a transplantation is done

Preparation of donor

Suitable donors are tested for hepatitis B, C, human immunodeficiency virus (HIV) and CMV. Blood is also taken to determine ABO blood group and HLA tissue type. The relative shortage of suitable donors means that it is rarely possible to achieve close HLA matching. Ideally, if the recipient is CMV-negative they should receive a graft from a CMV-negative donor. After brain death has been confirmed for the second time and if serological tests for hepatitis B, C and HIV are negative, then consent is obtained from a relative.

If the donor is not already receiving broad-spectrum antibiotics a suitable combination of drugs covering both aerobes and anaerobes will be given before starting the graft retrieval procedure. The donor is given muscle relaxants and the whole small bowel is removed with a vascular pedicle including the superior mesenteric artery on an aortic patch and the portal vein divided close to its junction with the superior mesenteric vein. A segment of donor iliac artery may have to be resected to provide an additional vascular conduit to allow the graft arterial circulation to be linked to the recipient without the vessels being under tension. If a combined liver and small bowel graft is being performed the aortic patch will include the coeliac axis in addition to the superior mesenteric artery and the superior mesenteric vein and portal vein will be retrieved in continuity. After retrieval the superior mesenteric artery is perfused with a preservation solution at 4°C. University of Wisconsin solution is the preparation used by virtually all centres. It is a specially formulated electrolyte solution aimed at maintaining the integrity of the graft cells. It is high in sodium and low in potassium, buffered to prevent intra-cellular acidosis and contains imperiments to prevent cell swelling. It therefore reduces many of the deleterious effects of I/R injury. The lumen of the graft can be filled with a saline solution containing antibiotics to reduce reperfusion endotoxaemia and the open ends stapled across. Lavage of the graft in an attempt to reduce the bacterial load is counter productive as it may damage the protective mucus layer covering the villous epithelium. The graft is placed in a large sterile plastic bag surrounded by cold preservation solution. It is stored on melting ice and satisfactory graft function is possible with cold ischaemic times of up to 10 hours.[75]

Preparation of recipient

Blood group matching is the best that can be achieved for the majority of patients receiving a small bowel graft. Good HLA matching would almost certainly be a benefit, but the shortage of suitable donors, the small numbers of patients on waiting lists and the need to keep the cold storage time as short as possible render this unachievable. Size matching is important, especially in paediatric transplantation, to ensure that the grafted intestine will fit into a peritoneal cavity that has often shrunk down in size as a result of previous extensive resection of diseased bowel. Broad-spectrum prophylactic antibiotics are administered immediately pre-operatively.

The transplantation

The patch of aorta around the superior mesenteric artery is anastomosed to the infra-renal aorta either directly or using a conduit of donor iliac artery (Fig. 34.2). Ideally the donor portal vein should be drained into the recipient portal vein, but if this is not technically possible the donor portal vein can be sutured end-to-side to the recipient IVC.[76] The proximal end of the graft bowel is now connected to the duodenum or residual jejunum of the recipient. A variety of different anatomical configurations are possible in dealing with the distal end of the graft. Most authorities favour either a loop ileostomy or an end

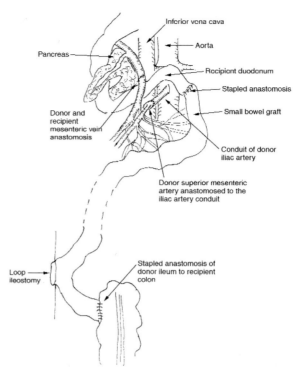

Figure 34.2 – Diagram of an isolated small bowel transplant in man.

external ileal stoma with connection of the recipient colon end-to-side. This situation allows regular endo-scopic biopsies to be obtained. The graft is not put into continuity with the recipient intestine until 2–3 months after the transplant.[77]

Immunosuppression and postoperative care

Tacrolimus is currently the mainstay of immuno-suppressive treatment. The drug has to be given by intravenous infusion until there is evidence of absorption by the transplanted intestine. Initial tacrolimus therapy is usually 0.1–0.15 mg/kg/day. As soon as possible the patient should be converted to an oral regimen of around 0.3 mg/kg/day in two divided doses. A whole blood trough level of 25–35 ng/ml in the first week after transplantation is the aim with the dose adjusted to give levels of 10–20 ng/ml in the long-term. Most patients have been given steroids in an initial dose of 200 mg/day with a rapid taper to 10–20 mg/day by the end of the first month.

Additional immunosuppression during the first month with either azathioprine (2 mg/kg/day) or MMF (2 g/day) has been common practice in most units. In the first few days after a transplant the graft hypersecretes fluid (about 2 litres a day) and is hypermotile possibly due to neural disruption, but these problems usually resolve steadily after the first week.

Monitoring and diagnosis of rejection

Routine biopsies of the transplanted bowel via a distal stoma have been the corner stone of rejection diagnosis in clinical transplantation.[78] However, the rejection response can be patchy and collection of appropriate biopsies relies heavily on the ability of the endoscopist to recognize inflamed areas. As there are usually many lymphocytes in the bowel mucosa the slight increase that is the first sign of early rejection is difficult to identify histologically. Sub-mucosal oedema with excess numbers of macrophages and neutrophils has been the main indicator of rejection, although immunohistochemical analysis of the infiltrating cell populations has also proved useful.[79] Acute rejection is associated with pericryptic infiltration of CD3[+] lymphocytes with clusters of CD8[+] and CD25[+] cells and a prominent presence of CD68[+] macrophages. The mucosa can be stained for the brush border enzyme maltase and its disappearance from the enterocytes has been found to be a reliable sign of early rejection.[80] A rise in blood procoagulant activity has also been reported in rejection.[81] In more severe cases, the sub-mucosal blood vessels show evidence of damage with intimal thickening and a loss of villus tips. In this situation breaches occur in the mucosal barrier and there may be signs of sepsis with positive blood cultures.[82]

Monitoring absorptive function has also been attempted in both experimental and clinical transplantation. In the Pittsburgh series, D-xylose absorption tests were used on a regular basis and of 43 long-term patients with functioning transplants, only 50% had normal D-xylose absorption when assessed more than 18 months post-transplantation. Faecal fat absorption remained abnormal for more than a year in some patients.[83] Gut integrity and barrier function can be assessed using [51]chromium-labelled ethylenediaminetetraacetic acid (^{51}Cr-EDTA). If the mucosa is damaged increased amounts of ^{51}Cr EDTA are absorbed and excreted in the urine.[84] Although this test has been used by the London, Ontario group as an aid to diagnosing rejection,[69] biopsy remains the most important means of patient monitoring as absorption tests can also be affected by ischaemia and gastroenteritis.[85]

INTESTINAL TRANSPLANT REGISTRY RESULTS

The International Intestinal Transplant Registry based in London, Ontario and organized by Grant and his colleagues (http://www.lhsc.on.ca/itr/) shows that only small advances have been made in improving the outcome of small bowel transplantation during the late 1990s (Fig. 34.3). By 1997, a total of 273 transplants in 260 patients had been registered by 33 centres worldwide (Table 34.2) for a number of indications (Fig. 34.4). Of these grafts 130 were combined liver and small bowel transplants, almost all of which had been performed in paediatric recipients. The demographics show roughly equal numbers of male and female patients and a preponderance of recipients in the paediatric age group (Fig. 34.5). Sepsis remains a major problem and accounts for 47% of deaths (Table 34.1). Graft survival with tacrolimus immunosuppression is clearly superior to that achieved with cyclosporin in both isolated and combined liver/small bowel grafts; however, the effects of repeated late rejection are responsible for the substantial rate of graft failure in years 2 and 3 after transplantation. This is in sharp contrast to graft survival after other forms of transplantation where, beyond the first post-transplant year, the attrition rate from chronic rejection is only around 2–3% per year.

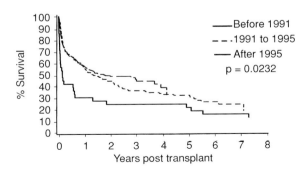

Figure 34.3 – Small intestinal graft survival by era (as at February 1999). The majority of transplants performed since 1993 have used tacrolimus as the primary immunosuppressant. Data were reprinted with permission from the Intestinal Transplant Registry (© 1999 Intestinal Transplant Registry).

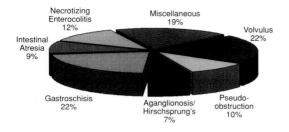

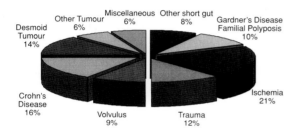

Figure 34.4 – Indications for small bowel transplantation in paediatric (upper) and adult (lower) patients (as at February 1999). Data were reprinted with permission from the Intestinal Transplant Registry (© 1999 Intestinal Transplant Registry).

Table 34.2 – International Intestinal Transplant Registry Database (as at February 1999). Data were reprinted with permission from the Intestinal Transplant Registry (© 1999 Intestinal Transplant Registry).

	Total
Number of centres	46
Number of patients	446
Number of transplants	474
Types of transplant	
Intestine	216
Intestine/liver	186
Multi-organ	72
Maintenance immunosuppression	
Prednisone	408
Tacrolimus	376
Myophenolate Mofetil	94
Azathioprine	61
Cyclosporin	37
Rapamycin	7
None (twin or triplet donor)	3
No treatment (early failure)	48
Other	29

THE FUTURE

Good HLA matching should lead to an improvement in graft outcome. However, the need for a short preservation time dictates that this is currently only a realistic proposition in live-related transplantation. Parent to child grafting is guaranteed to have at least a

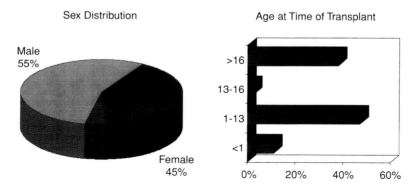

Figure 34.5 – Demographics of patients that have undergone small intestine, combined liver/small intestine or multi-organ transplantation (as at February 1999). Data were reprinted with permission from the Intestinal Transplant Registry (© 1999 Intestinal Transplant Registry).

one haplotype match and in large families it may be possible to identify an HLA identical sibling. The use of sufficient baseline immunosuppression to prevent acute rejection is the most important immediate challenge and the judicious use of new agents may offer a realistic prospect for improvement in graft outcome. In addition, reducing I/R injury using some of the strategies discussed earlier in this chapter may be beneficial. In particular, preventing endothelial cell activation and leucocyte-endothelial interactions are likely to reduce early immune activation. Agents to block cytokine responses will help reduce rejection-mediated damage to the bowel wall and lessen the risk of bacterial translocation and life-threatening sepsis.

SUMMARY

Currently 40–47% of patients having a small bowel transplant will be alive 3 years later if tacrolimus is used for immunosuppression and 29–38% will have a functioning graft. However, only 78% of those who survive with the transplant in place are able to stop parenteral nutrition altogether.[86] Although there are problems with rejection and occasionally GVHD, most deaths are related to the side-effects and complications of immunosuppression.[86] The transplant survival figures contrast to those for adult patients on home parenteral nutrition for non-malignant conditions who can expect to have a relatively good quality of life[5] and a survival rate of 70% at 3 years.

In addition, many patients currently receiving home parenteral nutrition for intestinal failure are unlikely to be good candidates for transplantation owing to the complexity of the underlying disease and previous surgical procedures.[87] Surgery may be technically difficult in an abdomen that has already been the site of many operations and immunosuppression may be unwise when there have been previous problems with intra-abdominal sepsis. There is a risk that the underlying disease process such as Crohn's disease can recur in the transplanted bowel.[88]

Before transplantation can be recommended to all patients with intestinal failure the procedure needs to have a much lower mortality rate and a higher chance that the graft will function well enough for parenteral nutrition to be stopped completely.

RECOMMENDED FURTHER READING

Bach FH, Auchincloss H Jr (eds) *Transplantation Immunology*. Wiley-Liss Inc: New York, 1995.

Grant DR, Wood RFM (eds) *Small Bowel Transplantation*. Edward Arnold: London, 1994.

Solez K, Racusen LC, Billingham ME (eds) *Solid Organ Transplant Rejection*. Marcel Dekker Inc: New York, 1996.

REFERENCES

1. Bienenstock J, Befus AD. Mucosal Immunology. *Immunology* 1980; **41**: 249–270.

2. Lear PA, Cunningham AJ, Crane PW, Wood RFM. Lymphocyte migration patterns in small bowel transplantation. *Transplant Proc* 1989; **21**: 2881–2882.

3. Ingham Clark CL, Price BA, Malcolm P, Lear PA, Wood RFM. Graft-versus-host disease in small bowel transplantation. *Br J Surg* 1991; **78**: 1077–1079.

4. Ingham Clark CL, Price BA, Crane PW, Lear PA, Wood RFM. Persistence of allogeneic cells in graft and host tissues following small bowel transplantation. *Br J Surg* 1992; **79**: 424–426.

5. Lear PA, Ingham Clark CL, Crane PW, Pockley AG, Wood RFM. Donor cell infiltration of recipient tissue as an indicator of small bowel allograft rejection in the rat. *Transplant Int* 1993; **6**: 85–88.

6. Webster GA, Wood RFM, Pockley AG. Identification of migratory graft and host cell populations after allogeneic rat small bowel transplantation. *Immunol Invest* 1996; **25**: 435–436.

7. Grover R, Lear PA, Ingham Clark CL, Pockley AG, Wood RFM. Method for diagnosing rejection in small bowel transplantation. *Br J Surg* 1993; **80**: 1024–1026.

8. Iwaki Y, Starzl TE, Yagihashi A, *et al.* Replacement of donor lymphoid tissue in small-bowel transplants. *Lancet* 1991; **337**: 818–819.

9. Starzl TE, Demetris AJ, Murase N, Thomson AW, Trucco M, Ricordi C. Donor cell chimerism permitted by immunosuppressive drugs: a new view of organ transplantation. *Immunol Today* 1993; **14**: 326–332.

10. De Bruin RWF, Heineman E, Marquet RL. Small bowel transplantation: an overview. *Transplant Int* 1994; **7**: 47–61.

11. Bernstein CN. Small bowel transplantation. *Scand J Gast* 1995; **208**(Suppl 30): 118–124.

12. Starzl TE, Demetris AJ, Murase N, Ildstad S, Ricordi C, Trucco M. Cell migration, chimerism, and graft acceptance. *Lancet* 1992; **339**: 1610–1611.

13. Springer TA. Adhesion receptors of the immune system. *Nature* 1990; **346**: 425–434.

14. Dustin ML, Springer TA. Role of lymphocyte adhesion receptors in transient interactions and cell locomotion. *Ann Rev Immunol* 1991; **9**: 27–66.

15. Dustin ML, Carpen O, Springer TA. Regulation of locomotion and cell-cell contact area by the LFA-1 and ICAM-1 adhesion receptors. *J Immunol* 1992; **148**: 2654–2663.

16. Harding FA, McArthur JG, Gross JA, Raulet DH, Allison JP. CD28-mediated signalling co-stimulates murine T-cells and prevents induction of anergy in T-cell clones. *Nature* 1992; **356**: 607–609.

17. Harding FA, Allison JP. CD28-B7 interactions allow the induction of CD8+ cytotoxic T lymphocytes in the absence of exogenous help. *J Exp Med* 1993; **177**: 1791–1796.

18. Funayama Y, Sasaki I, Masuda T, Nagura H, Matsuno S. Changes in cell adhesion molecule expression after small bowel transplantation in rats. *Transplant Proc* 1995; **27**: 595–596.

19. Reid SD, Uff CR, Saeed I, Ross J, Wood RFM, Pockley AG. Differential adhesion molecule expression in rat small bowel allograft rejection. *Transplantation* 1995; **60**: 989–992.

20. Uff CR, Reid SD, Wood RFM, Pockley AG. CD44 expression in rejecting rat small bowel allografts. *Transplantation* 1995; **60**: 985–989.

21. Thomas EL, Lehrer RI, Rest RF. Human neutrophil antimicrobial activity. *Rev Infect Dis* 1988; **10**: S450–S456.

22. van Kessel KP, Verhoef J. A view to a kill: cytotoxic mechanisms of human polymorphonuclear leukocytes compared with monocytes and natural killer cells. *Pathobiology* 1990; **58**: 249–264.

23. Lloyd AR, Oppenheim JJ. Poly's lament: The neglected role of the polymorphonuclear neutrophil in the afferent limb of the immune response. *Immunol Today* 1992; **13**: 169–172.

24. Wei S, Blanchard DK, Liu JH, Leonard WJ, Djeu JY. Activation of tumour necrosis factor-α production from human neutrophils by IL-2 via IL-2-Rβ. *J Immunol* 1993; **150**: 1979–1987.

25. Adams DH, Wang LF, Burnett D, Stockley RA, Neuberger JM. Neutrophil activation – An important cause of tissue damage during liver allograft rejection. *Transplantation* 1990; **50**: 86–91.

26. Scott JP, Holt DW, Wallwork J. Neutrophil elastase and obliterative bronchiolitis. *Transplant Int* 1994; **7** (Suppl 1): S402–S403.

27. Webster GA, Bowles MJ, Karim MS, Wood RFM, Pockley AG. Activation antigen expression on peripheral blood neutrophils following rat small bowel transplantation: NKR-P1 is a novel antigen preferentially expressed during allograft rejection. *Transplantation* 1994; **58**: 707–712.

28. Farmer DG, McDiarmid SV, Kuniyoshi J, Robert ME, Shaked A, Busuttil RW. Intragraft expression of messenger RNA for interleukin-6 and tumor necrosis factor-alpha is a predictor of rat small intestine transplant rejection. *J Surg Res* 1994; **57**: 138–142.

29. McDiarmid SV, Farmer DG, Kuniyoshi JS, Robert M, Khadavi A, Shaked A, Busuttil RW. The correlation of intragraft cytokine expression with rejection in rat small intestine transplantation. *Transplantation* 1994; **58**: 690–697.

30. Quan D, Grant DR, Zhong RZ, Zhang Z, Garcia BM, Jevnikar AM. Altered gene expression of cytokine, ICAM-1, and class II molecules precedes mouse intestinal allograft rejection. *Transplantation* 1994; **58**: 808–816.

31. Toogood GJ, Rankin AM, Tam PK, Morris PJ, Dallman MJ. The immune response following small bowel transplantation: I. An unusual pattern of cytokine expression. *Transplantation* 1996; **62**: 851–855.

32. Toogood GJ, Rankin AM, Tam PK, Morris PJ, Dallman MJ. The immune response following small bowel transplantation. II. A very early cytokine response in the gut-associated lymphoid tissue. *Transplantation* 1997; **63**: 1118–1123.

33. Webster GA, Wood RFM, Pockley AG. Identification of localized anti-host responses in the graft mesenteric lymph node and Peyer's patches after rat small bowel transplantation. *Immunol Invest* 1997; **26**: 517–529.

34. Almond PS, Matas A, Gillingham K, Dunn DL, Payne PG, Gruessner R, Najarian JS. Risk factors for chronic rejection in renal allograft recipients. *Transplantation* 1993; **55**: 752–757.

35. Furukawa H, Abu-Elmagd K, Reyes J, *et al*. Intestinal transplantation in 31 adults. *Transplant Proc* 1996; **28**: 2753–2754.

36. Goulet O, Jan D, Sarnacki S, *et al*. Isolated and combined liver-small bowel transplantation in Paris: 1987–1995. *Transplant Proc* 1996; **28**: 2750.

37. Lee RG, Nakamura K, Tsamandas AC, *et al*. Pathology of human intestinal transplantation. *Gastroenterology* 1996; **110**: 1820–1834.

38. Land W, Messmer K. The impact of ischemia reperfusion injury on specific and non-specific early and late chronic events after organ transplantation. *Transplant Rev* 1996; **10**: 108–127.

39. Cicalese L, Caraceni P, Nalesnik MA, Borle AB, Schraut WH. Oxygen free radical content and neutrophil infiltration are important determinants in mucosal injury after rat small bowel transplantation. *Transplantation* 1996; **62**: 161–166.

40. Katz SM, Sun S, Schechner RS, Tellis VA, Alt ER, Greenstein SM. Improved small intestinal preservation after lazaroid U74389G treatment and cold storage in University of Wisconsin solution. *Transplantation* 1995; **59**: 694–698.

41. Takada M, Nadeau KC, Shaw GD, Marquette KA, Tilney NL. The cytokine-adhesion molecule cascade in ischaemia/reperfusion injury of the rat kidney. Inhibition by a soluble P-selectin ligand. *J Clin Invest* 1997; **99**: 2682–2690.

42. Grant D, Hurlbut D, Zhong R, *et al.* Intestinal permeability and bacterial translocation following small bowel transplantation in the rat. *Transplantation* 1991; **52**: 221–224.

43. Price BA, Cumberland NS, Ingham Clark CL, Pockley AG, Lear PA, Wood RFM. The effect of rejection and graft-versus-host disease on small intestinal microflora and bacterial translocation after rat small bowel transplantation. *Transplantation* 1993; **56**: 1072–1076.

44. Price BA, Cumberland NS, Ingham Clark CL, Pockley AG, Lear PA, Wood RFM. Effect of small bowel transplantation, denervation and ischaemia on rat intestinal microflora. *Transplant Int* 1994; **7**: 334–339.

45. Price BA, Cumberland NS, Ingham Clark CL, Pockley AG, Wood RFM. Orthotopic transposition following rat heterotopic small bowel transplantation corrects overgrowth of potentially pathogenic bacteria. *Transplantation* 1996; **61**: 649–651.

46. Xia W, Kirkman RL. Immune function in transplanted small intestine. Total secretory IgA production and response against cholera toxin. *Transplantation* 1990; **49**: 277–280.

47. Schmid T, Korozsi G, Oberhuber G, Klima G, Margreiter R. Lymphatic regeneration after small-bowel transplantation. *Transplant Proc* 1990; **22**: 2446.

48. Lear PA. The physiology of transplanted small intestine. In: Grant DR, Wood RFM (eds) *Small Bowel Transplantation*. Edward Arnold: London, pp. 18–29.

49. Szymula von Richter TP, Baumeister RGH, Hammer C. Microsurgical reconstruction of the lymphatic and nerve system in small bowel transplantation: the rat model, first results. *Transplant Int* 1996; **9** (Suppl 1): S286–S289.

50. Szymula von Richter TP, Baumeister RG. Allograft survival prolongation after microsurgical lymphatic reconstruction in a short-term immunosuppressed rat small bowel transplantation model. *Transplant Proc* 1997; **29**: 1804–1806.

51. Watson AJM, Lear PA, Montgomery A, Elliot E, Dacre J, Farthing MJ, Wood RFM. Water, electrolyte, glucose, and glycine absorption in rat small intestinal transplants. *Gastroenterology* 1988; **94**: 863–869.

52. Schraut WH, Abraham VS, Lee KKW. Portal versus systemic drainage for small bowel allografts. *Surgery* 1985; **98**: 579–586.

53. Stepkowski SM, Kahan BD. Immunosuppression of small bowel allografts in experimental animals. In: Grant DR, Wood RFM (eds) *Small Bowel Transplantation*. Edward Arnold: London, pp. 78–87.

54. Alessiani M, Spada M, Dionigi P, Arbustini E, Regazzi M, Fossati GS, Zonta A. Combined immunosuppressive therapy with tacrolimus and mycophenolate mofetil for small bowel transplantation in pigs. *Transplantation* 1996; **62**: 563–567.

55. Soulillou JP. Relevant targets for therapy with monoclonal antibodies in allograft transplantation. *Kidney Int* 1994; **46**: 540–553.

56. Remuzzi G, Rossini M, Imberti O, Perico N. Kidney graft survival in rats without immunosuppressants after intrathymic glomerular transplantation. *Lancet* 1991; **337**: 750–752.

57. Campos L, Alfrey EJ, Posselt AM, Odorico JS, Barker CF, Naji A. Prolonged survival of rat orthotopic liver allografts after intrathymic inoculation of donor-strain cells. *Transplantation* 1993; **55**: 866–870.

58. Nakafusa Y, Goss JA, Mohanakumar T, Flye MW. Induction of donor-specific tolerance to cardiac but not skin or renal allografts by intrathymic injection of splenocyte antigen. *Transplantation* 1993; **55**: 877–882.

59. Bowles MJ, Webster GA, Wood RFM, Pockley AG. Effect of anti-CD4 monoclonal antibody therapy on rat small bowel allograft survival. *Transplant Proc* 1994; **26**: 1605.

60. Bowles MJ, Wood RFM, Pockley AG. Combined monoclonal antibody therapy in experimental small bowel transplantation. *Transplant Proc* 1996; **28**: 2510.

61. Karim MS, Webster GA, Wood RFM, Pockley AG. Effect of intrathymic injection of donor splenocytes on rat small bowel allograft survival. *Transplant Proc* 1994; **26**: 1583–1584.

62. Goss JA, Nakafusa Y, Flye MW. Prolongation of small bowel allografts after intrathymic injection of donor alloantigen and ALS. *J Surg Res* 1993; **54**: 494–498.

63. Yamataka T, Kobayashi H, Yagita H, Okumura K, Tamatani T, Miyasaka M. The effect of anti-ICAM-1 monoclonal antibody treatment on the transplantation of the small bowel in rats. *J Pediatr Surg* 1993; **28**: 1471–1477.

64. Tice DG, Bruch D, Ikramuddin S. Anti-VLA-4 and cyclosporine synergistically prolong rat heterotopic small bowel allografts. *Transplant Proc* 1996; **28**: 24.

65. Fortner JG, Sichuk G, Litwin SD, Beattie EJ. Immunological responses to an intestinal allograft with HLA identical donor-recipient. *Transplantation* 1972; **14**: 531–535.

66. Deltz E, Mengel W, Hamelmann H. Small bowel transplantation: report of a clinical case. *Prog Ped Surg* 1990; **25**: 90–96.

67. Goulet O, Revillon Y, Jan D, *et al.* Small bowel transplantation in children. *Transplant Proc* 1990; **22**: 2499–2500.

68. Calne RY, Sells RA, Pena JR, *et al.* Induction of immunological tolerance by porcine liver allografts. *Nature* 1969; **223**: 472–476.

69. Grant D, Wall W, Mimeault R, *et al.* Successful small bowel/liver transplantation. *Lancet* 1990; **335**: 181–184.

70. Todo S, Reyes J, Furukawa H, *et al.* Outcome analysis of 71 clinical intestinal transplantations. *Ann Surg* 1995; **222**: 270–280.

71. Reyes J, Tzakis AG, Bonet H, *et al.* Lymphoproliferative disease after intestinal transplantation under primary FK 506 immunosuppression. *Transplant Proc* 1994; **26**: 1426–1427.

72. Hashimoto T, Zhong R, Garcia B, *et al.* Ileocolic allotransplantation in rats. *Transplant Proc* 1994; **26**: 1533.

73. Todo S, Tzakis AG, Reyes J, *et al.* Small intestinal transplantation in humans with or without the colon. *Transplantation* 1994; **57**: 840–848.

74. Pirenne J, Benedetti E, Gruessner A, *et al.* Combined transplantation of small and large bowel. FK506 versus cyclosporine A in a porcine model. *Transplantation* 1996; **61**: 1685–1694.

75. Todo S, Tzakis AG, Abu-Elmagd K, *et al.* Cadaveric small bowel and small bowel-liver transplantation in humans. *Transplantation* 1992; **53**: 369–376.

76. Todo S, Murase N, Tzakis A, Starzl TE. Role of the liver and the portal circulation in intestinal grafting. In: Grant DR, Wood RFM (eds) *Small Bowel Transplantation*. Edward Arnold: London, 1996, pp. 101–111.

77. Watson AJM, Lear PA. Current status of intestinal transplantation. *Gut* 1989; **30**: 1771–1782.

78. Goulet O, Brousse N, Revillon Y, Ricour C. Pathology of human intestinal transplantation. In: Grant DR, Wood RFM (eds) *Small Bowel Transplantation*. Edward Arnold: London, 1996, pp. 112–120.

79. Fromont G, Cerf-Bensussan N, Patey N, *et al.* Small bowel transplantation in children: an immunohistochemical study of intestinal grafts. *Gut* 1995; **37**: 783–790.

80. Schroeder P, Schweizer E, Hansmann K, *et al.* Monitoring in small bowel transplantation using cytochemistry and immunochemistry: a comparison of different techniques. *Transplant Proc* 1991; **23**: 675–676.

81. Cohen Z, Silverman RE, Wassef R, *et al.* Small intestinal transplantation using cyclosporine. Report of a case. *Transplantation* 1986; **42**: 613–621.

82. Reyes J, Abu-Elmagd K, Tzakis A, *et al.* Infectious complications after human small bowel transplantation. *Transplant Proc* 1992; **24**: 1249–1250.

83. Todo S, Tzakis AG, Abu-Elmagd K, *et al.* Intestinal transplantation in composite visceral grafts or alone. *Ann Surg* 1992; **216**: 223–234.

84. Crissinger KD, Kvietys PR, Granger DN. Pathophysiology of gastrointestinal mucosal permeability. *J Int Med* 1990; **228** (Supp 1): 145–154.

85. Asfar S, Wood RFM, Grant DR. Clinical diagnosis in intestinal allograft rejection. In: Solez K, Racusen LC, Billingham ME (eds) *Solid Organ Transplant Rejection*. Marcel Dekker: New York, 1996, pp. 445–454.

86. Grant D. Current results of intestinal transplantation. *Lancet* 1996; **347**: 1801–1803.

87. Ingham Clark CL, Lear PA, Wood S, Lennard-Jones JE, Wood RFM. Potential candidates for small-bowel transplantation. *Br J Surg* 1992; **79**: 676–679.

88. Sustento-Reodica N, Ruiz P, Rogers A, Viciana AL, Conn HO, Tzakis AG. Recurrent Crohn's disease in transplanted bowel. *Lancet* 1997; **349**: 688–691.

GLOSSARY

This glossary provides definitions of immunological and transplant-related terms, which may be unfamiliar to some readers.

Allograft: Transplant between two genetically different members of the same species.

Allogeneic: Of different genetic make up and therefore capable of inducing rejection.

Antigen: A protein molecule that is capable of inducing an immune reaction. In transplantation antigens on the surface of graft cells are the trigger to the immune system of the recipient-inducing rejection.

Cell surface markers: Antigenic determinants on the surface of cells. In some circumstances these act as binding sites and linkage with a matching determinant is important to allow an immune reaction to proceed. Cell surface antigens have been defined by a number of international workshops that have generated the Cluster of Differentiation (CD) nomenclature.

CD3: The CD3 antigen is composed of five invariable chains and is closely associated with the T-cell antigen receptor. It is expressed on 70–80% of normal peripheral blood lymphocytes and plays a significant role in signal transduction during antigen recognition (see Cell surface markers).

CD4: The CD4 antigen is transmembrane glyco-protein expressed on T helper/inducer cell popula-tions. It is expressed on approximately 45% of peripheral blood lymphocytes and it is involved in the co-recognition of MHC class II antigens in association with the T-cell receptor (see Cell surface markers).

CD8: The CD8 antigen is a two-chain complex expressed on T cytotoxic/suppressor cell populations. It is expressed on 13–48% of peripheral blood lymphocytes and it is involved in the co-recognition of MHC class I antigens in association with the T-cell receptor (see Cell surface markers).

CD25: The CD25 antigen is the low affinity inter-leukin-2 receptor. It associates with the common (CD132) and high affinity (CD122) chains to form the high affinity IL-2 receptor complex. CD25 is expressed on activated T and B lymphocytes and activated macrophages and its expression on lymphocytes is upregulated on activation (see Cell surface markers).

CD28: The CD28 antigen is expressed on most mature T-cells and antibody-producing B-cells (plasma cells). It is involved in signal transduction and cell activation events (see Cell surface markers).

CD44: The CD44 antigen is expressed on leucocytes, erythrocytes and weakly on platelets. The molecule has a functional role in cell migration, leucocyte homing and adhesion during lymphocyte activation (see Cell surface markers).

CD68: The CD68 antigen is primarily expressed within lysosomal membranes inside cells, but can be detected in smaller amounts on the surface of activated monocytes, macrophages, neutrophils, eosinophils and two subpopulations of B-cells. It is involved in endocytosis and/or lysosomal traffic (see Cell surface markers).

CD80: The CD80 (B7.1) antigen is expressed on activated B-cells, macrophages and dendritic cells and activated CD4$^+$ and CD8$^+$ T-cells. It is the ligand for CD28 and its binding to CD28 delivers co-stimulatory signals and triggers T-cell activation.

CD86: The CD86 (B7.2) antigen is primarily expressed on monocytes, dendritic cells and activated B-cells and it is the second ligand for CD28. It may play an important role in co-stimulation of T-cells and the primary immune responses.

DA: (See In-bred rat strains).

Fischer: (See In-bred rat strains).

Graft-versus-host disease: A reaction in which lymphoid cells in a graft are capable of migrating to recipient tissues and stimulating an inflammatory immune reaction. This is an important feature in bone marrow transplantation but can also occur in intestinal trans-plantation because the gut contains large numbers of lymphoid cells capable of migrating.

Haplotype: A set of genetic determinants located on a single chromosome.

Heterotopic: A graft placed in an abnormal anatomical position. In experimental small bowel transplantation the term refers to a graft in which both the proximal and distal ends of the bowel are exteriorized as stomas on the skin surface.

In-bred rat strains: e.g. DA, PVG, Lewis, Fischer – These are strains of rats where every member of the strain is genetically identical. Transplants between members of the same strain (isografts, e.g. DA to DA) will not result in rejection. In transplants between different strains (allografts, e.g. DA to PVG) rejection occurs in a predictable manner.

Lewis: (See In-bred rat strains).

Micro-chimerism: The colonization of recipient tissues by graft cells. It has been proposed that the persistence of these cells is an indication of a degree of tolerance (permanent graft acceptance) by the recipient.

Natural killer cells: Cells capable of reacting against foreign proteins without undergoing prior sensitiza-tion. They act as immune scavengers and are important in both cancer (in eliminating abnormal cells) and in transplantation where they may be able to initiate rejection.

NKR-P1: Natural killer cell receptor protein 1. This is expressed at high levels on rat natural killer cells, sub-populations of T-cells and also on activated peripheral blood neutrophils in some species. It appears to be involved in natural killer cell target cell recognition, but its role in neutrophil function is currently unknown.

Orthotopic: A graft placed in its normal anatomical position. In intestinal transplantation the proximal end of the small bowel would therefore be connected to the duodenum and the distal end to the ilio-caecal junction.

PVG: (See In-bred rat strains).

Selectins: Selectins are a family of transmembrane molecules that are expressed on the surface of leuco-cytes and activated endothelium. L-selectin is expressed on the majority of leucocytes, P-selectin is expressed on activated platelets and endothelial cells and E-selectin is expressed on activated endothelial cells. The selectin molecules are involved in the early events associated with leucocyte capture and adhesion to vessel walls during the development of inflammatory responses.

VLA-4: Very late activation antigen 4. This is expressed on lymphocytes, monocytes, thymocytes, eosinophils and several B- and T-cell lines. It is involved in rolling and attachment of cells to the endothelium and the generation and localization of effector cells (for example neutrophils and macrophages) at inflammatory sites.

Appendices

Appendix 1

BODY MASS INDEX (BMI) kg/m^2

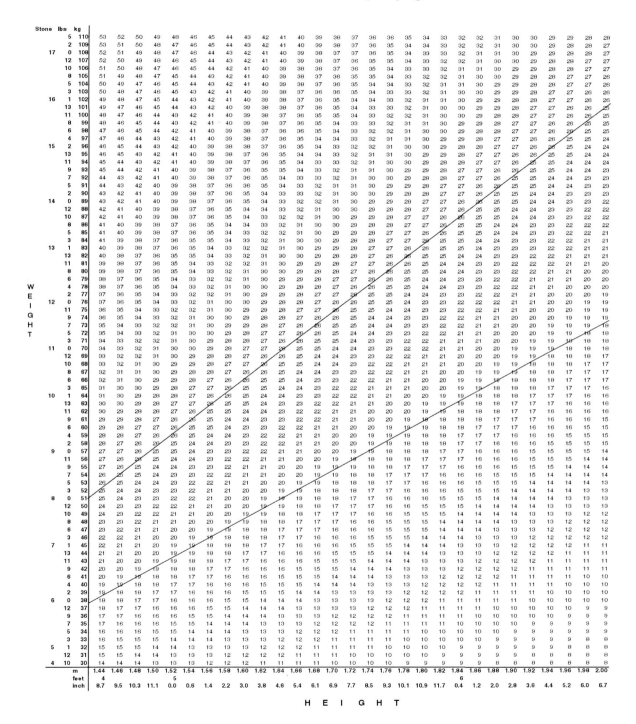

Appendix 2

PERCENTAGE WEIGHT LOSS

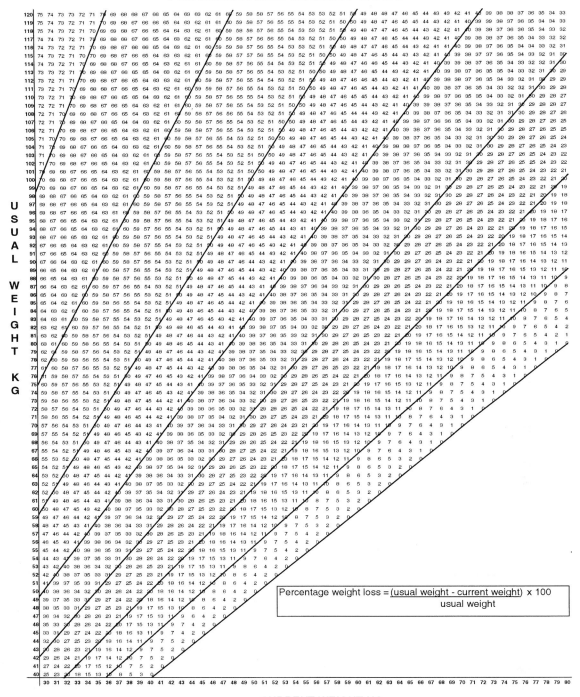

Percentage weight loss = (usual weight - current weight) x 100
                                    usual weight

CURRENT WEIGHT KG

Appendix 3
MID-ARM MUSCLE CIRCUMFERENCE (MAMC)

MID-ARM CIRCUMFERENCE CM	0.2	0.4	0.6	0.8	1.0	1.2	1.4	1.6	1.8	2.0	2.2	2.4	2.6	2.8	3.0
50	49	49	48	47	47	46	46	45	44	44	43	42	42	41	41
49	48	48	47	46	46	45	45	44	43	43	42	41	41	40	40
48	47	47	46	45	45	44	44	43	42	42	41	40	40	39	39
47	46	46	45	44	44	43	43	42	41	41	40	39	39	38	38
46	45	45	44	43	43	42	42	41	40	40	39	38	38	37	37
45	44	44	43	42	42	41	41	40	39	39	38	37	37	36	36
44	43	43	42	41	41	40	40	39	38	38	37	36	36	35	35
43	42	42	41	40	40	39	39	38	37	37	36	35	35	34	34
42	41	41	40	39	39	38	38	37	36	36	35	34	34	33	33
41	40	40	39	38	38	37	37	36	35	35	34	33	33	32	32
40	39	39	38	37	37	36	36	35	34	34	33	32	32	31	31
39	38	38	37	36	36	35	35	34	33	33	32	31	31	30	30
38	37	37	36	35	35	34	34	33	32	32	31	30	30	29	29
37	36	36	35	34	34	33	33	32	31	31	30	29	29	28	28
36	35	35	34	33	33	32	32	31	30	30	29	28	28	27	27
35	34	34	33	32	32	31	31	30	29	29	28	27	27	26	26
34	33	33	32	31	31	30	30	29	28	28	27	26	26	25	25
33	32	32	31	30	30	29	29	28	27	27	26	25	25	24	24
32	31	31	30	29	29	28	28	27	26	26	25	24	24	23	23
31	30	30	29	28	28	27	27	26	25	25	24	23	23	22	22
30	29	29	28	27	27	26	26	25	24	24	23	22	22	21	21
29	28	28	27	26	26	25	25	24	23	23	22	21	21	20	20
28	27	27	26	25	25	24	24	23	22	22	21	20	20	19	19
27	26	26	25	24	24	23	23	22	21	21	20	19	19	18	18
26	25	25	24	23	23	22	22	21	20	20	19	18	18	17	17
25	24	24	23	22	22	21	21	20	19	19	18	17	17	16	16
24	23	23	22	21	21	20	20	19	18	18	17	16	16	15	15
23	22	22	21	20	20	19	19	18	17	17	16	15	15	14	14
22	21	21	20	19	19	18	18	17	16	16	15	14	14	13	13
21	20	20	19	18	18	17	17	16	15	15	14	13	13	12	12
20	19	19	18	17	17	16	16	15	14	14	13	12	12	11	11
19	18	18	17	16	16	15	15	14	13	13	12	11	11	10	10
18	17	17	16	15	15	14	14	13	12	12	11	10	10	9	9
17	16	16	15	14	14	13	13	12	11	11	10	9	9	8	8
16	15	15	14	13	13	12	12	11	10	10	9	8	8	7	7
15	14	14	13	12	12	11	11	10	9	9	8	7	7	6	6
14	13	13	12	11	11	10	10	9	8	8	7	6	6	5	5
13	12	12	11	10	10	9	9	8	7	7	6	5	5	4	4
12	11	11	10	9	9	8	8	7	6	6	5	4	4	3	3
11	10	10	9	8	8	7	7	6	5	5	4	3	3	2	2
10	9	9	8	7	7	6	6	5	4	4	3	2	2	1	1

TRICEPS SKIN FOLD THICKNESS CM

MAMC = Mid-arm circumference - (3.14 x Triceps skin fold thickness)

The mid-arm circumference and triceps skin fold measurement are made mid-way between the tip of the acromion (shoulder tip) and the olecranon process (elbow) on the relaxed extended left (non-dominant) arm.

MID-ARM MUSCLE CIRCUMFERENCE (CM) PERCENTILES

cm

	Men				Women		
	5th	10th	15th		5th	10th	15th
Age (years)							
20–29	22	23	24		18	19	19
30–39	22	23	23		18	19	19
40–49	23	23	24		19	19	20
50–59	22	23	23		19	19	19
60–69	22	23	23		19	19	20
70–79	21	22	23		18	19	19
80–89	20	21	22		17	18	18
>90	20	20	21		17	17	18
All ages	22	22	23		18	19	19

This 'normal range' of mid-arm muscle circumference (MAMC) has been chosen as it includes a large age range (1). A MAMC of less than 19 cm in women and less than 21 cm in men of all ages, would detect most patients found to be undernourished by a loss of 10% body weight or a body mass index of less then 19 kg/m² (2).

The MAMC is useful for monitoring the progress of nutritional support especially in patients who cannot be weighed, have fluid retention or are obese.

1. Symreng T. Arm anthropometry in a large reference population and in surgical patients. *Clin Nutr* 1982; **1:** 211–219

2. Nightingale JMD, Walsh N, Bullock ME, Wicks AC. Comparison of three simple methods for the detection of malnutrition. *J R Soc Med* 1996; **89:** 144–148

APPENDIX 4

Useful Websites

American Dietetic Association
www.eatright.org/

American Society for Parenteral and Enteral Nutrition
– ASPEN
www.clinnutr.org

Arbor Nutrition Guide
www.arborcom.com

Australian Society for Parenteral and Enteral Nutrition
– AuSPEN
www.southcom.com.au/~hartley/home.htm

Bandolier
www.jr2.ox.ac.uk/Bandolier

British Association for Parenteral and Enteral Nutriton
– BAPEN
www.bapen.org.uk

British Dietetic Assocation
www.bda.uk.com/

British Medical Journal
www.bmj.com

Canadian Parenteral – Enteral Nutrition Association –
CPENA
www.magi.com/~epena

Dietitians of Canada
www.dietitians.ca/

Department of Health
www.doh.gov.uk

European Society of Parenteral and Enteral Nutriton –
ESPEN
www.hostindia.com/ispen
Italian Society of Parenteral and Enteral Nutrition –
SINPE
www.sameint.it/sinpe

Motor Neurone Disease Association
www.mndassociation.org

National Electronic Library for Health
www.nelh.nhs.uk/

National Library of Medicine – free Medline
www.nlm.nih.gov/

NHS Direct Online
www.nhsdirect.nhs.uk

Oley Foundation (home PEN organisation)
www.wizvax.net/oleyfdn

OMNI
www.omni.ac.uk

Parenteral and Enteral Nutrition Group of the British
Dietetic Assocation
www.peng.org.uk

Parenteral and Enteral Nutrition Society of Asia –
PENSA
www.pensa.org

Patients on Intravenous and Naso-gastric Nutrition
Therapy – PINNT
www.pinnt.com

Primary Care National Electronic Library for Health
www.nelh–pc.nhs.uk/

Scottish Intercollegiate Guidelines Network (SIGN)
www.show.scot.nhs.uk/sign/

South African Society for Parenteral and Enteral
Nutrition – SAPSEN
www.sapsen.com

The Cochrane Collaboration
www.cochrane.org/

The Swedish Association for Children with Home
Parenteral Nutrition
www.dataphone.se/~hpn

TPN Support (egroup support for parents of children
who require TPN)
www.eproups.com/group/tpnsupport

Index